Neurodegeneration: Advanced Researches

Neurodegeneration: Advanced Researches

Edited by Antonio Chavez

hayle medical

New York

Hayle Medical,
750 Third Avenue, 9th Floor,
New York, NY 10017, USA

Visit us on the World Wide Web at:
www.haylemedical.com

ISBN: 978-1-63241-682-7

Cataloging-in-Publication Data

Neurodegeneration : advanced researches / edited by Antonio Chavez.
    p. cm.
Includes bibliographical references and index.
ISBN 978-1-63241-682-7
1. Nervous system--Degeneration. 2. Neuroscience. 3. Degeneration (Pathology).
4. Nervous system--Diseases. I. Chavez, Antonio.
RC394.D35 N48 2019
616.804 7--dc23

Table of Contents

Preface

It is often said that books are a boon to mankind. They document every progress and pass on the knowledge from one generation to the other. They play a crucial role in our lives. Thus I was both excited and nervous while editing this book. I was pleased by the thought of being able to make a mark but I was also nervous to do it right because the future of students depends upon it. Hence, I took a few months to research further into the discipline, revise my knowledge and also explore some more aspects. Post this process, I begun with the editing of this book.

Neurodegeneration is a gradual but irreversible process of neuronal damage and neuronal death. It is a common characteristic of neurodegenerative disorders such as Alzheimer's disease and Parkinson's disease, among others. Research is being conducted to determine the underlying cause of this process. One of the strategies for this involves the study of neurodegenerative conditions and identifying similarities and parallels among these on a sub-cellular level. Finding such similarities allows the development of therapeutic strategies to combat these diseases and manage neural degeneration. Immunotherapy is another emerging area of research. Neurodegeneration is an active area of study that has undergone rapid advancement over the past few decades. It brings forth some of the most innovative concepts and elucidates the unexplored aspects of neurodegeneration. This book is appropriate for students seeking detailed information in this area as well as for experts.

I thank my publisher with all my heart for considering me worthy of this unparalleled opportunity and for showing unwavering faith in my skills. I would also like to thank the editorial team who worked closely with me at every step and contributed immensely towards the successful completion of this book. Last but not the least, I wish to thank my friends and colleagues for their support.

Editor

Wnt3a protects SH-SY5Y cells against 6-hydroxydopamine toxicity by restoration of mitochondria function

Lei Wei[1,2*], Li Ding[3], Ming-shu Mo[2], Ming Lei[2], Limin Zhang[2], Kang Chen[5] and Pingyi Xu[2,4*]

Abstract

Background: Wnt/β-catenin signal has been reported to exert cytoprotective effects in cellular models of several diseases, including Parkinson's disease (PD). This study aimed to investigate the neuroprotective effects of actived Wnt/β-catenin signal by Wnt3a on SH-SY5Y cells treated with 6-hydroxydopamine (6-OHDA).

Methods: Wnt3a-conditioned medium (Wnt3a-CM) was used to intervene dopaminegic SH-SY5Y cells treated with 6-OHDA. Cell toxicity was determined by cell viability and lactate dehydrogenase leakage (LDH) assay. The mitochondria function was measured by the mitochondrial membrane potential, while oxidative stress was monitored with intracellular reactive oxygen species (ROS). Western blot analysis was used to detect the expression of GSK3β, β-catenin as well as Akt.

Results: Our results showed that 100 μM 6-OHDA treated for 24 h significantly decreased cell viability and mitochondrial transmembrane potential, reduced the level of β-catenin and p-Akt, increased LDH leakage, ROS production and the ratio of p-GSK3β (Tyr216) to p-GSK3β (Ser9). However, Wnt3a-conditioned medium reversing SH-SY5Y cells against 6-OHDA-induced neurotoxicity by reversing these changes.

Conclusions: Activating of Wnt/β-catenin pathway by Wnt3a-CM attenuated 6-OHDA-induced neurotoxicity significantly, which related to the inhibition of oxidative stress and maintenance of normal mitochondrial function.

Keywords: Wnt3a, 6-OHDA, Mitochondria function, Parkinson's disease

Background

Parkinson's disease (PD), characterized by loss of dopaminergic neurons in substantia nigra, is the second most common neurodegenerative diseases in elderly people. Studies have shown that several mechanisms are involved in pathogenesis of PD including oxidative stress, mitochondrial dysfunction and elevated brain iron levels [1–3]. Although much research has helped to elucidate the pathogenesis of PD, the precise etiology and pathogenesis of the disease still remain unknown. Moreover, Current treatments for PD predominantly rely on pharmacotherapy to improve the symptoms of movement disorder, but little efficacy in preventing disease progression. Therefore neuroprotective therapy may play a key role in the therapeutic strategy of PD.

Wnt signaling pathway is an autocrine-paracrine signal transduction pathway which has been demonstrated to participate in embryonic development, cell differentiation and ontogenesis [4–7]. A main Wnt signaling pathway branch is the wnt/β-catenin pathway, which initiates with Wnt proteins binding to Frizzled receptors and activates Dishevelled. Activation of Dishevelled results in inhibition of glycogen synthase kinase-3β (GSK3β), which in turn causes stabilization of β-catenin. Stabilized β-catenin accumulates and is taken into the nucleus where it regulates expression of numerous genes [8]. Extensive research has confirmed the vital role of Wnt signaling in midbrain dopaminergic neuronal development [9, 10]. For example, Wnt1 and Wnt3a, which exert effects by Wnt/β-catenin pathway, are key regulators in the development of dopaminergic neurons [9].

The cellular protective effects of Wnt/β-catenin pathway have been demonstrated in animal and cellular

* Correspondence: weilei068@163.com; pingyixu@sina.com
[1]Department of Neurology, The Third Affiliated Hospital of Sun Yat-sen University, Guangzhou 510630, China
[2]Department of Neurology, The First Affiliated Hospital of Sun Yat-sen University, Guangzhou 510080, China
Full list of author information is available at the end of the article

models of Alzheimer's disease, retinal degeneration, cerebral ischemia as well as PD [11–14]. Our previous study hasdemonstrated that Wnt/β-catenin signal is inhibited in SH-SY5Y cells treated with 6-OHDA, a cellular model of PD, while activation of Wnt/β-catenin signal by exogenous Wnt1 could protect cells by restoring mitochondria and endoplasmic reticulum function [15]. However, the precise mechanism for the pathogenesis of the disease remains unknown. In this study, we report that Wnt3a-conditioned medium (Wnt3a-CM) protected cells from 6-OHDA neurotoxicity by a mechanism that involved maintenance of normal mitochondrial.

Methods
Cell culture
Human neuroblastoma SH-SY5Y cells were obtained from American Type Culture Collection (ATCC, Manassas, VA, U.S.A.), maintained in DMEM with high glucose (Invitrogen, USA) supplemented with 10 % fetal bovine serum (FBS, Invitrogen), and cultured in a humidified incubator with 5 % CO_2 at 37 °C. Cells with 20–30 passages were used. For experiments, cells were seeded at a density of 1×10^5 /cm^2 in the plastic flasks or plates. Conditioned media containing Wnt3a (Wnt3a-CM) were prepared from mouse L cells (ATCC) stably expressing Wnt3a. Control conditioned media were obtained from parental L cells (Ctrl-CM). Different proportions of Ctrl-CM or Wnt3a-CM were performed according to corresponding experiments.

Cell viability assay
SH-SY5Y cells were seeded in a 96-well plate at a density of 1×10^3 cells per well. After attachment, cells were treated with 100 μM 6-OHDA, Ctrl-CM (10–80 %) or Wnt3a-CM (10–80 %) for 24 h. After treatment, cells were incubated with 0.5 mg/mL MTT (Sigma-Aldrich, USA) for 4 h at 37 °C [16]. Following aspiration of the MTT solution, the same volume of DMSO was added

into each well to dissolve the purple formazan crystals. Absorbance was read in a microtiter plate reader at 490 nm. Cell viability was expressed as a percentage of the absorbance from control cells. The toxic effects of 6-OHDA to SH-SY5Y cells were also detected by measuring the leakage of the cytosolic enzyme LDH to the culture medium using a colorimetric LDH assay kit (KeyGen, China) according to the manufacturer's instructions [17]. Briefly, after 100 μM 6-OHDA added, 20 μl of cell medium were added into basic solution to measure extracellular LDH activity, which could catalyze the conversion of lactate to pyruvate, which then reacted with 2,4-dinitrophenylhydrazine to give the brownish red color. The absorbance was measured at a wavelength of 440 nm by colorimetric assay, and the LDH leakage was expressed as the percentage versus control cells.

Measurement of mitochondrial transmembrane potential (MMP) and intracellular ROS production
Changes in the mitochondrial membrane potential with various treatments in SH-SY5Y cells were measured by rhodamine-123 or DCFH-DA using a fluorescence spectrophotometer [18]. Briefly, cells were treated with 6-OHDA, Ctrl-CM and Wnt3a-CM for 24 h and then incubated with rhodamine-123 (Sigma-Aldrich, USA) or DCFH-DA (Sigma-Aldrich, USA) in a final concentration of 10 or 25 μmol/L respectively for 30 min at 37 °C. After washing twice with HEPES buffer saline (Invitrogen, USA), fluorescence was recorded at 488 nm excitation and 523 nm emission wave-lengths. Each field of cells was photographed using a fluorescence microscopy.

Western blot analysis
The immunoblotting was performed in accordance with a standard procedure [16, 19]. The following primary antibodies were used: rabbit anti-β-catenin (1:1000 dilution, Abcam, Cambridge, UK), rabbit anti-p-GSK3β (Ser9) (1:1000 dilution, CST, USA), rabbit anti-p-GSK3β

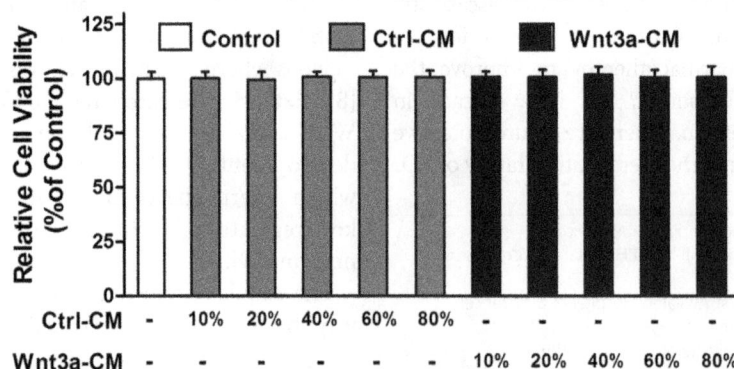

Fig. 1 Treatment with Wnt3a-CM or Ctrl-CM didn't change SH-SY5Y cell viability. SH-SY5Y cells were treated with different proportion of Ctrl-CM or Wnt3a-CM, cell viability was measured by MTT assay. Data were presented as mean ± SD from four independent experiments

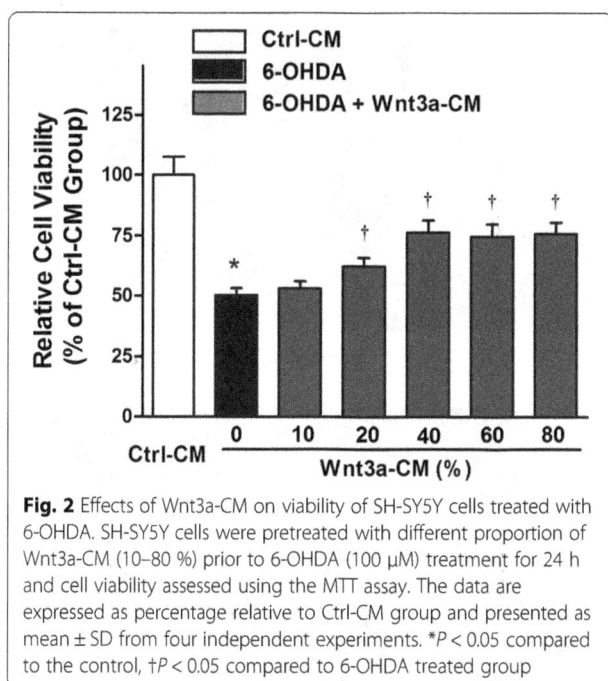

Fig. 2 Effects of Wnt3a-CM on viability of SH-SY5Y cells treated with 6-OHDA. SH-SY5Y cells were pretreated with different proportion of Wnt3a-CM (10–80 %) prior to 6-OHDA (100 μM) treatment for 24 h and cell viability assessed using the MTT assay. The data are expressed as percentage relative to Ctrl-CM group and presented as mean ± SD from four independent experiments. *$P < 0.05$ compared to the control, †$P < 0.05$ compared to 6-OHDA treated group

(Tyr216) (1:1000 dilution, CST, USA), rabbit anti-p-Akt (Ser473) (1:1000 dilution, Millipore, USA), mouse anti-β-actin (1:1000 dilution, Millipore, USA). Proteins were detected with the SuperSignal® West Pico Chemiluminescent Substrate (Thermo Fisher Scientific Inc., IL, USA) and membranes were exposed to X-ray films (Fujifilm Corporation, Japan), which were scanned and analyzed by using the Quantity One v4.62 for Windows software (Biorad, CA, USA).

Statistical analysis

Results were presented as mean ± SD. One-way analysis of variance (ANOVA) followed by Student–Newman–Keuls test was used to compare differences between means in more than two groups. The level of significance was set at $P < 0.05$. All the statistical analyses were performed with SPSS 12.0 for windows (SPSS Inc., Chicago, IL, USA).

Results

Wnt3a-CM attenuated 6-OHDA-induced cell injury

Our previous studies have confirmed that treatment with 6-OHDA for 24 h caused a concentration-dependent reduction in cell viability and a concentration-dependent increase in LDH release in dopaminergic SH-SY5Y cells [15]. According to our previous results, a 100 μM 6-OHDA was chosen for the following experiments.

We then tested the effect of Wnt3a-CM on SH-SY5Y cells, and found that treatment with Wnt3a-CM or Ctrl-CM at proportion of 10–80 % didn't obviously change the cell viability (Fig. 1). Thus, Ctrl-CM at a proportion of 40 % was used as control and we investigated whether

Wnt3a-CM could attenuate the toxic effect of 6-OHDA on SH-SY5Y cells. Wnt3a-CM was added to the cultures at different proportion 20 min prior to 6-OHDA. Cells pre-treated with Wnt3a-CM were partially protected against 6-OHDA toxicity. Treatment with 100 μM 6-OHDA for 24 h decreased the cell viability to ~50 % compared with Ctrl-CM group. However, when cells were pre-treated with Wnt3a-CM the reduction of cell viability was ameliorated. Specifically, the level of cell viability increased to 62.16 ± 3.71 % of the control value when 20 % of Wnt3a-CM was used and that was up to 76.35 ± 5.00 % when 40 % of Wnt3a-CM was added. Then the cell viability of higher proportion of Wnt3a-CM (60 and 80 %) was reduced to 74.64 ± 5.21 and 75.79 ± 4.71 respectively (Fig. 2). Similarly, pretreatment of 20, 40, 60 and 80 % Wnt3a-CM could significantly inhibit LDH release induced by 6-OHDA (Fig. 3).

Wnt3a-CM antagonized 6-OHDA-induced MMP and ROS production

It is generally accepted that the 6-OHDA-induced neuronal apoptosis is mediated by the mitochondrial dysfunction. Markers of mitochondria function, such as mitochondrial membrane potential are often used to monitor the cell apoptosis. In the experiment, there was a significant reduction of MMP in 6-OHDA-treated SH-SY5Y cells. However, a partial restoration of MMP was observed in the cells treated with Wnt3a-CM at a proportion of 40 % (Fig. 4a and 4c). In consideration of ROS

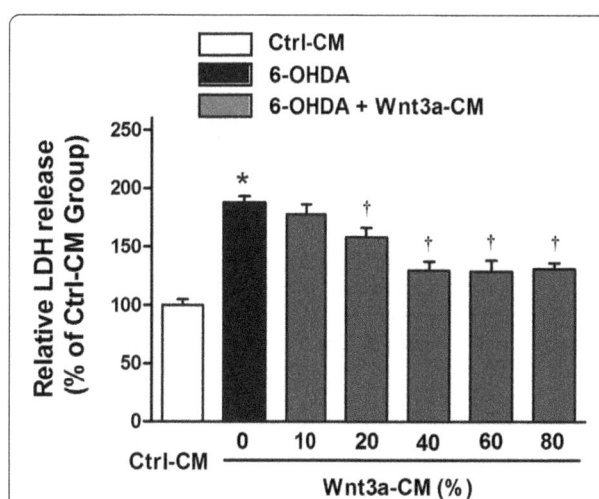

Fig. 3 Effects of Wnt3a-CM on LDH leakage of SH-SY5Y cells treated with 6-OHDA. SH-SY5Y cells were pretreated with different proportion of Wnt3a-CM (10–80 %) prior to 6-OHDA (100 μM) treatment for 24 h and LDH assay was performed to determine the degree of cell injury. The data are expressed as percentage relative to Ctrl-CM group and presented as mean ± SD from four independent experiments. *$P < 0.05$ compared to the control, †$P < 0.05$ compared to 6-OHDA treated group

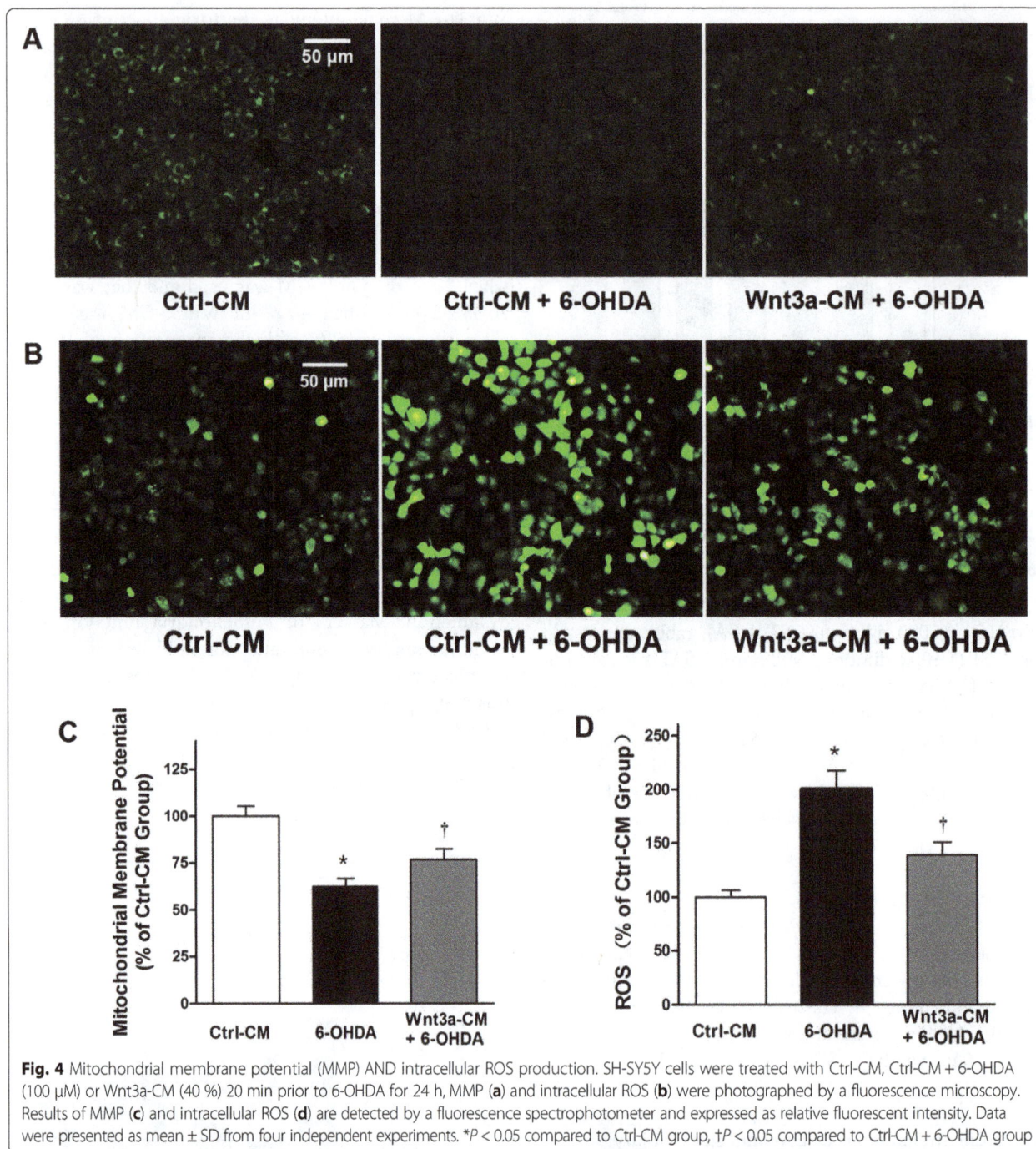

Fig. 4 Mitochondrial membrane potential (MMP) AND intracellular ROS production. SH-SY5Y cells were treated with Ctrl-CM, Ctrl-CM + 6-OHDA (100 μM) or Wnt3a-CM (40 %) 20 min prior to 6-OHDA for 24 h, MMP (**a**) and intracellular ROS (**b**) were photographed by a fluorescence microscopy. Results of MMP (**c**) and intracellular ROS (**d**) are detected by a fluorescence spectrophotometer and expressed as relative fluorescent intensity. Data were presented as mean ± SD from four independent experiments. *$P < 0.05$ compared to Ctrl-CM group, †$P < 0.05$ compared to Ctrl-CM + 6-OHDA group

elevation believed to initiate a neurotoxic cascade induced by 6-OHDA [20], we further examined if Wnt3a-CM inhibit 6-OHDA-induced cell apoptosis by suppressing ROS production. As shown in Fig. 4b and d, 6-OHDA treatment alone for 24 h induced about 2-fold increase in ROS level compared to the control group, whereas pre-treatment with 40 % Wnt3a-CM exhibited an inhibitive effect of ROS production from cells.

Wnt3a-CM activated Wnt/β-catenin pathway

To verify the activation effect of Wnt3a-CM on Wnt/β-catenin pathway, western blot was used to detect the expression of p-GSK3β (Ser9), p-GSK3β (Tyr216) and β-catenin in SH-SY5Y cells. Because the activity of GSK3β is regulated negatively by the phosphorylation of serine 9 (Ser9) and positively by the phosphorylation of tyrosine 216 (Tyr216) [21], the ratio of p-GSK3β (Tyr216) to p-GSK3β (Ser9) can be used to monitor the activity of GSK3β. We found that treatment of 100 μM 6-OHDA for 24 h increase the ratio of p-GSK3β (Tyr216) to p-GSK3β (Ser9), and decrease β-catenin level. However, pretreatment with Wnt3a-CM reverse these changes induced by 6-OHDA treatment (Fig. 5a, b and c).

Wnt3a-CM reversed 6-OHDA-induced Akt down-regulation

Investigation has documented that Wnt signal rely upon PI3K/Akt activation to support the cell survival [22]. Here we detected the level of p-Akt (Ser473) protein, an active form of Akt, in SH-SY5Y cells treated with

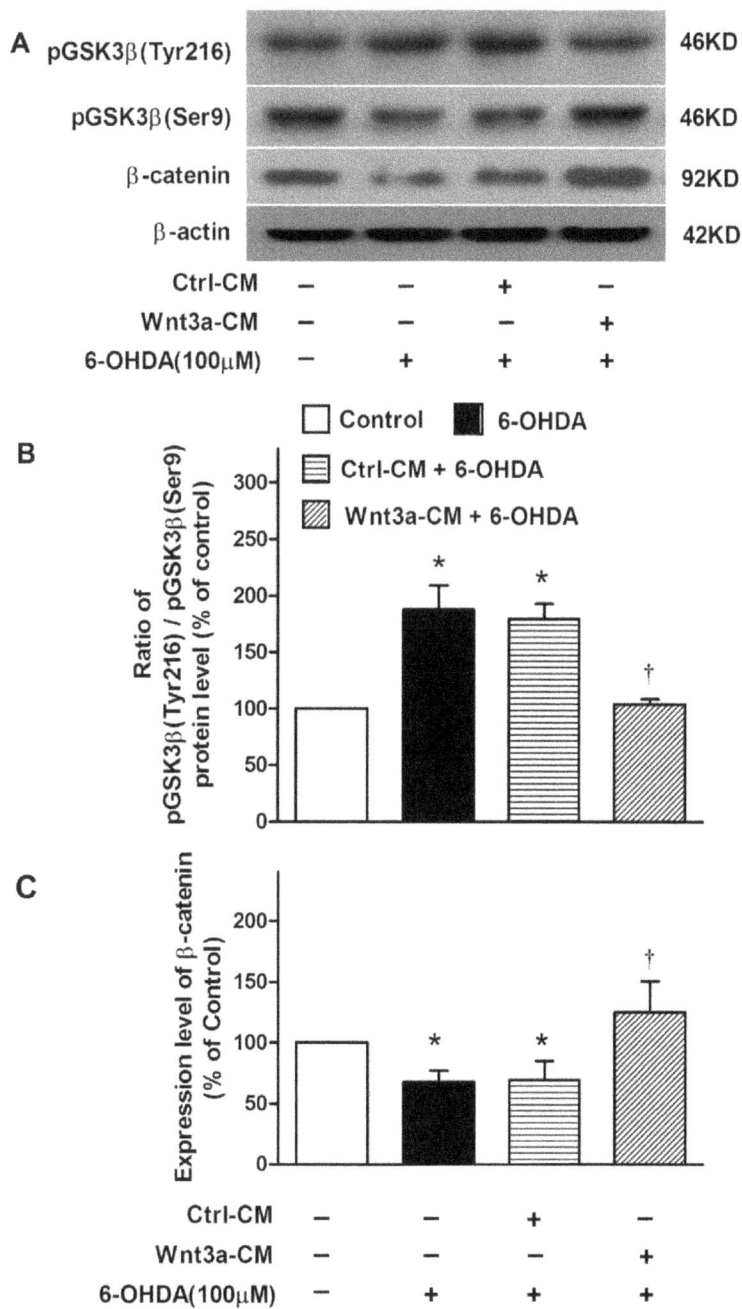

Fig. 5 Change of related signal proteins in the cytoprotective effect of Wnt3a-CM in Sh-SY5Y treated with 6-OHDA. SH-SY5Y cells were treated with vehicle, 6-OHDA (100 μM), Ctrl-CM, or Wnt3a-CM (40 %) 20 min prior to 6-OHDA for 24 h, the protein levels of 2 phosphorylation forms of GSK3β and β-catenin (**a**) were detected by Western blot with β-actin as internal control. The band intensities were measured by Quantity One software and normalized to the expression of β-actin in SHSY5Y cells. The ratio of p-GSK3β (Tyr216) to p-GSK3β (Ser9) (**b**) and the relative levels of β-catenin (**c**) were expressed in histogram. Data were presented as mean ± SD of 3 experiments. *$P < 0.05$ compared to the control, †$P < 0.05$ compared to Ctrl-CM + 6-OHDA group

6-OHDA or/and Wnt3a-CM. We found that the p-Akt protein level in 6-OHDA treated group were decreased to ~54 % compared with control group, while that in cells pretreatment of Wnt3a-CM was ~88 % (Fig. 6), which suggested that treatment of Wnt3a might reverse the down-regulation of PI3K/Akt pathway by 6-OHDA treatment.

Discussion

This study investigated the protective effects of Wnt3a-conditioned medium on a cellular model of PD and showed that Wnt/β-catenin pathway was inhibited after treatment of 100 μM 6-OHDA for 24 h, evidenced by the decreased β-catenin level and increased GSK3β activity. Moreover, activating Wnt/β-catenin pathway by Wnt3a-CM was found to attenuate 6-OHDA-induced neurotoxicity in SH-SY5Y cells through restoration of mitochondria transmembrane potential and reducing ROS production, indicating the Wnt/β-catenin pathway related to the maintenance of mitochondrial function.

SH-SY5Y cell line chosen in this study was considered for its expression of tyrosine hydroxylase (TH) simulating

to dopaminergic neurons [23]. As an endogenous oxidative metabolite of dopamine, 6-OHDA could inhibit the mitochondrial respiratory chain through inhibiting Complex I, uncoupling oxidative phosphorylation and collapsing mitochondrial membrane [24–26]. It is thought that 6-OHDA induces toxicity that mimics the neuropathological and biochemical characteristics of PD in SH-SY5Y cells [27].

Wnt3a is one of the Wnt ligands that activate the canonical Wnt pathway [28]. Because the purified Wnt3a is unstable, the Wnt3a conditioned medium is commonly used for the activation of the canonical Wnt pathway in in vitro experiments [29]. Recently, L'Episcopo et al. found the β-catenin protein acts as a pro-survival factor for mesencephalic TH+ neurons [14]. Meanwhile, Dickkopf-1 (DKK1), a negative regulator of the Wnt/β-catenin signaling pathway, was found to promote apoptosis of SH-SY5Y cells [30]. Dun Y and colleagues also found that induction of DKK1 contributes to the MPP+-induced neurotoxicity in PC12 cells via inhibition of the canonical Wnt pathway, and inhibition of DKK1 which could rescue the Wnt pathway might

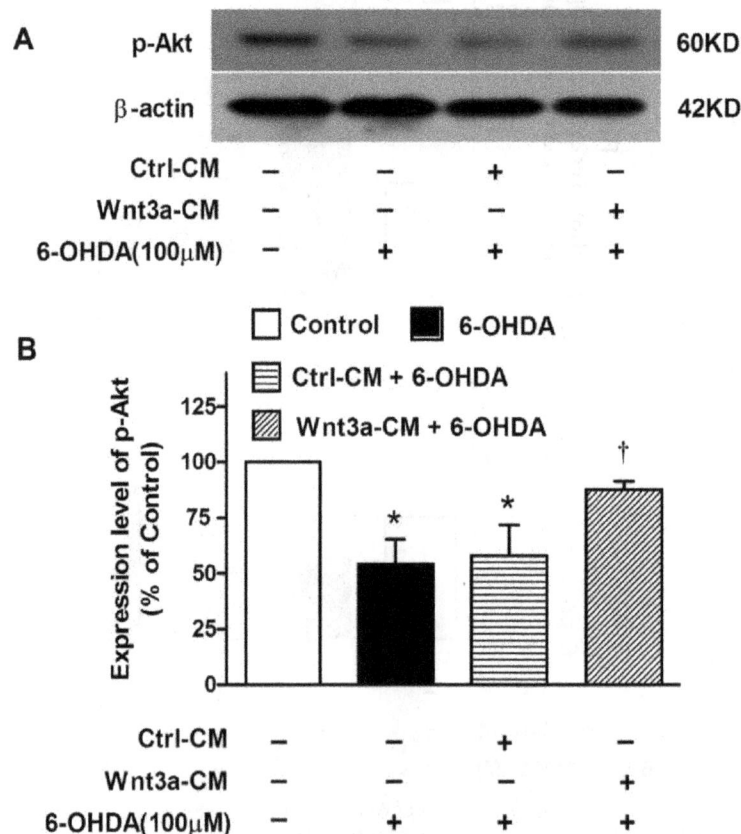

Fig. 6 Change of p-Akt level in the cytoprotective effect of Wnt3a-CM in Sh-SY5Y treated with 6-OHDA. SH-SY5Y cells were treated with vehicle, 6-OHDA (100 μM), Ctrl-CM, or Wnt3a-CM (40 %) 20 min prior to 6-OHDA for 24 h, the protein levels of p-Akt (a) were detected by Western blot with β-actin as internal control. The relative band intensities of p-Akt (b) were measured by Quantity One software and normalized to the expression of β-actin in SHSY5Y cells. Data were presented as mean ± SD of 3 experiments. *P < 0.05 compared to the control, †P < 0.05 compared to Ctrl-CM + 6-OHDA group

be neuroprotective in PD [31]. Our present study also confirmed that Wnt3a-CM increase the β-catenin protein level, which might contribute to the protective effect on cells. Moreover, our previous study uncovered that down-regulation of GSK3β, also a central component of the Wnt/β-catenin pathway, attenuate 6-OHDA-induced neuronal death and apoptosis [25]. The inhibition of GSK3β was reported to be linked with the attenuation of oxidative stress [32]. Data in this study confirmed that Wnt3a-CM inhibited the activity of GSK3β by increasing the phosphorylation at site Ser9 and decreasing the phosphorylation at site Tyr216.

Due to the mitochondrial dysfunction was considered a key factor in PD onset, we also measured MMP and ROS production from the SH-SY5Y cells in vitro. Mitochondria is the major site of ROS production and also prime target of oxidative molecular damage, the consequent formation of ROS further damages the mitochondrial membrane and such damages are implicated as key events in the pathogenic cascades leading to apoptosis [24, 33]. Shin SY and colleagues reported that stimulation of Wnt signaling by Wnt3a-CM inhibits H_2O_2-induced mitochondrial cytochrome C release and DNA fragmentation L1210 cells [34]. In this experiment, we found that Wnt3a-CM eliminated ROS production, stabilized mitochondrial transmembrane potential in SH-SY5Y cells.

PI3K and Akt are central to the regulation of cell growth and survival throughout the body [35, 36]. Akt, which is also known as protein kinase B (PKB), is a key molecule in growth factor signaling pathways mediating neuronal survival in both development and disease in multiple paradigms, including resistance against oxidative insults in the brain and protection of mitochondria function [37, 38]. Here our data showed that Wnt3a-CM reverse the down-regulation of p-Akt (Ser473) which is the active form of Akt caused by 6-OHDA treatment, clearly suggesting the mediation of the PI3K/Akt pathway in the protective effect of Wnt3a-CM on 6-OHDA-induced cell injury.

In conclusion, our data showed that activating of Wnt/β-catenin pathway by Wnt3a attenuated 6-OHDA-induced neurotoxicity, which involved in the mechanism about the inhibition of oxidative stress relate to the mitochondrial functional maintenance. These result may provide a new potential therapeutic target for Parkinson's diseases.

Competing interests
The authors declare that they have no competing interest and have approved the final article.

Authors' contributions
LW, LD, MSM, ML and LMZ performed the research; LW, KC and PYX participated in the design of the study and performed the statistical analysis. LW prepared the manuscript. All authors read and approved the final manuscript.

Acknowledgements
This work was supported by Nature Science Foundation of China (81401058, 81401645, 81271428 and 81471292), a grant from the State Key Development Program for Basic Research of China (2011CB510000), a grant from Medical Scientific Research Foundation of Guangdong Province (B2014139) and a grant supported by assisting research project of science and technology for Xinjiang (201591160).

Author details
[1]Department of Neurology, The Third Affiliated Hospital of Sun Yat-sen University, Guangzhou 510630, China. [2]Department of Neurology, The First Affiliated Hospital of Sun Yat-sen University, Guangzhou 510080, China. [3]Department of pathology, The First Affiliated Hospital of Sun Yat-sen University, Guangzhou 510080, China. [4]Department of Neurology, The First Affiliated Hospital of Guangzhou Medical University, Guangzhou 510120, China. [5]Division of Clinical Laboratory, Zhongshan Hospital of Sun Yat-sen University, Zhongshan 528403, China.

References
1. Andersen JK. Oxidative stress in neurodegeneration: cause or consequence? Nat Med. 2004;10(Suppl):S18–25. doi:10.1038/nrn1434.
2. Schapira AH, Gegg M. Mitochondrial contribution to Parkinson's disease pathogenesis. Parkinsons Dis. 2011;2011:159160. doi:10.4061/2011/159160.
3. Dexter DT, Carayon A, Javoy-Agid F, Agid Y, Wells FR, Daniel SE, et al. Alterations in the levels of iron, ferritin and other trace metals in Parkinson's disease and other neurodegenerative diseases affecting the basal ganglia. Brain. 1991;114(Pt 4):1953–75.
4. Li F, Chong ZZ, Maiese K. Winding through the WNT pathway during cellular development and demise. Histol Histopathol. 2006;21(1):103–24.
5. Yamaguchi TP. Heads or tails: Wnts and anterior-posterior patterning. Curr Biol. 2001;11(17):R713–24.
6. Mazemondet O, Hubner R, Frahm J, Koczan D, Bader BM, Weiss DG, et al. Quantitative and kinetic profile of Wnt/beta-catenin signaling components during human neural progenitor cell differentiation. Cell Mol Biol Lett. 2011;16(4):515–38. doi:10.2478/s11658-011-0021-0.
7. Vidya Priyadarsini R, Senthil Murugan R, Nagini S. Aberrant activation of Wnt/beta-catenin signaling pathway contributes to the sequential progression of DMBA-induced HBP carcinomas. Oral Oncol. 2012;48(1):33–9. doi:10.1016/j.oraloncology.2011.08.008.
8. Nusse R. WNT targets. Repression and activation. Trends Genet. 1999;15(1):1–3.
9. Castelo-Branco G, Wagner J, Rodriguez FJ, Kele J, Sousa K, Rawal N, et al. Differential regulation of midbrain dopaminergic neuron development by Wnt-1, Wnt-3a, and Wnt-5a. Proc Natl Acad Sci U S A. 2003;100(22):12747–52. doi:10.1073/pnas.1534900100.
10. Castelo-Branco G, Rawal N, Arenas E. GSK-3beta inhibition/beta-catenin stabilization in ventral midbrain precursors increases differentiation into dopamine neurons. J Cell Sci. 2004;117(Pt 24):5731–7.
11. De Ferrari GV, Chacon MA, Barria MI, Garrido JL, Godoy JA, Olivares G, et al. Activation of Wnt signaling rescues neurodegeneration and behavioral impairments induced by beta-amyloid fibrils. Mol Psychiatry. 2003;8(2):195–208. doi:10.1038/sj.mp.4001208.
12. Lin S, Cheng M, Dailey W, Drenser K, Chintala S. Norrin attenuates protease-mediated death of transformed retinal ganglion cells. Mol Vis. 2009;15:26–37.
13. Chong ZZ, Shang YC, Hou J, Maiese K. Wnt1 neuroprotection translates into improved neurological function during oxidant stress and cerebral ischemia through AKT1 and mitochondrial apoptotic pathways. Oxid Med Cell Longev. 2010;3(2):153–65. doi:10.4161/oxim.3.2.11758.
14. L'Episcopo F, Serapide MF, Tirolo C, Testa N, Caniglia S, Morale MC, et al. A Wnt1 regulated Frizzled-1/beta-Catenin signaling pathway as a candidate regulatory circuit controlling mesencephalic dopaminergic neuron-astrocyte crosstalk: Therapeutical relevance for neuron survival and neuroprotection. Mol Neurodegener. 2011;6:49. doi:10.1186/1750-1326-6-49.
15. Wei L, Sun C, Lei M, Li G, Yi L, Luo F, et al. Activation of Wnt/beta-catenin pathway by exogenous Wnt1 protects SH-SY5Y cells against 6-hydroxydopamine toxicity. J Mol Neurosci. 2013;49(1):105–15. doi:10.1007/s12031-012-9900-8.

16. Luo F, Wei L, Sun C, Chen X, Wang T, Li Y, et al. HtrA2/Omi is involved in 6-OHDA-induced endoplasmic reticulum stress in SH-SY5Y cells. J Mol Neurosci. 2012;47(1):120–7. doi:10.1007/s12031-011-9694-0.

17. Dong J, Song N, Xie J, Jiang H. Ghrelin antagonized 1-methyl-4-phenylpyridinium (MPP(+))-induced apoptosis in MES23.5 cells. J Mol Neurosci. 2009;37(2):182–9. doi:10.1007/s12031-008-9162-7.

18. Yu S, Liu M, Gu X, Ding F. Neuroprotective effects of salidroside in the PC12 cell model exposed to hypoglycemia and serum limitation. Cell Mol Neurobiol. 2008;28(8):1067–78. doi:10.1007/s10571-008-9284-z.

19. Zhang Z, Cao X, Xiong N, Wang H, Huang J, Sun S, et al. DNA polymerase-beta is required for 1-methyl-4-phenylpyridinium-induced apoptotic death in neurons. Apoptosis. 2010;15(1):105–15. doi:10.1007/s10495-009-0425-8.

20. Hwang CK, Chun HS. Isoliquiritigenin isolated from licorice Glycyrrhiza uralensis prevents 6-hydroxydopamine-induced apoptosis in dopaminergic neurons. Biosci Biotechnol Biochem. 2012;6(3):536–43.

21. Grimes CA, Jope RS. The multifaceted roles of glycogen synthase kinase 3beta in cellular signaling. Prog Neurobiol. 2001;65(4):391–426.

22. Sinha D, Wang Z, Ruchalski KL, Levine JS, Krishnan S, Lieberthal W. Lithium activates the Wnt and phosphatidylinositol 3-kinase Akt signaling pathways to promote cell survival in the absence of soluble survival factors. Am J Physiol Renal Physiol. 2005;288(4):F703–13. doi:10.1152/ajprenal.00189.2004.

23. Takahashi T, Deng Y, Maruyama W, Dostert P, Kawai M, Naoi M. Uptake of a neurotoxin-candidate, (R)-1,2-dimethyl-6,7-dihydroxy-1,2,3,4-tetrahydroisoquinoline into human dopaminergic neuroblastoma SH-SY5Y cells by dopamine transport system. J Neural Transm Gen Sect. 1994;98(2):107–18.

24. Blum D, Torch S, Nissou MF, Benabid AL, Verna JM. Extracellular toxicity of 6-hydroxydopamine on PC12 cells. Neurosci Lett. 2000;283(3):193–6.

25. Li Y, Luo F, Wei L, Liu Z, Xu P. Knockdown of glycogen synthase kinase 3 beta attenuates 6-hydroxydopamine-induced apoptosis in SH-SY5Y cells. Neurosci Lett. 2011;487(1):41–6. doi:10.1016/j.neulet.2010.09.070.

26. Soto-Otero R, Mendez-Alvarez E, Hermida-Ameijeiras A, Munoz-Patino AM, Labandeira-Garcia JL. Autoxidation and neurotoxicity of 6-hydroxydopamine in the presence of some antioxidants: potential implication in relation to the pathogenesis of Parkinson's disease. J Neurochem. 2000;74(4):1605–12.

27. Elkon H, Melamed E, Offen D. 6-Hydroxydopamine increases ubiquitin-conjugates and protein degradation: implications for the pathogenesis of Parkinson's disease. Cell Mol Neurobiol. 2001;21(6):771–81.

28. Wodarz A, Nusse R. Mechanisms of Wnt signaling in development. Annu Rev Cell Dev Biol. 1998;14:59–88. doi:10.1146/annurev.cellbio.14.1.59.

29. Zhou T, Hu Y, Chen Y, Zhou KK, Zhang B, Gao G, et al. The pathogenic role of the canonical Wnt pathway in age-related macular degeneration. Invest Ophthalmol Vis Sci. 2010;51(9):4371–9. doi:10.1167/iovs.09-4278.

30. Wang KP, Bai Y, Wang J, Zhang JZ. Morphine protects SH-SY5Y human neuroblastoma cells against Dickkopf1-induced apoptosis. Mol Med Rep. 2015;11(2):1174–80. doi:10.3892/mmr.2014.2832.

31. Dun Y, Yang Y, Xiong Z, Feng M, Zhang Y, Wang M, et al. Induction of Dickkopf-1 contributes to the neurotoxicity of MPP+ in PC12 cells via inhibition of the canonical Wnt signaling pathway. Neuropharmacology. 2013;67:168–75. doi:10.1016/j.neuropharm.2012.10.031.

32. Chen G, Bower KA, Ma C, Fang S, Thiele CJ, Luo J. Glycogen synthase kinase 3beta (GSK3beta) mediates 6-hydroxydopamine-induced neuronal death. FASEB J. 2004;18(10):1162–4. doi:10.1096/fj.04-1551fje.

33. Yao G, Yang L, Hu Y, Liang J, Hou Y. Nonylphenol-induced thymocyte apoptosis involved caspase-3 activation and mitochondrial depolarization. Mol Immunol. 2006;43(7):915–26. doi:10.1016/j.molimm.2005.06.031.

34. Shin SY, Kim CG, Jho EH, Rho MS, Kim YS, Kim YH, et al. Hydrogen peroxide negatively modulates Wnt signaling through downregulation of beta-catenin. Cancer Lett. 2004;212(2):225–31. doi:10.1016/j.canlet.2004.03.003.

35. Chong ZZ, Hou J, Shang YC, Wang S, Maiese K. EPO relies upon novel signaling of Wnt1 that requires Akt1, FoxO3a, GSK-3beta, and beta-catenin to foster vascular integrity during experimental diabetes. Curr Neurovasc Res. 2011;8(2):103–20.

36. Chong ZZ, Kang JQ, Maiese K. Erythropoietin is a novel vascular protectant through activation of Akt1 and mitochondrial modulation of cysteine proteases. Circulation. 2002;106(23):2973–9.

37. Rodriguez-Blanco J, Martin V, Herrera F, Garcia-Santos G, Antolin I, Rodriguez C. Intracellular signaling pathways involved in post-mitotic dopaminergic PC12 cell death induced by 6-hydroxydopamine. J Neurochem. 2008;107(1):127–40. doi:10.1111/j.1471-4159.2008.05588.x.

38. Johnson-Farley NN, Travkina T, Cowen DS. Cumulative activation of akt and consequent inhibition of glycogen synthase kinase-3 by brain-derived neurotrophic factor and insulin-like growth factor-1 in cultured hippocampal neurons. J Pharmacol Exp Ther. 2006;316(3):1062–9.

2

Roles of functional catechol-O-methyltransferase genotypes in Chinese patients with Parkinson's disease

Yiwei Qian, Jiujiang Liu, Shaoqing Xu, Xiaodong Yang and Qin Xiao[*]

Abstract

Background: Recent studies have found that the functional catechol-O-methyltransferase (COMT) gene may be associated with the susceptibility to and pharmacotherapy of Parkinson's disease (PD). In this case–control study, we investigated the most common functional COMT gene haplotypes that had been shown to influence COMT enzymatic activity and the association of the single and combined COMT haplotypes with clinical symptoms and pharmacotherapy in Chinese patients with PD.

Methods: One hundred forty-three patients with idiopathic PD and 157 healthy individuals were enrolled in this study. Four single nucleotide polymorphisms (SNPs) in the COMT gene (formed by SNPs) were genotyped in each participant: rs6269 A > G; rs4633 C > T; rs4818 C > G; and rs4680 G > A.

Results: The frequencies of rs4633 T carriers, rs4680 A carriers and the two linked rs4633-rs4680 T/A carriers were significantly higher in the early onset PD group than in the healthy controls (all $P < 0.05$). Homozygosity for rs4633 (TT), rs4680 (AA) and of the two linked rs4633-rs4680 (TT/AA) was significantly more frequent in patients who exhibited the "wearing-off" phenomenon, longer disease duration, higher levodopa equivalent doses (LED) and higher Unified Parkinson's Disease Rating Scale (UPDRS) scores ($P < 0.05$). No significant differences were observed in the clinical features of patients who carried individual rs6269 and rs4818, the two linked rs6269-rs4818 and the four combined COMT SNPs.

Conclusions: The results showed a possible association of combined functional COMT SNPs with PD risk, disease duration, the "wearing-off" phenomenon, daily LEDs and higher UPDRS scores, which may be useful in instituting individualized therapy for patients with PD.

Keywords: Parkinson's disease, COMT, SNP, Pharmacotherapy

Background

Parkinson's disease (PD) is a common progressive neurodegenerative disease in middle-aged and elderly people that consists of interactions between environmental and genetic factors and contributes to the dysfunction of dopaminergic neurotransmission in the central nervous system (CNS).

Genetic polymorphisms in enzymes, which regulate the biosynthesis or degradation of dopamine and its metabolites, may play a role in the susceptibility to PD and levodopa treatment. Catechol-O-methyltransferase (COMT) is one of the most important enzymes in the metabolism of drugs and neurotransmitters, such as L-dopa, dopamine, noradrenaline, etc. [1]; COMT-mediated O-methylation inactivates biologically active or toxic catechol and some hydroxylated metabolites [2]. Blocking of COMT activity further reduces peripheral levodopa degradation, as it prolongs plasma half-life of levodopa and elevates delivery of levodopa to the brain [3]. The human COMT gene is located on chromosome 22q11.21, and polymorphisms in COMT are associated with high, intermediate and low levels of enzyme activity, which might affect the risk and treatment of PD [4].

Most studies focused on the rs4680 single nucleotide polymorphisms (SNPs), which is a G to A substitution

* Correspondence: xiaoqin67@medmail.com.cn
Ruijin Hospital affiliated to Shanghai JiaoTong University School of Medicine, No. 197, Ruijin Er Road, Shanghai 200025, China

in the fourth exon of the COMT gene, leading to the substitution of valine 158 with a methionine (Val158-Met) and resulting in low COMT enzyme activity, which is regarded as the L (low activity) allele, in contrast to the H (high activity) allele [5]. The COMT protein encoded by the L allele is thermolabile, which influences individual variations in the therapeutic response to levodopa and susceptibility to PD [6–9]. Moreover, studies [1, 10–12] have focused on three other common haplotypes comprising combinations of four SNPs in the COMT gene: rs6269 A > G, rs4633 C > T (His62His), rs4818 C > G (Leu136Leu) and rs4680 G > A (Val158-Met). The haplotype structure formed by all four SNPs affects COMT enzymatic activity more than the single rs4680 SNP, which was regarded as a key determinant of COMT enzymatic activity in previous studies. COMT activity has been reported to depend on the presence of haplotypes formed by the four analyzed SNPs: A_C_C_G-low activity-L, A_T_C_A –medium activity-M, and G_C_G_G-high activity-H [11]. One study in Poland reported a high frequency of patients with late onset PD who were carriers of the G_C_G_G (high activity) haplotype, and the COMT haplotype seemed to have little influence on the development of levodopa-induced dyskinesia [1].

Additionally, some of the SNPs that have been studied with respect to PD risk exhibit linkage disequilibrium, although interethnic differences exist. According to the 1000 genome datasets (http://browser.1000genomes.org/Homo_-sapiens/Search/Results?site=ensembl&q=comt), Caucasian individuals show higher linkage values: the SNPs rs4680 and rs4633 exhibit complete linkage (D' = 1.00), the SNPs rs4680 and rs4818 exhibit partial linkage (D' = 0.685), and the SNPs rs4633 and rs4818 also exhibit partial linkage (D' = 0.685). However, for Oriental individuals, all linkages showed lower values: D' = 0.927 for the SNPs rs4680 and rs4633, D' = 0.240 for the SNPs rs4680 and rs4818, and D' = 0.223 for the SNPs rs4633 and rs4818 [4]. To our knowledge, no study has examined the associations between the two linked COMT SNPs (rs4680-rs4633 or rs6269-rs4818) with PD risk, clinical characteristics, and drug treatment. However, of the studies that have estimated the association between the combined two linked or four combined COMT SNPs and PD risk, the clinical symptoms and pharmacotherapy have not yet been investigated in China.

In this case–control study, we investigated the association of the most common functional COMT gene haplotypes (formed by SNPs: rs6269 A > G; rs4633C > T; rs4818 C > G; and rs4680 G > A), whether single, two linked or four combined SNPs, with PD risk in China. In addition, we examined the association of single, two linked or four combined COMT SNPs with the patients' clinical features and pharmacotherapy, particularly the complications of levodopa therapy in patients with PD.

Methods

Samples

We recruited 143 outpatients with idiopathic PD (79 males, 64 females, mean age (standard deviation [SD]) 65.1 (8.7)) as the PD group from the Movement Disorder Clinic at the Department of Neurology of Ruijin Hospital (affiliated with the Shanghai JiaoTong University School of Medicine, Shanghai, China) and 157 age- and gender-matched healthy individuals (88 males, 69 females, mean age (SD) 65.4 (7.2)) as the control group during the period from December 2013 to December 2014. All 143 patients with PD who were eligible for this study were diagnosed with idiopathic PD according to the UK brain bank criteria [13]. Among the 143 patients with PD, 24 were diagnosed with early onset PD (EOPD, onset before 50 years of age) and 119 were diagnosed with late onset PD (LOPD, onset after 50 years) [1]. All individuals who were diagnosed with atypical parkinsonism, including progressive supranuclear palsy (PSP), multiple system atrophy (MSA), vascular or drug-induced parkinsonism and severe dementia, characterized by a Mini Mental State Examination (MMSE) score <24 [14], were excluded from our study.

Each participant was informed of the purpose of this study and signed an informed consent form. This study was performed in accordance with The Code of Ethics of the World Medical Association (Declaration of Helsinki) for experiments involving humans and the protocol was approved by the Research Ethics Committee of Ruijin Hospital affiliated with the Shanghai Jiao Tong University School of Medicine.

Genotyping

Genomic DNA was extracted from peripheral blood samples collected from each individual using the standardized phenol/chlorine extraction method. Genotyping of rs6269 A > G was performed on a 456-bp DNA fragment amplified with the following primers: forward: CAACAGCCTGAGTCCGTGTC, reverse: TCCAGCC GATAAGGCACAGG. rs4680 G > A and rs4818 C > G were contained within the same 564-bp DNA fragment and amplified with the following primers: forward: ACCAGCGTGAGCATAGAGGC, reverse: GGTTTTC AGTGAACGTGGTGTG. rs4633C > T was genotyped using a 398-bp DNA fragment amplified with following pair of primers: forward: CTTGCCCCTCTGCAAA CAC, reverse: TTCTTGTCGCCCACGTTC. A 50 µl volume was used to conduct the polymerase chain reaction (PCR), which contained 1 µl of 100 ng/µl primer, 0.6 µl 5 of U/ml r-Taq DNA polymerase, 1 µl of 10 mM dNTPs, 5 µl of 10 × Buffer, 2.5 µl of genomic DNA and 38.9 µl of ddH2O. For rs6269, the PCR thermal profile consisted of initial denaturation at 95 °C for 5 min, 30 cycles at 95 °C, 58 °C and 72 °C (each step for 30 s) and a final elongation at 72 °C for 7 min. For rs4680 and rs4818, the PCR conditions included an initial step at 95 °C for 5 min, 30 cycles at 95 °C for 30 s, 58 °C for 30 s and 72 °C for 40 s and a final elongation at 72 °C for 7 min. For rs4633, the PCR conditions included an initial step at 95 °C for 5 min, 30 cycles at 95 °C, 56 °C and 72 °C (each step for 30 s) and a final elongation at 72 °C for 7 min. The PCR products were purified and sequenced on an ABI 3730xl automated sequencer (Applied Biosystems, Foster City, CA, USA).

Data collection

In this study, clinical data were collected through face-to-face interviews and questionnaires assessing demographic and clinical characteristics of patients with PD that were conducted by at least two movement disorder specialists. Demographic information included age, gender, and employment information; PD clinical characteristics included disease duration, onset condition (such as the age at diagnosis, the initial limb in which the PD symptoms were observed, and the first symptom of PD), drug treatment, and motor complications (mainly include "wearing-off" phenomenon, characterized by gradual expected re-emergence of parkinsonian symptoms at the end of an L-dopa dose, and L-dopa–induced dyskinesia, characterized by emergence of hyperkinetic involuntary movements). All patients were examined during the "on" state (improvement in symptoms after L-dopa administration is described as being "on") to determine their baseline motor function and activities of daily living using the Unified Parkinson's Disease Rating Scale (UPDRS), and disease severity was evaluated using the classification of Hoehn and Yahr stage (H&Y stage). The levodopa equivalent doses (LED) were calculated using a method reported in a previous study [15]. The PD-related non-motor symptoms were evaluated using the Non-Motor Symptoms questionnaire for Parkinson's disease (NMS-Quest), the Hamilton Anxiety Scale (HAMA), and the Hamilton Depression Scale (HAMD).

Statistical analysis

In this study, SPSS 17.0 software (SPSS Inc., Chicago, IL, USA) was used for the statistical analysis. In descriptive analyses, mean and standard deviation (mean ± SD) was used for normally distributed continuous variables, median and interquartile range (median ± IQ) for continuous variables with skewed distribution, and proportions for categorical variables. Concordance of genotype distribution with Hardy–Weinberg equilibrium was assessed using the Chi-square test. The Chi-square test and Fisher's exact test were used to compare the COMT allelic frequencies or genotype frequencies between the control group and PD group. Analysis of variance of

factorial design was used perform the association between COMT polymorphisms and clinical outcomes, adjusted age and sex as covariates. Binary logistic regression model was used to analyze the relation between SNP and motor complication (wearing-off phenomenon and dyskinesia), with age and sex as covariates. P-values were adjusted with Bonferroni correction. All statistically significant differences were considered P-value < 0.05.

Results

Linkage disequilibrium and haplotype analysis

In the pairwise analysis of the four COMT SNPs using the Haploview software, rs6269, rs4633, rs4818 and rs4680 showed strong linkage disequilibrium (LD) in both groups (Table 1), particularly rs6269-rs4818 and rs4633-rs4680. The LD of rs6269-rs4818 in the control group was D' = 0.94, LOD = 48.14, $r2$ = 0.85, whereas the LD in the PD group was D' = 0.98, LOD = 48.84, $r2$ = 0.92. The LD of rs4633-rs4680 in the control group was D' = 0.95, LOD = 41.80, $r2$ = 0.83, whereas the LD in the PD group was D' = 1.00, LOD = 49.53, $r2$ = 0.96. The patients with PD showed a stronger linkage in rs6269-rs4818 and rs4633-rs4680; therefore, we used the two linked SNPs rs6269-rs4818 and rs4633-rs4680 in the subsequent analysis.

Different COMT SNPs influenced the susceptibility to PD

The genotype and allele distributions of COMT SNPs were listed on Table 2. All the observed genotype or allele frequencies did not differ from the expected frequencies according to the Hardy-Weinberg equilibrium. For the single SNPs (rs6269A > G; rs4633C > T; rs4818C > G and rs4680G > A), no significant differences were found in the allele and genotype frequencies between the PD group and the control group. However, the frequency of rs6269 GG (P = 0.09) and

Table 1 Linkage disequilibrium (LD) of the combined studied SNPs in PD patients and healthy controls

		Control group			PD group		
		rs4633	rs4818	rs4680	rs4633	rs4818	rs4680
rs6269	D'	0.90	0.94	0.77	0.91	0.98	1.00
	LOD	8.05	48.14	4.84	4.43	48.84	5.49
	r^2	0.18	0.85	0.12	0.14	0.92	0.16
rs4633	D'	-	1.00	0.95	-	0.91	1.00
	LOD	-	10.20	41.80	-	3.85	49.53
	r^2	-	0.21	0.83	-	0.13	0.96
rs4818	D'	-	-	0.94	-	-	1.00
	LOD	-	-	7.47	-	-	4.88
	r^2	-	-	0.17	-	-	0.16

The LD pattern of the studied COMT SNPs was analyzed in Haploview. D' and r^2: measures of linkage disequilibrium between two genetic markers. *LOD* the logarithm of the odds for LD

Table 2 Frequencies of the studied SNPs in PD, EOPD and LOPD patients and healthy controls

	Control group n (%)	PD group n (%)	P	OR (95% CI)	EOPD n (%)	P	OR (95% CI)	LOPD n (%)	P	OR (95% CI)
rs6269 A > G										
AA	56 (35.0)	62 (43.4)	-	-	10 (41.7)	-	-	52 (43.7)	-	-
AG	77 (49.0)	67 (46.9)	0.33	0.79 (0.48–1.28)	12 (50.0)	0.77	0.87 (0.35–2.16)	55 (46.2)	0.32	0.77 (0.46–1.28)
GG	24 (15.9)	14 (9.9)	0.09	0.53 (0.25–1.12)	2 (8.3)	0.50	0.47 (0.10–2.29)	12 (10.1)	0.12	0.54 (0.25–1.19)
AG + GG	101 (65.0)	81 (56.6)	0.17	0.72 (0.46–1.15)	14 (58.3)	0.57	0.78 (0.32–1.86)	67 (56.3)	0.18	0.71 (0.44–1.16)
Major (A) allele frequency	189 (60.2)	191 (66.8)	-	-	32 (66.7)	-	-	159 (66.8)	-	-
Minor (G) allele frequency	125 (39.8)	95 (33.2)	0.09	0.75 (0.54–1.05)	16 (33.3)	0.29	0.71 (0.38–1.34)	79 (33.2)	0.11	0.75 (0.53–1.07)
rs4633 C > T										
CC	89 (55.4)	78 (54.6)	-	-	8 (33.3)	-	-	70 (58.8)	-	-
CT	57 (37.2)	56 (39.2)	0.64	1.12 (0.70–1.81)	15 (62.5)	0.02*	2.93 (1.17–7.35)	41 (34.5)	0.73	0.92 (0.55–1.52)
TT	11 (7.4)	9 (6.3)	0.89	0.94 (0.37–2.37)	1 (4.2)	1.00	1.01 (0.12–8.87)	8 (6.7)	0.87	0.93 (0.35–2.42)
CT + TT	68 (44.6)	65 (45.5)	0.71	1.09 (0.69–1.72)	16 (66.7)	0.03*	2.68 (1.06–6.47)	49 (41.2)	0.72	0.92 (0.57–1.49)
Major (C) allele frequency	235 (74.8)	212 (74.1)	-	-	31 (64.6)	-	-	181 (76.1)	-	-
Minor (T) allele frequency	79 (25.2)	74 (25.9)	0.84	1.04 (0.72–1.50)	17 (35.4)	0.13	1.63 (0.86–3.11)	57 (23.9)	0.75	0.94 (0.63–1.39)
rs4818 C > G										
CC	55 (35.0)	64 (44.8)	-	-	10 (41.7)	-	-	54 (45.4)	-	-
CG	82 (52.2)	66 (46.2)	0.14	0.69 (0.43–1.12)	12 (50.0)	0.64	0.81 (0.33–1.99)	54 (45.4)	0.12	0.67 (0.40–1.12)
GG	20 (12.7)	13 (9.1)	0.14	0.56 (0.26–1.23)	2 (8.3)	0.72	0.55 (0.11–2.73)	11 (9.2)	0.17	0.56 (0.25–1.28)
CG + GG	102 (65.0)	79 (55.3)	0.09	0.67 (0.42–1.06)	14 (58.3)	0.53	0.76 (0.32–1.81)	65 (54.6)	0.08	0.65 (0.40–1.06)
Major (C) allele frequency	192 (61.2)	194 (67.8)	-	-	32 (66.7)	-	-	162 (68.1)	-	-
Minor (G) allele frequency	122 (38.9)	92 (32.2)	0.09	0.75 (0.53–1.05)	16 (33.3)	0.46	0.79 (0.41–1.50)	76 (31.9)	0.09	0.74 (0.52–1.05)
rs4680 G > A										
GG	91 (58.0)	79 (55.2)	-	-	8 (33.3)	-	-	71 (59.7)	-	-
AG	57 (36.3)	56 (39.2)	0.61	1.13 (0.70–1.82)	15 (62.5)	0.02*	2.99 (1.19–7.51)	41 (34.5)	0.75	0.92 (0.56–1.53)
AA	9 (5.7)	8 (5.6)	0.96	1.02 (0.38–2.78)	1 (4.2)	0.59	1.26 (0.14–11.28)	7 (5.9)	1.00	1.00 (0.35–2.81)
AG + AA	66 (42.0)	64 (44.8)	0.64	1.12 (0.71–1.77)	16 (66.7)	0.02*	2.76 (1.12–6.82)	48 (40.3)	0.78	0.93 (0.57–1.51)
Major (G) allele frequency	239 (76.1)	214 (74.8)	-	-	31 (64.6)	-	-	183 (76.9)	-	-
Minor (A) allele frequency	75 (23. 9)	72 (25.2)	0.71	1.07 (0.74–1.56)	17 (35.4)	0.09	1.75 (0.92–3.33)	55 (23.1)	0.83	0.96 (0.64–1.43)
rs4633 C > T, rs4680 G > A										
CC/GG	86 (54.8)	78 (54.5)	-	-	8 (33.3)	-	-	70 (58.8)	-	-
Others	71 (45.2)	65 (45.5)	0.97	1.01 (0.64–1.59)	16 (66.7)	0.05	2.42 (0.98–5.99)	49 (41.2)	0.50	0.85 (0.52–1.37)
CC/GA	3 (1.9)	0	0.25	-	0	1.00	-	0	0.26	-
CT/GG	4 (2.6)	1 (0.7)	0.37	0.28 (0.03–2.52)	0	1.00	-	1 (0.8)	0.39	0.31 (0.03–2.81)

Table 2 Frequencies of the studied SNPs in PD, EOPD and LOPD patients and healthy controls (Continued)

	PD n (%)	EOPD n (%)	P	OR (95% CI)	LOPD n (%)	P	OR (95% CI)	Controls n (%)	P	OR (95% CI)
CT/GA	53 (33.8)	55 (38.5)	0.59	1.14 (0.70–1.86)	15 (62.5)	0.02*	3.04 (1.21–7.66)	40 (33.6)	0.78	0.93 (0.55–1.56)
TT/GG	1 (0.6)	0	1.00	-	0	1.00	-	0	1.00	-
TT/GA	1 (0.6)	1 (0.7)	1.00	1.10 (0.07–17.93)	0	1.00	-	1 (0.8)	1.00	1.23 (0.08–20.00)
TT/AA	9 (5.7)	8 (5.6)	0.97	0.98 (0.36–2.67)	1 (4.2)	1.00	1.19 (0.13–10.67)	7 (5.9)	0.93	0.96 (0.34–2.70)
rs6269 A > G; rs4818 C > G										
AA/CC	52 (33.1)	61 (42.7)	-	-	10 (41.7)	-	-	51 (42.9)	-	-
Others	105 (66.9)	82 (57.3)	0.09	0.67 (0.42–1.06)	14 (58.3)	0.41	0.69 (0.29–1.67)	68 (57.1)	0.10	0.66 (0.40–1.08)
AA/CG	4 (2.6)	1 (0.7)	0.19	0.21 (0.02–1.97)	0	1.00	-	1 (0.8)	0.37	0.26 (0.03–2.36)
AG/CG	76 (48.4)	64 (44.8)	0.19	0.72 (0.44–1.18)	12 (50.0)	0.67	0.82 (0.33–2.04)	52 (43.7)	0.18	0.70 (0.41–1.18)
AG/CC	1 (0.6)	3 (2.1)	0.63	2.56 (0.26–25.34)	0	1.00	-	3 (2.5)	0.62	3.06 (0.31–30.38)
GG/CC	2 (1.3)	0	0.22	-	0	1.00	-	0	0.50	-
GG/CG	2 (1.3)	1 (0.7)	0.60	0.43 (0.04–4.84)	0	1.00	-	1 (0.8)	1.00	0.51 (0.05–5.80)
GG/GG	20 (12.7)	13 (9.1)	0.14	0.55 (0.25–1.22)	2 (8.3)	0.72	0.52 (0.11–2.58)	11 (9.2)	0.17	0.56 (0.24–1.29)
6269 A > G; rs4633 C > T; rs4818 C > G; rs4680 G > A;										
1. L/L	20 (12.7)	29 (20.3)	0.10	0.47 (0.19–1.17)	2 (8.3)	1.00	1.05 (0.13–8.24)	27 (22.7)	0.11	0.47 (0.19–1.18)
2. L/M	20 (12.7)	23 (16.1)	0.27	0.60 (0.24–1.50)	7 (29.2)	0.26	0.30 (0.06–1.63)	16 (13.4)	0.64	0.79 (0.30–2.10)
3. M/M	9 (6.3)	8 (5.6)	0.67	0.77 (0.24–2.52)	1 (4.2)	1.00	0.95 (0.08–11.87)	7 (5.9)	0.74	0.81 (0.24–2.76)
4. H/L	45 (31.5)	33 (23.1)	0.87	0.93 (0.40–2.15)	4 (16.7)	1.00	1.18 (0.20–7.02)	29 (24.4)	0.96	0.98 (0.42–2.32)
5. H/M	29 (20.3)	30 (21.0)	0.35	0.66 (0.28–1.58)	8 (33.3)	0.30	0.38 (0.07–2.00)	22 (18.5)	0.70	0.83 (0.34–2.07)
6. H/H	19 (14.0)	13 (9.1)	-	-	2 (8.3)	-	-	12 (10.1)	-	-
7. Rare	15 (10.5)	7 (4.9)	0.51	0.68 (0.22–2.14)	0	0.50	-	6 (5.0)	0.45	0.63 (0.19–2.08)
8. H carrier (4 + 5 + 6)	93 (65.0)	76 (53.2)	-	-	14 (58.3)	-	-	63 (52.9)	-	-
9. L carrier (1 + 2 + 4)	85 (59.4)	85 (59.4)	0.35	1.22 (0.80–1.88)	13 (54.2)	0.97	1.02 (0.45–2.28)	72 (60.5)	0.33	1.25 (0.80–1.96)
10. other (1 + 2 + 3)	49 (31.2)	60 (41.6)	0.10	1.50 (0.92–2.43)	10 (41.7)	0.50	1.36 (0.56–3.28)	50 (42.0)	0.11	1.51 (0.91–2.50)

CI confidence interval, EOPD early onset PD, LOPD late onset PD, OR odds ratio

L low activity haplotype -A_C_C_G, M medium activity haplotype -A_T_C_A, H high activity haplotype -G_C_G_G; P values calculated in relation to each SNP normal genotype and allele frequency (rs6269 AA, allele A; rs4633 CC, allele C; rs4818 CC, allele C; rs4680 GG, allele G; rs4633-rs4680 CC/GG; rs6269-s4818 AA/CC) as a referent genotype; four SNPs: H/H (6) as a referent genotype [(1–5, 7), H carriers (8) as a referent genotype (9, 10); and L carriers (9) as a referent genotype (11). When more than 20% of the cell numbers were missing, or when the expected number of cases was less than 1.0 in a cell, Fisher's exact test was performed.

*P 0.05

allele G (*P* = 0.09), rs4818 CG + GG (*P* = 0.09) and allele G (*P* = 0.08) tended to be slightly lower among patients with PD than the controls. For the two linked SNPs (rs4633-rs4680 and rs6269-rs4818), there were also no significant differences in the allele and genotype frequencies between the PD group and control group. Moreover, no significant differences in the four combined SNPs (rs6269, rs4633, rs4818, and rs4680) were observed between the two groups. However, the frequency of the low (A_C_C_G) activity haplotypes (L) tended to be slightly higher among patients with PD (*P* = 0.10, G_C_G_G-high activity haplotype (H) as reference), and the frequency of the haplotypes without the H carrier tended to be higher in the PD group than in the controls (*P* = 0.10, H carrier was used as a reference).

In the subset analysis (Table 2), the frequencies of rs4633 T carriers (*P* = 0.03, odds ratio (OR) = 2.68, 95% confidence interval (CI): 1.06–6.47), rs4680 A carriers (*P* = 0.02, OR = 2.76, 95% CI: 1.12–6.82) and linked rs4633-rs4680 T/A carriers (*P* = 0.05, OR = 2.42, 95% CI: 0.98–5.99) were significantly higher in the EOPD group than in the control group. No significant difference in the SNPs or haplotypes was observed between the LOPD group and controls. No significant difference in the four combined SNPs was observed between the EOPD or LOPD groups and the control groups.

COMT SNPs influenced PD disease severity, levodopa treatment response and wearing-off phenomenon

The clinical characteristics of the patients with PD who were carriers of different SNPs are listed in Table 3. After adjusted for sex and gender, for rs4633, patients with the TT genotype had a higher H&Y stage (*P* = 0.007 among groups; *P* = 0.006 vs CC, *P* = 0.009 vs CT, respectively), younger age onset (*P* = 0.01 among groups; *P* = 0.03 vs CC), longer disease duration (*P* = 0.005 among groups; *P* = 0.005 vs CC), higher UPDRS scores (*P* = 0.006 among groups; *P* = 0.03 vs CC, *P* = 0.005 vs CT, respectively) (particularly on Part II (*P* = 0.002 among groups; *P* = 0.004 vs CC, *P* = 0.001 vs CT, respectively) and Part III, (*P* = 0.01 among groups; *P* = 0.02 vs CT), higher LED (*P* = 0.005 among groups; *P* = 0.009 vs CC) and more "wearing-off" symptoms (*P* = 0.008 among groups; *P* = 0.006 vs CC) than patients with the other genotypes, indicating that patients with the TT genotype of rs4633 presented more advanced disease stages, required higher dosages of drugs and had more fluctuations than patients with the other two genotypes. For rs4680, patients with the AA genotype also had a higher H&Y stage (*P* = 0.01 among groups; *P* = 0.01 vs GG, *P* = 0.02 vs GA, respectively), younger age onset (*P* = 0.01 among groups; *P* = 0.02 vs GG), longer disease duration (*P* = 0.005 among groups; *P* = 0.006 vs GG), higher LED (*P* = 0.007

among groups; *P* = 0.012 vs GG), higher UPDRS scores (*P* = 0.04 among groups; *P* = 0.03 vs GA) (particularly on Part II (*P* = 0.02 among groups; *P* = 0.02 vs GG, *P* = 0.02 vs GA, respectively)) and more "wearing-off" symptoms (*P* = 0.009 among groups; *P* = 0.008 vs GG) than patients with the other genotypes. These also suggested that the patients with the AA genotype of rs4680 may more easily develop a more severe form of the disease, require larger quantities of drugs and had more fluctuations. For rs4633-4680 (Table 4), patients with the TT/AA genotypes had a higher H&Y stage (*P* = 0.03 among groups; *P* = 0.02 vs CC/GG, *P* = 0.03 vs CT/GA, respectively), younger age onset (*P* = 0.03 among groups; *P* = 0.045 vs CC/GG), longer disease duration (*P* = 0.02 among groups; *P* = 0.01 vs CC/GG), higher UPDRS scores (*P* = 0.047 among groups; *P* = 0.046 vs CT/GA) (particularly on Part II, *P* = 0.03 among groups; *P* = 0.049 vs CC/GG, *P* = 0.02 vs CT/GA, respectively), more "wearing-off" symptoms (*P* = 0.02 among groups; *P* = 0.04 vs CC/GG) and higher LED (*P* = 0.01 among groups; *P* = 0.01 vs CC/GG) than patients without complete variants, indicating that patients who were simultaneous carriers of the TT genotype of rs4633 and AA genotype of rs4680 also showed the same tendency to develop a more severe illness and to experience poor drug treatment effects.

For rs6269, rs4818 and rs6269-rs4818 (Tables 3 and 4), no significant differences in clinical features, such as age of onset, duration of the disease, H&Y stage, LED, or the UPDRS, NMS, HAMA, HAMD and MMSE scores, were observed. For the four combined functional SNPs (rs6269, rs4633, rs4818, and rs4680) (data not shown), no significant differences in the clinical features, such as age of onset, duration of the disease, H&Y stage, LED, or the UPDRS, NMS, HAMA, HAMD and MMSE scores, were observed.

Discussion

The COMT enzyme is a natural candidate that has been implicated in the pathogenesis of PD. In this study, we investigated the association between functional COMT haplotypes and PD susceptibility. We found that the frequencies of rs4633 T carriers, rs4680 A carriers and rs4633-rs4680 T/A carriers were significantly higher in the EOPD group than in the healthy control group, suggesting that rs4633 and rs4680 polymorphisms are associated with susceptibility to EOPD. Considering the sample size is small, larger cohort studies focus EOPD patients are needed. However, no other significant difference in the risk of the individual COMT gene variants for PD pathogenesis was observed. The results of previous studies addressing the possible association between SNPs in the COMT gene and the risk of developing PD are controversial, particularly for rs4680, which primarily determines COMT activity. One meta-analysis examined 24 studies of 9,719 patients with PD and 14,634 controls

Table 3 Relationships between clinical features of patients and single SNPs

Characteristics	Total	rs4633 C > T				rs4680 G > A				rs6269 A > G				rs4818 C > G			
		CC	CT	TT	P	GG	GA	AA	P	AA	AG	GG	P	CC	CG	GG	P
n	143	78	56	9		79	56	8		62	67	14		64	66	13	
H&Y stage[b]	2.0±1.0	2.0±1.5	2.0±1.0	3.0±0.5	0.007**	2.0±1.5	2.0±1.0	2.8±0.5	0.01*	2.5±1.0	2.0±1.0	2.0±0.8	0.07	2.5±1.0	2.0±1.0	2.0±0.8	0.09
Age onset (years)[a]	59.2±9.2	60.7±9.2	57.5±5.6	57.3±5.6	0.01*	60.7±9.2	57.6±9.4	56.8±5.7	0.01*	59.5±9.5	58.8±2.6	60.3±10.6	0.80	59.6±9.5	58.6±8.6	60.8±10.9	0.89
Disease duration (years)[b]	6.0±5.0	6.0±4.0	6.0±5.8	9.0±7.5	0.005**	6.0±4.0	6.0±6.0	8.5±9.5	0.005**	6.0±5.3	6.0±5.0	7.5±7.3	0.73	6.0±5.0	6.0±5.0	8.0±8.5	0.75
LED (mg)[a]	448.8±327.4	386.2±287.5	496.8±358.0	693.2±322.6	0.005**	389.5±287.2	497.7±358.5	692.4±344.8	0.007**	475.3±399.2	425.0±241.7	445.5±346.5	0.56	469.7±396.5	435.0±243.6	416.4±342.2	0.59
Wearing-off (yes, %)	43 (30.1)	18 (23.1)	19 (33.9)	6 (66.7)	0.008**	18 (22.8)	20 (35.7)	5 (65.1)	0.009**	20 (32.3)	17 (25.4)	6 (42.9)	0.94	20 (31.3)	18 (27.3)	5 (38.5)	0.87
Dyskinesia (yes, %)[b]	18 (12.6)	7 (9.0)	9 (16.1)	2 (22.2)	0.12	7 (8.9)	9 (16.1)	2 (25.0)	0.09	8 (12.9)	7 (10.5)	3 (21.4)	0.76	8 (12.5)	7 (10.6)	3 (23.1)	0.67
UPDRS Part I score[b]	2.0±3.0	2.0±3.0	3.0±3.0	2.0±3.0	0.92	2.0±3.0	3.0±3.0	2.0±3.5	0.91	2.0±3.0	2.0±3.0	3.0±3.0	0.41	2.0±4.0	2.0±3.0	3.0±3.0	0.31
UPDRS Part II score[b]	8.0±7.0	8.5±9.0	8.0±7.3	13.0±10.0	0.002**	8.0±9.0	8.0±6.8	13.0±7.8	0.02*	8.0±7.0	8.0±8.0	11.0±7.3	0.48	8.0±7.0	9.0±7.0	9.0±7.5	0.70
UPDRS Part III score[a]	24.7±12.1	25.9±11.9	21.8±11.6	32.8±12.3	0.01*	25.8±11.9	22.4±12.1	31.0±11.9	0.06	25.3±12.3	24.2±12.1	24.6±11.6	0.82	24.8±12.3	24.4±12.3	26.2±10.3	0.96
UPDRS Part IV score[b]	3.0±2.0	3.0±2.0	2.0±3.0	5.0±3.0	0.10	3.0±2.0	2.0±3.8	4.5±4.0	0.13	3.0±4.0	2.0±3.0	3.0±2.0	0.98	3.0±4.0	2.5±3.0	3.0±2.0	0.96
UPDRS total score[a]	40.0±17.7	41.0±17.4	36.3±16.5	54.8±20.2	0.006**	40.8±17.3	37.1±17.3	52.0±19.7	0.04*	40.7±18.4	38.8±17.4	42.6±15.8	0.79	40.2±18.8	39.0±17.1	44.1±15.5	0.81
NMS score[b]	6.0±6.0	6.0±6.0	6.0±4.8	7.0±9.5	0.60	6.0±6.0	6.5±4.8	6.5±10.8	0.68	7.0±6.3	6.0±6.0	6.5±5.5	0.57	7.0±7.8	6.0±5.3	6.0±6.0	0.38
HAMA score[b]	4.0±6.0	4.0±6.0	5.0±4.5	4.0±14.0	0.48	4.0±6.0	5.0±4.8	4.5±13.3	0.40	5.0±6.0	4.0±4.0	6.0±7.0	0.85	5.0±6.0	4.0±4.0	6.0±6.0	0.93
HAMD score[b]	3.0=4.0	2.0±5.0	4.0±4.0	4.0±6.0	0.40	2.0±5.0	4.0±4.0	3.0±6.5	0.20	2.0±6.3	3.0±4.0	2.0±3.8	0.14	2.0±7.0	3.0±4.0	2.0±2.0	0.41
MMSE score[b]	28.0±3.0	28.0±3.0	28.0±3.0	27.0±4.0	0.49	28.0±3.0	28.0±3.0	27.5±3.0	0.54	28.0±3.0	28.0±3.0	28.0±3.5	0.12	28.0±3.0	28.0±3.0	28.0±3.5	0.13

Data were analyzed with analysis of variance of factorial design with age and sex as covariates

Binary logistic regression model was used to analyze the relation between SNP and motor complication (wearing-off phenomenon and dyskinesia), with age and sex as covariates

*P < 0.05 **P < 0.01

[a]Values are expressed as the mean ±SD

[b]Values are expressed as the median ±IQ

Table 4 Demographic and clinical features of patients with two combined SNPs

Characteristics	rs4633 C > T; rs4680 G > A					rs6269 A > G; rs4818 C > G				
	CC/GG	CT/GA	TT/AA	Rare	P	AA/CC	AG/CG	GG/GG	Rare	P
n	78	55	8	2		61	64	13	5	
H&Y stage[b]	2.0±1.5	2.0±1.0	2.8±0.5	2.50±1.0	0.03*	2.5±1.0	2.0±1.0	2.0±0.8	2.0±1.5	0.12
Age onset (years)[a]	60.7±9.2	57.5±9.5	56.8±5.7	58.0±5.7	0.03*	59.4±9.6	58.6±8.8	60.8±10.9	60.8±5.1	0.71
Disease duration (years)[b]	6.0±4.0	6.0±6.0	8.5±9.5	9.0±4.0	0.02*	6.0±5.5	6.0±5.3	8.0±8.5	4.0±3.5	0.67
LED (mg)[a]	386.2±287.5	494.0±360.7	692.4±344.8	675.0±35.4	0.01*	479.0±401.5	431.8±241.4	416.4±342.2	448.8±327.4	0.67
Wearing-off (yes, %)	18 (23.1)	19 (34.6)	5 (62.5)	1(50.0)	0.02*	20 (32.8)	17 (26.6)	5 (38.5)	1 (20.0)	0.87
Dyskinesia (yes, %)	7 (9.0)	9 (16.4)	2 (25.0)	0	0.07	8 (13.1)	7 (10.9)	3 (23.1)	0	0.52
UPDRS Part I score[b]	2.0±3.0	3.0±3.0	2.0±3.5	3.0±0.0	0.98	2.0±4.0	2.0±3.0	3.0±3.0	3.0±5.5	0.50
UPDRS Part II score[b]	8.5±9.0	8.0±6.0	13.0±7.8	13.5±17.0	0.03*	8.0±7.0	8.5±7.0	9.0±7.5	10.0±13.0	0.77
UPDRS Part III score[a]	25.9±11.9	21.9±11.7	31.0±11.9	32.0±21.2	0.08	25.1±12.3	24.5±12.2	26.2±10.3	19.4±14.9	0.83
UPDRS Part IV score[b]	3.0±2.0	2.0±3.0	4.5±4.0	4.0±2.0	0.24	3.0±3.5	2.0±2.8	3.0±2.0	2.0±4.0	0.78
UPDRS total score[a]	41.0±17.4	36.4±16.6	52.0±19.7	52.5±34.7	0.047*	40.5±18.6	39.1±17.2	44.1±15.5	34.6±20.4	0.86
NMS score[b]	6.0±6.0	6.0±4.0	6.5±10.8	6.5±9.0	0.85	7.0±6.5	6.0±5.75	6.0±6.0	9.0±11.0	0.46
HAMA score[b]	4.0±6.0	5.0±5.0	4.5±13.3	3.0±4.0	0.29	5.0±6.0	4.0±4.0	6.0±6.0	8.0±12.5	0.20
HAMD score[b]	2.0±5.0	4.0±4.0	3.0±6.5	2.0±4.0	0.56	2.0±6.5	3.0±4.0	2.0±2.0	7.0±7.5	0.86
MMSE score[b]	28.0±3.0	28.0±3.0	27.5±3.0	26.5±3.0	0.72	28.0±3.0	28.0±3.0	28.0±3.0	29.0±2.0	0.37

Data were analyzed with analysis of variance of factorial design with age and sex as covariates
Binary logistic regression model was used to analyze the relation between SNP and motor complication (wearing-off phenomenon and dyskinesia), with age and sex as covariates
*P < 0.05, [a]Values are expressed as the mean ± SD; [b]Values are expressed as the median ± IQ

and concluded that the rs4680 polymorphism is not a major determinant of the risk for PD [4]. Based on another meta-analysis, the Val158Met polymorphism may be a risk factor associated with Parkinson's disease in Asian rather than Caucasian populations [16]. Chuan, Gao [17] examined 13 studies including 1,834 patients and 2,298 controls and showed that the Val158Met polymorphism may be associated with PD in Japanese rather than Chinese populations. In conclusion, there is a remarkable heterogeneity in COMT gene variants in different ethnic groups.

Moreover, one study identified a decreased risk for PD in homozygous carriers of the COMT rs4680G and rs4633C alleles [12], whereas other studies focusing on the rs6269 [1], rs4818 [1, 18] and rs4633 SNPs [1, 19] did not detect a significant influence on PD susceptibility. However, Kimchi-Sarfaty [20] suggested that the determination of haplotypes is more appropriate than SNPs for the analysis of genetic variations in patients with pain, and Nackley, Shabalina [11] found that COMT haplotypes might have more influence on COMT activity than single SNPs. Few studies have focused on the four linked SNPs (rs6269, rs4818, rs4680 and rs4633) regarding pain intensity [21] or cognitive impairment in patients with PD [12]. Studies from Portland [1, 12] (including 322 patients with PD and 357 controls) did not demonstrate an association between functional COMT haplotypes in patients with PD and the controls; the frequencies of low (A_C_C_G) and medium (A_T_C_A) or without high (G_C_G_G) activity haplotypes tended to be slightly lower among patients with PD than among the controls. Unfortunately, our results did not identify an association of the four-combined functional COMT SNPs with patients and controls. The frequencies of low and without high haplotypes tended to be slightly higher among patients with PD, although the difference was not significant. Considering the ethnic factors, this result requires further evaluation.

In our results, both the linkage of rs6269-rs4818 and rs4680-rs4633 in the PD group were higher than that in the control group, such as D' = 1.00 for rs4680 and rs4633 in control group, D' = 0.91 for rs4680 and rs4633 in PD group. While according to the online data from the International HapMap Project (http://hapmap.nc-bi.nlm.nih.gov/index.html.en) in 2016, the linkages of rs4633 with rs4680 are D' = 1.0, LOD = 14.07, $r2 = 0.887$, and the linkage of rs6269 with rs4818 has not been shown in Chinese people. In particular, our results were different from data of Oriental individuals concluded from 1000 genome datasets in 2015 [4]. These data of the Oriental individuals were concluded from the northern and southern part in China (Beijing, Yunnan, Hunan and Fujian), while Shanghai, as the eastern part of China,

was not involved in that program (http://www.interna-tionalgenome.org/cell-lines-and-dna-coriell). According to the different geographic and host genetic factors, larger sample sizes and multi-center studies are needed in the future. Although no report has yet addressed the issue of dopamine catabolism in relation to the PD risk using a two-SNP model, we speculated that the difference might be associated with PD progression.

The patients with the T allele of rs4633 or the A allele of rs4680 and the TT/AA alleles of the two linked SNPs rs4633-rs4680 had a tendency to experience the "wearing-off" phenomenon, had a longer disease duration and larger daily LED and had higher UPDRS scores, suggesting that patients with rs4633 and rs4680 polymorphisms had more severe disease. Only one study focused on the association of rs4633 with medication and reported that the rs4633 polymorphism was associated with the UPDRS score but not with L-dopa medication [19]. Both rs4633 TT and rs4680 AA encode the low activity COMT enzyme, which may decrease COMT activity and dopamine degradation [8, 22]. The rs4680 SNP has been an area of intense research for several years. Our results were similar to those of other studies. A meta-analysis published in 2015 concluded that allele A of rs4680 was correlated with a risk of PD "wearing-off" [23]. As shown in the study by Watanabe, Harada [22], the "wearing-off" phenomenon tended to occur in patients with PD carrying the COMT rs4680 (AA) SNP. The authors proposed that decreased COMT activity might result in increased neuromelanin metabolism, which might subsequently promote the formation of cytotoxic radicals released upon neuromelanin interactions, contributing to neuronal degeneration. The possible effects of COMT SNPs on PD-correlated neuropharmacological variables are controversial. Bialecka, Kurzawski [1] reported a study of COMT haplotypes in Poland that did not identify a significant impact of COMT haplotypes on the development of the "wearing-off" phenomenon, longer disease duration and larger LED. Hao, Shao [9] found that the rs4680 GG allele may be a risk factor for the "wearing-off" phenomenon. The reasons for the discrepancy with our results may be that the patients involved in our study presented different disease severities. The mean disease duration of our patients was 6.0 years, which was longer than the 3 years of the patients in the study of Hao, Shao [9]. The mean disease duration of the patients in the study by Watanabe, Harada [22] was 9.4 years, which established the same conclusion as our study. In patients with low COMT activity, the prolonged duration and increased quantities of levodopa and dopamine in the plasma may lead to an increased accumulation, which may accelerate the neurodegenerative process. In addition to the "wearing-off" phenomenon, a recent prospective study showed that the homozygosity in the AA allele of the COMT Val158-Met polymorphism increases the risk of dyskinesia, which also suggests that the AA genotype may decrease L-dopa metabolism [24]. Our study did not arrive at the same conclusion because of the limited number of patients who presented dyskinesia. Finally, there were no significant effects of rs6269 and rs4818 on the morbidity and pharmacotherapy of PD, and the results are consistent with other currently available studies [4].

However, our results concerning the association of COMT SNPs with PD susceptibility and medication were based on a small sample size, and further investigations, particularly a larger cohort study including patients with different disease severities, should investigate the role of combined functional COMT haplotypes in Chinese Han patients. Additionally, the limitation of technology (e.g., low throughput, only sequenced by segments, needed manual comparison) used in this research could not be ignored, and the novel technologies of high-throughput sequencing become more popular and easily available in the future.

Conclusions

In conclusion, we provide the first report highlighting the possible association of functional COMT haplotypes with the risk of PD in Chinese patients. The combined COMT genotype also showed a possible influence on the motor response to levodopa and disease severity, particularly the duration, the "wearing-off" phenomenon, daily LED and UPDRS in patients with PD, which may be useful in instituting individualized therapy for patients with PD.

Abbreviations

CNS: Central nervous system; COMT: Catechol-O-methyltransferase; EOPD: Early onset PD; H&Y stage: Hoehn and Yahr stage; HAMA: Hamilton Anxiety Scale; HAMD: Hamilton Depression Scale; LD: Linkage disequilibrium; LED: Levodopa equivalent doses; LOPD: Late onset PD; MMSE: Mini Mental State Examination; MSA: Multiple system atrophy; NMS-Quest: Non-Motor Symptoms questionnaire; OR: Odds ratio; PCR: Polymerase chain reaction; PD: Parkinson's disease; PSP: Progressive supranuclear palsy; SD: Standard deviation; SNP: Single nucleotide polymorphisms; UPDRS: Unified Parkinson's Disease Rating Scale

Acknowledgments

We thank all the patients and healthy subjects for their generous donations of blood samples.

Funding

This work was supported by the National Natural Science Foundation of China (Grant No. 81071023) and the Natural Science Foundation of Shanghai (Grant No. 14ZR1425700).

Competing interests

We state explicitly that there are no potential competing interests.

Authors' contributions

QYW: study design and data collection. LJJ: data collection. XSQ: statistical analysis and interpretation. YXD: critical revision of the manuscript for important intellectual content. QX: study supervision and manuscript revision. All authors read and approved the final manuscript.

References

1. Bialecka M, Kurzawski M, Klodowska-Duda G, Opala G, Tan EK, Drozdzik M. The association of functional catechol-O-methyltransferase haplotypes with risk of Parkinson's disease, levodopa treatment response, and complications. Pharmacogenet Genom. 2008;18:815–21.
2. Torkaman-Boutorabi A, Shahidi GA, Choopani S, Zarrindast MR. Original article association of monoamine oxidase B and catechol-O-methyltransferase polymorphisms with sporadic Parkinson's disease in an Iranian population. Folia Neuropathol. 2012;4:382–9.
3. Muller T. Drug therapy in patients with Parkinson's disease. Transl Neurodegener. 2012;1:10.
4. Jimenez-Jimenez FJ, Alonso-Navarro H, Garcia-Martin E, Agundez JA. COMT gene and risk for Parkinson's disease: a systematic review and meta-analysis. Pharmacogenet Genom. 2014;24:331–9.
5. Hosak L. Role of the COMT gene Val158Met polymorphism in mental disorders: a review. Eur Psychiatry. 2007;22:276–81.
6. Corvol JC, Bonnet C, Charbonnier-Beaupel F, Bonnet AM, Fievet MH, Bellanger A, Roze E, Meliksetyan G, Ben Djebara M, Hartmann A, Lacomblez L, Vrignaud C, Zahr N, Agid Y, Costentin J, Hulot JS, Vidailhet M. The COMT Val158Met polymorphism affects the response to entacapone in Parkinson's disease: a randomized crossover clinical trial. Ann Neurol. 2011;69:111–8.
7. Torkaman-Boutorabi A, Shahidi GA, Choopani S, Rezvani M, Pourkosary K, Golkar M, Zarrindast MR. The catechol-O-methyltransferase and monoamine oxidase B polymorphisms and levodopa therapy in the Iranian patients with sporadic Parkinson's disease. Acta Neurobiol Exp (Wars). 2012;72:272–82.
8. Wu H, Dong F, Wang Y, Xiao Q, Yang Q, Zhao J, Quinn TJ, Chen SD, Liu J. Catechol-O-methyltransferase Val158Met polymorphism: modulation of wearing-off susceptibility in a Chinese cohort of Parkinson's disease. Parkinsonism Relat Disord. 2014;20:1094–6.
9. Hao H, Shao M, An J, Chen C, Feng X, Xie S, Gu Z, Chan P, Chinese Parkinson Study Group. Association of Catechol-O-Methyltransferase and monoamine oxidase B gene polymorphisms with motor complications in parkinson's disease in a Chinese population. Parkinsonism Relat Disord. 2014;20:1041–5.
10. Diatchenko L, Slade GD, Nackley AG, Bhalang K, Sigurdsson A, Belfer I, Goldman D, Xu K, Shabalina SA, Shagin D, Max MB, Makarov SS, Maixner W. Genetic basis for individual variations in pain perception and the development of a chronic pain condition. Hum Mol Genet. 2005;14:135–43.
11. Nackley AG, Shabalina SA, Tchivileva IE, Satterfield K, Korchynskyi O, Makarov SS, Maixner W, Diatchenko L. Human catechol-O-methyltransferase haplotypes modulate protein expression by altering mRNA secondary structure. Science. 2006;314:1930–3.
12. Bialecka M, Kurzawski M, Roszmann A, Robowski P, Sitek EJ, Honczarenko K, Gorzkowska A, Budrewicz S, Mak M, Jarosz M, Golab-Janowska M, Koziorowska-Gawron E, Drozdzik M, Slawek J. Association of COMT, MTHFR, and SLC19A1(RFC-1) polymorphisms with homocysteine blood levels and cognitive impairment in Parkinson's disease. Pharmacogenet Genom. 2012;22:716–24.
13. Daniel SE, Lees AJ. Parkinson's disease society brain bank, London: overview and research. J Neural Transm Suppl. 1993;39:165–72.
14. Fereshtehnejad SM, Ghazi L, Sadeghi M, Khaefpanah D, Shahidi GA, Delbari A, Lokk J. Prevalence of malnutrition in patients with Parkinson's disease: a comparative study with healthy controls using Mini Nutritional Assessment (MNA) questionnaire. J Parkinsons Dis. 2014;4:473–81.
15. Tomlinson CL, Stowe R, Patel S, Rick C, Gray R, Clarke CE. Systematic review of levodopa dose equivalency reporting in Parkinson's disease. Mov Disord. 2010;25:2649–53.
16. Lechun L, Yu S, Pengling H, Changqi H. The COMT Val158Met polymorphism as an associated risk factor for Parkinson's disease in Asian rather than Caucasian populations. Neurol India. 2013;61:12–6.
17. Chuan L, Gao J, Lei Y, Wang R, Lu L, Zhang X. Val158Met polymorphism of COMT gene and Parkinson's disease risk in Asians. Neurol Sci. 2015;36:109–15.

18. Punia S, Das M, Behari M, Mishra BK, Sahani AK, Govindappa ST, Jayaram S, Muthane UB, Thelma BK, Juyal RC. Role of polymorphisms in dopamine synthesis and metabolism genes and association of DBH haplotypes with Parkinson's disease among North Indians. Pharmacogenet Genom. 2010;20:435–41.

19. Yin B, Chen Y, Zhang L. Association between Catechol-O-Methyltransferase (COMT) gene polymorphisms, Parkinson's disease, and levodopa efficacy. Mol Diagn Ther. 2013;18:253–60.

20. Kimchi-Sarfaty C. A 'silent' polymorphism in the MDR1 gene changes substrate specificity. Science. 2007;315:525–8.

21. Zhang F, Tong J, Hu J, Zhang H, Ouyang W, Huang D, Tang Q, Liao Q. COMT gene haplotypes are closely associated with postoperative fentanyl dose in patients. Anesth Analg. 2015;120:933–40.

22. Watanabe M, Harada S, Nakamura T, Ohkoshi N, Yoshizawa K, Hayashi A, Shoji S. Association between Catechol-O-Methyltransferase gene polymorphisms and wearing-off and dyskinesia in Parkinson's disease. Neuropsychobiology. 2003;48:190–3.

23. Liu J, Chen P, Guo M, Lu L, Li L. Association of COMT Val158Met polymorphism with wearing-off susceptibility in Parkinson's disease. Neurol Sci. 2015;36:621–3.

24. de Lau LM, Verbaan D, Marinus J, Heutink P, van Hilten JJ. Catechol-O-methyltransferase Val158Met and the risk of dyskinesias in Parkinson's disease. Mov Disord. 2012;27:132–5.

3

Dysregulation of autophagy and mitochondrial function in Parkinson's disease

Bao Wang[1,2], Neeta Abraham[2], Guodong Gao[1] and Qian Yang[1*]

Abstract

Parkinson's disease (PD) is the second most common neurodegenerative disease. Increasing evidence supports that dysregulation of autophagy and mitochondrial function are closely related with PD pathogenesis. In this review, we briefly summarized autophagy pathway, which consists of macroautophagy, microautophagy and chaperone-mediated autophagy (CMA). Then, we discussed the involvement of mitochondrial dysfunction in PD pathogenesis. We specifically reviewed the recent developments in the relationship among several PD related genes, autophagy and mitochondrial dysfunction, followed by the therapeutic implications of these pathways. In conclusion, we propose that autophagy activity and mitochondrial homeostasis are of high importance in the pathogenesis of PD. Better understanding of these pathways can shed light on the novel therapeutic methods for PD prevention and amelioration.

Keywords: Parkinson's disease, Autophagy, Macroautophagy, Mitophagy, Chaperone-mediated autophagy, Mitochondria,α-synuclein, PINK/Parkin, LRRK2, DJ-1

Background

Parkinson's disease (PD) is the second most common neurodegenerative disease. Although most of PD cases are sporadic, more than 5 % are inherited [1]. The PD related genes mainly include (1) *SNCA*, the gene encoding α-synuclein, which is the main component of Lewy bodies [2]; (2) *LRRK2*, which encodes a multi-domain large protein. Variable LRRK2 mutants contribute to over 10 % of familial and about 3 % of sporadic PD cases [3]; (3) *PINK1* and *Parkin*, which are genes involved in mitochondrial turnover and maintenance. Their mutations are associated with early-onset PD [4]. (4) *DJ-1*, whose mutants contribute to 1–2 % of autosomal recessive PD [5].

Given the role of autophagy in the elimination of cellular dysfunctional proteins/organelles, the contribution of impaired autphagy to PD has attracted increasing interest. Accumulating evidence indicates autophagy defects are involved in the PD pathogenesis. PD related VPS35

D620N mutant inhibits autophagy and impairs the trafficking of the autophagy protein ATG9A [6]. In addition, in the substantia nigra (SN) of PD patients, aberrant autophagy activity is identified [7]. Inducing autophagy by manipulating Polo-like kinase 2 or activiting chaperone-mediated autophagy (CMA) can reduce α-synuclein aggregation [8, 9]. Finally, PD related neurotoxin 1-methyl-4-phenyl-1,2,3,6-tetrahydropyridine (MPTP) can induce autophagy through CDK5-mediated phosphorylation of endophilin B1 [10]. Rotenone could impair mitophagy to damage neurons which can be rescued by DJ-1 overexpression [11].

Recently, increasing reports support the role of mitochondrial dysfunction in the degeneration of DA neurons during PD initiation and progression. Mitochondria are double membrane organelles and participate in multiple cellular processes, including calcium homeostasis, energy supply, metabolic synthesis and apoptosis [12]. Mutations in mtDNA are more frequent in PD patients when compared with the age-matched population [13]. Interestingly, one recent study reports that α-synuclein overexpression augments mitochondrial Ca^{2+} transient by enhancing endoplasmic reticulum-mitochondria interactions and

* Correspondence: qianyang@fmmu.edu.cn
[1]Department of Neurosurgery, Tangdu Hospital, The Fourth Military Medical University, No. 569 Xinsi Road, Baqiao District, Xi'an 710038, Shaanxi Province, China
Full list of author information is available at the end of the article

physiological levels of α-synuclein are essential to maintain mitochondrial function and morphology [14]. MPTP and rotenone can disturb mitochondrial function, impair respiratory chain complex and induce oxidative stress [15, 16]. Thus, excessive mitochondrial stress in response to environmental toxins or impaired capability of neurons to remove damaged mitochondria through mitophagy may result in the death of neurons.

This review discussed the recent findings in the relationship among several PD related genes, autophagy and mitochondrial dysfunction (Table 1).

Autophagy

Autophagy, which derived from the Greek words for "self-digesting", refers to the cellular catabolic process to remove the cytosolic components, including mainly dysfunctional organelles, misfolded proteins, and surplus or unnecessary cytoplasmic contents to lysosome for digestion [17].

Autophagy can be divided into three major types: macroautophagy, microautophagy and chaperone-mediated autophagy (CMA). This classification is dictated by the way in which the cellular components are being delivered to lysosomes [17].

Macroautophagy (MA) is the most common and well conserved form of autophagy, and enables the bulk degradation of cellular contents [18]. It mainly involves five steps: initiation, nucleation, elongation, fusion, and degradation [19]. In this process, the pre-autophagosomal structure (PAS) elongates from membrane of Golgi, mitochondria or endoplasmic reticulum and sequesters the cullular contents or organelles to form the autophagosome. Subsequently, the autophagosome fuses with lysosomes to allow the cargo to be degraded [20]. Mitophagy describes the clearance of damaged mitochondria by macroautophagy. Increasing evidence prove that dysregulation of mitophagy play important roles in neurodegenerative diseases [21].

Microautophagy is the process in which cytoplastic contents are directly engulfed into lysosomes for degradation without an intermediate autophagosome [22]. Also, microautophagy is constitutionally active under normal conditions and maintains the turnover of cellular nutrients via selective degradation of proteins and organelles [23]. Unlike macroautophagy, nutritional deprivation or stress cannot activate microautphagy [24]. Currently, knowledge about the role and function of microautophagy, especially in neurodegenerative disease, is limited and further studies are needed.

CMA is characterized by the high selectivity in substrates targeting [25]. The substrates for CMA present a unique pentapeptide motif, which is known as KFERQ. Notably, this motif is a pattern recognition motif associated with the hydrophobicity and charge of amino acid residues, rather than 100 % compliance with specific amino acid residues [26]. Interestingly, post-translational modification could perfect some KFERQ-similar motif for CMA through changing the hydrophobicity and charge of amino acid residues [27]. Briefly, CMA can be divided into four main steps: recognition, unfolding, translocation and degradation [28]. Cytoplastic heat shock cognate protein 70 (Hsc70) binds to the substrates after recognizing the KFERQ motif and delivers it to lysosomal surface, where the substrates could be unfolded with the help of Hsc70 and other chaperons. Afer that, the unfolded substrate is translocated into lysosome via lysosome associated membrane protein type 2A (LAMP2A) for degradation under the lysosomal acid environment.

Mitochondrial dysfunction in Parkinson's disease

Although the mechanism underlying PD pathogenesis is still unclear, mitochondrial dysfunction has been increasingly confirmed to be a vital contributor. The main characterizations of mitochondrial dysfunction include ROS overproduction, ATP depletion, mitochondrial DNA depletion, caspase release and electron transport complex (ETC.) enzyme defection [29]. Neurotoxins applied to establish PD models, including MPTP and rotenone, damage mitochondrial function by inhibiting complex I activity [30]. One recent study specifically knockouts *Ndufs4* gene in mice midbrain DA neurons and reports significant compromise in complex I activity. However, *Ndufs4* deficit mice show no obvious neurodegeneration, no loss of striatal innervation and no movement impairment, but with increased vulnerability to MPTP, suggesting that impaired complex I activity is involved in the pathogenesis of PD [31]. Another study shows that complex I inhibition can lead to abnormal oxidition of optic atrophy 1 (OPA1), which in turn results in mitochondrial structural abnormalities and dopaminergic neurodegeneration. All these pathogenic changes are abolished by OPA1 upregulation, hinting that OPA1 is a novel therapeutic target for PD [32].

Table 1 PD-related genes are involved in dysregulation of autophagy and mitochondria

α-synuclein	Macroautophagy
	Mitophagy
	CMA
PINK1/Parkin	Mitophagy
LRRK2	Macroautophagy
	CMA
	Mitochondria
DJ-1	Macroautophagy
	CMA
	Mitochondria

Mitophagy means the way in which damaged mitochondria are eliminated by autophagy. Through mitophagy, cells regulate both the number and quality of mitochondria in response to the metabolic stress. One recent study using genome-wide RNAi screen identifies *sterol regulatory element binding transcription factor 1* (*SREBF1*), *F-box* and *WD40 domain protein 7* (*FBXW7*) as key regulators for PINK/Parkin pathway, which is reponsible for mitophagy activation [33]. Moreover, SREBF1 is considered as a risk locus for sporadic PD [34]. Thus, this study hints that mitophagy may act as a common mechanistic link between sporadic and autosomal recessive PD. Mutation in F-box domain-containing protein Fbxo7 is related with early-onset autosomal recessive PD. One study reports that Fbox7 is involved in mitochondrial maintainance via directly interaction with Parkin to induce mitophagy, which further confirms the importance of mitophagy in PD pathogenesis [35].

Our study shows that the myocyte enhancer factor 2D (MEF2D) is present in neuronal mitochondria and heat shock protein 70 (Hsp70) interacts with MEF2D and mediates its mitochondrial translocation. Mitochondrial MEF2D is responsible for the expression of the gene NADH dehydrogenase 6 (ND6), which encodes an essential component of the complex I. Blocking MEF2D function leads to impaired complex I activity, oxidative stress and neuronal death. More importantly, in the postmortem PD brain samples, both mitochondrial MEF2D and ND6 levels are decreased compared with age-matched controls [36]. Our further study shows that MPTP caused a significant decrease in the half-life and total level of MEF2D mRNA. Down-regulation of MEF2D mRNA alone can reduces the viability of SN4741 cells and sensitizes the cells to neurotoxin [37].

PD-related genes are involved in dysregulation of autophagy and mitochondria
α-synuclein

α-synuclein is encoded by *SNCA* and its fibrillar form is the major component of Lowy bodies [38]. Existence of hydrophobic non-amyloid β component domain endows α-synuclein with the propensity to aggregate [39]. Aggregated α-synuclein can trigger neuronal death in PD [40]. Thus, intensive researches focus on how to prevent or eliminate the aggregation of α-synuclein. Study show that ubiquitin proteasome system (UPS) is responsible for degrading monoubiquitinated α-synuclein, while macroautophagy is for removing deubiquitinated α-synuclein [41, 42]. Further study demonstrates, in normal condition, α-synuclein is mainly degraded by UPS [43]. Macroautophagy pathway can be activated in response to increased level of wild type or A53T mutant α-synuclein [44, 45]. However, some studies show that

increased α-synuclein can impair autophagosome synthesis by inhibiting Rab1a [46]. Also, pre-formed α-synuclein aggregates compromise autophagosome clearance and are resistant to degradation by autophagy [47]. The difference may be derived from the variability of models or different levels of α-synuclein. Further studies are warranted to address such discrepancy.

Abnormal α-synuclein level can also disrupt mitophagy. In PD postmortem brain tissues, α-synuclein accumulation increases oxidative stress and disturbs mitochondrial function [48]. Moreover, both in vivo and in vitro, expression of α-isoforms of α-synuclein in neurons causes the fragmentation of mitochondria, which will eventually leads to the decline in respiration and neuronal death [49]. Over-expression of α-synuclein can occur in mitochondria and disrupt mitochondrial membrane potential by opening the mitochondrial permeability transition pore (mPTP), thereby initiating mitophagy [45]. α-synuclein can activate mPTP via interacting with either adenylate translocator (ANT) or voltage dependent anion channel (VDAC) [50, 51]. Further study found that A53T mutant could impair mitochondrial function by residing in mitochondria membrane as monomers and oligomers [52].

Increasing evidence confirms α-synuclein as a target of chaperone mediated autophagy (CMA). Hsc70 can recognize soluble α-synuclein and the affinity between Hsc70 and α-synuclein fibrils is 5-fold tighter compared with soluble α-synuclein [53]. One recent study showed that Hsc70 and Ssa1p work like a tweezer to bind two domains within α-synuclein [54]. Also, in vitro, one study shows the uptake of extracellular α-synuclein by neurons and their retrograde axonal transportation to neuronal soma. However, Hsc70 chaperones α-synuclein in the extracellular space and alleviates α-synuclein oligomer formation [55]. Activating CMA activity via up-regulating LAMP2A decreases α-synuclein turnover and protects against α-synuclein over-expression induced neurotoxicity [9]. Our study showed MEF2D, a transcription activator identified as neuronal survival factor, is the substrate of CMA. Wild type or mutant α-synuclein accumulation compromises normal turnover of MEF2D by CMA and leads to decrease in the MEF2D DNA binding ability and neuronal stress, which underlies the neuronal loss of PD [56]. Thus, enhancing CMA pathway could be a promising therapeutic strategy for PD treatment.

PINK1/Parkin

PINK1 is a serine/threonine kinase protein and mutations in PINK1 cause a rare form of autosomal recessive PD [57]. Parkin containing ubiquitin E3 ligase can ubiquitinate multiple substrates for degradation. Mutations of Parkin lead to accumulation of its substrates and are related with early onset juvenile autosomal recessive PD [58].

Increasing evidence suggests the PINK1/Parkin pathway is essential for mitochondrial quality control. One recent study shows that Parkin ubiquitinates dynamin-related protein 1 (Drp1) to promote its degradation. Disruption of this interaction by Parkin mutation leads to the accumulation of Drp1 and mitochondrial fragmentation [59]. In *Drosophila*, both Parkin and PINK null mutants show a significant overall slowing of motichondrial protein turnover and mitophagy. Failure to remove the damaged mitochondrial proteins plays an important role in PD pathogenesis [60]. PINK1 mutation affects mitochondrial complex I activity and the maintainance of the electron transport chain, which disturbs the mitochondrial membrane potential [61]. Upregulation of Parkin protects cells against multiple stresses, including endoplasmic reticulum stress, mitochondrial stress, proteotoxicity and excitotoxicity [62, 63]. By contrast, loss of Parkin results in mitochondrial fragmentation, decreased cellular Ca^{2+} handling capability and increased cellular vulnerability to stress [64]. All the above findings demonstrate that deficiency in PINK1/Parkin pathway leads to mitochondrial dysregulation.

Recent researches on PINK1/Parkin pathway have revealed molecular details for mitochondria protection. Once the mitochondria are impaired and the membrane potential gets depolarized, PINK1 will accumulate on the outer membrane of mitochondria (OMM). A study showed dimeric PINK1 on OMM can recruit Parkin and thereby phosphorylates Parkin at Ser65 [65]. Research using mass spectrometry identified VDACs as the docking site for Parkin recruitment to the OMM [66]. After Parkin translocation to mitochondria, many OMM proteins are ubiquitinated by Parkin and in turn recruited other proteins to initiate mitophagy. Then, these Parkin labeled mitochondria are brought to lysosomes for degradation. This PINK1/Parkin signaling pathway can be positively modulated by AF-6, which is lacked in caudate/putamen and SN of sporadic PD patients [67]. Moreover, up-regulation of translocation of the OMM (TOMM) can rescue mitophagy impaired by Parkin mutations, hinting that TOMM acts as an important regulator in PINK1/Parkin mediated mitophagy [68]. Despite extensive research, how autophagy related proteins are recruited during mitophagy process is still unclear and to what extent mitophagy dysregulation contributes to PD pathogenesis remains to be investigated.

LRRK2

Leucine-rich repeat kinase 2 (LRRK2) is one of the generic contributors to PD. As estimated, variable LRRK2 mutants contribute to over 10 % of familial and about 3 % of sporadic PD cases [69]. So far, over 50 LRRK2 mutations have been identified in PD patients. Among these, the G2019S mutation is the most common cause of autosomal

dominant familial PD cases [70]. Also, G2019S mutation can be found in about 2 % sporadic PD. Thus, exploring LRRK2 pathogenicity is essential to understand the molecular mechanisms of PD.

Many reports show a relationship between LRRK2 and macroautophagy. In kidney of mouse, loss of LRRK2 leads to age-dependent bi-phasic alteration of macroautophagy activity [71]. In human neuroglioma cells, inhibition of LRRK2 kinase activity can stimulate macroautophagy in the absence of any alteration in mTOR pathway, suggesting that LRRK2 regulates autophagic activity independent of mTOR signalings [72]. Consistently, LRRK2 activates a persistent increase in autophagosome formation through a calcium associated pathway. Simultaneously, LRKR2 upregulation increases p62 and decreases the number of acidic lysosomes [73]. Moreover, G2019S mutation increases autophagic vacuoles and shortens neurite length [74]. The effects of G2019S on neurite length can be abolished by down-regulation of LC3 or Atg7 and enhanced by autophagy inducer rapamycin, hinting that autophagy plays an important role in regulation of neurite length [75]. In fibroblasts, G2019S LRRK2 mutant exacerbates MPTP-induced cell death dependent of autophagic activity [76]. Furthermore, a study showed that LRRK2 increases the number of autophagosomes by activating CaMKK/AMPK pathway [73]. In addition, G2019S mutation augments autophagic flux by MEK/ERK signaling [77].

LRRK2 and the PD-associated mutations can be degraded by CMA. In normal condition, both UPS and CMA are responsible for the degradation of wild-type LRRK2. However, G2019S LRRK2 disrupts degradation by these pathways [78, 79]. In addition, both wild-type LRRK2 up-regulation and its mutations inhibit formation of the CMA translocation complex, thereby suppressing CMA activity [80, 81]. Subsequently, the normal turnover of CMA substrates is disrupted. Although LRRK2 mutants damage CMA process, the detailed relationship with neuronal loss, especially in animal models, still needs to be further explored.

In physiological conditions, about 10 % of LRRK2 can present in the OMM, giving rise to the hypothesis that LRRK2 mutations might have influence over mitochondrial function. Study showed LRRK2 G2019S could lead to mitochondrial fragments by enhancing mitochondrial fission via phosphorylating decaprenyl diphosphate synthase subunit 2 Dlp1(Dlp1) [82]. Also, LRRK2 mutants activate dendritic mitochondrial clearance by autophagy in neurons [83].

DJ-1

DJ-1 belongs to the peptidase C56 family and acts as a redox-responsive cytoprotective protein. PD-related DJ-1 mutants are rare and contribute to 1–2 % of autosomal recessive PD [84].

DJ-1 can serve as a regulator of autophagy. The effect of DJ-1 up-regulation on macroautophagy depends on cell type. In dopaminergic neurons, DJ-1 overexpression induces ERK-dependent mitophagy and protects against neurotoxin induced apoptosis [11]. Also, in mouse embryonic fibroblasts, loss of DJ-1 suppresses basal autophagy and disrupts mitochondrial dynamics [85]. However, in some cancer cells, DJ-1 deficiency activates autophagy via JNK signaling [86]. Further studies are needed to address the relationship between DJ-1/autophagy and DA neuronal loss in the context of PD.

As an anti-oxidative protein, DJ-1 also plays an important role in regulating mitochondrial function. In human neuroblastoma M17 cells, DJ-1 wild-type overexpression induces elongated mitochondria while DJ-1 mutants overexpression causes mitochondrial fragmentation. Interestingly, DLP1 knockdown in these mutant DJ-1 cells rescues mitochondrial morphology and function [87]. Also, in DJ-1 knockout cells, autophagy degradation was impaired and defective mitochondria accumulated [88]. Loss of DJ-1 leads to mitochondrial phenotypes including reduced membrane potential, increased fragmentation and accumulation of autophagic markers. Supplementing DJ-1-deficient cells with glutathione reverses both mitochondrial and autophagic changes suggesting that DJ-1 may act to maintain mitochondrial function during oxidative stress [89].

In our recent study [90], we found that DJ-1, harboring CMA specific motif, is a direct substrate of CMA and mutation inside the motif can disturb the degradation of DJ-1 through CMA. In addition, we showed UPS is not the primary mechanism responsible for DJ-1 degradation. More interestingly, CMA preferentially clears the oxidatively injured DJ-1 and the extensive accumulation of the oxidized DJ-1 monomer following a reduction of lysosomal and CMA activity affects the formation or alters the balance of DJ-1 dimer. Furthermore, CMA-DJ-1 pathway plays a critical role in maintaining mitochondrial morphology and function under stress and protects against PD related neurotoxins induced cytoxicity. Our findings suggest that CMA/DJ-1 pathway is vital for mitochondrial homeostasis and dysregulation of this pathway may explain the neuronal loss during PD pathogenesis.

Recent findings on autophagy from PD human tissues

Compared with age-matched AD and control brain samples, CMA markers LAMP2A and Hsc70 are significantly decreased in SN and amygdala of PD brains, hinting the role of autophagy in PD pathogenesis [91]. Furthermore, in peripheral blood mononuclear cells from PD patients, Hsc70 protein level is decreased in all PD groups, while glucocerebrosidase protein level is reduced only in the genetic PD groups [92]. This study suggests that Hsc70

and glucocerebrosidase may serve as a screening tool for PD diagnosis. In addition, lysosomal glucocerebrosidase protein level and enzyme activity are selectively reduced in the region with increased α-synuclein inside the PD brain of early stage. The loss of lysosomal glucocerebrosidase is directly related to reduced lysosomal CMA activity, increased α-synuclein and decreased ceramide, which suggests that compromise in lysosomal function contributes to PD pathology [93]. One study also shows that the fibroblasts from PD patients with the mutation G2019S have higher level of autophagy compared with wild type fibroblasts, which contributes to the more vulnerability to MPP+ [76]. However, another study using the primary cultured fibroblasts from sporadic PD patients detects no changes in autophagy [94]. Further, one study uses iPSC-derived DA neurons from PD patients with GBA1 mutation and finds that these neurons has autophagic and lysosomal defects as well as increase in glucosylceramide and α-synuclein levels [95]. Together, these findings provide evidence for a link between autophagic/lysosomal system and PD pathogenesis.

Therapeutic implications

Currently, there is no effective treatment to halt the progression of neuronal loss in PD. Thus, developing effective therapeutic strategy will be of great importance and will likely result from a better understanding the relationship between macroautophagy, CMA, mitochondrial homeostasis and PD pathogenesis.

First, since PD is characterized by the presence of abnormal protein aggregation, enhancing macroautophagy to remove the redundant proteins and/or dysfunctional organelles is being considered as a potential therapeutic strategy. In vivo, enhancing autophagic activity through TFEB or Beclin-1 overexpression protects nigral neurons against α-synuclein-induced toxicity [96]. Coexpression of beclin-1 activated autophagy, reduced accumulation of α-synulein, and ameliorated associated neuritic alterations. The above data support that beclin-1 could be a promising molecular target for PD treatment. In addition, some autophagy-inducing chemical agents have been shown to decrease α-synuclein levels in cell and animal PD models [97, 98].

Furthermore, modulating CMA activity could provide benefits for PD treatment. In SH-SY5Y cells, generic overexpression of LAMP2A induces CMA activity and protectes DA neurons against α-synuclein neurotoxicity [9]. Moreover, in rat SN, overexpression of LAMP2A via lentivirus can reduce total levels of α-synuclein and ameliorate α-synuclein induced neuronal degeneration and stratal terminal loss [9]. Also, our data demonstrated restoration of CMA activity is essential to maintain the normal function of neuronal survival factor MEF2D, thereby regulating ND6 transcription and promoting mitochondrial complex I activity, which protect DA neurons from MPTP induced neurotoxicity [36, 37]. Furthermore, retinoic acid derivatives can activate CMA to protect cells against proteotoxicity and oxidative stress [99].

Finally, considering the contribution of mitochondrial dysfunction to the pathogenesis of PD, restoring it might be a way to prevent or treat PD. The first attempt is to enhance mitophagy. In drosophila, overexpression of Parkin increases mitochondrial activity, reduces proteotoxicity and extends lifespan [100]. Also, another possible way is modulate mitochondrial biogenesis, which would rejuvenate mitochondrial pool. The peroxisome proliferator-activated receptor gamma, coactivator 1 alpha (PGC-1α) is a potential target. PGC-1α positively regulates the expression of genes required for mitochondrial biogenesis and the cellular antioxidant responses. Also, expression of PGC-1α-regulated genes is low in SN neurons in early PD and overexpression of PGC-1α could suppress ROS and neurodegeneration [101]. Thus upregulation of PGC-1α is a candidate neuroprotective strategy in PD. However, targeted up-regulation of PGC-1α via adeno-associated virus (AAV) in SN region of mice showed detrimental effect [102, 103]. Thus, further studies need to clarify this discrepancy.

Conclusion

Future challenges

In our opinion, autophagy activity and mitochondrial homeostasis are of high importance in the pathogenesis of PD. Better understanding of the molecular interaction between autophagy and mitochondria function can give rise to novel therapeutic methods for PD prevention and amelioration. Since hypofunctional autophagy lead to protein/organelles accumulation while excessive autophagy activation can cause cell damage even autophagic cell death. The future challenges are to determine how to optimize autophagic activity to protect neurons during PD treatment. Also, challenges exist in identifying the common molecular pathway underlying the pathogenesis of multiple neurodegenerative diseases as well as the detailed molecular interaction between autophagy and mitochondrial dysfunction, especially in PD.

Abbreviations

ANT: Adenylate translocator; CMA: Chaperone-mediated autophagy; DA: Dopaminergic; DRP1: GTPase dynamic related protein 1; ETC.: Electron transport complex; LAMP2A: Lysosome associated membrane protein type 2A; LRRK2: Leucine-rich repeat kinase 2; MA: Macroautophagy; MFN1/2: Mitofusins 1/2; Miro: Mitochondrial Rho GTPases; MPP: Mitochondrial processing protease; MPTP: 1-methyl-4-phenyl-1,2,3,6-tetrahydropyridine; mPTP: Mitochondrial permeability transition pore; mtDNA: Mitochondrial DNA; ND6: NADH dehydrogenase 6; OMM: Outer membrane of mitochondria; PARL: Presenilin-associated rhomboid-like protease; PAS: Pre-autophagosomal structure; PD: Parkinson's disease; PGC-1α: peroxisome proliferator-activated receptor gamma, coactivator 1 alpha; PINK1: PTEN induced putative kinase 1; ROS: Reactive oxygen species; SN: Substantia nigra; UPS: Ubiquitin proteasome system; VDAC: Voltage dependent anion channel; VTA: Ventral segmental area

Acknowledgements
Not applicable.

Funding
The works were supported by National Natural Science Foundation of China (Grant No. 31371400) (Q.Y) and (Grant No. 31671060) (Q.Y).

Authors' contributions
BW made substantial contributions to design and draft the manuscript; NA and G-DG were involved in revising it critically; QY designed, revised the muscript; All the authors read and gave final approval of the manuscript to be published.

Competing interests
The authors declare that they have no competing interests.

Author details
[1]Department of Neurosurgery, Tangdu Hospital, The Fourth Military Medical University, No. 569 Xinsi Road, Baqiao District, Xi'an 710038, Shaanxi Province, China. [2]Department of Neurology, Beth Isreal Deaconess Medical Center, Harvard Medical School, 330 Brookline Ave, Boston 02215, MA, USA.

References

1. Klein C, Westenberger A. Genetics of Parkinson's disease. Cold Spring Harb Perspect Med. 2012;2:a008888.
2. Recasens A, Dehay B, Bove J, Carballo-Carbajal I, Dovero S, Perez-Villalba A, Fernagut PO, Blesa J, Parent A, Perier C, et al. Lewy body extracts from Parkinson disease brains trigger alpha-synuclein pathology and neurodegeneration in mice and monkeys. Ann Neurol. 2014;75:351–62.
3. Puschmann A. Monogenic Parkinson's disease and parkinsonism: clinical phenotypes and frequencies of known mutations. Parkinsonism Relat Disord. 2013;19:407–15.
4. Kilarski LL, Pearson JP, Newsway V, Majounie E, Knipe MD, Misbahuddin A, Chinnery PF, Burn DJ, Clarke CE, Marion MH, et al. Systematic review and UK-based study of PARK2 (parkin), PINK1, PARK7 (DJ-1) and LRRK2 in early-onset Parkinson's disease. Mov Disord. 2012;27:1522–9.
5. Ariga H, Takahashi-Niki K, Kato I, Maita H, Niki T, Iguchi-Ariga SM. Neuroprotective function of DJ-1 in Parkinson's disease. Oxid Med Cell Longev. 2013;2013:683920.
6. Zavodszky E, Seaman MN, Moreau K, Jimenez-Sanchez M, Breusegem SY, Harbour ME, Rubinsztein DC. Mutation in VPS35 associated with Parkinson's disease impairs WASH complex association and inhibits autophagy. Nat Commun. 2014;5:3828.
7. Nixon RA. The role of autophagy in neurodegenerative disease. Nat Med. 2013;19:983–97.
8. Oueslati A, Schneider BL, Aebischer P, Lashuel HA. Polo-like kinase 2 regulates selective autophagic alpha-synuclein clearance and suppresses its toxicity in vivo. Proc Natl Acad Sci U S A. 2013;110:E3945–54.
9. Xilouri M, Brekk OR, Landeck N, Pitychoutis PM, Papasilekas T, Papadopoulou-Daifoti Z, Kirik D, Stefanis L. Boosting chaperone-mediated autophagy in vivo mitigates alpha-synuclein-induced neurodegeneration. Brain. 2013;136:2130–46.
10. Wong AS, Lee RH, Cheung AY, Yeung PK, Chung SK, Cheung ZH, Ip NY. Cdk5-mediated phosphorylation of endophilin B1 is required for induced autophagy in models of Parkinson's disease. Nat Cell Biol. 2011;13:568–79.
11. Gao H, Yang W, Qi Z, Lu L, Duan C, Zhao C, Yang H. DJ-1 protects dopaminergic neurons against rotenone-induced apoptosis by enhancing ERK-dependent mitophagy. J Mol Biol. 2012;423:232–48.
12. Osellame LD, Blacker TS, Duchen MR. Cellular and molecular mechanisms of mitochondrial function. Best Pract Res Clin Endocrinol Metab. 2012;26:711–23.

13. Lin MT, Cantuti-Castelvetri I, Zheng K, Jackson KE, Tan YB, Arzberger T, Lees AJ, Betensky RA, Beal MF, Simon DK. Somatic mitochondrial DNA mutations in early Parkinson and incidental Lewy body disease. Ann Neurol. 2012;71:850–4.

14. Cali T, Ottolini D, Negro A, Brini M. alpha-Synuclein controls mitochondrial calcium homeostasis by enhancing endoplasmic reticulum-mitochondria interactions. J Biol Chem. 2012;287:17914–29.

15. Lee DH, Kim CS, Lee YJ. Astaxanthin protects against MPTP/MPP + –induced mitochondrial dysfunction and ROS production in vivo and in vitro. Food Chem Toxicol. 2011;49:271–80.

16. Karuppagounder SS, Madathil SK, Pandey M, Haobam R, Rajamma U, Mohanakumar KP. Quercetin up-regulates mitochondrial complex-I activity to protect against programmed cell death in rotenone model of Parkinson's disease in rats. Neuroscience. 2013;236:136–48.

17. Klionsky DJ, Abdelmohsen K, Abe A, Abedin MJ, Abeliovich H, Acevedo Arozena A, Adachi H, Adams CM, Adams PD, Adeli K, et al. Guidelines for the use and interpretation of assays for monitoring autophagy (3rd edition). Autophagy. 2016;12:1–222.

18. Rabinowitz JD, White E. Autophagy and metabolism. Science. 2010;330:1344–8.

19. Pyo JO, Nah J, Jung YK. Molecules and their functions in autophagy. Exp Mol Med. 2012;44:73–80.

20. Wong AS, Cheung ZH, Ip NY. Molecular machinery of macroautophagy and its deregulation in diseases. Biochim Biophys Acta. 2011;1812:1490–7.

21. Vives-Bauza C, Przedborski S. Mitophagy: the latest problem for Parkinson's disease. Trends Mol Med. 2011;17:158–65.

22. Mijaljica D, Prescott M, Devenish RJ. Microautophagy in mammalian cells: revisiting a 40-year-old conundrum. Autophagy. 2011;7:673–82.

23. Li WW, Li J, Bao JK. Microautophagy: lesser-known self-eating. Cell Mol Life Sci. 2012;69:1125–36.

24. Petrovski G, Das DK. Does autophagy take a front seat in lifespan extension? J Cell Mol Med. 2010;14:2543–51.

25. Kaushik S, Cuervo AM. Chaperone-mediated autophagy: a unique way to enter the lysosome world. Trends Cell Biol. 2012;22:407–17.

26. Cuervo AM. Chaperone-mediated autophagy: selectivity pays off. Trends Endocrinol Metab. 2010;21:142–50.

27. Ali AB, Nin DS, Tam J, Khan M. Role of chaperone mediated autophagy (CMA) in the degradation of misfolded N-CoR protein in non-small cell lung cancer (NSCLC) cells. PLoS One. 2011;6:e25268.

28. Cai Z, Zeng W, Tao K, E Z, Wang X, Yang Q. Chaperone-mediated autophagy: roles in neuroprotection. Neurosci Bull. 2015;31:452–8.

29. Exner N, Lutz AK, Haass C, Winklhofer KF. Mitochondrial dysfunction in Parkinson's disease: molecular mechanisms and pathophysiological consequences. EMBO J. 2012;31:3038–62.

30. Martinez TN, Greenamyre JT. Toxin models of mitochondrial dysfunction in Parkinson's disease. Antioxid Redox Signal. 2012;16:920–34.

31. Sterky FH, Hoffman AF, Milenkovic D, Bao B, Paganelli A, Edgar D, Wibom R, Lupica CR, Olson L, Larsson NG. Altered dopamine metabolism and increased vulnerability to MPTP in mice with partial deficiency of mitochondrial complex I in dopamine neurons. Hum Mol Genet. 2012;21:1078–89.

32. Ramonet D, Perier C, Recasens A, Dehay B, Bove J, Costa V, Scorrano L, Vila M. Optic atrophy 1 mediates mitochondria remodeling and dopaminergic neurodegeneration linked to complex I deficiency. Cell Death Differ. 2013;20:77–85.

33. Ivatt RM, Sanchez-Martinez A, Godena VK, Brown S, Ziviani E, Whitworth AJ. Genome-wide RNAi screen identifies the Parkinson disease GWAS risk locus SREBF1 as a regulator of mitophagy. Proc Natl Acad Sci U S A. 2014;111:8494–9.

34. Do CB, Tung JY, Dorfman E, Kiefer AK, Drabant EM, Francke U, Mountain JL, Goldman SM, Tanner CM, Langston JW, et al. Web-based genome-wide association study identifies two novel loci and a substantial genetic component for Parkinson's disease. PLoS Genet. 2011;7:e1002141.

35. Burchell VS, Nelson DE, Sanchez-Martinez A, Delgado-Camprubi M, Ivatt RM, Pogson JH, Randle SJ, Wray S, Lewis PA, Houlden H, et al. The Parkinson's disease-linked proteins Fbxo7 and Parkin interact to mediate mitophagy. Nat Neurosci. 2013;16:1257–65.

36. She H, Yang Q, Shepherd K, Smith Y, Miller G, Testa C, Mao Z. Direct regulation of complex I by mitochondrial MEF2D is disrupted in a mouse model of Parkinson disease and in human patients. J Clin Invest. 2011;121:930–40.

37. Wang B, Cai Z, Lu F, Li C, Zhu X, Su L, Gao G, Yang Q. Destabilization of survival factor MEF2D mRNA by neurotoxin in models of Parkinson's disease. J Neurochem. 2014;130:720–8.

38. Volpicelli-Daley LA, Luk KC, Patel TP, Tanik SA, Riddle DM, Stieber A, Meaney DF, Trojanowski JQ, Lee VM. Exogenous alpha-synuclein fibrils induce Lewy body pathology leading to synaptic dysfunction and neuron death. Neuron. 2011;72:57–71.

39. Horvath I, Weise CF, Andersson EK, Chorell E, Sellstedt M, Bengtsson C, Olofsson A, Hultgren SJ, Chapman M, Wolf-Watz M, et al. Mechanisms of protein oligomerization: inhibitor of functional amyloids templates alpha-synuclein fibrillation. J Am Chem Soc. 2012;134:3439–44.

40. Hansen C, Angot E, Bergstrom AL, Steiner JA, Pieri L, Paul G, Outeiro TF, Melki R, Kallunki P, Fog K, et al. alpha-Synuclein propagates from mouse brain to grafted dopaminergic neurons and seeds aggregation in cultured human cells. J Clin Invest. 2011;121:715–25.

41. Rott R, Szargel R, Shani V, Bisharat S, Engelender S. alpha-Synuclein ubiquitination and novel therapeutic targets for Parkinson's disease. CNS Neurol Disord Drug Targets. 2014;13:630–7.

42. Popova B, Kleinknecht A, Braus GH. Posttranslational Modifications and Clearing of alpha-Synuclein Aggregates in Yeast. Biomolecules. 2015;5:617–34.

43. Ebrahimi-Fakhari D, Cantuti-Castelvetri I, Fan Z, Rockenstein E, Masliah E, Hyman BT, McLean PJ, Unni VK. Distinct roles in vivo for the ubiquitin-proteasome system and the autophagy-lysosomal pathway in the degradation of alpha-synuclein. J Neurosci. 2011;31:14508–20.

44. Vogiatzi T, Xilouri M, Vekrellis K, Stefanis L. Wild type alpha-synuclein is degraded by chaperone-mediated autophagy and macroautophagy in neuronal cells. J Biol Chem. 2008;283:23542–56.

45. Choubey V, Safiulina D, Vaarmann A, Cagalinec M, Wareski P, Kuum M, Zharkovsky A, Kaasik A. Mutant A53T alpha-synuclein induces neuronal death by increasing mitochondrial autophagy. J Biol Chem. 2011;286:10814–24.

46. Winslow AR, Rubinsztein DC. The Parkinson disease protein alpha-synuclein inhibits autophagy. Autophagy. 2011;7:429–31.

47. Tanik SA, Schultheiss CE, Volpicelli-Daley LA, Brunden KR, Lee VM. Lewy body-like alpha-synuclein aggregates resist degradation and impair macroautophagy. J Biol Chem. 2013;288:15194–210.

48. Imaizumi Y, Okada Y, Akamatsu W, Koike M, Kuzumaki N, Hayakawa H, Nihira T, Kobayashi T, Ohyama M, Sato S, et al. Mitochondrial dysfunction associated with increased oxidative stress and alpha-synuclein accumulation in PARK2 iPSC-derived neurons and postmortem brain tissue. Mol Brain. 2012;5:35.

49. Nakamura K, Nemani VM, Azarbal F, Skibinski G, Levy JM, Egami K, Munishkina L, Zhang J, Gardner B, Wakabayashi J, et al. Direct membrane association drives mitochondrial fission by the Parkinson disease-associated protein alpha-synuclein. J Biol Chem. 2011;286:20710–26.

50. Zhu Y, Duan C, Lu L, Gao H, Zhao C, Yu S, Ueda K, Chan P, Yang H. alpha-Synuclein overexpression impairs mitochondrial function by associating with adenylate translocator. Int J Biochem Cell Biol. 2011;43:732–41.

51. Lu L, Zhang C, Cai Q, Lu Q, Duan C, Zhu Y, Yang H. Voltage-dependent anion channel involved in the alpha-synuclein-induced dopaminergic neuron toxicity in rats. Acta Biochim Biophys Sin Shanghai. 2013;45:170–8.

52. Auluck PK, Caraveo G, Lindquist S. alpha-Synuclein: membrane interactions and toxicity in Parkinson's disease. Annu Rev Cell Dev Biol. 2010;26:211–33.

53. Pemberton S, Madiona K, Pieri L, Kabani M, Bousset L, Melki R. Hsc70 protein interaction with soluble and fibrillar alpha-synuclein. J Biol Chem. 2011;286:34690–9.

54. Redeker V, Pemberton S, Bienvenut W, Bousset L, Melki R. Identification of protein interfaces between alpha-synuclein, the principal component of Lewy bodies in Parkinson disease, and the molecular chaperones human Hsc70 and the yeast Ssa1p. J Biol Chem. 2012;287:32630–9.

55. Danzer KM, Ruf WP, Putcha P, Joyner D, Hashimoto T, Glabe C, Hyman BT, McLean PJ. Heat-shock protein 70 modulates toxic extracellular alpha-synuclein oligomers and rescues trans-synaptic toxicity. FASEB J. 2011;25:326–36.

56. Yang Q, She H, Gearing M, Colla E, Lee M, Shacka JJ, Mao Z. Regulation of neuronal survival factor MEF2D by chaperone-mediated autophagy. Science. 2009;323:124–7.

57. Singleton AB, Farrer MJ, Bonifati V. The genetics of Parkinson's disease: progress and therapeutic implications. Mov Disord. 2013;28:14–23.

58. Rakovic A, Grunewald A, Kottwitz J, Bruggemann N, Pramstaller PP, Lohmann K, Klein C. Mutations in PINK1 and Parkin impair ubiquitination of Mitofusins in human fibroblasts. PLoS One. 2011;6:e16746.

59. Wang H, Song P, Du L, Tian W, Yue W, Liu M, Li D, Wang B, Zhu Y, Cao C, et al. Parkin ubiquitinates Drp1 for proteasome-dependent degradation: implication of dysregulated mitochondrial dynamics in Parkinson disease. J Biol Chem. 2011;286:11649–58.

60. Vincow ES, Merrihew G, Thomas RE, Shulman NJ, Beyer RP, MacCoss MJ, Pallanck LJ. The PINK1-Parkin pathway promotes both mitophagy and

selective respiratory chain turnover in vivo. Proc Natl Acad Sci U S A. 2013;110:6400–5.

61. Morais VA, Haddad D, Craessaerts K, De Bock PJ, Swerts J, Vilain S, Aerts L, Overbergh L, Grunewald A, Seibler P, et al. PINK1 loss-of-function mutations affect mitochondrial complex I activity via NdufA10 ubiquinone uncoupling. Science. 2014;344:203–7.

62. Bouman L, Schlierf A, Lutz AK, Shan J, Deinlein A, Kast J, Galehdar Z, Palmisano V, Patenge N, Berg D, et al. Parkin is transcriptionally regulated by ATF4: evidence for an interconnection between mitochondrial stress and ER stress. Cell Death Differ. 2011;18:769–82.

63. Van Laar VS, Roy N, Liu A, Rajprohat S, Arnold B, Dukes AA, Holbein CD, Berman SB. Glutamate excitotoxicity in neurons triggers mitochondrial and endoplasmic reticulum accumulation of Parkin, and in the presence of N-acetyl cysteine, mitophagy. Neurobiol Dis. 2015;74:180–93.

64. Cali T, Ottolini D, Negro A, Brini M. Enhanced parkin levels favor ER-mitochondria crosstalk and guarantee Ca(2+) transfer to sustain cell bioenergetics. Biochim Biophys Acta. 2013;1832:495–508.

65. Pickrell AM, Youle RJ. The roles of PINK1, parkin, and mitochondrial fidelity in Parkinson's disease. Neuron. 2015;85:257–73.

66. Scarffe LA, Stevens DA, Dawson VL, Dawson TM. Parkin and PINK1: much more than mitophagy. Trends Neurosci. 2014;37:315–24.

67. Haskin J, Szargel R, Shani V, Mekies LN, Rott R, Lim GG, Lim KL, Bandopadhyay R, Wolosker H, Engelender S. AF-6 is a positive modulator of the PINK1/parkin pathway and is deficient in Parkinson's disease. Hum Mol Genet. 2013;22:2083–96.

68. Lazarou M, Jin SM, Kane LA, Youle RJ. Role of PINK1 binding to the TOM complex and alternate intracellular membranes in recruitment and activation of the E3 ligase Parkin. Dev Cell. 2012;22:320–33.

69. Lubbe S, Morris HR. Recent advances in Parkinson's disease genetics. J Neurol. 2014;261:259–66.

70. Dusonchet J, Kochubey O, Stafa K, Young Jr SM, Zufferey R, Moore DJ, Schneider BL, Aebischer P. A rat model of progressive nigral neurodegeneration induced by the Parkinson's disease-associated G2019S mutation in LRRK2. J Neurosci. 2011;31:907–12.

71. Tong Y, Giaime E, Yamaguchi H, Ichimura T, Liu Y, Si H, Cai H, Bonventre JV, Shen J. Loss of leucine-rich repeat kinase 2 causes age-dependent bi-phasic alterations of the autophagy pathway. Mol Neurodegener. 2012;7:2.

72. Manzoni C, Mamais A, Dihanich S, Abeti R, Soutar MP, Plun-Favreau H, Giunti P, Tooze SA, Bandopadhyay R, Lewis PA. Inhibition of LRRK2 kinase activity stimulates macroautophagy. Biochim Biophys Acta. 2013;1833:2900–10.

73. Gomez-Suaga P, Luzon-Toro B, Churamani D, Zhang L, Bloor-Young D, Patel S, Woodman PG, Churchill GC, Hilfiker S. Leucine-rich repeat kinase 2 regulates autophagy through a calcium-dependent pathway involving NAADP. Hum Mol Genet. 2012;21:511–25.

74. Ramonet D, Daher JP, Lin BM, Stafa K, Kim J, Banerjee R, Westerlund M, Pletnikova O, Glauser L, Yang L, et al. Dopaminergic neuronal loss, reduced neurite complexity and autophagic abnormalities in transgenic mice expressing G2019S mutant LRRK2. PLoS One. 2011;6:e18568.

75. Winner B, Melrose HL, Zhao C, Hinkle KM, Yue M, Kent C, Braithwaite AT, Ogholikhan S, Aigner R, Winkler J, et al. Adult neurogenesis and neurite outgrowth are impaired in LRRK2 G2019S mice. Neurobiol Dis. 2011;41:706–16.

76. Yakhine-Diop SM, Bravo-San Pedro JM, Gomez-Sanchez R, Pizarro-Estrella E, Rodriguez-Arribas M, Climent V, Aiastui A, Lopez de Munain A, Fuentes JM, Gonzalez-Polo RA. G2019S LRRK2 mutant fibroblasts from Parkinson's disease patients show increased sensitivity to neurotoxin 1-methyl-4-phenylpyridinium dependent of autophagy. Toxicology. 2014;324:1–9.

77. Bravo-San Pedro JM, Niso-Santano M, Gomez-Sanchez R, Pizarro-Estrella E, Aiastui-Pujana A, Gorostidi A, Climent V, Lopez de Maturana R, Sanchez-Pernaute R, Lopez de Munain A, et al. The LRRK2 G2019S mutant exacerbates basal autophagy through activation of the MEK/ERK pathway. Cell Mol Life Sci. 2013;70:121–36.

78. Orenstein SJ, Kuo SH, Tasset I, Arias E, Koga H, Fernandez-Carasa I, Cortes E, Honig LS, Dauer W, Consiglio A, et al. Interplay of LRRK2 with chaperone-mediated autophagy. Nat Neurosci. 2013;16:394–406.

79. Lichtenberg M, Mansilla A, Zecchini VR, Fleming A, Rubinsztein DC. The Parkinson's disease protein LRRK2 impairs proteasome substrate clearance without affecting proteasome catalytic activity. Cell Death Dis. 2011;2:e196.

80. Yue Z, Yang XW. Dangerous duet: LRRK2 and alpha-synuclein jam at CMA. Nat Neurosci. 2013;16:375–7.

81. Sweet ES, Saunier-Rebori B, Yue Z, Blitzer RD. The Parkinson's Disease-Associated Mutation LRRK2-G2019S Impairs Synaptic Plasticity in Mouse Hippocampus. J Neurosci. 2015;35:11190–5.

82. Niu J, Yu M, Wang C, Xu Z. Leucine-rich repeat kinase 2 disturbs mitochondrial dynamics via Dynamin-like protein. J Neurochem. 2012;122:650–8.

83. Cherra 3rd SJ, Steer E, Gusdon AM, Kiselyov K, Chu CT. Mutant LRRK2 elicits calcium imbalance and depletion of dendritic mitochondria in neurons. Am J Pathol. 2013;182:474–84.

84. Rochet JC, Hay BA, Guo M. Molecular insights into Parkinson's disease. Prog Mol Biol Transl Sci. 2012;107:125–88.

85. Krebiehl G, Ruckerbauer S, Burbulla LF, Kieper N, Maurer B, Waak J, Wolburg H, Gizatullina Z, Gellerich FN, Woitalla D, et al. Reduced basal autophagy and impaired mitochondrial dynamics due to loss of Parkinson's disease-associated protein DJ-1. PLoS One. 2010;5:e9367.

86. Ren H, Fu K, Mu C, Li B, Wang D, Wang G. DJ-1, a cancer and Parkinson's disease associated protein, regulates autophagy through JNK pathway in cancer cells. Cancer Lett. 2010;297:101–8.

87. Wang X, Petrie TG, Liu Y, Liu J, Fujioka H, Zhu X. Parkinson's disease-associated DJ-1 mutations impair mitochondrial dynamics and cause mitochondrial dysfunction. J Neurochem. 2012;121:830–9.

88. Thomas KJ, McCoy MK, Blackinton J, Beilina A, van der Brug M, Sandebring A, Miller D, Maric D, Cedazo-Minguez A, Cookson MR. DJ-1 acts in parallel to the PINK1/parkin pathway to control mitochondrial function and autophagy. Hum Mol Genet. 2011;20:40–50.

89. McCoy MK, Cookson MR. DJ-1 regulation of mitochondrial function and autophagy through oxidative stress. Autophagy. 2011;7:531–2.

90. Wang B, Cai Z, Tao K, Zeng W, Lu F, Yang R, Feng D, Gao G, Yang Q. Essential control of mitochondrial morphology and function by chaperone-mediated autophagy through degradation of PARK7. Autophagy. 2016;12:1215–28.

91. Alvarez-Erviti L, Rodriguez-Oroz MC, Cooper JM, Caballero C, Ferrer I, Obeso JA, Schapira AH. Chaperone-mediated autophagy markers in Parkinson disease brains. Arch Neurol. 2010;67:1464–72.

92. Papagiannakis N, Xilouri M, Koros C, Stamelou M, Antonelou R, Maniati M, Papadimitriou D, Moraitou M, Michelakakis H, Stefanis L. Lysosomal alterations in peripheral blood mononuclear cells of Parkinson's disease patients. Mov Disord. 2015;30:1830–4.

93. Murphy KE, Gysbers AM, Abbott SK, Tayebi N, Kim WS, Sidransky E, Cooper A, Garner B, Halliday GM. Reduced glucocerebrosidase is associated with increased alpha-synuclein in sporadic Parkinson's disease. Brain. 2014;137:834–48.

94. Ambrosi G, Ghezzi C, Sepe S, Milanese C, Payan-Gomez C, Bombardieri CR, Armentero MT, Zangaglia R, Pacchetti C, Mastroberardino PG, et al. Bioenergetic and proteolytic defects in fibroblasts from patients with sporadic Parkinson's disease. Biochim Biophys Acta. 2014;1842:1385–94.

95. Schondorf DC, Aureli M, McAllister FE, Hindley CJ, Mayer F, Schmid B, Sardi SP, Valsecchi M, Hoffmann S, Schwarz LK, et al. iPSC-derived neurons from GBA1-associated Parkinson's disease patients show autophagic defects and impaired calcium homeostasis. Nat Commun. 2014;5:4028.

96. Decressac M, Mattsson B, Weikop P, Lundblad M, Jakobsson J, Bjorklund A. TFEB-mediated autophagy rescues midbrain dopamine neurons from alpha-synuclein toxicity. Proc Natl Acad Sci U S A. 2013;110:E1817–26.

97. Shoji-Kawata S, Sumpter R, Leveno M, Campbell GR, Zou Z, Kinch L, Wilkins AD, Sun Q, Pallauf K, MacDuff D, et al. Identification of a candidate therapeutic autophagy-inducing peptide. Nature. 2013;494:201–6.

98. Steele JW, Ju S, Lachenmayer ML, Liken J, Stock A, Kim SH, Delgado LM, Alfaro IE, Bernales S, Verdile G, et al. Latrepirdine stimulates autophagy and reduces accumulation of alpha-synuclein in cells and in mouse brain. Mol Psychiatry. 2013;18:882–8.

99. Anguiano J, Garner TP, Mahalingam M, Das BC, Gavathiotis E, Cuervo AM. Chemical modulation of chaperone-mediated autophagy by retinoic acid derivatives. Nat Chem Biol. 2013;9:374–82.

100. Rana A, Rera M, Walker DW. Parkin overexpression during aging reduces proteotoxicity, alters mitochondrial dynamics, and extends lifespan. Proc Natl Acad Sci U S A. 2013;110:8638–43.

101. St-Pierre J, Drori S, Uldry M, Silvaggi JM, Rhee J, Jager S, Handschin C, Zheng K, Lin J, Yang W, et al. Suppression of reactive oxygen species and neurodegeneration by the PGC-1 transcriptional coactivators. Cell. 2006;127:397–408.

102. Clark J, Silvaggi JM, Kiselak T, Zheng K, Clore EL, Dai Y, Bass CE, Simon DK. Pgc-1alpha overexpression downregulates Pitx3 and increases susceptibility to MPTP toxicity associated with decreased Bdnf. PLoS One. 2012;7:e48925.
103. Ciron C, Lengacher S, Dusonchet J, Aebischer P, Schneider BL. Sustained expression of PGC-1alpha in the rat nigrostriatal system selectively impairs dopaminergic function. Hum Mol Genet. 2012;21:1861–76.

4

Opioid system in L-DOPA-induced dyskinesia

Jing Pan and Huaibin Cai*

Abstract

L-3, 4-Dihydroxyphenylalanine (L-DOPA)-induced dyskinesia (LID) is a major clinical complication in the treatment of Parkinson's disease (PD). This debilitating side effect likely reflects aberrant compensatory responses for a combination of dopaminergic neuron denervation and repeated L-DOPA administration. Abnormal endogenous opioid signal transduction pathways in basal ganglia have been well documented in LID. Opioid receptors have been targeted to alleviate the dyskinesia. However, the exact role of this altered opioid activity is remains under active investigation. In the present review, we discuss the current understanding of opioid signal transduction in the basal ganglia and how the malfunction of opioid signaling contributes to the pathophysiology of LID. Further study of the opioid system in LID may lead to new therapeutic targets and improved treatment of PD patients.

Background

Parkinson's disease (PD) is the most common degenerative movement disorder clinically manifested with resting tremor, bradykinesia, rigidity and posture instability, resulting from impairments of dopamine transmission in the basal ganglia [1]. Pathologically, PD is marked by the substantial degeneration of dopamine-producing neurons in the substantia nigra pars compacta (SNc) and the presence of intracellular protein aggregates named Lewy bodies and neurites [2]. PD medications are mostly targeted at symptom relief. Since its initial prescription in 1960s, dopamine precursor L-DOPA remains the most effective drug for treating the movement abnormalities [3]. However, from the very beginning, it has been noticed that repeated administration of L-DOPA can induce motor fluctuations as well as impulsive control disorders [4]. Involuntary movements, also called L-DOPA induced dyskinesia (LID), is the most disturbing motor fluctuation. LID can be disabling and interfere with daily living. On average, about half of the patients develop LID after treated with L-DOPA for five years [5]. Although intensive studies have been carried out to understand the underlying molecular, cellular, and circuit mechanisms of LID, there still lack agents that can effectively ameliorate LID. Therefore, it remains critical to develop novel therapeutic strategies to reduce LID and improve the treatment and life quality of PD patients.

Denervation of dopaminergic neurons and repeated L-DOPA treatment might act together to cause LID [6]. The development of LID reflects multiplex compensatory reactions of nervous system in response to innate dopamine transmission deficiency and excessive supply of L-DOPA as discussed comprehensively in a recent review [7]. Here we paid special attention to the opioid receptor-mediated neurotransmission. Endogenous opioid peptides are dopamine co-transmitters that modulate various neural transmissions in basal ganglia. Alterations of opioid peptide expression and opioid receptor-mediated intracellular signal transduction have been reported in PD patients and animal models that develop dyskinesia [8]. Targeting opioid signaling in the basal ganglia may provide an additional avenue for the treatment of LID in PD.

Endogenous opioid peptides and receptors

There are three families of endogenous opioid peptides and three families of opioid receptors, comprising the so-called endogenous opioid system in the brain [9]. Endogenous opioid peptides consist of β-endorphin, enkephalins, and dynorphins, which are derived from precursor proteins encoded by pre-proopiomelanocortin (POMC), preproenkephalin (PENK), and pre-prodynorphin (PDYN), respectively [10]. Each precursor undergoes complex post-translational

* Correspondence: caih@mail.nih.gov
Transgenics Section, Laboratory of Neurogenetics, National Institute on Aging, National Institutes of Health, Building 35, Room 1A112, MSC 3707, 35 Convent Drive, Bethesda, MD 20892-3707, USA

modifications and proteolytic cleavage, giving rise to multiple active peptides [11, 12]. For instance, PENK is the precursor for two extended forms of Methionine (Met)-enkephalin and a single form of Leucine (Leu)-enkephalin. Opioid receptors can be divided into µ, δ, and κ three families, encoded by OPRM, OPRD, and OPRK genes [4, 13, 14]. While they are all G protein–coupled receptors, their extracellular loops are less conserved and responsible for the differential binding affinities to different opioid peptides [4, 13, 15–17]. All three subtypes of opioid receptors are coupling with the downstream G_i or G_o-mediated inhibitory intracellular signaling transduction pathways [18]. Furthermore, endogenous opioid peptides and receptors exhibit uneven distribution in different brain regions and cell types, and can act either pre- or post-synaptically. Therefore, the opioid system exerts a variety of modulatory roles in multiple neural processes, including pain sensation, reward and drug addiction, as well as seizure and PD [11].

Functional organization of basal ganglia

Increasing evidence suggests that well-coordinated direct and indirect striatal outputs in the basal ganglia are essential for the proper motor control [19]. On the other hand, a disruption of the coordination may cause parkinsonian as well as dyskinetic states [20]. The dopamine receptor D1 (DRD1)-expressing striatal projection neurons (dSPNs) form the direct pathway and project to the globus pallidus internal segment (GPi) as well as the substantia nigra pars reticulata (SNr) and SNc, while the dopamine receptor D2 (DRD2)-expressing SPNs (iSPNs) make up the indirect pathway and innervate the globus pallidus external segment (GPe) and the subthalamic nucleus (STh), where the GPe and STh neurons target their axons to the SNr (Fig. 1) [19, 20]. The direct pathway is used to be regarded as a promoter of movement, in opposite to the indirect pathway that inhibits the motor activity [19]. Along this line of thinking, PD weakens the direct pathway and potentiates the indirect pathway, resulting in impairments of movement [19, 21]. However, the recent live imaging studies of SPNs in free moving rodents argue against this binary "to go or not to go" model, and suggest a concerted activity of direct and indirect pathway SPNs is essential for the proper motor control in both moving and resting states [22–24]. In addition, the latest neuron tracing studies reveal a much more complicated and diverse connectivity of SNPs, as well as the midbrain dopaminergic neurons (Fig. 1) [25–27]. Further dissecting the local circuits and functional modalities of basal ganglia neurons will likely redraw the wiring of neural network that underlies the critical motor control of vertebrates.

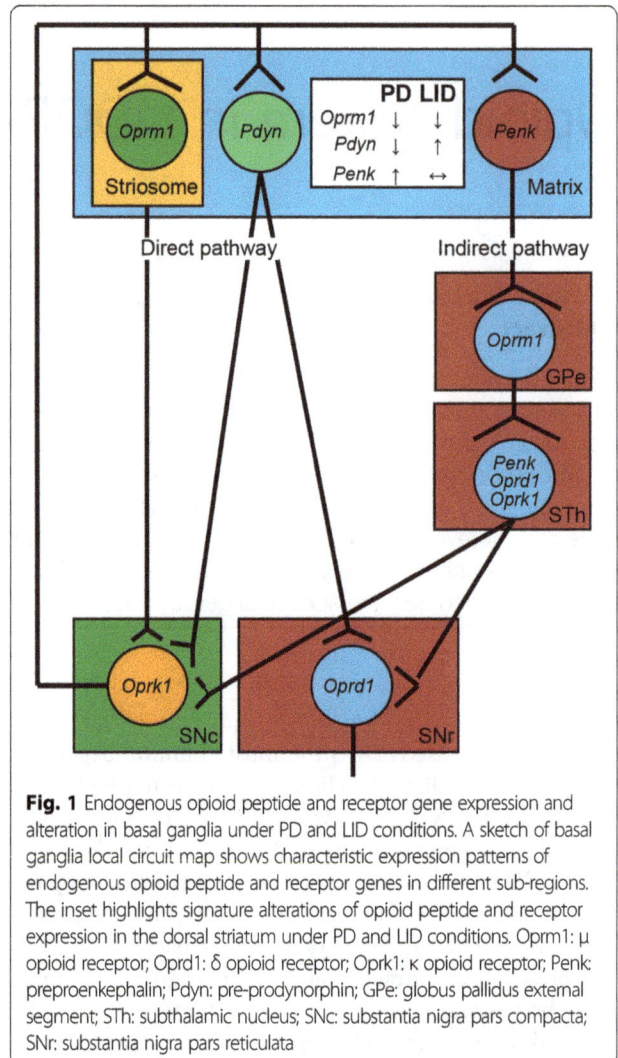

Fig. 1 Endogenous opioid peptide and receptor gene expression and alteration in basal ganglia under PD and LID conditions. A sketch of basal ganglia local circuit map shows characteristic expression patterns of endogenous opioid peptide and receptor genes in different sub-regions. The inset highlights signature alterations of opioid peptide and receptor expression in the dorsal striatum under PD and LID conditions. Oprm1: µ opioid receptor; Oprd1: δ opioid receptor; Oprk1: κ opioid receptor; Penk: preproenkephalin; Pdyn: pre-prodynorphin; GPe: globus pallidus external segment; STh: subthalamic nucleus; SNc: substantia nigra pars compacta; SNr: substantia nigra pars reticulata

Opioid system in basal ganglia

High levels of endogenous opioid peptides and opioid receptors are present in the basal ganglia [11]. Because the wide distribution of opioid peptides and receptors in the brain, it is difficult to determine whether the sources of these peptides and receptors are inside or outside of basal ganglia based on studying the protein expression using western blot and immunostaining. By contrast, the distribution of mRNAs determined by in situ hybridization serves a better indicator to the patterns of opioid peptide and receptor expression in basal ganglia (Fig. 1). The endogenous opioid peptide precursor PENK mRNAs are predominantly expressed by the iSNPs, whereas PDYN mRNAs are more abundant in the dSNPs [8, 28]. By contrast, the expression of POMC mRNAs is restricted to hypothalamus. *Penk* but not *Pdyn* mRNAs can also be detected in neuronal subpopulations in subthalamic nucleus and zona incerta in rodent brains (Allen Brain Atlas), regions targeted for deep brain stimulation (DBS) in treatment of PD and LID [29]. All three types of opioid receptors express in the striatum, but display distinct distribution patterns. The μ opioid receptors (OPRM1) are selectively expressed by the SPNs located in the striosome compartments in the rodent brains [30]. Correlatively, Oprm1 mRNAs also show a similar patchy distribution pattern in rodent dorsal striatum (Allen). In addition, Oprm1 mRNAs appear at ventral striatum and GPe (Allen Brain Atlas). δ-opioid receptors (Oprd1) mRNA-expressing cells sparsely distribute at dorsal striatum, GPe, GPi, and SNr, while more cells express Oprd1 in STh and ZI. κ-opioid receptors (Oprk1) mRNAs are mainly detected in cells distributed at ventral striatum and STh. Of interest, Oprk1 mRNAs are more enriched in SNc and ventral tegmental area (VTA) compared to other opioid peptides and receptors (Allen Brain Atlas). These distinct sub-regional localizations of opioid peptides and receptors underlie the diverse and complex functions of endogenous opioid system in the basal ganglia [10].

Alterations of striatal opioid peptide and receptor expression in LID

The expression levels of striatal PENK mRNAs correlate with the severity of LID, suggesting a causal role of increased opioid transmission in the development of LID [17, 31]. However, the pathophysiological impact of these alterations remains debatable [32]. Dopamine depletion as occurred in the parkinsonian states leads to increased expression of PENK mRNA in the iSPNs and decreased expression of PDYN mRNAs in the dSPNs (Fig. 1) [33, 34]. At the peak of LID, the expression of PDYN mRNAs increases, while the expression of PENK does not change (Fig. 1) [8, 33–35]. The expression of PDYN mRNAs and peptides also elevates in STh neurons in LID [34, 36]. However, such alterations of opioid peptide expression may not cause LID, but rather reflect an adaptive response compensating for the prolonged L-DOPA treatment [37, 38].

Correlated with the alterations of opioid peptide expression, opioid receptor levels also change in PD and LID (Fig. 1) [39]. Dopamine depletion causes an overall reduction of opioid receptor bindings, while LID leads to a further reduction [34]. OPRM1 binding levels are decreased in both the caudate and putamen of PD patients under chronic L-DOPA administration [40, 41]. OPRM1 levels are also suppressed in putamen and GPi of monkey LID models [42]. On the other hand, OPRM1 expression is increased in the premotor and motor cortex of rat LID models [43]. Therefore, it is important to investigate the differential alterations of opioid peptide and receptor expression in different brain regions in PD and LID.

Opioid signaling in the pathogenesis of LID

While OPRM1 cell surface presentation is decreased in LID, OPRM1-mediated signal transduction is enhanced in the striatum and GPi of LID models [44], suggesting increased sensitivity of OPRM1 in the dyskinetic states. Consistent with this notion, OPRM1 antagonists cyprodine and ADL5510 effectively reduce dyskinesia but preserve the anti-parkinsonian efficacy of L-DOPA in the monkey models [38, 45]. Moreover, a combination of both OPRM1 and OPRD1 antagonists appear more effective in reducing LID in animal models [46]. The anti-LID efficacy of OPRM1 and OPRD1 antagonists remains to be validated in PD patients, especially considering an earlier failed attempt with the non-selective opioid receptor antagonist naloxone [47, 48]. In addition, the diverse expression patterns of opioid receptors in different brain regions and their differential responses in the dyskinesia states may demand regional application of either receptor subtype-selective agonists or antagonists to effectively alleviate LID.

The underlying molecular mechanisms of LID remain under intensive investigation [49]. Dysregulation of cAMP and ERK signaling pathways has been reported in PD and LID models [50]. Opioid receptors relay opioid stimulation through G_i or G_o-mediated inhibitory intracellular signal transduction pathways [18], which may suppress G_{olf} or G_s-induced cAMP signaling in cells. For example, pharmacological activation of OPRM1 and OPRD1 blocks dopamine DRD1- or adenosine A2A-receptor-induced activation of adenylyl cyclase and reduces the production of cAMP in SPNs [51]. A reduction of cAMP levels may suppress protein kinase A (PKA) activity and leads to an aberrant activation of extracellular signal-regulated kinases (ERK1/2) in the generation of LID [52, 53]. ERK activation may play a causal role in the development of LID, as inhibition of ERK activity alleviates dyskinesia phenotypes [54]. Opioid receptor antagonists may achieve the anti-dyskinesia effects through negatively regulating ERK1/2 signaling [55]. Further studies, however, will be required to improve current understanding of the complex interplays between various signaling pathways critical in the formation of abnormal synaptic transmission and plasticity in LID.

Conclusions

LID represents an erratic adaptive response to dopamine denervation and repeated L-DOPA treatment. Although selective opioid receptor antagonists can effectively alleviate LID in animal models, the underlying molecular, cellular and circuit mechanisms remain to be characterized. The latest advance of next generation sequencing, gene editing, opt genetics, and live imaging technologies may greatly facilitate the inquiry of opioid signaling in the basal ganglia under normal and PD-like conditions. Modulation of opioid receptor activity may provide an effective means to reduce LID and optimize the dopamine-replacement therapy.

Acknowledgements
We appreciate the inputs and discussions from Cai lab for studying opioid system in Parkinson's disease.

Funding
This review was supported by the intramural research programs of National Institute on Aging (HC, AG000928).

Authors' contributions
Both authors read and approved the final manuscript. JP and HBC conceived and wrote the manuscript.

Competing interests
The authors declare that they have no competing interests.

References
1. Langston JW. Parkinson's disease: current and future challenges. Neurotoxicology. 2002;23:443–50.
2. Trojanowski JQ, Lee VM. Parkinson's disease and related synucleinopathies are a new class of nervous system amyloidoses. Neurotoxicology. 2002;23:457–60.
3. Mercuri NB, Bernardi G. The 'magic' of L-dopa: why is it the gold standard Parkinson's disease therapy? Trends Pharmacol Sci. 2005;26:341–4.
4. Vijayakumar D, Jankovic J. Drug-induced dyskinesia, Part 1: treatment of levodopa-induced dyskinesia. Drugs. 2016;76:759–77.
5. Cenci MA. Presynaptic mechanisms of l-DOPA-induced dyskinesia: the findings, the debate, and the therapeutic implications. Front Neurol. 2014;5:242.
6. Belujon P, Lodge DJ, Grace AA. Aberrant striatal plasticity is specifically associated with dyskinesia following levodopa treatment. Mov Disord. 2010;25:1568–76.
7. Bastide MF, Meissner WG, Picconi B, Fasano S, Fernagut PO, Feyder M, Francardo V, Alcacer C, Ding Y, Brambilla R, et al. Pathophysiology of L-dopa-induced motor and non-motor complications in Parkinson's disease. Prog Neurobiol. 2015;132:96–168.
8. Ravenscroft P, Chalon S, Brotchie JM, Crossman AR. Ropinirole versus L-DOPA effects on striatal opioid peptide precursors in a rodent model of Parkinson's disease: implications for dyskinesia. Exp Neurol. 2004;185:36–46.
9. Benarroch EE. Endogenous opioid systems: current concepts and clinical correlations. Neurology. 2012;79:807–14.
10. Samadi P, Bedard PJ, Rouillard C. Opioids and motor complications in Parkinson's disease. Trends Pharmacol Sci. 2006;27:512–7.
11. Hadjiconstantinou M, Neff NH. Nicotine and endogenous opioids: neurochemical and pharmacological evidence. Neuropharmacology. 2011;60:1209–20.
12. Le Merrer J, Becker JA, Befort K, Kieffer BL. Reward processing by the opioid system in the brain. Physiol Rev. 2009;89:1379–412.
13. Wei LN, Loh HH. Transcriptional and epigenetic regulation of opioid receptor genes: present and future. Annu Rev Pharmacol Toxicol. 2011;51:75–97.
14. Stein C. Opioid receptors. Annu Rev Med. 2016;67:433–51.
15. Chavkin C, Koob GF. Dynorphin, dysphoria, and dependence: the stress of addiction. Neuropsychopharmacology. 2016;41:373–4.
16. Zimprich A, Biskup S, Leitner P, Lichtner P, Farrer M, Lincoln S, Kachergus J, Hulihan M, Uitti RJ, Calne DB, et al. Mutations in LRRK2 cause autosomal-dominant parkinsonism with pleomorphic pathology. Neuron. 2004;44:601–7.
17. Pasternak GW, Pan YX. Mu opioids and their receptors: evolution of a concept. Pharmacol Rev. 2013;65:1257–317.
18. Cheng KC, Asakawa A, Li YX, Liu IM, Amitani H, Cheng JT, Inui A. Opioid mu-receptors as new target for insulin resistance. Pharmacol Ther. 2013;139:334–40.
19. Gerfen CR, Surmeier DJ. Modulation of striatal projection systems by dopamine. Annu Rev Neurosci. 2011;34:441–66.
20. Macpherson T, Morita M, Hikida T. Striatal direct and indirect pathways control decision-making behavior. Front Psychol. 2014;5:1301.
21. Surmeier DJ, Graves SM, Shen W. Dopaminergic modulation of striatal networks in health and Parkinson's disease. Curr Opin Neurobiol. 2014;29:109–17.
22. Surmeier DJ. Neuroscience: to go or not to go. Nature. 2013;494:178–9.
23. Cui G, Jun SB, Jin X, Pham MD, Vogel SS, Lovinger DM, Costa RM. Concurrent activation of striatal direct and indirect pathways during action initiation. Nature. 2013;494:238–42.
24. Barbera G, Liang B, Zhang L, Gerfen CR, Culurciello E, Chen R, Li Y, Lin DT. Spatially compact neural clusters in the dorsal striatum encode locomotion relevant information. Neuron. 2016;92:202–13.
25. Watabe-Uchida M, Zhu L, Ogawa SK, Vamanrao A, Uchida N. Whole-brain mapping of direct inputs to midbrain dopamine neurons. Neuron. 2012;74:858–73.
26. Menegas W, Bergan JF, Ogawa SK, Isogai Y, Umadevi Venkataraju K, Osten P, Uchida N, Watabe-Uchida M. Dopamine neurons projecting to the posterior striatum form an anatomically distinct subclass. Elife. 2015;4:e10032.
27. Lerner TN, Shilyansky C, Davidson TJ, Evans KE, Beier KT, Zalocusky KA, Crow AK, Malenka RC, Luo L, Tomer R, et al. Intact-brain analyses reveal distinct information carried by SNc dopamine subcircuits. Cell. 2015;162:635–47.
28. Gross CE, Ravenscroft P, Dovero S, Jaber M, Bioulac B, Bezard E. Pattern of levodopa-induced striatal changes is different in normal and MPTP-lesioned mice. J Neurochem. 2003;84:1246–55.
29. Hickey P, Stacy M. Deep brain stimulation: a paradigm shifting approach to treat Parkinson's disease. Front Neurosci. 2016;10:173.
30. Pert CB, Kuhar MJ, Snyder SH. Opiate receptor: autoradiographic localization in rat brain. Proc Natl Acad Sci U S A. 1976;73:3729–33.
31. Winkler C, Kirik D, Bjorklund A, Cenci MA. L-DOPA-induced dyskinesia in the intrastriatal 6-hydroxydopamine model of Parkinson's disease: relation to motor and cellular parameters of nigrostriatal function. Neurobiol Dis. 2002;10:165–86.
32. Mazzucchelli C, Vantaggiato C, Ciamei A, Fasano S, Pakhotin P, Krezel W, Welzl H, Wolfer DP, Pages G, Valverde O, et al. Knockout of ERK1 MAP kinase enhances synaptic plasticity in the striatum and facilitates striatal-mediated learning and memory. Neuron. 2002;34:807–20.
33. Calon F, Birdi S, Rajput AH, Hornykiewicz O, Bedard PJ, Di Paolo T. Increase of preproenkephalin mRNA levels in the putamen of Parkinson disease patients with levodopa-induced dyskinesias. J Neuropathol Exp Neurol. 2002;61:186–96.
34. Aubert I, Guigoni C, Li Q, Dovero S, Bioulac BH, Gross CE, Crossman AR, Bloch B, Bezard E. Enhanced preproenkephalin-B-derived opioid transmission in striatum and subthalamic nucleus converges upon globus pallidus internalis in L-3,4-dihydroxyphenylalanine-induced dyskinesia. Biol Psychiatry. 2007;61:836–44.
35. McGinty JF. Co-localization of GABA with other neuroactive substances in the basal ganglia. Prog Brain Res. 2007;160:273–84.
36. Bourdenx M, Nilsson A, Wadensten H, Falth M, Li Q, Crossman AR, Andren PE, Bezard E. Abnormal structure-specific peptide transmission and processing in a primate model of Parkinson's disease and l-DOPA-induced dyskinesia. Neurobiol Dis. 2014;62:307–12.
37. Huot P, Johnston TH, Winkelmolen L, Fox SH, Brotchie JM. 5-HT2A receptor levels increase in MPTP-lesioned macaques treated chronically with L-DOPA. Neurobiol Aging. 2012;33(194):e195–115.
38. Henry B, Fox SH, Crossman AR, Brotchie JM. Mu- and delta-opioid receptor antagonists reduce levodopa-induced dyskinesia in the MPTP-lesioned primate model of Parkinson's disease. Exp Neurol. 2001;171:139–46.
39. Laureano DP, Dalle Molle R, Alves MB, Luft C, Desai M, Ross MG, Silveira PP. Intrauterine growth restriction modifies the hedonic response to sweet

taste in newborn pups - Role of the accumbal mu-opioid receptors. Neuroscience. 2016;322:500–8.

40. Fernandez A, de Ceballos ML, Jenner P, Marsden CD. Neurotensin, substance P, delta and mu opioid receptors are decreased in basal ganglia of Parkinson's disease patients. Neuroscience. 1994;61:73–9.

41. Chen L, Togasaki DM, Langston JW, Di Monte DA, Quik M. Enhanced striatal opioid receptor-mediated G-protein activation in L-DOPA-treated dyskinetic monkeys. Neuroscience. 2005;132:409–20.

42. Aubert I, Guigoni C, Hakansson K, Li Q, Dovero S, Barthe N, Bioulac BH, Gross CE, Fisone G, Bloch B, et al. Increased D1 dopamine receptor signaling in levodopa-induced dyskinesia. Ann Neurol. 2005;57:17–26.

43. Johansson PA, Andersson M, Andersson KE, Cenci MA. Alterations in cortical and basal ganglia levels of opioid receptor binding in a rat model of l-DOPA-induced dyskinesia. Neurobiol Dis. 2001;8:220–39.

44. Hanrieder J, Ljungdahl A, Falth M, Mammo SE, Bergquist J, Andersson M. L-DOPA-induced dyskinesia is associated with regional increase of striatal dynorphin peptides as elucidated by imaging mass spectrometry. Mol Cell Proteomics. 2011;10(M111):009308.

45. Koprich JB, Fox SH, Johnston TH, Goodman A, Le Bourdonnec B, Dolle RE, DeHaven RN, DeHaven-Hudkins DL, Little PJ, Brotchie JM. The selective mu-opioid receptor antagonist ADL5510 reduces levodopa-induced dyskinesia without affecting antiparkinsonian action in MPTP-lesioned macaque model of Parkinson's disease. Mov Disord. 2011;26:1225–33.

46. Lundblad M, Andersson M, Winkler C, Kirik D, Wierup N, Cenci MA. Pharmacological validation of behavioural measures of akinesia and dyskinesia in a rat model of Parkinson's disease. Eur J Neurosci. 2002;15:120–32.

47. Manson AJ, Katzenschlager R, Hobart J, Lees AJ. High dose naltrexone for dyskinesias induced by levodopa. J Neurol Neurosurg Psychiatry. 2001;70:554–6.

48. Fox S, Silverdale M, Kellett M, Davies R, Steiger M, Fletcher N, Crossman A, Brotchie J. Non-subtype-selective opioid receptor antagonism in treatment of levodopa-induced motor complications in Parkinson's disease. Mov Disord. 2004;19:554–60.

49. Feyder M, Bonito-Oliva A, Fisone G. L-DOPA-induced dyskinesia and abnormal signaling in striatal medium spiny neurons: focus on dopamine D1 receptor-mediated transmission. Front Behav Neurosci. 2011;5:71.

50. Gerfen CR. D1 dopamine receptor supersensitivity in the dopamine-depleted striatum animal model of Parkinson's disease. Neuroscientist. 2003;9:455–62.

51. Ross CL, Teli T, Harrison BS. Effect of electromagnetic field on cyclic adenosine monophosphate (cAMP) in a human mu-opioid receptor cell model. Electromagn Biol Med. 2016;35:206–13.

52. Bjork K, Terasmaa A, Sun H, Thorsell A, Sommer WH, Heilig M. Ethanol-induced activation of AKT and DARPP-32 in the mouse striatum mediated by opioid receptors. Addict Biol. 2010;15:299–303.

53. Ramos-Miguel A, Garcia-Sevilla JA. Crosstalk between cdk5 and MEK-ERK signalling upon opioid receptor stimulation leads to upregulation of activator p25 and MEK1 inhibition in rat brain. Neuroscience. 2012;215:17–30.

54. Santini E, Valjent E, Usiello A, Carta M, Borgkvist A, Girault JA, Herve D, Greengard P, Fisone G. Critical involvement of cAMP/DARPP-32 and extracellular signal-regulated protein kinase signaling in L-DOPA-induced dyskinesia. J Neurosci. 2007;27:6995–7005.

55. Beaudry H, Mercier-Blais AA, Delaygue C, Lavoie C, Parent JL, Neugebauer W, Gendron L. Regulation of mu and delta opioid receptor functions: involvement of cyclin-dependent kinase 5. Br J Pharmacol. 2015;172:2573–87.

5

The role of cognitive activity in cognition protection: from Bedside to Bench

Bin-Yin Li[†], Ying Wang[†], Hui-dong Tang and Sheng-Di Chen[*]

Abstract

Background: Cognitive decline poses a great concern to elderly people and their families. In addition to pharmacological therapies, several varieties of nonpharmacological intervention have been developed. Most training trials proved that a well-organized task is clinically effective in cognition improvement.

Main body: We will first review clinical trials of cognitive training for healthy elders, MCI and AD patients, respectively. Besides, potential neuroprotective and compensatory mechanisms in animal models of AD are discussed. Despite controversy, cognitive training has promising effect on cognitive ability. In animal model of AD, environmental enrichment showed beneficial effect for cognitive ability, as well as neuronal plasticity. Neurotrophin, neurotransmitter and neuromodulator signaling pathway were also involved in the process. Well-designed cognitive activity could benefit cognitive function, and thus life quality of patients and their families.

Conclusion: The positive effects of cognitive activity is closely related with neural plasticity, neurotrophin, neurotransmitter and neuromodulator signaling pathway changes.

Background

Cognitive decline and its burden

Cognitive decline is age-specific or related with dementia. Alzheimer disease (AD) was the most common types of dementia. In 2006, the global prevalence of AD was 26.6 million [1]. It is estimated that the one in 85 persons worldwide will suffer from the disease by 2050. In the United States, AD causes estimated health-care costs of $172 billion per year [2]. It was reported that average total costs for AD patients were more than five-fold higher compared with matched controls [3]. If interventions could delay disease onset and slow its progression by a modest 1 year, there would be much fewer cases of the disease in 2050 with reduction by nearly 9.2 million, and thus fewer expenditure on care and treatment [1]. As a continuous course, Alzheimer's disease (AD) gradually develops from preclinical state, mild cognitive impairment (MCI) to dementia. MCI can thus be regarded as a transitional state between normal aging and AD.

Aging and aging-related diseases pose a major threat to individuals' life quality, and cause high economic burden on families and the whole society. Prevalence of MCI in population-based epidemiological studies ranges from 3 to 20% in adults older than 60 or 65 years old [4–7]. Some people with MCI seem to remain stable or return to normal over time [5]. However, approximately 50% of patients with MCI (roughly 12% per year) will progress to AD over 4–5 years.

Unfortunately, there is no cure or robust pharmacologic treatment for AD. So far, the primary focus is slowing down the decline of neurological and associated behavioral functions, by providing medications, training and caregiver support.

Pharmacological and non-pharmacological therapies

Due to the increasing prevalence of MCI and AD, pharmacological and non-pharmacological treatments have been greatly concerned about their effects. Donepezil, rivastigmine, galantamine, and memantine are the drugs presently approved by the Food and Drug Administration (FDA) for treatment of AD. Meta-analysis of cholinesterase inhibitors (ChEIs) showed their effects by a small improvement in activities of daily living [8]. Antiglutamatergic treatment (memantine) reduced

* Correspondence: chen_sd@medmail.com.cn
[†]Equal contributors
Department of Neurology, Institute of Neurology and the Collaborative Innovation Center for Brain Science, Rui Jin Hospital affiliated to Shanghai Jiao Tong University School of Medicine, Shanghai 200025, China

clinical deterioration in moderate-to-severe Alzheimer's disease [9]. In addition, it is still doubted that whether these drugs significantly improve long-term outcomes, such as the need for nursing home admission [10, 11]. Both ChEIs and antiglutamatergic treatment are not indicated for MCI patients. A review and meta-analysis concluded that treatment with cholinesterase inhibitors merely affected MCI progression to dementia or improved cognitive test scores [12]. In one study of data from Alzheimer's Disease Neuroimaging Initiative, MCI patients who received ChEIs with or without memantine were more impaired, showed greater decline in scores, and progressed to dementia sooner than patients who did not receive ChEIs [13].

As well as medications, non-pharmacological interventions also aim to delay the loss of cognitive abilities, to help people stay independent in everyday life as long as possible, and to increase their well-being and quality of life. Because of its readiness and few side effects, not only AD or MCI patients, healthy elder adults can also participate at home or in the community. There are various approaches, including mental exercise, diet control and physical exercises [14, 15]. However, their effect remains controversial in different clinical trials. Other interventions include art therapy, aromatherapy, music therapy, animal-assisted therapy and caregiver education programs.

From bedside to bench

There have been a large number of clinical trials and reviews about the effect of cognitive therapy for aging populations [16–18]. Computerized cognitive training showed its modest effect on cognitive performance in healthy older adults [19], and the effect of cognitive training was equivocal for AD patients [20]. Effective forms of training for AD patients included errorless learning, spaced retrieval, vanishing cues techniques, and the dyadic approach [21]. However, few of these reviews covered clinical outcomes and their underlying mechanisms together.

In this paper, we first review clinical trials of cognitive training for people with different extent of cognitive ability. The characteristics and special outcomes of the clinical trials of cognitive intervention were discussed, as well as shortcomes of clinical studies. Then, much attention was devoted to neural mechanisms of these training, exploring valuable information from animal studies.

Cognitive activity for human beings
Method for literature review of clinical trials
We take two steps in the literature review. In step one, we searched relevant meta-analysis for a quick look at the effect of cognitive intervention. In step two, we selected consolidated clinical trials for detailed analysis and discussion.

Step One: Several systemic reviews and meta-analysis have summarized cognitive training trials. Firstly, we selected the work which fully complies with the Preferred Reporting Items for Systematic Reviews and Meta-Analysis (PRISMA) or Delphi list. We searched PubMed- and PsycINFO-based literature for relevant meta-analysis using the following Boolean strategy: "cognitive stimulation" OR "cognitive rehabilitation" OR "cognitive activity" OR "cognitive intervention" OR "training" OR "memory training" OR "mnemonic training". After screened by title and abstract, meta analysis studies were included if they enrolled latest clinical trials that evaluated the effect of the cognitive intervention by assessing cognitive changes before and after intervention (Table 1).

Step Two: In order to further take a close look at the entire literature and details, we manually searched consolidated evidence from the references of selected articles and earlier review [16]. We also searched for published intervention studies in latest 5 years, limiting to English language, human and peer reviewed articles.

The search strategy in PubMed (clinical trials as article type) was shown as an example: ("Dementia"[Mesh] OR "Alzheimer Disease"[Mesh] OR "mild cognitive impairment"[Mesh] OR aging OR elder) AND (cognitive training OR mental training OR train*) AND (Intervention Studies OR intervention study OR intervention OR interventions OR interventional OR experimental)

We selected studies by three steps based on eligibility criteria of PRISMA checklist : the title and abstract screening, full-text assessment for rationale and eligibility of methodology, and final evaluation of results. Two reviewers (L, BY and W, Y) independently checked the following factors before inclusion, and discrepancy was discussed to arrive at agreement: subjects, study design, blinding, withdrawals and dropouts, intervention method and duration. Studies were excluded if they only enrolled participants with other dementias or no clearly intervention description. Eligible studies were classified by cognition level of subjects, in order to find out training effect on people of different cognitive ability.

Impact of cognitive activity for healthy older adults
Studies description
Normal aging causes natural decline in multiple cognitive domains, and thus poses threat to maintaining independence and quality of life. Researchers tended to develop methods to slow down the speed of cognitive decline, based on the theory that brain retains some plasticity. Since 1980s, a number of studies had tried cognitive interventions for healthy older adults, in order to improve cognitive performance and quality of life [22–25]. These interventions included both laboratory-based and community-based cognitive trainings for healthy older adults.

Table 1 Meta-analysis studies for cognitive training in healthy elders, MCI and AD patients

Reference	Participants	Training	Trials	Positive outcomes	Negative outcomes
Lampit, et al., 2014 [19]	Healthy elders	Computerized cognitive training	51	Overall effect; nonverbal, verbal and working memory; processing speed	EF and attention
Toril, P. et al., 2014 [200]	Healthy elders	Vedio game training	20	Reaction time, attention, memory, and global cognition	EF
Kelly, ME et al., 2014 [192]	Healthy elders	Memory-based intervention/diverse stimulations.	31	Executive function/global cognition—compared with active control. Memory/subjective cognition—compared with no training group	WM,recall, recognition Recall, attention
Papp, K. et al., 2009 [201]	Healthy elders	Multi-domain training	10	All outcome measures[c]	-
Li, H. et al., 2011 [202]	MCI	Multi-domain training	17	Overall cognition, self-ratings, EM, WM, EF	SM, PS, attention, VS
Martin, M. et al., 2011 [203]	Healthy elders	Multi-domain training	11	Immediate recall[a]	-
			6	Delayed recall[a]	-
			2	-	VS
			5	-	Short-term memory
			1	EF[a]	-
Bahar-F. et al., 2013 [204]	AD + VD	Multi-domain training	11	-	Any reported outcomes
Aquirre, E . et al., 2013 [205]	Dementia [b]	Cognitive and social function	7	ADAS-Cog	-
Sitzer, Dl. et al., 2006 [206]	AD	At least one domain cognitive function	17	Overall cognitive ability	-
Woods, B. et al., 2012 [207]	Dementia [b]	Cognitive stimulation	7	ADAS-Cog	-

EF executive function, *WM* working memory, *MCI* mild cognitive impairment, *EM* episodic memory, *PS* processing speed, *VS* visual-spatial ability, *VD* vascular dementia

[a]Improvements observed did not exceed the improvement in the active control condition
[b]Alzheimer's disease, vascular dementia mixed Alzheimer's and vascular dementia, other types of dementia. ADAS-Cog was applied only in AD patients
[c]Significant but negligible

Models of intervention

As memory loss is the major and early complaint from older adults, memory training was dominantly adopted in a number of studies as early as 1980s [26–29]. Working memory training was conducted in 39 80-year-old healthy adults, including visual free-recall tasks [30]. Both training effect (working memory ability) and transfer effect were found improved immediately after training. Nevertheless, after 1-year follow up, both effects were not significant. The pooled data also found its controversial or negligible effect [31, 32]. Spatial working memory task with 2 levels of processing demands helped older adults (70–80 years old) to gain substantial performance on the practiced task. The effects transferred to a more demanding spatial n-back task and to numerical n-back tasks. Both benefits lasted for 3 months, while no evidence was found for far transfer to complex span tasks [33]. Perceptual and verbal working memory training also showed their promising transfer and maintenance effects [34, 35].

More studies paid attention to comprehensive training covering more cognitive domains. Jobe et al. conducted a famous large-scale, randomized, controlled, single-masked trial (ACTIVE study) in 2001, which was designed to determine whether cognitive interventions could affect cognition-based daily functioning and basic trained abilities served as mediators [36]. The ACTIVE study has three models of intervention: speed of processing, memory and reasoning. Each intervention improved the targeted cognitive ability compared with baseline, durable to 2 years. If individuals received booster training 11 months after initial training (2 to 3 weeks), training gains were enhanced and maintained at 2-year follow-up. However, training effect did not transfer to other untrained cognitive skills. In addition, the authors also estimated training effects (cognitive change), compared with expected decline in elderly persons without dementia. The effects from speed of processing, memory and reasoning training were respectively of a magnitude equivalent to the amount of 2-, 7- and 14-year cognitive decline expected in elderly persons without dementia. The study did not find the changes of activities of daily living. The authors attributed it to minimal functional decline across all groups [37]. The study continued and showed improvement of targeted cognitive abilities for 10 years by reasoning and speed, but not memory [38]. Speed of processing training was also believed to be useful in helping driving mobility [39], though its effect was doubted in a new large-sample trials when compared with crossword puzzle game [40].

Donostia Longitudinal Study aimed at all cognitive functions. The authors compared structured training program with unstructured one and control in a 2-year time span. Each participant in experimental groups received 180 ninety-minute sessions (every session per week). Structured intervention covered the cognitive functions of attention and orientation, memory, language, visuoconstructive ability, executive functions, visuomanual coordination and praxia. Only the group that received structured intervention got higher scores in nearly all cognitive tests [41]. Similar computerized cognitive training also boosted memory/attention improvement in the experimental group (word list total score, word list delayed recall, digits backwards, letter-number sequencing) [42], as well as better mood and sleep [43].

In addition to these training programs for particular one or more cognitive domains, social activities or everyday activity were also evaluated as a kind of intervention [44]. Some manipulations included social communication, making sense of figures, drawing activities, and even word-logic puzzles in the community or nursing home [45]. Some training also covered problem-realization and strategy-seeking, helping develop personal strategies for each participant [46]. A large-scale RCT (FINGER study) combined diet, exercise, cognitive training and vascular risk monitoring for improvement or maintenance of cognitive functioning. The results suggested that 2-year multi-domain intervention could improve or maintain cognitive functioning in at-risk elderly people [47].

Cognitive activity for mild cognitive impairment patients
Studies description
Studies varied in the interventions, study design, duration of sessions and sample size. All programs mainly aimed at explicit memory because individuals with MCI suffered from memory deficiency. Similarly to intervention for healthy old adults, attention, speed of processing, language, visual-spatial abilities and executive functions were also adopted [48–51], while others only combined attention and memory training [52, 53]. Computerized cognitive training was also introduced here for some multifaceted interventions [48, 49, 53]. It could facilitate the individual's approach but did not show increased improvement when compared to non-computerized training, independent of participants' computer familiarity [54].

Interventions for one or more multiple cognitive domains
In the early 2000s, Rapp et al. tried multi-component memory interventions. Patients received education about symptoms of memory loss, memory skills training, and memory-related beliefs. Treated group did better in memory assessment at the end of treatment and at a 6-month follow-up [55].

In a prospective study, Rozzini et al. used training covered different cognitive functions for patients with MCI. After 1-year follow-up, subjects treated with training and cholinesterase inhibitors (ChEIs) medication showed significant improvements in memory, abstract reasoning and in behavioral disturbances. The combined treatment group showed its advantage over ChEIs group [48]. Wenisch et al. administered a cognitive stimulation program (both memory manipulation and information about memory functioning) for cognitive performance. It revealed a larger intervention benefits in MCI than in normal elders' performances on the associative learning task [56].

In addition to memory, behavior rehabilitation was once believed to be a potential cognitive helper. Nevertheless, it is a bit controversial of its effect in MCI patients. Greenaway et al. tested a calendar/notebook system, including three sections: appointments; daily "to do" items and important events that happened that day. Patients compliant with the system had a medium effect size for improvement in functional ability. Subjects further reported improved independence, self-confidence, and mood [52]. By contrast, Talassi et al. provided a combined cognitive program training and found an improvement in cognitive and affective status of patients with MCI, while no effects were observed in a rehabilitation program not providing a punctual stimulation of cognitive functions [49].

Memory strategy intervention
Another critical factor in cognitive training is the use of strategy. Strategy acts as a compensator in functioning. Belleville et al. focused on episodic memory strategies by comparing pre-and post-intervention difference. Progress was remarkable in delayed list recall and face-name association tasks of strategy-intervention group, while no improvement was observed in MCI individuals without receiving the intervention [57]. Hampstead et al. taught MCI patients the use of explicit memory strategies in classic face-name association tasks. Significant improvement was also found on both trained and untrained stimuli, raising the possibility of generalization of training strategies [58].

After being taught with memory strategies based on meta-memory, old adults had training-related gains in a recall task, as well as transfer benefits in short-term memory, long-term memory, working memory and motivation [59]. Strategy-based tasks can be viewed as the acquisition of knowledge that capitalizes on flexibility to improve performance [60]. Performance may increase because the person has acquired knowledge relevant for the particular task.

Londos et al. also aimed at developing compensatory memory strategies that can improve their cognition, as well as occupational performance and quality of life. The study compared cognitive function, occupational performance, and self-perceived quality of life before and after intervention. Significant improvements were seen in cognitive processing speed, occupational performance after participation in the program 2 days per week for 8 weeks [61]. Troyer et al. evaluated the effectiveness of a multidisciplinary intervention, providing evidenced-based memory training and lifestyle education to optimize memory behavior. After treatment, patients had increased memory-strategy knowledge that could change their everyday memory behavior by putting this knowledge into practice. Interestingly, no improvement of objective memory performance was observed [62].

Cognitive activity for AD patients
Studies descriptions
Since publication in the early 1980s by Zarit et al., much work has been done for cognitive stimulation in populations suffering from dementia, especially AD. The early detection and diagnosis of AD raised the importance of effective psychological intervention in the early stage. Types of stimulation programs covered all cognitive domains. Similarly to interventions for normal older adults and MCI patients, memory is the main target, as well as memory strategies and external memory aids. However, due to poor cooperation of AD patients, more delicate techniques were adopted.

Memory interventions
In contrary to its general application in MCI patients, memory intervention was questioned when it is applied in AD patients. Quayhagen et al. compared cognitive stimulation with other non-pharmacological interventions (dyadic counseling, dual supportive seminar, and early-stage day care). Cognitive stimulation group demonstrated more improvement over time only in cognitive outcomes [63].

Zarit et al. tried visual imagery for overcoming memory loss in senile dementia patients in community. Though recall performance (imagery techniques were taught) was improved for subjects in the intervention group, the author claimed its little practical value for caregivers [64]. Imaginary memory task (classic face-name association training) was also tried for AD. In a study of 7 AD patients, only one AD patient increased the time during which face-name associations could be held in memory. No training gains were observed for the

remaining six patients, thus questioning the generalizability of this method in enhancing memory in dementia [65].

In a combined intervention consisting of face-name associations, spaced retrieval, and cognitive stimulation, 37 patients with probable AD were enrolled for 5 weeks. AD patients who received stimulation showed significant improvement in trained tasks, while no benefit was observed in the additional neuropsychological measures of dementia severity, verbal memory, visual memory, word generation, motor speed, or caregiver-assessed patient quality of life [66].

Errorless learning and spaced retrieval
Errorless learning was an instructional design introduced in the 1930s in order to create the most effective learning environment. Errors are once regarded as a function of learning and vice-versa. However, in the errorful learning, people with amnesia much more easily remember their own mistakes than they remember the correction (which is usually the answer they hear from someone else). Errorless learning is an alternative way to get someone to learn something without the opportunity to make a mistake.

In addition to traditional memory or cognitive intervention, errorless learning provides a useful additional strategy. Patients should be tailored to interventions, based on errorless learning principles and specific cognitive problems. In one study, five of the six participants showed significant improvement on the target measures, and maintained this improvement up to 6 months later [67].

Spaced retrieval requires users to rehearse learned information at a certain time. Each new rehearsal is done with a longer or equal interval between itself and the previous rehearsal. At the end of every trial period there is a test phase [68]. Landauer and Bjork first described five types of this learning technique in 1978, and the effectiveness of the rehearsal types was measured by seeing how accurately participants responded during a test phase [69].

Schacter et al. applied the technique to people suffering from amnesia and other memory disorders. Participants were asked to remember some fact with increasing intervals. If the subject is able to recall the information correctly the time is doubled to further help them keep the information fresh in their mind to recall in the future. The findings showed that using spaced retrieval help name face association of young students, as well as individuals with memory disorders [70]. The technique helped demented patients able to place the information in their long-term memory, remembering particular objects names, daily tasks, name face association, information about themselves, and many other facts and behaviors [71]. Spaced retrieval also showed advantage in long-term outcome, which lasted weeks even months later [71].

Spaced-retrieval method was combined with traditional memory stimulation tasks. The term "prospective memory" refers to the timely execution of a previously formed intention. In 1991, it was used for training four AD patients to remember and to implement an intention for future action. All participants were able to shift to new task requirement, and all learned three successive coupon colors successfully [72]. A pilot study designed similar prospective memory tasks, consisting of errorless learning and spaced retrieval techniques. Results showed that AD patients who received prospective memory training performed another similar task successfully across 7 weeks post-treatment [73].

Training effect on brain activity from clinical perspectives
Neuronal mechanisms underlying the effects of these interventions were investigated by functional magnetic resonance imaging (fMRI) and electroencephalography (EEG). When training and tasks in the fMRI were the same (name-face association) for 6 MCI patients, increased activation was observed in the medial frontal cortex, parietal and occipital lobes neighboring the temporal-parietal junction, left frontal operculum and some areas of the left temporal cortex. It also revealed increased generally connectivity after training, particularly involving the medial temporal gyrus and foci in the occipital and precuneus cortices [74]. In a control study, 2-month verbal memory training improved left hippocampal activation [75], suggesting neuroplasticity related with cognitive training in the hippocampus in MCI.

Cortex also involves in memory trainings, especially when training and tests in fMRI involved different cognitive processes. A combination of specialized areas (activated areas during pre-training and new areas during post-training) was activated in the frontal, temporal and occipital areas. Right inferior parietal lobe was the only activated area that correlated with performance [76]. When tasks were visuospatial mnemonic, occipito-parietal and frontal brain regions had increased activity in younger adults. In older adults, only those that showed increased occipito-parietal activity benefited from the mnemonic. In the next section, more evidence suggested connectivity changes between different brain regions in combined cognitive training.

In gist reasoning training, higher fractional anisotrophy was found after 1-year training using diffusion tensor imaging (DTI) MRI [77]. DTI also revealed microstructural changes of limbic system structures (hippocampus and para-hippocampus) among young adults after a 2-h spatial learning and memory task [78]. A review of 20 research articles indicated that the most robust evidence among elderly adults was a change in anterior hippocampal volume with cognitive activities [79].

Connectivity between different brain areas may change during and after some specific cognitive manipulations. A 6-week training program for healthy older adults on Brain Fitness (an adaptive auditory perception computer game) showed improvement in the activities of daily living (a transfer effect from sensory processing to everyday problem solving). It also selectively increased the integrity of occipito-temporal white matter in the ventral attention network, and decreased connectivity between superior parietal cortex and inferior temporal lobe [80]. This indicates that top-down sensory processing training is associated with improvements in untrained everyday problem solving, depending on changes in the ventral attention network, rather than on the connectivity between the parietal cortex and the temporal lobe.

Neurons interaction could also be evaluated by EEG performance, taking its advantage of high temporal resolution. EEG coherence indicates synchronization between different cortical areas [81, 82]. After training of attention maintenance for 1 month, healthy elder participants demonstrated better performance, with remarkable increase in theta power and long-rang theta coherence between frontal and posterior brain regions [83]. EEG was used to evaluate participants before and after training in one study and revealed neural evidence of functional plasticity in older adult brains. The training-induced modifications in early visual processing during stimulus encoding predicted working memory accuracy improvements [34]. However, cognitive process could not be evaluated by EEG, since it is usually done when patients are under resting state.

Event-related potentials (ERP) [84] were used to find task-related neural discharges. An ERP study for visual search task showed that 10-week training improved attention resource allocation and capacity, by increasing N2pc and P3b amplitudes [85].

Despite the methodological limitations in both fMRI and EEG studies, such as small sample sizes and lack of control groups, these evidence suggested that elder individuals exhibit high plasticity, which can be used as a clue to understand the effects of cognitive interventions.

Why we turn to bench for more help?
Trials above provided exciting results for clinical practice. However, there are several problems confusing and unsolved. We raise the following reasons that make us turn to laboratory for more help.

At first, the selection and publication bias of clinical trials could not be ignored. AD has its owe pathological characteristics, and preclinical AD happened without any symptoms. Most of the clinical trials only lasted for a relatively short period and only evaluated participants by neuropsychological assessment. It is not sure that they enrolled participants of the correct diagnosis. Besides, some "normal aging" or MCI participants at baseline might progress to AD during follow-up, but few trial corrected the bias when enrollment. In this way, classic animal models of AD may help to find more consolidated evidence for cognitive intervention.

We once reviewed and concluded several principles for an effective training program [86], based on current clinical trials. However, before we design a training program, it is more important to find subjects who really have the indication. One of the most controversial issues of cognitive intervention is its various effect on patients with different level of cognitive ability. Some large-scale studies, such as ACTIVE study, did not precisely differentiate their participants. Positive effect was not proved to retain in participants with or without risk of AD. Though less side effect, cognitive intervention still has costs and is time-consuming. The duration of interventions varies among all studies. In some studies for normal older adults, participants attended the training for as long as 2 years, with a total of 270 h. In more studies, the training period ranged from 3 h to more than 100 h. Every session varied from 30 to 90 min in different studies. What is the relationship between training effect and the duration of intervention? Unfortunately, no one observed the quantitative interaction between duration and extent of improvement. Regarding these uncertainty, it is necessary to figure out who do need and could benefit from such interventions. A retrospective study suggested that neuropsychological profile helped differentiate subjects who respond better [87]. More neurobiological markers might make the intervention a more precise therapy.

Another problem is the duration of effect since intervention ends. The benefits of name-face association training were observed after 1 week [88], or after 1 month [89], and the participants could recognize the training material faster and with fewer errors [58]. Moreover, benefits of speed processing training were observed after 2 years with booster sessions over the course of 11 months [90]. Memory strategy worked as an enhancer of effect sustainment [55, 91], and it was not maintained after three [62] and four [91] months. Goal-oriented cognitive rehabilitation brought increase in self-performance and quality of life, which remained for 6 months [61]. However, the potential mechanisms of the prolonged effect are still unclear. The clarification of neurobiological changes stimulated by cognitive intervention might help a better design of cognitive program.

Finally, though functional MRI provided some evidence for brain activity changes, it has own methodological limitations. Blood oxygenation level dependent contrast (BOLD) in resting or task-related fMRI were mainly used to reflect brain activity. Various statistical methods were adopt to analyze BOLD data. Regional homogeneity, amplitude of low-frequency fluctuation (ALFF), fractional ALFF (fALFF) were once used as representation of regional activities in AD [92, 93], while some used Independent Component Analysis and Granger Causality Analysis to evaluate connectivity [94, 95]. Recently, fMRI validity was seriously questioned for its high false-positive rate from generally used software packages (SPM, FSL, AFNI) [96].

Cognitive stimulation for animals

Studies above have shown that the progression of dementia could be slowed down in the patients who have cognitively stimulating activities. These discoveries point to the conclusion that cognitive interventions intellectually may not only improve memory performance but also prevent future cognitive decline. Some difficulties met in clinical trials above asked for further exploration in neurobiological way.

Early experimental studies of brain stimulation on laboratory rodents

We now manipulate mental exercise as stimulating brain which acts a positive role on AD and other forms of dementias via neuroprotective and compensatory mechanism. Existing animal models that are most relevant to our understanding of non-pharmacological therapy include those which utilize environmental or cognitive stimulation as experimental paradigms to alter levels of cognitive activity. In order to attempt to investigate the mechanistic underpinnings of mental exercise in cognitive function, we should first understand early experimental studies of brain stimulation- environmental enrichment (EE) on animal models. EE has defined broadly as the use of housing conditions that offer enhanced sensory, motor, and cognitive stimulation of brain in comparison with standard caging [97]. In the late 1940s, Donald O. Hebb [98] was the first to propose the "enriched environment" as an experimental concept and reported anecdotally that the laboratory rats that he took home as pets solved test problems more easily than the rats kept at the laboratory. While his research did not investigate the brain nor use standardized and enriched environments. More quantitative and controlled EE studies needed to be conducted to test this paradigm systematically. In 1960, Mark Rosenzweig found the rats growing up in the cages with toys, ladders and tunnels showed higher enzyme cholinesterase activity [99]. The following work reported that living in enriched environment altered the function and structure of the brain, and increased cerebral cortex volume [100], thickness [101] and wet weight [102], greater synapse and glial numbers [103]. At that time brain weight and structure were considered a stable characteristic not subject to environmental influences.

From these early conclusions regarding the effects of EE, increasingly refined studies have progressed to showing effects at the cell and molecular levels. Adult rats were placed into enriched housing conditions for 1 year and showed significantly higher levels of nerve growth factor [104]. Another study reported the increased NGF, BDNF and NT-3 protein levels of EE adult rats compared with age-matched isolated condition ones [105]. Researchers also found EE affected the expression levels of a number of genes (microfibrilar protein, microtubule- associated protein 4, PSD-95/SAP90A, Bcl2/Bax, synaptobrevin, for example) involved in neuronal structure, synaptic signaling, and plasticity [106]. As research deepened, investigators have found that EE facilitated repair to the brain in a variety of situations, including severe traumatic brain injury [107, 108], developmental lead exposure [109], and stroke [110] prenatal stress [111], dark rearing [112], and even aging [113].

Numerous cognitive studies about how EE affected the brain had been also proposed. In the intact animals, EE could dramatically improve cognitive abilities [113–115]. In the brain-lesioned animals, EE was beneficial in attenuating cognitive deficits caused by cerebral contusion [107, 110, 116, 117]. Since then, a large volume of literature has evolved describing the effects of EE in a number of different transgenic mouse models of AD (Table 2).

Environmental enrichment-cognitive stimulation on animal models of AD

Many studies had shown that placing animals in complex environments for extended period improved their cognitive performance and brain activity in normal mice and rats. Whether did EE show beneficial effects on behavior and cognition in an animal model of AD? There were several mouse models of neurodegeneration like AD studying the modulating effects of environmental factors: transgenic mice overexpressing amyloid precursor protein (APP) and/or presenilin (PS)-1, AD11 mice expressing anti-nerve growth factor (NGF) antibodies and double transgenic TgCRND8 mice overexpressing the Swedish and Indiana mutations in the human APP. In these researches, the mouse models were given extensive enrichment such as cognitive stimulation or complex housing condition. Cognitive impairment and neuronal alterations elicited by neurodegenerative pathologies were evaluated to determine if they had been ameliorated or rescued by EE. If a long-lasting exposure to EE, the mouse model should display a delayed onset or progression of cognitive impairment.

Before the onset of amyloid formation, APP/PS1 transgenic mice exposed to the long term of EE from 2 to 8 months of age would show mitigated learning and memory deficits. For example, long term EE led to improvement in cognitive function but without decreasing brain beta-amyloid deposition in the aged APPsw mice [118]. Jankowsky, J. L reported that 2-month-old APP/PS1 mice were placed into enriched environment for 6 months, and they swam shorter distances to reach the hidden platform in water maze and more efficiently remembered the platform position. The performance of learning and memory were both normalized to the level of standard-housed non-transgenic mice [119]. Lazarov et al. found pronounced reduction in the levels of cerebral beta-amyloid peptides and amyloid deposits in the same EE APP/PS1 mice [120].

AD11 mice developed age-dependent neurodegeneration including hallmarks of human AD and exhibited progressive memory impairment [121, 122]. Exposed to EE before the onset of behavior deficits for a long time in AD11 mice resulted in preserved visual recognition memory and spatial memory in comparison to non-EE AD11 mice. EE AD11 mice displayed a stronger curiosity when faced a novel object than a familiar object and showed the same ability with wild-type mice on a water maze task [123].

In the TgCRND8 mice, EE had increased exploratory behavior and decreased anxiety-related behavior but could not clearly ameliorate deficits in learning and memory performance [124]. More recent evidence also suggested EE may reduce the cerebral oxidative stress [125], compensate for the effects of stress on disease progression [126], prevent astroglial pathological changes [127] and lessen the cognitive decline [128]. In the Tau-Tg transgenic mice, the NFTs decreased in EE mice [129]. In senescence-accelerated prone mice (SAM-P8),EE gave rise to significant beneficial effects at the molecular, cellular, and behavioral levels during brain development, particularly in the hippocampus [130]. In this part, EE provided animals with more novel and complex environment, and thus stimulated cognitive processes, particularly learning and memory. This evidence in AD mice indicated that enhanced cognitive stimulation of EE played a pivotal role in the protection from cognitive impairment.

What are the mechanisms for the effect of cognitive activity?
Neuronal circuits
Adult neurogenesis
Adult neurogenesis is shown to continue in two parts of brains: the subventricular zone (SVZ) lining the lateral ventricles and subgranular zone (SGZ). In fully adult mammals, new neurons born in SVZ migrate anteriorly into the olfactory bulb (OB), where they mature into local interneurons [131–133]. Adult-generated olfactory interneurons contribute to odor discrimination and

Table 2 Cognitive activity effects of enriched environment in animal models

References	Animal models	Age (weeks)	EE Duration (weeks)	Behavior effects	Morphological effects	Molecular effects
Kempermann et al., 2002 [149]	wild type, C57BL	40	40	Behavioral performance↑	Hippocampal neurogenesis↑	
Veyrac et al., 2008 [157]	wild type, C57BL	8 - 12	7	Short-term olfactory memory ↑	Neurogenesis↑	Noradrenalin levels↑
Frick KM et al., 2003 [113]	wild type, C57BL	12, 104- 108	3	spatial learning task in water maze task ↑		synaptophysin levels↑
Polito L et al., 2014 [128]	APP23, C57BL	12	20, 60	behavioral performance in Water Maze and visual novel Object Recognition Test ↑	Aβ 40/42, pGlu-Aβ 3-40/3-42, or Aβ oligomer level→	BDNF expression↑, sirtuin mRNA and protein levels→
Jeong et al., 2011 [126]	APP, C57BL	12	12 or 24	Cognitive performance↑	Hippocampal neurogensis↑, P-tau at AT8 and AT180 sites ↓, Aβ plaque and levels ↓	
Valero et al., 2011 [154]	APP, C57BL	12	7	Learning and memory↑	neurogenesis ↑, the number of DCX-positive cells↑	
Wolf et al., 2006 [151]	APP23, C57BL	10	34	Water maze performance↑	Hippocampal neurogenesis↑, Aβ plaque ↓	NT-3, BDNF levels↑
Costa et al., 2007 [152]	PDGF-hAPP, C57BL	3	18-22	performance of multiple behavioral tasks and memory ↑	Total Aβ and amyloid plaque levels↓	Hippocampal gene expression changed
Jankowsky JL et al.,2005 [119]	APP/PS1, C57BL	8	24	Cognitive function↑	Hippocampal Aβ levels ↑	
Berardi et al., 2007 [123]	AD11, C57BL	8	20	Spatial and visual recognition memory ↑	Aβ burdens↓	Cholinergic deficits↓
Dong et al., 2007 [153]	PS1/2 CKO, B6CBA	4	20	memory performance↑	less enlargement of the lateral ventricles ↑	inflammation-related genes↓
Varman et al., 2013 [174]	Mus booduga	12	4	anxiety-like behavior↓	miR-183 expression↑	acetylcholinesterase level in amygdala of mice ↓
Durairaj et al., 2014 [175]	Mus booduga	12	4	anxiety-like behavioral↓	Hippocampal neurogenesis↑	Dicer, Ago-2 and microRNA-124a expression↑

Aβ amyloid beta protein, P-tau phosphorylated tau, pGlu-Aβ 3-40/3-42 Human pGlu-amyloidβ3-40 and human pGlu-amyloidβ3-42, AT8 specifically recognizing phospho Ser202/Thr205 tau, AT180 monoclonal raised against residue Thr231 of PHF-tau, NT-3 Neurotrophin-3, BDNF Brain-derived neurotrophic factor, Dicer argonaute RISC catalytic component 2, Ago-2 argonaute RISC catalytic component 2

olfactory memory [134–136]. It has long been convinced that the hippocampus plays critical role in learning and memory [137], so the production of neurons in the adult hippocampal dentate gyrus (DG) has introduced the possibility of a new form of plasticity that could sustain memory processes. A growing body of evidence support that hippocampal neurogenesis improves pattern separation and spatial memory [138, 139].

Hippocampal neurogenesis could be influenced by several environmental factors and stimuli [140, 141]. While aging was the greatest environmental risk factor, increasing evidence showed noteworthy alteration in neurogenesis took place much earlier than the onset of hallmark lesions or neuronal loss in AD [142, 143]. In aged and AD brains, the proliferation of progenitor cells and their numbers were significantly declined (for review see [144]). The levels of stem cell factor (SCF) which supported neurogenesis in the brain were reduced in the plasma and cerebrospinal fluid of AD patients [145]. In WT mice, EE could enhance hippocampal cell proliferation [146, 147]. And transient receptor potential-canonical 1(TRPC1) was indispensable for the EE-induced hippocampal neurogenesis [148].

Previous studies in transgenic models of AD had generated mounting evidence supporting alterations in neurogenesis. Short-term exposure to EE led to a striking increase in new neurons and a substantial improvement in behavior performance [149]. Studies in several transgenic mice expressing AD-linked gene suggested that adult neurogenesis could be altered by external neurogenic stimulus- enriched environment. EE was reported to increase hippocampal DG neurogenesis and improve their water maze performance in APP23 mice [150, 151]. Enriched housing environment could also improve cognitive performance in PS1/PDAPP transgenic mouse models [152]. In PS1 and PS2 conditional double knockout mice, EE had been shown to be able to induce neurogenesis and effectively enhance memory of the brain [153]. In APP/PS1 double transgenic mice, EE for 7 weeks efficiently ameliorated early hippocampal-dependent spatial learning and memory deficits [154]. Complex environment had been reported to rescue impaired neurogenesis, reduce Aβ levels and amyloid deposition, and significantly enhance hippocampal LTP in APP/PS1 mice [120, 155]. EE applied to SAMP8 at young ages resulted in an increase in NeuN and Ki67 expression [130]. Thus, the proliferation of new neurons which had a reciprocal connection with AD pathogenesis would provide new opportunities for cell therapy for AD.

Although there are lots of studies reporting that EE could increase neurogenesis in DG of the adult hippocampus, neurogenesis in other parts of the brain- the subventricular zone(SVZ) or olfactory bulb (OB) system may be affected by other forms of enhanced stimulation significantly [156]. Olfactory enrichment- a specific form of enhanced sensory stimulation, does appear to increase neurogenesis in the OB [157] and additionally the piriform cortex [158].

Neuronal and glial developments

Neurons, neuroglia (including astrocytes, oligodendrocytes and microglia) and ependymal cells make up the complex structure of the adult central nervous system (CNS). Adult neurogenesis bridges between neuronal and glial neurobiology in an intriguing way. When the enrichment environment altered the neurogenesis, the differentiation and development of neuron and glial were always changed at the same time. Increased neuronal differentiation in DG was observed in the EE treated rats and the density of NeuN positive cells was enhanced without new neurons [159]. As many as 90% of cells in the brain are thought to be glial, therefore it is not difficult to understand that the beneficial effects of EE involve glial cell types. There is in fact evidence that EE could alter the numbers of glial in specific brain regions. EE could lead to a significant increase in the number of new astrocytes in layer 1 of the motor cortex [160]. In CA1 region, environmental condition increased the number of astrocytes [161] and stimulated astrocytes to acquire a more stellate morphology [162]. Two months old rats enriched for 7 weeks showed increased antigen expression of both astrocytes and microglia within DG [163]. Glia cells are known to interact extensively with neuron in the brain. Astrocytes secrete factors that promote neuron survival and provide crucial support to neurons. Oligodendrocytes are essential regulators of neurotransmission along myelinated axons. These reports of neuronal effects or non-neuronal effects of EE were interesting in light of evidence that EE plays an important role in modulating neurogenesis and cognition in AD.

Molecular mechanisms improving cognitive activity

We have now outlined various important structural and cellular changes that have been observed to occur in the animal brain exposure to EE. Evidence in support of such behavioral and cellular effects on molecular mechanisms has been gathered using a range of approaches. Examples of such molecular classes including specific neurotrophins, neurotransmitters and neuromodulator receptors, and synaptic signaling pathways have been validated via gene/protein studies.

Activity dependent modulation of gene expression

One early study demonstrated the attenuated expression of AP-2 in the CA2 and CA3 subfield of hippocampus after exposure to EE for 30 days [164]. In adult rats, EE has been shown to upregulate 3H-AMPA binding in the hippocampus by decreasing the capacity of calcium or phosphatidylserine without changes in mRNAs for AMPA receptors [165]. Male rats exposed to EE for 30 days could result in significant higher expression of 5-HT1A receptor mRNA in the hippocampus [166], decreased level of EAAC1 mRNA and increased level of NMDA mRNA specifically in the hippocampus [167]. EE could also increase the mRNA expression levels of 5α-reductase-1 and 3α-hydroxysteroid dehydrogenase, which catalyze synthesis of allopregnanolone from progesterone [168].

A more detailed research analyzed gene expression changes in the cortex of mice and found a large number of genes changed in response to enrichment [106]. Another study analyzed the effects of enriched surroundings with DNA microarrays and found the hippocampus was more responsive to environment stimuli than sensorimotor cortex [169]. Others have also shown the expression of immediate-early gene (IEG) Zif268 could be induced to higher level in the CA3/CA4 region which was associated with enhanced spatial learning task [170]. In NMDAR1-Knockout mice which showed memory impairment, the expression levels of 104 genes involved in multiple signal pathways could be recovered or reversed by EE [171]. Similarly, levels of CREB were increased following EE [172]. With the growing knowledge regarding environment and gene interactions, the framework has been built by an association between gene-environment interactions and disease [173].

Furthermore, there are still numbers of evidence that non-coding RNA species such as microRNAs (MiR) could also be modulated by EE. For example, MiR-183 expression could be upregulated by EE and reduce anxiety-like behavior in mice [174]. MiR-124a showed a similar performance following enriched environment condition [175]. MiR-325 was downregulated in 3 × Tg AD mice but upregulated by EE, which may open new avenues for the studies of treating AD [176]. Until now, this field of exploration is now relatively new, therefore many questions regarding the epigenetic impacts of EE remain unsolved. While the genomic and biochemical tools available are evolving rapidly, there will no doubt be great progress in the near future.

Oxidative stress

Previous studies have demonstrated that oxidative stress is an important factor contributing to the onset and progression of AD and the brain is sensitive to oxidative imbalance. Oxidative stress results from increased production of reactive oxygen species (ROS) and reactive nitrogen species (RNS) [177] and possibly precedes Aβ and tau aggregation. The exact mechanisms by how EE provides protection against oxidative damage in the

brain with AD remain speculative. In aged rats, complex EE modifies exploration activity, cognition and biochemical markers which may be mediated by oxidative stress levels [178]. Long term exposure to EE from adult age would increase life span in mice [179]. EE rats showed higher values for antioxidant measures and lower values for oxidative stress parameters than control animals [180]. In transgenic mice with Alzheimer-like pathology, cognitive stimulation in the form of EE attenuated pro-oxidative processes and triggered anti-oxidative defense mechanisms by diminishing reactive oxygen and nitrogen species, downregulating pro-inflammatory and pro-oxidative mediators, decreasing expression of pro-apoptotic caspases, and increasing the activities of SOD1 and SOD2 [125]. In another study, EE increased anti-oxidative SOD1 protein and decreased the levels of nitro-tyrosine- a prominent biomarker for oxidative damage [181].

Neurotrophin, neurotransmitter and neuromodulator signaling pathway

Modulation of neurotrophin expression and changes in neurotransmitters and neuromodulators are related to EE according to extensive findings. The primary effect of increased cognitive activity must be via enhanced synaptic and neuronal activity in the relevant neural circuitry. So, it is not difficult to image that molecular effects induced by EE have been shown to involve changes in neurotransmitters. Numbers of studies have shown that EE in animals increased the expression levels of brain-derived neurotrophic factor (BDNF), nerve growth factor (NGF) and vascular endothelial growth factor (VEGF) [182].

In rats with cognitive impairment, the levels of BDNF decreased in the hippocampus and EE exposure could up-regulate the decreased protein levels of BDNF [183]. More studies explained that the enhancement of learning and memory observed after treatment of EE is causally dependent on increased neurogenesis in DG. And BDNF was required for neurogenesis in the adult hippocampus [184] and might be responsible for learning and memory enhancement [185]. EE could significantly increase hippocampal BDNF levels accompanied by increased astrocytes (GFAP+) and microglia (Iba1+) antigen expression [163]. As BDNF supports hippocampal long-term potentiation (LTP), EE also improved synaptic plasticity and cognition through increased levels of BDNF [186].

The experience of APP/PS1 mice in EE would upregulate critical signaling that plays a major role in learning and memory, such as BDNF, IGF-1, N-methyl-D-aspartic acid receptor (NMDAR) and CREB transcripts [187]. NGF is another intensively investigated neurotrophin, when exposed to EE, the levels of NGF was increased either [188, 189] in the cerebral cortex, hippocampal formation, basal forebrain, and hindbrain in EE mice [105]. The levels of NGF mRNA were significant higher in rats housed in a stimulus-rich environment than those in single cages [190]. Short-term EE also increased NGF concentration and improved memory, early neuronal survival in DG [191]. Researchers draw attention to BDNF and NGF mostly because they appeared to be most labile in their expression dynamics and they are important in brain development, function and disease.

Conclusion and perspectives for the future

As one of non-pharmacological therapies, cognitive activity could benefit cognitive function, and thus life quality of patients and their families. These reviewed clinical studies above highlighted the positive effects of cognitive activity on cognitive ability, well-beings, behavior, and mood in older adults or patients with cognitive decline. We also reviewed the molecular and cellular mechanisms underlying this non-pharmacological therapy.

Based on these clinical trials and meta analysis, we recommend some key features of training that often associated with positive outcomes. Firstly, multi-domain tasks contribute more to cognition [19, 192]. As trained effect could hardly transfer to untrained domains, multi-domain trainings are generally adopted and recommended. Evidence from neuroimaging and animal research suggested that transfer effect could be maximized when tasks are designed to stimulate common brain regions (e.g., hippocampus, striatum) [193, 194]. Besides, challenging tasks for individuals are much more helpful in promoting cognitive ability: training is not learning until the participant can complete the task perfectly. During this period, challenging tasks are helpful for the survival of new neurons [193]. Computerized cognitive training is a lucrative and expanding business. It could easily offer standard and self-adaptive tasks with various levels of difficulty. At the end of training, performance could be evaluated and participants know how well they did. It brings more convenience, as well as less supervision. The researchers identified small but significant effect, while "do-it-yourself" training at home did not produce cognitive improvements [19]. Motivational strategies also can be applied to increase treatment adherence. As described above, training package is recommended, which composes cognitive training package, behavioral therapy for hopelessness and low expectations of success, and a motivational milieu [195]. Compared with control group, AD patients receiving the training package reported fewer depressive symptoms. Fewer depression also leads to better memory improvement and better quality of life [196, 197]. Errorless learning has its special advantage in mild to moderate AD patients. It provides more clues and leads to the only correct answer, which lessens confusion from the difference between correct answer and incorrect response. More importantly, this training process encourages elders to learn by clues in daily life [89, 198].

However, the heterogeneity of cognitive intervention poses great difficulty for a safe conclusion. Combining data from trials of different sample size can result in overestimating the precision of smaller studies. Because of limitation in clinical trials mentioned in Section Why we turn to bench for more help?, we turn to animal studies for more help.

Evidence from epidemiology and animal model studies suggests that the onset of neurodegenerative diseases could be modulated by environmental factors [199]. However, understanding the mechanism of EE requires animal models showing both behavioral and intrinsic changes which could link data from molecular through to systems levels. The studies compared the behavioral, cellular and molecular data on animal models under EE versus standard conditions. The positive effects of EE include increased adult neurogenesis, elevated or declined gene expression, reduced oxidative stress and subsequently reduced anxiety-like behaviors and improved cognitive performance. This enhanced understanding of EE may provide insight into the mechanistic basis and lead to novel therapeutic approaches which boost endogenous cognitive activity, and thus delay onset of a range of devastating AD and other dementias (Fig. 1).

We find EE has positive influence on normal aging and transgenic AD mouse, which could induce brain structure to produce a variety of changes. The change on anatomy includes the increases of brain weight, thickening of cerebral cortex and enlargement of hippocampus volume, etc. On cellular levels, EE could increase the proliferation of neural progenitor cells, production of newly generated neurons, the dendritic branches and tree density and the number of neuronal synapsis. These changes are most obvious in hippocampus and cerebral cortex. EE also could change the morphology of glia cells (including astrocyte and oligodendroglia cell) and promote the glial cell proliferation in the brain and cerebellum. EE could also induce various neural active substance changes, BDNF, VEGF, NGF and so on. These growth factors play important role on neurogenesis and neural network, which helps neuron development, differentiation and survival. In these ways, EE could improve the learning ability and cognition.

Several questions remain unclear. Classic water maze was usually applied in mice around 8 months old. However, most EE studies used transgenic AD mice of relative young age, about 2–3 month-old. Thus, the effect of EE in elder mice was still unclarified. Maybe older mice should be used on EE in the following days. Besides, few study concerns how EE influence neuronal death and

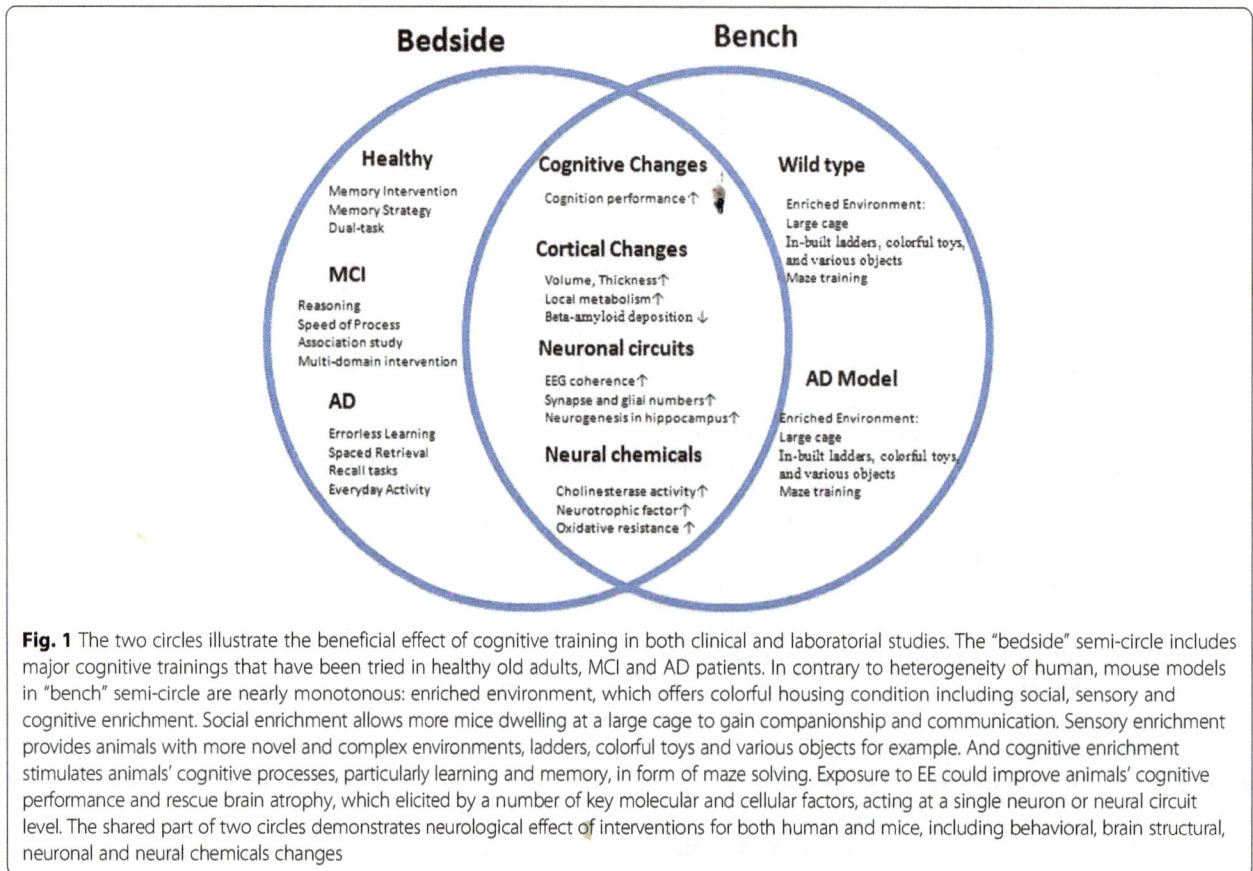

Fig. 1 The two circles illustrate the beneficial effect of cognitive training in both clinical and laboratorial studies. The "bedside" semi-circle includes major cognitive trainings that have been tried in healthy old adults, MCI and AD patients. In contrary to heterogeneity of human, mouse models in "bench" semi-circle are nearly monotonous: enriched environment, which offers colorful housing condition including social, sensory and cognitive enrichment. Social enrichment allows more mice dwelling at a large cage to gain companionship and communication. Sensory enrichment provides animals with more novel and complex environments, ladders, colorful toys and various objects for example. And cognitive enrichment stimulates animals' cognitive processes, particularly learning and memory, in form of maze solving. Exposure to EE could improve animals' cognitive performance and rescue brain atrophy, which elicited by a number of key molecular and cellular factors, acting at a single neuron or neural circuit level. The shared part of two circles demonstrates neurological effect of interventions for both human and mice, including behavioral, brain structural, neuronal and neural chemicals changes

related mechanism for its non-ignorable role in neural circuit. A more difficult challenge is linking animal model data with clinical studies. Finally, the questions we raised in Section Why we turn to bench for more help? were only partly answered in animal studies. We could conclude that the pathological changes in AD model could be modified by cognitive interventions. The best duration and long-term effect of these intervention still remain unclear. An overall systematic explanation for the internal mechanism of EE should be given in further studies.

Abbreviations
AD: Alzheimer's disease; APP: Myloid precursor protein; BDNF: Brain-derived neurotrophic factor; BOLD: Blood oxygenation level dependent contrast; ChEIs: Cholinesterase inhibitors; CNS: Central nervous system; CREB: cAMP-response element binding protein; DG: Dentate gyrus; DTI: Diffusion tensor imaging; EE: Environmental enrichment; EEG: Electroencephalography; ERP: Event-related potentials; FDA: Food and drug administration; fMRI: Functional magnetic resonance imaging; IEG: Immediate-early gene; IGF: IGF nsulin-like growth factor; MCI: Mild cognitive impairment; MiR: microRNAs; NGF: Nerve growth factor; NMDAR: N-methyl-D-aspartic acid receptor; OB: Olfactory bulb; PRISMA: Preferred Reporting Items for Systematic Reviews and Meta-Analysis; PS: Presenilin; RNS: Reactive nitrogen species; ROS: Reactive oxygen species; SAMP8: Senescence-accelerated prone mice; SCF: Stem cell factor; SOD: Superoxide Dismutase; SVZ: Subventricular zone; TRPC1: Transient receptor potential-canonical 1; VEGF: Vascular endothelial growth factor; WT: Wild type

Acknowledgements
Not applicable.

Funding
This work (information collection) was supported by grants from the National Natural Science Foundation of China [81400888] and Clinical Research Center, Shanghai Jiao Tong University School of Medicine [DLY201603].

Authors' contributions
BL searched and collected clinical information and drafted the manuscript. YW searched data and studies of animal models and thus drafted the lab part. HT and SC conceived of the review, and participated in its structure and helped to draft the manuscript. All authors read and approved the final manuscript.

Competing interests

The corresponding author, Dr Shengdi Chen, is the Editor in Chief for this journal.

References

1. Brookmeyer R, et al. Forecasting the global burden of Alzheimer's disease. Alzheimers Dement. 2007;3(3):186–91.
2. Reitz C, Mayeux R. Alzheimer disease: epidemiology, diagnostic criteria, risk factors and biomarkers. Biochem Pharmacol. 2014;88(4):640–51.
3. Joyce AT, et al. Burden of illness among commercially insured patients with Alzheimer's disease. Alzheimers Dement. 2007;3(3):204–10.
4. Ding D, et al. Prevalence of mild cognitive impairment in an urban community in China: A cross-sectional analysis of the Shanghai Aging Study. Alzheimers Dement. 2014;11(3):300–9.e2.
5. Gauthier S, et al. Mild cognitive impairment. Lancet. 2006;367(9518):1262–70.
6. Jia J, et al. The prevalence of mild cognitive impairment and its etiological subtypes in elderly Chinese. Alzheimers Dement. 2014;10(4):439–47.
7. Ravaglia G, et al. Mild cognitive impairment: epidemiology and dementia risk in an elderly Italian population. J Am Geriatr Soc. 2008;56(1):51–8.
8. Trinh NH, et al. Efficacy of cholinesterase inhibitors in the treatment of neuropsychiatric symptoms and functional impairment in Alzheimer disease: a meta-analysis. JAMA. 2003;289(2):210–6.
9. Reisberg B, et al. Memantine in moderate-to-severe Alzheimer's disease. N Engl J Med. 2003;348(14):1333–41.
10. Raina P, et al. Effectiveness of cholinesterase inhibitors and memantine for treating dementia: evidence review for a clinical practice guideline. Ann Intern Med. 2008;148(5):379–97.
11. Courtney C, et al. Long-term donepezil treatment in 565 patients with Alzheimer's disease (AD2000): randomised double-blind trial. Lancet. 2004; 363(9427):2105–15.
12. Russ TC, Morling JR. Cholinesterase inhibitors for mild cognitive impairment. Cochrane Database Syst Rev. 2012;9:CD009132.
13. Schneider LS, et al. Treatment with cholinesterase inhibitors and memantine of patients in the Alzheimer's Disease Neuroimaging Initiative. Arch Neurol. 2011;68(1):58–66.
14. Olazaran J, et al. Nonpharmacological therapies in Alzheimer's disease: a systematic review of efficacy. Dement Geriatr Cogn Disord. 2010;30(2):161–78.
15. Buschert V, Bokde AL, Hampel H. Cognitive intervention in Alzheimer disease. Nat Rev Neurol. 2010;6(9):508–17.
16. Reijnders J, van Heugten C, van Boxtel M. Cognitive interventions in healthy older adults and people with mild cognitive impairment: a systematic review. Ageing Res Rev. 2013;12(1):263–75.
17. Jean L, et al. Cognitive intervention programs for individuals with mild cognitive impairment: systematic review of the literature. Am J Geriatr Psychiatry. 2010;18(4):281–96.
18. Simon SS, Yokomizo JE, Bottino CM. Cognitive intervention in amnestic Mild Cognitive Impairment: a systematic review. Neurosci Biobehav Rev. 2012;36(4):1163–78.
19. Lampit A, Hallock H, Valenzuela M. Computerized cognitive training in cognitively healthy older adults: a systematic review and meta-analysis of effect modifiers. PLoS Med. 2014;11(11):e1001756.
20. Clare L, et al. Cognitive rehabilitation and cognitive training for early-stage Alzheimer's disease and vascular dementia. Cochrane Database Syst Rev. 2003;4:CD003260.
21. Grandmaison E, Simard M. A critical review of memory stimulation programs in Alzheimer's disease. J Neuropsychiatry Clin Neurosci. 2003;15(2):130–44.
22. Baltes, P. B. and S. L. Willis. Plasticity and Enhancement of Intellectual Functioning in Old Age. Aging and Cognitive Processes. F. I. M. Craik and S. Trehub. Boston, MA: Springer US; 1982: 353-89.
23. Yesavage JA. Nonpharmacologic treatments for memory losses with normal aging. Am J Psychiatry. 1985; 142(5):600-5.
24. Greenberg C, Powers SM. Memory improvement among adult learners. Educ Gerontol. 1987;13(3):263–80.
25. Rebok GW, Balcerak LJ. Memory self-efficacy and performance differences in young and old adults: The effect of mnemonic training. Dev Psychol. 1989;25(5):714.
26. Rebok GW, Rasmusson D, Brandt J. Prospects for computerized memory training in normal elderly: Effects of practice on explicit and implicit memory tasks. Appl Cogn Psychol. 1996;10(3):211–23.
27. Rasmusson DX, et al. Effects of three types of memory training in normal elderly. Aging Neuropsychol Cogn. 1999;6(1):56–66.
28. Fairchild JK, Scogin FR. Training to Enhance Adult Memory (TEAM): an investigation of the effectiveness of a memory training program with older adults. Aging Ment Health. 2010;14(3):364–73.
29. McDougall Jr GJ, et al. The SeniorWISE study: improving everyday memory in older adults. Arch Psychiatr Nurs. 2010;24(5):291–306.
30. Buschkuehl M, et al. Impact of working memory training on memory performance in old-old adults. Psychol Aging. 2008;23(4):743–53.
31. Melby-Lervag M, Hulme C. There is no convincing evidence that working memory training is effective: A reply to Au et al. (2014) and Karbach and Verhaeghen (2014). Psychon Bull Rev. 2016; 23(1):324-30.
32. Karbach J, Verhaeghen P. Making working memory work: a meta-analysis of executive-control and working memory training in older adults. Psychol Sci. 2014;25(11):2027–37.
33. Li SC, et al. Working memory plasticity in old age: practice gain, transfer, and maintenance. Psychol Aging. 2008;23(4):731–42.
34. Berry AS, et al. The influence of perceptual training on working memory in older adults. PLoS ONE. 2010;5(7):e11537.
35. Borella E, et al. Working memory training in older adults: evidence of transfer and maintenance effects. Psychol Aging. 2010;25(4):767–78.
36. Jobe JB, et al. ACTIVE: a cognitive intervention trial to promote independence in older adults. Control Clin Trials. 2001;22(4):453–79.
37. Ball K, et al. Effects of cognitive training interventions with older adults: a randomized controlled trial. JAMA. 2002;288(18):2271–81.
38. Rebok GW, et al. Ten-year effects of the advanced cognitive training for independent and vital elderly cognitive training trial on cognition and everyday functioning in older adults. J Am Geriatr Soc. 2014;62(1):16–24.
39. Ross LA, et al. The Transfer of Cognitive Speed of Processing Training to Older Adults' Driving Mobility Across 5 Years. J Gerontol B Psychol Sci Soc Sci. 2016;71(1):87–97.
40. Wolinsky FD, et al. Effects of cognitive speed of processing training on a composite neuropsychological outcome: results at one-year from the IHAMS randomized controlled trial. Int Psychogeriatr. 2016;28(2):317–30.
41. Buiza C, et al. A randomized, two-year study of the efficacy of cognitive intervention on elderly people: the Donostia Longitudinal Study. Int J Geriatr Psychiatry. 2008;23(1):85–94.
42. Smith GE, et al. A cognitive training program based on principles of brain plasticity: results from the Improvement in Memory with Plasticity-based Adaptive Cognitive Training (IMPACT) study. J Am Geriatr Soc. 2009;57(4):594–603.
43. Diamond K, et al. Randomized controlled trial of a healthy brain ageing cognitive training program: effects on memory, mood, and sleep. J Alzheimers Dis. 2015;44(4):1181–91.
44. Carlson MC, et al. Exploring the effects of an "everyday" activity program on executive function and memory in older adults: Experience Corps. Gerontologist. 2008;48(6):793–801.
45. Tranter LJ, Koutstaal W. Age and flexible thinking: an experimental demonstration of the beneficial effects of increased cognitively stimulating activity on fluid intelligence in healthy older adults. Neuropsychol Dev Cogn B Aging Neuropsychol Cogn. 2008;15(2):184–207.
46. Wagner S, et al. Does a cognitive-training programme improve the performance of middle-aged employees undergoing in-patient psychosomatic treatment? Disabil Rehabil. 2008;30(23):1786–93.
47. Ngandu T, et al. A 2 year multidomain intervention of diet, exercise, cognitive training, and vascular risk monitoring versus control to prevent cognitive decline in at-risk elderly people (FINGER): a randomised controlled trial. Lancet. 2015;385(9984):2255-63.
48. Rozzini L, et al. Efficacy of cognitive rehabilitation in patients with mild cognitive impairment treated with cholinesterase inhibitors. Int J Geriatr Psychiatry. 2007;22(4):356–60.
49. Talassi E, et al. Effectiveness of a cognitive rehabilitation program in mild dementia (MD) and mild cognitive impairment (MCI): a case control study. Arch Gerontol Geriatr. 2007;44 Suppl 1:391–9.
50. Wenisch E, et al. Cognitive stimulation intervention for elders with mild cognitive impairment compared with normal aged subjects: preliminary results. Aging Clin Exp Res. 2007;19(4):316–22.
51. Kurz A, et al. Cognitive rehabilitation in patients with mild cognitive impairment. 2009. p. 163–8.
52. Greenaway MC, et al. A behavioral rehabilitation intervention for amnestic mild cognitive impairment. Am J Alzheimers Dis Other Demen. 2008;23(5):451–61.
53. Barnes DE, et al. Computer-based cognitive training for mild cognitive impairment: results from a pilot randomized, controlled trial. Alzheimer Dis Assoc Disord. 2009;23(3):205–10.

54. Bottiroli S, Cavallini E. Can computer familiarity regulate the benefits of computer-based memory training in normal aging? A study with an Italian sample of older adults. Neuropsychol Dev Cogn B Aging Neuropsychol Cogn. 2009;16(4):401–18.

55. Rapp S, Brenes G, Marsh AP. Memory enhancement training for older adults with mild cognitive impairment: a preliminary study. Aging Ment Health. 2002;6(1):5–11.

56. Cappelletti M, et al. Transfer of Cognitive Training across Magnitude Dimensions Achieved with Concurrent Brain Stimulation of the Parietal Lobe. J Neurosci. 2013;33(37):14899–907.

57. Belleville S, et al. Improvement of episodic memory in persons with mild cognitive impairment and healthy older adults: evidence from a cognitive intervention program. Dement Geriatr Cogn Disord. 2006;22(5–6):486–99.

58. Hampstead BM, et al. Explicit memory training leads to improved memory for face-name pairs in patients with mild cognitive impairment: results of a pilot investigation. J Int Neuropsychol Soc. 2008;14(5):883–9.

59. Vranic A, et al. The efficacy of a multifactorial memory training in older adults living in residential care settings. Int Psychogeriatr. 2013;25(11):1885-97.

60. Lovden M, et al. A theoretical framework for the study of adult cognitive plasticity. Psychol Bull. 2010;136(4):659–76.

61. Londos E, et al. Effects of a goal-oriented rehabilitation program in mild cognitive impairment: a pilot study. Am J Alzheimers Dis Other Demen. 2008;23(2):177–83.

62. Troyer AK, et al. Changing everyday memory behaviour in amnestic mild cognitive impairment: a randomised controlled trial. Neuropsychol Rehabil. 2008;18(1):65–88.

63. Quayhagen MP, et al. Coping with dementia: evaluation of four nonpharmacologic interventions. Int Psychogeriatr. 2000;12(2):249–65.

64. Zarit SH, Zarit JM, Reever KE. Memory training for severe memory loss: effects on senile dementia patients and their families. Gerontologist. 1982;22(4):373–7.

65. Backman L, et al. The generalizability of training gains in dementia: effects of an imagery-based mnemonic on face-name retention duration. Psychol Aging. 1991;6(3):489–92.

66. Davis RN, Massman PJ, Doody RS. Cognitive intervention in Alzheimer disease: a randomized placebo-controlled study. Alzheimer Dis Assoc Disord. 2001;15(1):1–9.

67. Clare L, et al. Intervening with everyday memory problems in dementia of Alzheimer type: an errorless learning approach. J Clin Exp Neuropsychol. 2000;22(1):132–46.

68. Haslam C, Hodder KI, Yates PJ. Errorless learning and spaced retrieval: how do these methods fare in healthy and clinical populations? J Clin Exp Neuropsychol. 2011;33(4):432–47.

69. Landauer TK, Bjork RA. Optimum rehearsal patterns and name learning. Pract Asp Mem. 1978;1:625–32.

70. Hawley KS, et al. A comparison of adjusted spaced retrieval versus a uniform expanded retrieval schedule for learning a name-face association in older adults with probable Alzheimer's disease. J Clin Exp Neuropsychol. 2008;30(6):639–49.

71. Small JA. A new frontier in spaced retrieval memory training for persons with Alzheimer's disease. Neuropsychol Rehabil. 2012;22(3):329–61.

72. McKitrick LA, Camp CJ, Black FW. Prospective memory intervention in Alzheimer's disease. J Gerontol. 1992;47(5):P337–43.

73. Kixmiller JS. Evaluation of prospective memory training for individuals with mild Alzheimer's disease. Brain Cogn. 2002;49(2):237–41.

74. Hampstead BM, et al. Activation and effective connectivity changes following explicit-memory training for face-name pairs in patients with mild cognitive impairment: a pilot study. Neurorehabil Neural Repair. 2011;25(3):210–22.

75. Rosen AC, et al. Cognitive training changes hippocampal function in mild cognitive impairment: a pilot study. J Alzheimers Dis. 2011;26 Suppl 3:349–57.

76. Belleville S, et al. Training-related brain plasticity in subjects at risk of developing Alzheimer's disease. Brain. 2011;134(6):1623–34.

77. Chapman SB. et al. Neural Mechanisms of Brain Plasticity with Complex Cognitive Training in Healthy Seniors. Cereb Cortex. 2013;25(2):396-405.

78. Sagi Y, et al. Learning in the fast lane: new insights into neuroplasticity. Neuron. 2012;73(6):1195–203.

79. Thomas C, Baker CI. Teaching an adult brain new tricks: a critical review of evidence for training-dependent structural plasticity in humans. Neuroimage. 2013;73:225–36.

80. Strenziok M. et al. Neurocognitive enhancement in older adults: Comparison of three cognitive training tasks to test a hypothesis of training transfer in brain connectivity. Neuroimage. 2014;15;85Pt 3: 1027-39.

81. Sauseng P, et al. Dissociation of sustained attention from central executive functions: local activity and interregional connectivity in the theta range. Eur J Neurosci. 2007;25(2):587–93.

82. Onton J, Delorme A, Makeig S. Frontal midline EEG dynamics during working memory. Neuroimage. 2005;27(2):341–56.

83. Anguera JA, et al. Video game training enhances cognitive control in older adults. Nature. 2013;501(7465):97–101.

84. Albouy G, et al. Neural correlates of performance variability during motor sequence acquisition. Neuroimage. 2012;60(1):324–31.

85. O'Brien JL. et al. Cognitive training and selective attention in the aging brain: An electrophysiological study. Clin Neurophysiol. 2013;124(11):2198-208.

86. Li BY, et al. Mental Training for Cognitive Improvement in Elderly People: What have We Learned from Clinical and Neurophysiologic Studies? Curr Alzheimer Res. 2015;12(6):543–52.

87. Martinez-Moreno M., et al. Comparison of neuropsychological and functional outcomes in Alzheimer's disease patients with good or bad response to a cognitive stimulation treatment: a retrospective analysis. Int Psychogeriatr. 2016;28(11):1–13.

88. Jean L, et al. Towards a cognitive stimulation program using an errorless learning paradigm in amnestic mild cognitive impairment. Neuropsychiatr Dis Treat. 2007;3(6):975–85.

89. Jean L, et al. Efficacy of a cognitive training programme for mild cognitive impairment: results of a randomised controlled study. Neuropsychol Rehabil. 2010;20(3):377–405.

90. Unverzagt FW, et al. Effect of memory impairment on training outcomes in ACTIVE. J Int Neuropsychol Soc. 2007;13(6):953–60.

91. Kinsella GJ, et al. Early intervention for mild cognitive impairment: a randomised controlled trial. J Neurol Neurosurg Psychiatry. 2009;80(7):730–6.

92. He Y, et al. Regional coherence changes in the early stages of Alzheimer's disease: a combined structural and resting-state functional MRI study. Neuroimage. 2007;35(2):488–500.

93. Cha J, et al. Assessment of Functional Characteristics of Amnestic Mild Cognitive Impairment and Alzheimer's Disease Using Various Methods of Resting-State FMRI Analysis. Biomed Res Int. 2015;2015:907464.

94. Chen Y, et al. Functional Activity and Connectivity Differences of Five Resting-State Networks in Patients with Alzheimer's Disease or Mild Cognitive Impairment. Curr Alzheimer Res. 2016;13(3):234–42.

95. Whitwell JL, et al. Working memory and language network dysfunctions in logopenic aphasia: a task-free fMRI comparison with Alzheimer's dementia. Neurobiol Aging. 2015;36(3):1245–52.

96. Eklund A, Nichols TE, Knutsson H. Cluster failure: Why fMRI inferences for spatial extent have inflated false-positive rates. Proc Natl Acad Sci U S A. 2016;113(28):7900–5.

97. Toth LA, et al. Environmental enrichment of laboratory rodents: the answer depends on the question. Comp Med. 2011;61(4):314–21.

98. Hebb DO. The effects of early experience on problem solving at maturity. Am Psychol. 1947;2:306–7.

99. Krech D, Rosenzweig MR, Bennett EL. Effects of environmental complexity and training on brain chemistry. J Comp Physiol Psychol. 1960;53:509–19.

100. Rosenzweig MR, et al. Effects of environmental complexity and training on brain chemistry and anatomy: a replication and extension. J Comp Physiol Psychol. 1962;55:429–37.

101. Diamond MC, Krech D, Rosenzweig MR. The Effects of an Enriched Environment on the Histology of the Rat Cerebral Cortex. J Comp Neurol. 1964;123:111–20.

102. Bennett EL, Rosenzweig MR, Diamond MC. Rat brain: effects of environmental enrichment on wet and dry weights. Science. 1969;163(3869):825–6.

103. Altman J, Das GD. Autoradiographic Examination of the Effects of Enriched Environment on the Rate of Glial Multiplication in the Adult Rat Brain. Nature. 1964;204:1161–3.

104. Pham TM, et al. Changes in brain nerve growth factor levels and nerve growth factor receptors in rats exposed to environmental enrichment for one year. Neuroscience. 1999;94(1):279–86.

105. Ickes BR, et al. Long-term environmental enrichment leads to regional increases in neurotrophin levels in rat brain. Exp Neurol. 2000;164(1):45–52.

106. Rampon C, et al. Effects of environmental enrichment on gene expression in the brain. Proc Natl Acad Sci U S A. 2000;97(23):12880–4.

107. Passineau MJ, Green EJ, Dietrich WD. Therapeutic effects of environmental enrichment on cognitive function and tissue integrity following severe traumatic brain injury in rats. Exp Neurol. 2001;168(2):373–84.

108. Xerri C, Zennou-Azougui Y, Coq JO. Neuroprotective effects on somatotopic maps resulting from piracetam treatment and environmental enrichment after focal cortical injury. ILAR J. 2003;44(2):110–24.

109. Guilarte TR, et al. Environmental enrichment reverses cognitive and molecular deficits induced by developmental lead exposure. Ann Neurol. 2003;53(1):50–6.

110. Dahlqvist P, et al. Environmental enrichment reverses learning impairment in the Morris water maze after focal cerebral ischemia in rats. Eur J Neurosci. 2004;19(8):2288–98.

111. Morley-Fletcher S, et al. Environmental enrichment during adolescence reverses the effects of prenatal stress on play behaviour and HPA axis reactivity in rats. Eur J Neurosci. 2003;18(12):3367–74.

112. Bartoletti A, et al. Environmental enrichment prevents effects of dark-rearing in the rat visual cortex. Nat Neurosci. 2004;7(3):215–6.

113. Frick KM, Fernandez SM. Enrichment enhances spatial memory and increases synaptophysin levels in aged female mice. Neurobiol Aging. 2003;24(4):615–26.

114. Duffy SN, et al. Environmental enrichment modifies the PKA-dependence of hippocampal LTP and improves hippocampus-dependent memory. Learn Mem. 2001;8(1):26–34.

115. Leggio MG, et al. Environmental enrichment promotes improved spatial abilities and enhanced dendritic growth in the rat. Behav Brain Res. 2005;163(1):78–90.

116. Hicks RR, et al. Environmental enrichment attenuates cognitive deficits, but does not alter neurotrophin gene expression in the hippocampus following lateral fluid percussion brain injury. Neuroscience. 2002;112(3):631–7.

117. Dobrossy MD, Dunnett SB. Environmental enrichment affects striatal graft morphology and functional recovery. Eur J Neurosci. 2004;19(1):159–68.

118. Arendash GW, et al. Environmental enrichment improves cognition in aged Alzheimer's transgenic mice despite stable beta-amyloid deposition. Neuroreport. 2004;15(11):1751–4.

119. Jankowsky JL, et al. Environmental enrichment mitigates cognitive deficits in a mouse model of Alzheimer's disease. J Neurosci. 2005;25(21):5217–24.

120. Lazarov O, et al. Environmental enrichment reduces Abeta levels and amyloid deposition in transgenic mice. Cell. 2005;120(5):701–13.

121. De Rosa R, et al. Intranasal administration of nerve growth factor (NGF) rescues recognition memory deficits in AD11 anti-NGF transgenic mice. Proc Natl Acad Sci U S A. 2005;102(10):3811–6.

122. Capsoni S, et al. Alzheimer-like neurodegeneration in aged antinerve growth factor transgenic mice. Proc Natl Acad Sci U S A. 2000;97(12):6826–31.

123. Berardi N, et al. Environmental enrichment delays the onset of memory deficits and reduces neuropathological hallmarks in a mouse model of Alzheimer-like neurodegeneration. J Alzheimers Dis. 2007;11(3):359–70.

124. Gortz N, et al. Effects of environmental enrichment on exploration, anxiety, and memory in female TgCRND8 Alzheimer mice. Behav Brain Res. 2008;191(1):43–8.

125. Herring A, et al. Reduction of cerebral oxidative stress following environmental enrichment in mice with Alzheimer-like pathology. Brain Pathol. 2010;20(1):166–75.

126. Jeong YH, et al. Environmental enrichment compensates for the effects of stress on disease progression in Tg2576 mice, an Alzheimer's disease model. J Neurochem. 2011;119(6):1282–93.

127. Beauquis J, et al. Environmental enrichment prevents astroglial pathological changes in the hippocampus of APP transgenic mice, model of Alzheimer's disease. Exp Neurol. 2013;239:28–37.

128. Polito L, et al. Environmental enrichment lessens cognitive decline in APP23 mice without affecting brain sirtuin expression. J Alzheimers Dis. 2014;42(3):851–64.

129. Lahiani-Cohen I, et al. Moderate environmental enrichment mitigates tauopathy in a neurofibrillary tangle mouse model. J Neuropathol Exp Neurol. 2011;70(7):610–21.

130. Grinan-Ferre C, et al. Environmental Enrichment Improves Behavior, Cognition, and Brain Functional Markers in Young Senescence-Accelerated Prone Mice (SAMP8). Mol Neurobiol. 2016;53(4):2435–50.

131. Altman J, Das GD. Autoradiographic and histological studies of postnatal neurogenesis. I. A longitudinal investigation of the kinetics, migration and transformation of cells incorporating tritiated thymidine in neonate rats,

with special reference to postnatal neurogenesis in some brain regions. J Comp Neurol. 1966;126(3):337–89.

132. Lois C, Alvarez-Buylla A. Long-distance neuronal migration in the adult mammalian brain. Science. 1994;264(5162):1145–8.

133. Kornack DR, Rakic P. The generation, migration, and differentiation of olfactory neurons in the adult primate brain. Proc Natl Acad Sci U S A. 2001;98(8):4752–7.

134. Mouret A, et al. Turnover of newborn olfactory bulb neurons optimizes olfaction. J Neurosci. 2009;29(39):12302–14.

135. Kageyama R, Imayoshi I, Sakamoto M. The role of neurogenesis in olfaction-dependent behaviors. Behav Brain Res. 2012;227(2):459–63.

136. Sakamoto M, et al. Continuous neurogenesis in the adult forebrain is required for innate olfactory responses. Proc Natl Acad Sci U S A. 2011;108(20):8479–84.

137. Squire LR. Memory and the hippocampus: a synthesis from findings with rats, monkeys, and humans. Psychol Rev. 1992;99(2):195–231.

138. Sahay A, et al. Increasing adult hippocampal neurogenesis is sufficient to improve pattern separation. Nature. 2011;472(7344):466–U539.

139. Stone SS, et al. Stimulation of entorhinal cortex promotes adult neurogenesis and facilitates spatial memory. J Neurosci. 2011;31(38):13469–84.

140. Kuhn HG, Dickinson-Anson H, Gage FH. Neurogenesis in the dentate gyrus of the adult rat: age-related decrease of neuronal progenitor proliferation. J Neurosci. 1996;16(6):2027–33.

141. Kempermann G, Kuhn HG, Gage FH. More hippocampal neurons in adult mice living in an enriched environment. Nature. 1997;386(6624):493–5.

142. Lazarov O, Marr RA. Neurogenesis and Alzheimer's disease: at the crossroads. Exp Neurol. 2010;223(2):267–81.

143. Lopez-Toledano MA, et al. Adult neurogenesis: a potential tool for early diagnosis in Alzheimer's disease? J Alzheimers Dis. 2010;20(2):395–408.

144. Brinton RD, Wang JM. Therapeutic potential of neurogenesis for prevention and recovery from Alzheimer's disease: allopregnanolone as a proof of concept neurogenic agent. Curr Alzheimer Res. 2006;3(3):185–90.

145. Donovan MH, et al. Decreased adult hippocampal neurogenesis in the PDAPP mouse model of Alzheimer's disease. J Comp Neurol. 2006;495(1):70–83.

146. Rogers J, et al. Dissociating the therapeutic effects of environmental enrichment and exercise in a mouse model of anxiety with cognitive impairment. Transl Psychiatry. 2016;6:e794.

147. Leger M, et al. Environmental Enrichment Duration Differentially Affects Behavior and Neuroplasticity in Adult Mice. Cereb Cortex. 2015;25(11):4048–61.

148. Du LL, et al. Transient Receptor Potential-canonical 1 is Essential for Environmental Enrichment-Induced Cognitive Enhancement and Neurogenesis. Mol Neurobiol. 2017;54(3):1992-2002.

149. Kempermann G, Gast D, Gage FH. Neuroplasticity in old age: sustained fivefold induction of hippocampal neurogenesis by long-term environmental enrichment. Ann Neurol. 2002;52(2):135–43.

150. Mirochnic S, et al. Age effects on the regulation of adult hippocampal neurogenesis by physical activity and environmental enrichment in the APP23 mouse model of Alzheimer disease. Hippocampus. 2009;19(10):1008–18.

151. Wolf SA, et al. Cognitive and physical activity differently modulate disease progression in the amyloid precursor protein (APP)-23 model of Alzheimer's disease. Biol Psychiatry. 2006;60(12):1314–23.

152. Costa DA, et al. Enrichment improves cognition in AD mice by amyloid-related and unrelated mechanisms. Neurobiol Aging. 2007;28(6):831–44.

153. Dong S, et al. Environment enrichment rescues the neurodegenerative phenotypes in presenilins-deficient mice. Eur J Neurosci. 2007;26(1):101–12.

154. Valero J, et al. Short-term environmental enrichment rescues adult neurogenesis and memory deficits in APP(Sw, Ind) transgenic mice. PLoS ONE. 2011;6(2):e16832.

155. Hu YS, et al. Complex environment experience rescues impaired neurogenesis, enhances synaptic plasticity, and attenuates neuropathology in familial Alzheimer's disease-linked APPswe/PS1DeltaE9 mice. FASEB J. 2010;24(6):1667–81.

156. Brown J, et al. Enriched environment and physical activity stimulate hippocampal but not olfactory bulb neurogenesis. Eur J Neurosci. 2003;17(10):2042–6.

157. Veyrac A, et al. Novelty determines the effects of olfactory enrichment on memory and neurogenesis through noradrenergic mechanisms. Neuropsychopharmacology. 2009;34(3):786–95.

158. Shapiro LA, et al. Olfactory enrichment enhances the survival of newly born cortical neurons in adult mice. Neuroreport. 2007;18(10):981–5.

159. Matsumori Y, et al. Enriched environment and spatial learning enhance hippocampal neurogenesis and salvages ischemic penumbra after focal cerebral ischemia. Neurobiol Dis. 2006;22(1):187–98.

160. Ehninger D, Kempermann G. Regional effects of wheel running and environmental enrichment on cell genesis and microglia proliferation in the adult murine neocortex. Cereb Cortex. 2003;13(8):845–51.

161. Kronenberg G, et al. Local origin and activity-dependent generation of nestin-expressing protoplasmic astrocytes in CA1. Brain Struct Funct. 2007;212(1):19–35.

162. Viola GG, et al. Morphological changes in hippocampal astrocytes induced by environmental enrichment in mice. Brain Res. 2009;1274:47–54.

163. Williamson LL, Chao A, Bilbo SD. Environmental enrichment alters glial antigen expression and neuroimmune function in the adult rat hippocampus. Brain Behav Immun. 2012;26(3):500–10.

164. Olsson T, et al. Transcription factor AP-2 gene expression in adult rat hippocampal regions: effects of environmental manipulations. Neurosci Lett. 1995;189(2):113–6.

165. Gagne J, et al. AMPA receptor properties in adult rat hippocampus following environmental enrichment. Brain Res. 1998;799(1):16–25.

166. Rasmuson S, et al. Environmental enrichment selectively increases 5-HT1A receptor mRNA expression and binding in the rat hippocampus. Brain Res Mol Brain Res. 1998;53(1–2):285–90.

167. Andin J, et al. Influence of environmental enrichment on steady-state mRNA levels for EAAC1, AMPA1 and NMDA2A receptor subunits in rat hippocampus. Brain Res. 2007;1174:18–27.

168. Munetsuna E, et al. Environmental enrichment alters gene expression of steroidogenic enzymes in the rat hippocampus. Gen Comp Endocrinol. 2011;171(1):28–32.

169. Keyvani K, et al. Gene expression profiling in the intact and injured brain following environmental enrichment. J Neuropathol Exp Neurol. 2004;63(6):598–609.

170. Toscano CD, McGlothan JL, Guilarte TR. Experience-dependent regulation of zif268 gene expression and spatial learning. Exp Neurol. 2006;200(1):209–15.

171. Li C, et al. Effects of enriched environment on gene expression and signal pathways in cortex of hippocampal CA1 specific NMDAR1 knockout mice. Brain Res Bull. 2007;71(6):568–77.

172. Huang FL, Huang KP, Boucheron C. Long-term enrichment enhances the cognitive behavior of the aging neurogranin null mice without affecting their hippocampal LTP. Learn Mem. 2007;14(8):512–9.

173. Patel CJ, Butte AJ. Predicting environmental chemical factors associated with disease-related gene expression data. BMC Med Genomics. 2010;3:17.

174. Ragu Varman D, Marimuthu G, Rajan KE. Environmental enrichment upregulates micro-RNA-183 and alters acetylcholinesterase splice variants to reduce anxiety-like behavior in the little Indian field mouse (Mus booduga). J Neurosci Res. 2013;91(3):426–35.

175. Durairaj RV, Koilmani ER. Environmental enrichment modulates glucocorticoid receptor expression and reduces anxiety in Indian field male mouse Mus booduga through up-regulation of microRNA-124a. Gen Comp Endocrinol. 2014;199:26–32.

176. Barak B, et al. Opposing actions of environmental enrichment and Alzheimer's disease on the expression of hippocampal microRNAs in mouse models. Transl Psychiatry. 2013;3:e304.

177. Miranda S, et al. The role of oxidative stress in the toxicity induced by amyloid beta-peptide in Alzheimer's disease. Prog Neurobiol. 2000;62(6):633–48.

178. Fernandez CI, et al. Environmental enrichment-behavior-oxidative stress interactions in the aged rat: issues for a therapeutic approach in human aging. Ann N Y Acad Sci. 2004;1019:53–7.

179. Arranz L, et al. Environmental enrichment improves age-related immune system impairment: long-term exposure since adulthood increases life span in mice. Rejuvenation Res. 2010;13(4):415–28.

180. Marmol F, et al. Anti-oxidative effects produced by environmental enrichment in the hippocampus and cerebral cortex of male and female rats. Brain Res. 2015;1613:120–9.

181. Herring A, et al. Preventive and therapeutic types of environmental enrichment counteract beta amyloid pathology by different molecular mechanisms. Neurobiol Dis. 2011;42(3):530–8.

182. Goshen I, et al. Environmental enrichment restores memory functioning in mice with impaired IL-1 signaling via reinstatement of long-term potentiation and spine size enlargement. J Neurosci. 2009;29(11):3395–403.

183. Sun H, et al. Environmental enrichment influences BDNF and NR1 levels in the hippocampus and restores cognitive impairment in chronic cerebral hypoperfused rats. Curr Neurovasc Res. 2010;7(4):268–80.

184. Rossi C, et al. Brain-derived neurotrophic factor (BDNF) is required for the enhancement of hippocampal neurogenesis following environmental enrichment. Eur J Neurosci. 2006;24(7):1850–6.

185. Bekinschtein P, et al. Effects of environmental enrichment and voluntary exercise on neurogenesis, learning and memory, and pattern separation: BDNF as a critical variable? Semin Cell Dev Biol. 2011;22(5):536–42.

186. Novkovic T, Mittmann T, Manahan-Vaughan D. BDNF contributes to the facilitation of hippocampal synaptic plasticity and learning enabled by environmental enrichment. Hippocampus. 2015;25(1):1–15.

187. Hu YS, et al. Molecular mechanisms of environmental enrichment: impairments in Akt/GSK3beta, neurotrophin-3 and CREB signaling. PLoS ONE. 2013;8(5):e64460.

188. Pham TM, et al. Effects of environmental enrichment on cognitive function and hippocampal NGF in the non-handled rats. Behav Brain Res. 1999;103(1):63–70.

189. Angelucci F, et al. Increased concentrations of nerve growth factor and brain-derived neurotrophic factor in the rat cerebellum after exposure to environmental enrichment. Cerebellum. 2009;8(4):499–506.

190. Torasdotter M, et al. Environmental enrichment results in higher levels of nerve growth factor mRNA in the rat visual cortex and hippocampus. Behav Brain Res. 1998;93(1–2):83–90.

191. Birch AM, McGarry NB, Kelly AM. Short-term environmental enrichment, in the absence of exercise, improves memory, and increases NGF concentration, early neuronal survival, and synaptogenesis in the dentate gyrus in a time-dependent manner. Hippocampus. 2013;23(6):437–50.

192. Kelly ME, et al. The impact of cognitive training and mental stimulation on cognitive and everyday functioning of healthy older adults: a systematic review and meta-analysis. Ageing Res Rev. 2014;15:28–43.

193. Curlik DM, Shors TJ. Learning Increases the Survival of Newborn Neurons Provided That Learning Is Difficult to Achieve and Successful. J Cogn Neurosci. 2011;23(9):2159–70.

194. Dahlin E, et al. Transfer of learning after updating training mediated by the striatum. Science. 2008;320(5882):1510–2.

195. Mahncke HW, Bronstone A, Merzenich MM. Brain plasticity and functional losses in the aged: scientific bases for a novel intervention. Prog Brain Res. 2006;157:81–109.

196. Logsdon RG, et al. Assessing quality of life in older adults with cognitive impairment. Psychosom Med. 2002;64(3):510–9.

197. Alexopoulos GS, et al. Cornell Scale for Depression in Dementia. Biol Psychiatry. 1988;23(3):271–84.

198. Thivierge S, Jean L, Simard M. A Randomized Cross-over Controlled Study on Cognitive Rehabilitation of Instrumental Activities of Daily Living in Alzheimer Disease. Am J Geriatr Psychiatry. 2014;22(11):1188–99.

199. Mayeux R. Epidemiology of neurodegeneration. Annu Rev Neurosci. 2003;26:81–104.

200. Toril P, Reales JM, Ballesteros S. Video game training enhances cognition of older adults: a meta-analytic study. Psychol Aging. 2014;29(3):706–16.

201. Papp KV, Walsh SJ, Snyder PJ. Immediate and delayed effects of cognitive interventions in healthy elderly: a review of current literature and future directions. Alzheimers Dement. 2009;5(1):50–60.

202. Li H, Li J, Li N, Li B, Wang P, Zhou T. Cognitive intervention for persons with mild cognitive impairment: A meta-analysis. Ageing Res Rev. 2011;10(2):285–96.

203. Martin M, Clare L, Altgassen AM, Cameron MH, Zehnder F. Cognition-based interventions for healthy older people and people with mild cognitive impairment. Cochrane Database Syst Rev. 2011;1:CD006220.

204. Bahar-Fuchs A, Clare L, Woods B. Cognitive training and cognitive rehabilitation for mild to moderate Alzheimer's disease and vascular dementia. Cochrane Database Syst Rev. 2013;6:CD003260.

205. Aguirre E, Woods RT, Spector A, Orrell M. Cognitive stimulation for dementia: a systematic review of the evidence of effectiveness from randomised controlled trials. Ageing Res Rev. 2013;12(1):253–62.

206. Sitzer DI, Twamley EW, Jeste DV. Cognitive training in Alzheimer's disease: a meta-analysis of the literature. Acta Psychiatr Scand. 2006;114(2):75–90.

207. Woods B, Aguirre E, Spector AE, Orrell M. Cognitive stimulation to improve cognitive functioning in people with dementia. Cochrane Database Syst Rev. 2012;2:CD005562.

6

Clinical characteristics of fatigued Parkinson's patients and the response to dopaminergic treatment

Rao Fu, Xiao-Guang Luo[*], Yan Ren, Zhi-Yi He and Hong Lv

Abstract

Background: Fatigue, which is commonly observed in Parkinson's disease (PD), can greatly reduce quality of life and is difficult to treat. We here aimed to investigate the prevalence and characteristics of fatigue among PD patients and to explore an effective strategy to treat PD fatigue.

Method: This was an observational cross-sectional study conducted in northeastern China. We examined fatigue in 222 PD patients from northeastern China using the Parkinson Fatigue Scale-16 (PFS-16). The disease severity, depression, sleep and cognitive functioning were assessed with the Hoehn & Yahr staging (H-Y stage), Unified Parkinson's Disease Rating Scale (UPDRS), Hamilton Depression Scale (HAMD), Parkinson's Disease Sleep Scale (PDSS) and Montreal Cognitive Assessment (MoCA) by interview.

Results: The frequency of fatigue in PD patients was 59.46 %. Fatigued patients had longer disease durations and greater disease severity than nonfatigued patients. Additionally, fatigued PD patients scored significantly higher for all motor symptoms, except for tremor, and had more serious depressive symptoms and sleep disturbances than nonfatigued PD patients did. The sleep disturbance severity was an independent factor for fatigue. Furthermore, 43.04 % of fatigued patients taking dopaminergic drugs had fatigue remission. Depression severity was identified as an independent factor for dopaminergic drug non-responsive fatigue.

Conclusions: PD patients with severe sleep disturbances tend to suffer from fatigue. Levodopa improved fatigue only in PD patients with mild depression or no depression, implying that dopaminergic medication is required, but not sufficient, for fatigue suppression in PD patients with moderate or severe depression. Thus, restoring serotonergic neurotransmission as a combination therapy may offer a better strategy for the treatment of fatigue in these patients.

Keywords: Parkinson's disease, Fatigue, Sleep disorder, Depression, Dopaminergic drugs

Background

Fatigue is one of the most common non-motor symptoms in Parkinson disease (PD). Currently, there is no universally accepted definition of fatigue in PD. PD patients complaining about fatigue describe it as a sensation of tiredness, lack of energy, or exhaustion. These states are experienced as abnormally severe. It is often unpredictable in its onset and duration, often attributable to activity levels [1]. According to a recent study in PD, fatigue is one of the most bothersome problems [2], which has been confirmed as the most disabling symptom by 15–33 % of PD patients [3, 4]. Despite its high prevalence and negative impact on life quality, fatigue in PD remains an under-recognized problem in routine clinical practice [5].

Most of the published investigations have focused on prevalence and clinical characteristics of PD related fatigue, and found the close relationship between fatigue, sleep disturbance, depression and anxiety [6–8]. However few of them explored the prevalence and profiles of dopaminergic-responsive fatigue in fatigued PD patients on dopaminergic treatment. Previous studies have shown that dopamine is involved in the development of exercise-

* Correspondence: grace_shenyang@163.com
Neurology Department, Outpatient of Parkinson's Disease, First Affiliated Hospital of China Medical University, 155# Nanjing bei streetHeping District, Shenyang 110001, P R China

induced fatigue [9, 10]. Decreased dopamine levels were detected in the brain using a rat model of exercise-induced fatigue [11], indicating that the shortage of dopamine contributed to the occurrence of fatigue. This is consistent with the ELLDOPA Trial [12], which noted improved fatigue with levodopa treatment, even though the benefit was minimal. However, a recent meta-analysis of the intervention for fatigue in PD concluded [13] that currently there is insufficient evidence to support the effective treatment of fatigue in PD with any drug. Clinically, we do have some patients whose fatigue can be relieved with levodopa treatment, in our personal experience. Therefore, in the present study, we specifically examined fatigue and fatigue-related clinical features in patients with PD to determine the clinical characteristics of fatigue in PD patients. More importantly, we aimed to clarify the profile of dopaminergic-responsive fatigue and its associated factors.

Methods

Subjects and demographic data

This was an observational cross-sectional study. Two hundred and twenty-two PD patients, diagnosed according to the UK PD Brain Bank criteria [14], were recruited between December 2012 and April 2014 from the outpatient Department of Neurology of the First Affiliated Hospital of China Medical University (Shenyang, China). Patients with other forms of parkinsonism were excluded. Patients with dementia or fatigue related to a disease other than PD were excluded (e.g., peripheral circulatory disorders, such as ischemic heart disease and left ventricular failure, or acute and chronic inflammatory demyelinating polyneuropathies, such as Guillain-Barre syndrome). All patients enrolled in the study gave written informed consent. The Ethics Review Board of First Affiliated Hospital of China Medical University (Shenyang, China) approved the protocol of the study. Demographic data were collected for all PD patients. The total amount of dopaminergic medication was expressed as the levodopa equivalent daily dosage (LEDD), which was determined using methods previously reported in a systematic review of LEDD [15].

Assessments

Disease severity was evaluated during the on phase using the Unified Parkinson's Disease Rating Scale (UPDRS) and Hoehn & Yahr staging (H-Y stage) [16]. As previously described [17], the following sub-scores obtained from specific items of UPDRS III were calculated as following: tremor (items 20 and 21), rigidity (item 22), bradykinesia (items 23–26 and 31) and posture/gait (items 27–30).

Fatigue was assessed using the Parkinson Fatigue Scale-16 (PFS-16). The PFS-16 is a 16-item self-report scale that is specifically designed to assess the physical aspects of fatigue in PD patients [1]. The item response options

range from 1 ("strongly disagree") to 5 ("strongly agree"). The total PFS-16 score ranges from 1 to 5 and is obtained by dividing the sum of all item scores by 16 [18]. A cut-off score of 3.3 was used to indicate the presence of fatigue [1]. Subjects with a PFS-16 score <3.3 were classified as nonfatigued, and those scoring ≥3.3 were classified as fatigued.

The Montreal Cognitive Assessment (MoCA) Beijing version was used to evaluate cognitive functioning. Because depression and sleep disturbances have been reported to affect fatigue, we revised our study protocol during the study. The 17-item Hamilton Depression Scale [19] (HAMD) and Parkinson's Disease Sleep Scale (PDSS) [20] were administered to 177 of the 222 patients to assess depression and sleep disturbance, respectively. In the 17-item HAMD, a higher score indicates severe depression, and depression was classified as follows: no depression (0–7); mild depression (8–16); moderate depression (17–23); and severe depression (≥24) [21]. The range of PDSS score was 0–150, and a lower score indicated a higher number of sleep disturbances.

Statistical analysis

All continuous data are presented as the mean ± standard deviation (SD). Categorical variables were compared with chi-square tests; the Mann-Whitney U test was used for continuous variables. Correlations were assessed using Spearman rank order correlation coefficients. The odds ratios were calculated using logistic regression and chi-square tests. All data analyses were performed using SPSS software. A value of $P < 0.05$ was considered statistically significant.

Results

Comparison of demography and clinical profiles between the fatigued and nonfatigued groups

According to the suggested cut-off score for the PFS-16 (≥3.3), fatigue was present in 132 (59.46 %) patients. Comparisons of the demographic and clinical characteristics between the fatigued and nonfatigued groups are listed in Table 1. The mean disease duration in the nonfatigued group was significantly shorter than that in the fatigued group (3.75 ± 3.26 years vs. 4.61 ± 2.99 years, $p = 0.046$). There were no significant differences between the two groups in other clinical characteristics, including sex, age, onset age and education.

Disease severity, as determined by H-Y stage and the total UPDRS score and all subscales, was more serious in the fatigued group than in the nonfatigued group (Table 1). Further analysis of the individual motor symptoms revealed that except for tremor, most motor symptoms, including rigidity, bradykinesia and posture/gait, were more serious (higher scores) in the fatigued group than in the nonfatigued group (Table 1). Similarly, the fatigued group

Table 1 Demographic and clinical characteristics of fatigued vs. nonfatigued subjects

Characteristic	Nonfatigued	Fatigued	P-value
Male (n= 222)	54 (60.00 %)	64 (48.48 %)	0.101
Age, y	61.63 ± 9.49	62.50 ± 10.21	0.524
Onset age, y (n= 222)	57.88 ± 9.77	57.89 ± 10.51	0.992
Duration of disease, y (n= 222)	3.75 ± 3.26	4.61 ± 2.99	0.046*
Education, y (n= 222)	10.61 ± 3.12	9.80 ± 3.69	0.09
LEDD (mg/day) (n= 222)	211.19 ± 263.18	280.24 ± 304.04	0.081
H-Y stage (n= 222)	1.73 ± 0.78	2.00 ± 0.76	0.009*
UPDRS total score (n= 222)	39.43 ± 20.26	52.39 ± 20.19	<0.001*
UPDRS part I (n= 222)	2.93 ± 1.93	4.19 ± 2.26	<0.001*
UPDRS part II (n= 222)	9.88 ± 4.80	12.57 ± 5.72	<0.001*
UPDRS part III (n= 222)	25.76 ± 15.37	33.53 ± 14.66	<0.001*
Postural/gait (sum of UPDRS item 27–30)	3.28 ± 2.80	4.80 ± 3.07	<0.001*
Bradykinesia (sum of UPDRS item 23–26,31)	12.30 ± 7.98	15.9 ± 7.35	0.001*
Rigidity (UPDRS item 22)	4.87 ± 4.23	6.45 ± 4.36	0.008*
Tremor (sum of UPDRS item20 and item21)	3.36 ± 3.26	3.78 ± 3.88	0.391
UPDRS IV (n= 222)	0.86 ± 1.65	1.70 ± 2.57	0.007*
MoCA (n= 222)	22.87 ± 4.59	21.85 ± 4.27	0.066
HAMD (n= 177)	7.26 ± 5.47	9.32 ± 5.17	0.006*
PDSS (n= 177)	119.10 ± 23.65	98.82 ± 25.74	<0.001*

Data are expressed as numbers, with percentages in parentheses, or as mean ± SD. *Significant difference. *H-Y stage* Hoehn & Yahr staging, *LEDD* levodopa equivalent daily dosage, *UPDRS* Unified Parkinson' Disease Rating Scale, *MoCA* Montreal Cognitive Assessment, *HAMD* Hamilton Depression Scale score, *PDSS* Parkinson's Disease Sleep Scale

had significantly worse scores for depressive symptoms and sleep disturbance than the nonfatigued group had (Table 1).

The LEDD and MoCA scores tended to be higher in the fatigued group than in the nonfatigued group, but this was not significant.

Independent risk factors related to fatigue

As shown in Table 2, the univariate logistic regression revealed that longer disease duration, a greater disease severity (H-Y stage, total UPDRS score and all subscales), depression and sleep disturbances were associated with fatigue ($p < 0.05$). Other clinical variables, including gender, age onset age, education, LEDD and MoCA score were not significantly associated with fatigue.

We further explored the independent risk factors of fatigue in PD patients using multivariate logistic regression. Only sleep disturbance (odds ratio = 0.974, 95%CI 0.959–0.989, $P = 0.001$) remained an independent risk factor for fatigue (Table 2). Disease duration, disease severity (H-Y stage, total UPDRS score and all subscales) and depression were not associated with fatigue (Table 2).

Comparison of clinical variables between the dopaminergic responsive fatigue and dopaminergic non-responsive fatigue groups

To further explore the clinical profiles of dopaminergic drug responsive fatigue, we examined the data of 79 patients in the fatigued group with complaints of fatigue and who were treated with dopaminergic drugs. We defined the fatigue amelioration rate between 0 % and 100 %, and assigned fatigue remission rate into 4 level (level 0: no remission, remission rate <25 %; level 1: mild remission, remission rate between 25 % and 50 %; level 2: moderate remission, remission rate between 50 % and 75 %; level 3: obvious remission, remission rate over 75 %) with a lower level indicating less responsiveness to dopaminergic medication. According to their response to dopaminergic drugs the 79 patients were assigned to either the dopaminergic drug responsive fatigued (DDRF) group (fatigue amelioration rate > level 0) or the dopaminergic drug non-responsive fatigued (DDNRF) group (fatigue amelioration rate = level 0).

The demographic and clinical profiles were compared between the DDRF and DDRNF groups; the results of these comparisons are shown in Table 3. There were 34 (43.04 %) patients in the DDRF group and 45 (56.96 %) patients in the DDNRF group. Onset age was significantly higher in the DDNRF group than in the DDRF group, and significantly more severe depression was found in the DDNRF group. There were no significant differences between the two groups in age, sex, disease duration, education, disease severity (H-Y stage, UPDRS total score and all subscores), individual motor symptoms, sleep disturbance or cognitive functioning (Table 3).

Depression severity is an independent risk factor for dopaminergic drug non-responsive fatigue

As shown in Table 4, the Spearman rank order correlation coefficients revealed significant correlations between fatigue remission rate and age, onset age, and depression

Table 2 Logistic regression modal of the association between fatigue and clinical characteristics in PD patients

Variable	Univariate analysis		Multivariate analysis	
	odds ratio	P-value	odds ratio	P-value
Female sex (n= 222)	1.594 (0.926–2.742)	0.092		
Age, y (n= 222)	1.009 (0.982–1.037)	0.522		
Onset age, y (n= 222)	1.000 (0.974–1.027)	0.992		
Duration of disease, y (n= 222)	1.100 (1.000–1.208)	0.049*		
Education, y (n= 222)	0.935 (0.864–1.011)	0.091		
LEDD (mg/day) (n= 222)	1.001 (1.000–1.002)	0.083		
H-Y stage (n= 222)	1.578 (1.102–2.258)	0.013*		
UPDRS total score (n= 222)	1.033 (1.018–1.048)	<0.001*		
UPDRS part I (n= 222)	1.333 (1.159–1.533)	<0.001*		
UPDRS part II (n= 222)	1.122 (1.059–1.189)	<0.001*		
UPDRS part III (n= 222)	1.036 (1.016–1.056)	<0.001*		
UPDRS part IV (n= 222)	1.210 (1.049–1.396)	0.009*		
HAMD score (n= 177)	1.079 (1.016–1.146)	0.013*		
PDSS (n= 177)	0.967 (0.954–0.981)	<0.001*	0.974 (0.959–0.989)	0.001
MoCA score (n= 222)	0.948 (0.890–1.009)	0.094		

Figures in parentheses indicate 95 % confidence intervals. *Significant difference. *H-Y* stage Hoehn & Yahr staging, *LEDD* levodopa equivalent daily dosage, *UPDRS* Unified Parkinson' Disease Rating Scale, *MoCA* Montreal Cognitive Assessment, *HAMD* Hamilton Depression Scale score, *PDSS* Parkinson's Disease Sleep Scale

severity. Other factors including sex, education, LEDD, disease severity (H-Y stage, UPDRS total score and all subscales) and cognitive functioning were not associated with the fatigue remission rate.

To identify independent factors influencing dopaminergic responsive fatigue, variables significantly associated with fatigue remission rate in the bivariate correlation analyses (Table 4) were entered as independent variables into a logistic regression model. Only depression severity (odds ratio = 1.182, 95%CI 1.044–1.338, P = 0.008) was identified as an independent risk factor for dopaminergic drug non-responsive fatigue.

Discussion

In the present study, fatigue problems were found in more than half of the PD patients (59.46 %) in northeastern China, which is consistent with previous reports [3, 22–24]. Moreover, fatigue appeared to be related with prolonged disease duration, increased disease severity, enhanced depressive symptoms, serious sleep disturbance, and the development of motor symptoms, except tremors. A univariate logistic regression analysis demonstrated that fatigue was significantly associated with several clinical characteristics of PD patients. Among the variables examined, only sleep disturbance was identified as an independent risk factor for fatigue. In addition, fatigue remission was found in 43.04 % of fatigued patients taking dopaminergic drugs. The development of DDNRF was associated with an older age and depressive symptoms, and depression severity was an independent risk factor for dopaminergic drug non-responsive fatigue. Our findings provide basic evidence for understanding the clinical significance of the non-motor symptom of fatigue in PD.

Sleep disturbance is an independent risk factor for fatigue in PD patients

Sleep is necessary for the maintenance of mammalian homeostasis. Additionally, sleep is one of the most crucial determinants of fatigue severity [25]. In the general population, high-quality sleep is associated with less fatigue [26, 27]. Sleep disturbance has been associated with fatigue in several disorders, including cancer [28], multiple sclerosis [29] and traumatic brain injury [30]. In addition, it was reported that dissatisfaction with sleep, and not sleep itself, was associated with fatigue in psychotic patients [31].

Although the mechanisms of sleep abnormalities and fatigue have not yet been clarified, increased inflammatory cytokine release has been associated with poor sleep conditions and fatigue [32]. Specifically, the production of interleukin (IL)-1β and tumor necrosis factor (TNF)-α promotes non-rapid eye movement sleep (NREMS) under physiological and inflammatory conditions. Disturbed NREMS is associated with abnormal cyclic alternating pattern (CAP) rates and electroencephalogram arousals, and it is correlated with fatigue and sleepiness [33]. IL-1β and TNF-α alter neuronal excitability and induce symptoms associated with sleep loss by binding to their neural receptors, which subsequently regulate neurotransmitters or neuromodulators [34]. Moreover, the neurotransmitter serotonin governs sleep-wake behavior [35], and a reduction of serotonin transporters was found in subjects with fatigue syndrome [36]. These findings suggest that serotoninergic functions may play pivotal roles in controlling sleep and fatigue.

Table 3 Comparison between dopaminergic drug responsive fatigue (DDRF) and dopaminergic drug non-responsive fatigue (DDNRF)

Variable	DDRF	DDNRF	p
Male (n= 79)	13 (38.24 %)	24 (53.33 %)	0.354
Age, y (n= 79)	59.59 ± 8.89	63.64 ± 11.80	0.074
Onset age, y (n= 79)	54.24 ± 8.95	58.82 ± 11.93	0.040*
Duration of disease (n= 79)	5.35 ± 3.02	4.82 ± 3.24	0.276
Education, y (n= 79)	10.03 ± 2.93	9.36 ± 4.23	0.681
LEDD (mg/day) (n= 79)	473.38 ± 281.42	438.26 ± 271.25	0.804
H-Ystage (n= 79)	2.15 ± 0.82	2.04 ± 0.74	0.526
UPDRS total (n= 79)	55.94 ± 21.46	52.91 ± 20.22	0.674
UPDRS I (n= 79)	4.06 ± 2.15	3.87 ± 2.61	0.506
UPDRS II (n= 79)	13.00 ± 5.65	13.59 ± 6.36	0.67
UPDRS III (n= 79)	36.76 ± 15.50	33.63 ± 14.67	0.362
Gait (n= 79)	5.12 ± 3.15	5.26 ± 3.41	0.843
Tremor (n= 79)	4.32 ± 4.20	320 ± 3.89	0.19
Rigidity (n= 79)	7.56 ± 4.59	6.20 ± 4.19	0.198
Bradykinesia (n= 79)	16.94 ± 7.50	16.38 ± 7.47	0.741
UPDRS IV (n= 79)	2.11 ± 2.77	1.82 ± 2.70	0.541
HAMD (n= 70)	7.66 ± 4.51 (N= 32)	10.66 ± 4.70 (N= 38)	0.006*
PDSS (n= 70)	107.81 ± 25.33 (N= 32)	97.26 ± 25.98 (N= 38)	0.073
MoCA (n= 79)	22.47 ± 4.14	21.42 ± 4.59	0.353

Data are expressed as numbers, with percentages in parentheses, or as mean ± SD. *Significant difference. *DDRF* dopaminergic drug responsive fatigue, *DDNRF* dopaminergic drug non-responsive fatigueH-Y stage: Hoehn & Yahr staging, *LEDD* levodopa equivalent daily dosage, *UPDRS* Unified Parkinson' Disease Rating Scale, *MoCA* Montreal Cognitive Assessment, *HAMD* Hamilton Depression Scale score, *PDSS* Parkinson's Disease Sleep Scale

Table 4 Correlations between fatigue remission rate and clinical characteristics of the patients with fatigue

Variables	Spearman's rank-order Correlation coefficient	p
Gender	0.119	0.297
Age, y	−0.223	0.049*
Onset age, y	−0.250	0.026*
Duration of disease	0.123	0.282
Education, y	0.010	0.929
LEDD	0.003	0.976
PFS total score	−0.155	0.173
H-Y stage	0.089	0.436
UPDRS total score	0.033	0.772
UPDRS part I	0.053	0.645
UPDRS part II	−0.029	0.798
UPDRS part III	0.074	0.515
UPDRS part IV	0.032	0.781
HAMD	−0.318	0.007*
PDSS	0.120	0.324
MoCA	0.123	0.280

*Significant difference. *H-Y* stage Hoehn & Yahr staging, *LEDD* levodopa equivalent daily dosage, *UPDRS* Unified Parkinson' Disease Rating Scale, *MoCA* Montreal Cognitive Assessment, *HAMD* Hamilton Depression Scale score, *PDSS* Parkinson's Disease Sleep Scale

Fatigue, sleep disturbance and depression are the primary neuropsychiatric manifestations of PD, and they are related to patient quality of life [37, 38]. In this study, a logistic regression analysis revealed that sleep disturbance is the only independent factor for fatigue in PD patients, which is in accordance with the findings of a previous study [6]. Emerging lines of evidence indicate that sleep disorder treatment is effective for improving fatigue in patients with multiple sclerosis [39, 40]. Similarly, the management of sleep loss may provide a valuable approach for improving fatigue in PD patients. It has been proposed that fatigue stems at least in part from disturbed cytokine production in diseases such as PD [41]. Indeed, elevated secretion of IL-1β and TNF-α have been detected in the cerebrospinal fluid (CSF) of PD patients with sleep problems [42]. The circulating level of IL-1β is also increased in PD patients with fatigue [43]. Pavese et al. indicated that in addition to increased inflammatory cytokine production, fatigue in PD patients might result from serotonergic (5-hydroxytryptamine, 5-HT) dysfunction in the basal ganglia and limbic circuitry [44]. Considering the crucial roles that cytokine release and serotonergic functioning play in regulating sleep and fatigue, we hypothesize that sleep disturbance and fatigue may share a similar mechanism in the pathogenesis of PD, with abnormal cytokine release and serotonergic dysfunction being the primary components of this mechanism. Future studies should explore the molecular mechanisms involved in this process.

Dopamine imbalance is associated with fatigue in PD patients

Another important finding of the current study was that dopaminergic medication improved fatigue in 43.04 % of PD patients with fatigue problems, whereas more than half of the fatigued patients were not responsive to dopaminergic medication. This result is consistent with ELLDOPA study [45], which showed that levodopa/carbidopa is effective in reducing the progression of fatigue in drug naïve PD patients [12]. Moreover, the study of ADAGIO [46] also showed that rasagiline was associated with significantly less progression of fatigue compared with placebo over a 9-month period in drug naïve patients with PD [47]. Both carbidopa/levodopa and rasagiline are dopaminergic drugs, which increase the extracellular levels of dopamine. Thus, we infer dopamine dysfunction may involve in the pathogenesis of fatigue in PD. The effects we observed might be due to enhanced dopaminergic neurotransmission, indicating the therapeutic value of dopaminergic treatment for fatigue relief in PD. However, according to the univariate logistic regression and correlation analysis performed in our study, there are no significant associations among fatigue, fatigue severity, remission rate, and dopaminergic medication dosage because a no dose-effect correlation was detected between levodopa and fatigue. Hence, levodopa may play a role in the mechanism underlying the development of fatigue, which is consistent with other current results. The dopamine imbalance hypothesis of fatigue was recently presented in multiple sclerosis and other neurological disorders [48]. Thus, restoring dopamine levels in the CNS by means of dopaminergic medication, such as levodopa, might be an essential strategy for the treatment of fatigue in PD.

Depression is an independent risk factor for dopaminergic drug non-responsive fatigue

Depression is another prominent non-motor symptom in PD [49]. Fatigue in PD is often associated with depression, using a logistic regression model, we further demonstrated that depression was the only independent factor for the efficacy of dopaminergic medication in treating fatigue in PD patients, which might imply crosstalk between depression, fatigue and dopamine insufficiency.

Pavese et al. found that compared with patients without fatigue, PD patients with fatigue showed greatly reduced serotonin transporter binding in the basal ganglia and limbic circuitry, as well as a significant reduction in dopamine uptake in the caudate and insula [44]. These results demonstrate that even though a dysfunctional serotonergic pathway plays a predominant role in fatigue, reduced dopaminergic functioning also contributes to the incidence of fatigue [44]. Hence, both dopaminergic and serotonergic pathways contribute to fatigue in PD patients. Interestingly, other studies have indicated that excessive 5-HT also induced fatigue. Indeed, increased 5-HT and decreased dopamine concentrations were detected in the brain in a rat model of exercise-induced fatigue [50]. These findings imply that the level of 5-HT may not be a determinant, and maintaining the balance between serotonergic and dopaminergic function is key for fatigue relief. Hence, dopamine administration may improve fatigue only in PD patients who have a functional serotonergic system with normal 5-HT concentrations and receptor functioning, which is consistent with our results. In other words, functional serotonergic pathway is necessary for dopamine to alleviate fatigue. Therefore, both 5-HT and dopamine should be considered during the treatment of PD fatigue. For instance, in the early stage of PD, a supplement of only 5-HT without levodopa medication may be

insufficient for relieving fatigue, as levodopa is usually not prescribed early in PD due to the absence of obvious motor symptoms. Similarly, when fatigue is present with no obvious depression, a combined administration of levodopa with 5-HT, but not levodopa alone, may provide greater relief from fatigue. Thus, we hypothesize that dopaminergic medication is required, but not sufficient, for fatigue suppression in fatigued PD patients with moderate depression, and such treatment can restore serotonergic neurotransmission and serve as a combination therapy. This may offer an ideal strategy for the treatment of fatigue in PD patients.

Conclusions

In the present study, we found that fatigue is common in PD patients. PD patients with severe sleep disturbances tend to suffer from fatigue. Levodopa improved fatigue only in PD patients with mild depression or no depression, restoring serotonergic neurotransmission as a combination therapy may offer a better strategy for the treatment of fatigue in these patients.

Consent

Written informed consent was obtained from the patient for the publication of this report and any accompanying images.

Competing interests
The authors declare that they have no competing interests.

Authors' contributions
RF: study design and data collection. XGL: statistical analysis and interpretation. YR: critical revision of the manuscript for important intellectual content. ZYH: study supervision. HL: manuscript revision. All authors read and approved the final manuscript.

Acknowledgments
This work was funded by the China National Nature Science Fund (no.30973153), Liaoning Doctoral Starting Fund (20071042) and the Foundation of the Liaoning Educational Committee (L202013136, L2010560)

References
1. Brown RG, Dittner A, Findley L, Wessely SC. The Parkinson fatigue scale. Parkinsonism Relat Disord. 2005;11:49–55.
2. Uebelacker LA, Epstein-Lubow G, Lewis T, Broughton MK, Friedman JH. A Survey of Parkinson's Disease Patients: Most Bothersome Symptoms and Coping Preferences. J Parkinsons Dis. 2014;4:717–23.
3. Friedman J, Friedman H. Fatigue in Parkinson's disease. Neurology. 1993;43:2016–8.
4. van Hilten JJ, Weggeman M, van der Velde EA, Kerkhof GA, van Dijk JG, Roos RA. Sleep, excessive daytime sleepiness and fatigue in Parkinson's disease. J Neural Transm Park Dis Dement Sect. 1993;5:235–44.
5. Shulman LM, Taback RL, Rabinstein AA, Weiner WJ. Non-recognition of depression and other non-motor symptoms in Parkinson's disease. Parkinsonism Relat Disord. 2002;8:193–7.
6. Okuma Y, Kamei S, Morita A, Yoshii F, Yamamoto T, Hashimoto S, Utsumi H, Hatano T, Hattori N, Matsumura M, Takahashi K, Nogawa S, Watanabe Y, Miyamoto T, Miyamoto M, Hirata K. Fatigue in Japanese patients with Parkinson's disease: a study using Parkinson fatigue scale. Mov Disord. 2009;24:1977–83.

7. Zuo LJ, Yu SY, Wang F, Hu Y, Piao YS, Du Y, Lian TH, Wang RD, Yu QJ, Wang YJ, Wang XM, Chan P, Chen SD, Wang Y, Zhang W. Parkinson's Disease with Fatigue: Clinical Characteristics and Potential Mechanisms Relevant to alpha-Synuclein Oligomer. J Clin Neurol. 2016;12(2):172–80.

8. Kang SY, Ma HI, Lim YM, Hwang SH, Kim YJ. Fatigue in drug-naive Parkinson's disease. Eur Neurol. 2013;70:59–64.

9. Heyes MP, Garnett ES, Coates G. Central dopaminergic activity influences rats ability to exercise. Life Sci. 1985;36:671–7.

10. Chaouloff F, Laude D, Merino D, Serrurrier B, Guezennec Y, Elghozi JL. Amphetamine and alpha-methyl-p-tyrosine affect the exercise-induced imbalance between the availability of tryptophan and synthesis of serotonin in the brain of the rat. Neuropharmacology. 1987;26:1099–106.

11. Tanaka M. Establishment and assessment of a rat model of fatigue. Neurosci Lett. 2003;352(3):159–62.

12. Schifitto G, Friedman JH, Oakes D, Shulman L, Comella CL, Marek K, Fahn S. Fatigue in levodopa-naive subjects with Parkinson disease. Neurology. 2008;71:481–5.

13. Franssen M, Winward C, Collett J, Wade D, Dawes H. Interventions for fatigue in Parkinson's disease: A systematic review and meta-analysis. Mov Disord. 2014;29:1675–8.

14. Hughes AJ, Daniel SE, Kilford L, Lees AJ. Accuracy of clinical diagnosis of idiopathic Parkinson's disease: a clinico-pathological study of 100 cases. J Neurol Neurosurg Psychiatry. 1992;55:181–4.

15. Tomlinson CL, Stowe R, Patel S, Rick C, Gray R, Clarke CE. Systematic review of levodopa dose equivalency reporting in Parkinson's disease. Mov Disord. 2010;25:2649–53.

16. Hoehn MM, Yahr MD. Parkinsonism: onset, progression and mortality. Neurology. 1967;17:427–42.

17. Solla P, Cannas A, Mulas CS, Perra S, Corona A, Bassareo PP, Marrosu F. Association between fatigue and other motor and non-motor symptoms in Parkinson's disease patients. J Neurol. 2014;261:382–91.

18. Friedman JH, Alves G, Hagell P, Marinus J, Marsh L, Martinez-Martin P, Goetz CG, Poewe W, Rascol O, Sampaio C, Stebbins G, Schrag A. Fatigue rating scales critique and recommendations by the Movement Disorders Society task force on rating scales for Parkinson's disease. Mov Disord. 2010;25:805–22.

19. Hamilton M. A rating scale for depression. J Neurol Neurosurg Psychiatry. 1960;23:56–62.

20. Chaudhuri KR, Pal S, DiMarco A, Whately-Smith C, Bridgman K, Mathew R, Pezzela FR, Forbes A, Hogl B, Trenkwalder C. The Parkinson's disease sleep scale: a new instrument for assessing sleep and nocturnal disability in Parkinson's disease. J Neurol Neurosurg Psychiatry. 2002;73:629–35.

21. Zimmerman M, Martinez JH, Young D, Chelminski I, Dalrymple K. Severity classification on the Hamilton Depression Rating Scale. J Affect Disord. 2013;150:384–8.

22. Herlofson K, Larsen JP. The influence of fatigue on health-related quality of life in patients with Parkinson's disease. Acta Neurol Scand. 2003;107:1–6.

23. Shulman LM, Taback RL, Bean J, Weiner WJ. Comorbidity of the nonmotor symptoms of Parkinson's disease. Mov Disord. 2001;16:507–10.

24. Alves G, Wentzel-Larsen T, Larsen JP. Is fatigue an independent and persistent symptom in patients with Parkinson disease? Neurology. 2004;63:1908–11.

25. Ferentinos P, Kontaxakis V, Havaki-Kontaxaki B, Paparrigopoulos T, Dikeos D, Ktonas P, Soldatos C. Sleep disturbances in relation to fatigue in major depression. J Psychosom Res. 2009;66:37–42.

26. Alapin I, Fichten CS, Libman E, Creti L, Bailes S, Wright J. How is good and poor sleep in older adults and college students related to daytime sleepiness, fatigue, and ability to concentrate? J Psychosom Res. 2000;49:381–90.

27. Pilcher JJ, Ginter DR, Sadowsky B. Sleep quality versus sleep quantity: relationships between sleep and measures of health, well-being and sleepiness in college students. J Psychosom Res. 1997;42:583–96.

28. Olson K. Sleep-related disturbances among adolescents with cancer: a systematic review. Sleep Med. 2014;15:496–501.

29. Veauthier C, Radbruch H, Gaede G, Pfueller CF, Dorr J, Bellmann-Strobl J, Wernecke KD, Zipp F, Paul F, Sieb JP. Fatigue in multiple sclerosis is closely related to sleep disorders: a polysomnographic cross-sectional study. Mult Scler. 2011;17:613–22.

30. Gardani M, Morfiri E, Thomson A, O'Neill B, McMillan TM. Evaluation of Sleep Disorders in Patients With Severe Traumatic Brain Injury During Rehabilitation. Arch Phys Med Rehabil. 2015;96(9):1691–7.

31. Waters F, Naik N, Rock D. Sleep, fatigue, and functional health in psychotic patients. Schizophr Res Treatment. 2013;2013:425826.

32. Chrousos G, Vgontzas AN, Kritikou I. HPA Axis and Sleep. In: De Groot LJ, Beck-Peccoz P, Chrousos G, Dungan K, Grossman A, Hershman JM, editors. Endotext. South Dartmouth: MDText.com, Inc.; 2000.

33. Guilleminault C, Lopes MC, Hagen CC, da Rosa A. The cyclic alternating pattern demonstrates increased sleep instability and correlates with fatigue and sleepiness in adults with upper airway resistance syndrome. Sleep. 2007;30:641–7.

34. Jewett KA, Krueger JM. Humoral sleep regulation; interleukin-1 and tumor necrosis factor. Vitam Horm. 2012;89:241–57.

35. Monti JM. Serotonin control of sleep-wake behavior. Sleep Med Rev. 2011;15:269–81.

36. Yamamoto S, Ouchi Y, Onoe H, Yoshikawa E, Tsukada H, Takahashi H, Iwase M, Yamaguti K, Kuratsune H, Watanabe Y. Reduction of serotonin transporters of patients with chronic fatigue syndrome. Neuroreport. 2004;15:2571–4.

37. Dogan VB, Koksal A, Dirican A, Baybas S, Dogan GB. Independent effect of fatigue on health-related quality of life in patients with idiopathic Parkinson's disease. Neurol Sci. 2015;36(12):2221–6.

38. Oikonomou E, Paparrigopoulos T. Neuropsychiatric manifestations in Parkinson's disease. Psychiatriki. 2015;26:116–30.

39. Veauthier C, Gaede G, Radbruch H, Gottschalk S, Wernecke KD, Paul F. Treatment of sleep disorders may improve fatigue in multiple sclerosis. Clin Neurol Neurosurg. 2013;115:1826–30.

40. Cote I, Trojan DA, Kaminska M, Cardoso M, Benedetti A, Weiss D, Robinson A, Bar-Or A, Lapierre Y, Kimoff RJ. Impact of sleep disorder treatment on fatigue in multiple sclerosis. Mult Scler. 2013;19:480–9.

41. Scalzo P, Kummer A, Cardoso F, Teixeira AL. Increased serum levels of soluble tumor necrosis factor-alpha receptor-1 in patients with Parkinson's disease. J Neuroimmunol. 2009;216:122–5.

42. Hu Y, Yu SY, Zuo LJ, Cao CJ, Wang F, Chen ZJ, Du Y, Lian TH, Wang YJ, Chan P, Chen SD, Wang XM, Zhang W. Parkinson disease with REM sleep behavior disorder: features, alpha-synuclein, and inflammation. Neurology. 2015;84:888–94.

43. Katsarou Z, Bostantjopoulou S, Hatzizisi O, Giza E, Soler-Cardona A, Kyriazis G. Immune factors or depression? Fatigue correlates in Parkinson's disease. Rev Neurol. 2007;45:725–8.

44. Pavese N, Metta V, Bose SK, Chaudhuri KR, Brooks DJ. Fatigue in Parkinson's disease is linked to striatal and limbic serotonergic dysfunction. Brain. 2010;133:3434–43.

45. Fahn S, Oakes D, Shoulson I, Kieburtz K, Rudolph A, Lang A, Ianow CW, Tanner C, Marek K. Levodopa and the progression of Parkinson's disease. N Engl J Med. 2004;351:2498–508.

46. Olanow CW, Rascol O, Hauser R, Feigin PD, Jankovic J, Lang A, Langston W, Melamed E, Poewe W, Stocchi F, Tolosa E. A double-blind, delayed-start trial of rasagiline in Parkinson's disease. N Engl J Med. 2009;361:1268–78.

47. Stocchi F. Benefits of treatment with rasagiline for fatigue symptoms in patients with early Parkinson's disease. Eur J Neurol. 2013;21(2):357–60.

48. Dobryakova E, Genova HM, DeLuca J, Wylie GR. The dopamine imbalance hypothesis of fatigue in multiple sclerosis and other neurological disorders. Front Neurol. 2015;6:52.

49. Aarsland D, Marsh L, Schrag A. Neuropsychiatric symptoms in Parkinson's disease. Mov Disord. 2009;24:2175–86.

50. Bailey SP, Davis JM, Ahlborn EN. Neuroendocrine and substrate responses to altered brain 5-HT activity during prolonged exercise to fatigue. J Appl Physiol. 1993;74:3006–12.

7

Mesencephalic astrocyte-derived neurotrophic factor reduces cell apoptosis via upregulating HSP70 in SHSY-5Y cells

Hui Sun[1†], Ming Jiang[2,3†], Xing Fu[3], Qiong Cai[1], Jingxing Zhang[1], Yanxin Yin[3], Jia Guo[3], Lihua Yu[3], Yun Jiang[3], Yigang Liu[1], Liang Feng[1], Zhiyu Nie[1], Jianmin Fang[2*] and Lingjing Jin[1*]

Abstract

Background: Mesencephalic astrocyte-derived neurotrophic factor (MANF) is a new candidate growth factor for dopaminergic neurons against endoplasmic reticulum stress (ER stress). HSP70 family, a chaperon like heat shock protein family, was proved to be involved in the MANF induced survival pathway in 6-OHDA treated SHSY-5Y cells. However, the ER stress relative transcriptome, in MANF signaling cascades is still investigated. The involvement of HSP70, a 70kd member of HSP70 family, need further to be verified.

Methods: The cell apoptosis was assayed by MTT, TUNEL staining and western blot of cleaved Caspase-3. The differentially expressed genes in SHSY-5Y cells under different conditions (control, 6-OHDA, 6-OHDA + MANF) were investigated by RNA-seq. Expression of HSP70 was further confirmed by real-time PCR. RNAi knockdown for HSP70 was performed to investigate the role of HSP70 in the MANF signaling pathway.

Results: MANF inhibits 6-OHDA-induced apoptosis in SHSY-5Y cells. Six ER stress relative genes (HSP70, GRP78, xbp-1, ATF-4, ATF-6, MAPK) were found enriched in 6-OHDA + MANF treatment group. HSP70 was the most significantly up-regulated gene under 6-OHDA + MANF treatment in SHSY-5Y cells. RNAi knockdown for HSP70 inhibits the protective effects of MANF against 6-OHDA toxicity in SHSY-5Y cells.

Conclusion: MANF exerts a protective role against 6-OHDA induced apoptosis in SHSY-5Y cells via up-regulating some ER stress genes, including HSP70 family members. The HSP70 expression level plays a key role in MANF-mediated survival pathway.

Keywords: HSP70, MANF, Parkinson's disease, SHSY-5Y cell

Background

Parkinson's disease (PD) is one of the most common neurodegenerative disorders of the central nervous system. It is characterized by chronic and progressive loss of midbrain dopaminergic (DA) neurons. Over the past years, the precise etiology and disease pathogenesis are mostly unknown. Current therapy strategies aim at symptomatic relief rather than preventing disease progression. The use of neurotrophic factors represents a potential treatment strategy, which is essential to neuronal differentiation and maturation during development and adulthood.

The newest candidate growth factor for dopaminergic neurons is mesencephalic astrocyte-derived neurotrophic factor (MANF), a kind of evolutionarily conserved neurotrophic factor. It was described few years ago as a survival promoting factor for embryonic midbrain dopaminergic neurons in vitro [1]. The protective effect of MANF is specific for dopaminergic neurons, and no effects on GABAergic or serotonergic neurons are detected [1].

Some studies have shown that MANF selectively protects dopaminergic neurons by inhibiting the neurotoxicity induced by unfolded protein response(UPR) [2, 3]. Additionally, MANF has been shown to regulate the

* Correspondence: jfang@tongji.edu.cn; lingjingjin@163.com
†Equal contributors
2School of Life Science and Technology, Tongji University, 1239 Siping Road, Shanghai 200092, People's Republic of China
1Department of Neurology, Shanghai Tongji Hospital, Tongji University School of Medicine, 389 Xincun Road, Shanghai 200065, People's Republic of China
Full list of author information is available at the end of the article

endoplasmic reticulum stress (ER stress) induced gene transcription, such as HSP70 family, ATF family, xbp-1 and MAPK [4–6]. In our previous studies, we found that the expression level of HSP70 family, which is considered as a chaperon like heat shock protein family, play key roles in neuroprotection process. In SHSY-5Y cells treated with 6-OHDA or overexpressed α-synuclein, the expression of GRP78, a 78kd member of HSP70 family, is up-regulated under the treatment of MANF [7]. In PC12 cell line, the transcription level and protein level of HSP70 is up-regulated under 6-OHDA treatment [8]. GRP78 and HSP70 share a high degree of homology with HSP70 family [9]. They are considered to be involved in the survival pathway after ER stress [10]. Whether HSP70 is also involved in MANF signaling pathway is still unknown.

RNA sequencing (RNA-seq) is an unbiased sequencing tool that allows transcriptome profiling to detect gene expression changes in a cell or tissue sample. In this study, we aim to comprehensively investigate the expression level of ER stress relative genes in response to MANF treatment. For in vitro study, a DA neurons like cell line, SHSY-5Y cells [11], was employed and cell apoptosis was detected to verify the function of HSP70, which was found significantly changed in the transcriptome in response to MANF treatment. And we also found that MANF/HSP70 is 6-OHDA specific. Hydrogen peroxide solution (H_2O_2), tunicamycin (TM) and thapsigargin (TG) have been used as normal models for ER stress induced apoptosis. In TM, TG and H_2O_2-induced ER stress, the expression of HSP70 was not changed under MANF treatment.

Methods

SHSY-5Y cell culture

The human neuroblastoma cell line, SHSY-5Y, was cultured in DMEM/F-12 medium (life technologies, Carlsbad, CA, USA) containing L-Glutamine 300 mg/L, 10%FBS (fetal bovine serum) and kept at 37 °C in a humidified 5% CO2 incubator. 150 μM 6-OHDA (Sigma, St.Louis, MO) was used to induce apoptosis, leading to 50% reduction of viability after 24 h as measured with MTT assay.

RNA-Seq

SHSY-5Y cells were harvested and total RNA was extracted using the TRIzol (Life Technologies) method. mRNA was further enriched from the total RNA using oligo dT magnetic beads (Life Technologies). Then, the mRNA was fragmented into short fragments (200–500 bp) using an RNA fragmentation kit (Ambion, Austin, TX). First strand cDNA was synthesized by random primers, followed by the synthesis of second strand cDNA. Double stranded cDNA was purified using a QIAquick PCR extraction kit (Qiagen, Hilden, Germany) and used for end repair and base A addition. For high throughput sequencing library constructed according to the manufacture's instructions of BGI-Shenzhen (Beijing Genomics Institute, Shenzhen, China). Paired-end sequence reads were generated utilizing an illumina HiSeq 2000 instrument with TruSeq v3 reagents at BGI-Shenzhen.

RNA Seq data analyses

For RNA Seq sequence reads, one base was trimmed from the 5'end and then the reads aligned to the human genome (hsa, NCBI) and transcriptome using TopHat [12]. The Refseq gene annotation file was provided for TopHat using the default parameters. Only uniquely and properly aligned read pairs were used for downstream analysis. The Cuffdiff program was used to calculate the relative abundance of each gene. A gene was defined to be differentially expressed with statistical significance if it met either of the following conditions: the fragments per kilobase of exon model per million fragments mapped (FPKM) value was zero in one sample and not less than 0.05 in the other, or the q-value calculated by Cuffdiff was less than 0.05. Gene ontology (GO) analysis was performed using the online program DAVID.

Quantitative real-time PCR

To analyze HSP70 transcription by quantitative real-time PCR (qPCR), total RNA was extracted as described above and reverse-transcribed to cDNA using oligo-dT primer and Superscript II reverse transcriptase (Invitrogen, Darmstadt). The genetic expression of HSP70 was normalized to the internal reference control gene, β-actin. The following primer pairs were used: β-actin, forward primer: 5'- CCCAGATCATGTTTGAGACCT-3' and reverse primer: 5'- CAGAGGCGTACAGGGATAG C-3'; human HSP70, forward primer: 5'- TAACCCCAT-CATCAGCGGAC -3' and reverse primer: 5'-GAAGCT CCAAAACAAAAACAGCA -3'. human GRP78, forward primer:: 5'- AGACGGGCAAAGATGTCAGG -3'and reverse primer: 5'- GCCCGTTTGGCCTTTTCT AC -3'; human Xbp1, forward primer: 5'- CTGAGTC CGCAGCAGGTG -3'and reverse primer: 5'- TGTCCA-GAATGCCCAACAGG -3'; human ATF4, forward primer: 5'- CTTGATGTCCCCCTTCGACC-3', reverse primer: 5'- CTTGTCGCTGGAGAACCCAT-3'; human ATF6, forward primer: 5'- GAGTATTTTGTCCGCCTG CC -3'; reverse primer: 5'- GGCTCCCCCATTTCA-CAAGT -3'; human MAPK, forward primer: 5'- CAG-GACTGCAGGAACGAGT -3', Reverse primer: 5'-TTCCTTGTAGCCCATGCCAA -3'; GAPDH, forward primer:5'- GTCAAGGCTGAGAACGGGAA -3', reverse primer:5'- TCGCCCCACTTGATTTTGGA -3'.

The relative gene expression was calculated via the comparative Ct method.

RNAi of HSP70

For hsp70 RNAi knockdown experiment in SH-SY5Y cells, we design the target site of small hairpin RNAs (shRNA) for hsp70 from 3476 to 3494 cDNA (NM_005347). 2 independent shRNAs (shHSP70-3 and shHSP70-4) is as follows. Synthesized shRNA template oligonucleotides were phosphorylated, annealed, and then ligated into linearized PLV-shRNA clotech vector digested with EcoRI/BamHI. SHSY-5Y were transfected with shRNA plasmid by Lipofectamine 3000 reagent (Invitrogen) and then were treated with drugs.

Western blot analysis

Cells were homogenized in RIPA lysis buffer. Lysates were centrifuged at 14,000 rpm for 3 min, and protein concentrations in the supernatant were analyzed using a BCA Protein Quantitation Kit. Proteins (30 μg) were loaded to each lane and separated by electrophoresis on SDS–PAGE gels, followed by transferring to PVDF membranes. Membranes were incubated with 5% BSA for 1 h. Then, membranes were incubated with primary antibodies against hsp70 (4872; Cell Signaling Technology, USA), PERK(MA5–15033, Thermo Fisher, USA), caspase-3 (9579; Cell Signaling Technology, USA), and MANF (H00007873-M01; Abnova, USA), overnight at 4 °C. Membranes were incubated with horseradish-linked secondary antibodies (7074; Cell Signaling Technology, USA) for 2 h at 37 °C. Bands were visualized using an ECL detection system.

TUNEL staining

TUNEL staining was performed according to manufacturer's protocols. Briefly, cells were washed with PBS three times and fixed in 4% paraformaldehyde in PBS. Cells were treated with 50 μL of TUNEL reaction mixture for 1 h at 37 °C, then washed three times with PBS. Cells were counterstained with DAPI for 5 min and examined under a fluorescence microscope.

Statistical analysis

All results were expressed as mean ± SEM. GraphPad Prism 5.0 software was used for statistical evaluation. Comparisons among different conditions were performed using one-way ANOVA and two-way ANOVA with Bonferroni post-test, and unpaired, two-tailed t test.

Results

6-OHDA has neurotoxic effects on SHSY-5Y cells

To induce excitotoxicity, SHSY-5Y cells were exposed to 6-OHDA in concentrations ranging from 25 to 150 μM

for 24 h. A significant reduction in SHSY-5Y cell number was observed following incubation with 75-150 μM 6-OHDA, as determined by MTT assay (Fig. 1).

MANF inhibits 6-OHDA-induced apoptosis in SHSY-5Y cells

TUNEL staining significantly increased in SHSY-5Y cells treated with 6-OHDA, compared with control cells (Fig. 2a). Forty-eight hours of MANF (4 μg/ml) treatment significantly inhibited the increase in TUNEL staining induced by 6-OHDA treatment (Fig. 2a). These results suggest that MANF inhibited 6-OHDA-induced cell apoptosis. Cleaved caspase-3 level was significantly increased in SHSY-5Y cells under 6-OHDA treatment, compared with control cells (Fig. 6c). Forty-eight hours of MANF (4 μg) treatment significantly inhibited the increase in cleaved caspase-3 level induced by 6-OHDA (Fig. 6c). These results suggest that MANF inhibited 6-OHDA-induced cell apoptosis.

Up-regulation of ER stress relative genes under MANF treatment

To gain insight into the molecular mechanism underlying the protective effect of MANF against 6-OHDA-induced apoptosis, we performed whole transcriptome profiling using RNA-seq. For each condition (control, MANF, 6-OHDA, 6-OHDA + MANF), total RNA was isolated. Then, mRNA was further purified and processed for next-generation sequencing. The difference in the read coverage of gene expression between the 6-OHDA and 6-OHDA + MANF is shown in Fig. 3a. These analyses identified 4763 genes with statistically significant differences in gene expression levels between the two samples; 2027 genes were up-regulated and 2736 were down-regulated in 6-OHDA + MANF group relative to the 6-OHDA group. GO analysis showed that the

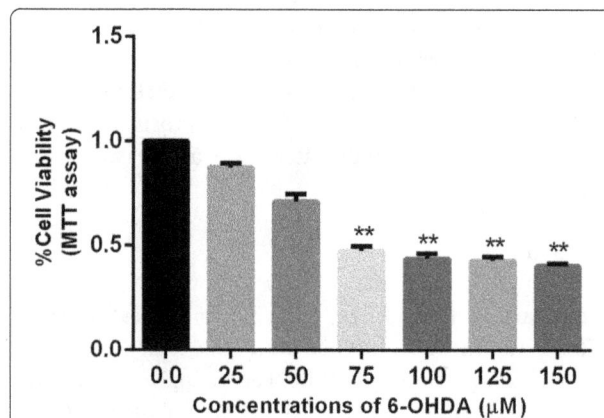

Fig. 1 Assessment of 6-OHDA-induced toxicity in SHSY-5Y cells. Dose dependent neurotoxic effects of 6-OHDA in SHSY-5Y cells as detected by MTT assay. Values represent mean ± SEM, ***p < 0.001,*p < 0.05. One-way ANOVA

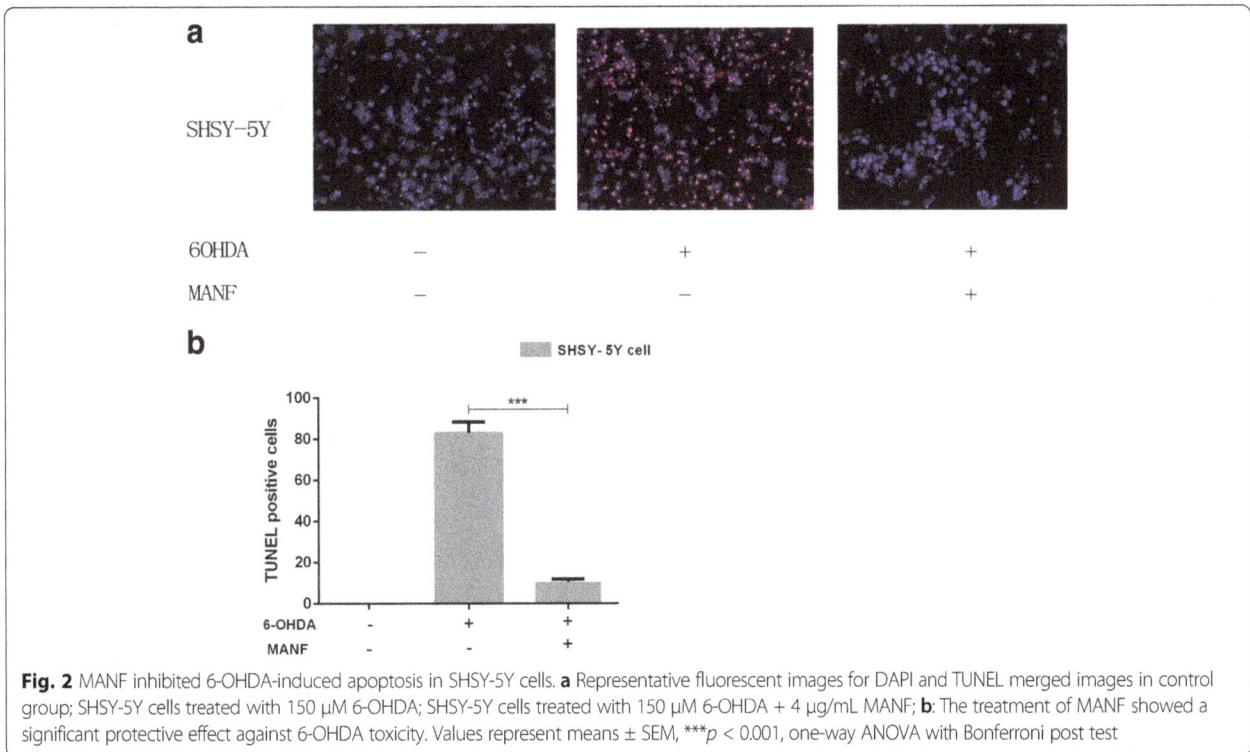

Fig. 2 MANF inhibited 6-OHDA-induced apoptosis in SHSY-5Y cells. **a** Representative fluorescent images for DAPI and TUNEL merged images in control group; SHSY-5Y cells treated with 150 μM 6-OHDA; SHSY-5Y cells treated with 150 μM 6-OHDA + 4 μg/mL MANF; **b**: The treatment of MANF showed a significant protective effect against 6-OHDA toxicity. Values represent means ± SEM, ***$p < 0.001$, one-way ANOVA with Bonferroni post test

up-regulated genes in the *6-OHDA + MANF* samples were enriched in cellular process (Fig. 3b). Strikingly, two ER stress genes (HSP70, xbp-1) were down-regulated and four ER stress genes (GRP78, ATF4, ATF6, MAPK) were up-regulated under 6-OHDA treatment. Six ER stress relative genes (HSP70, GRP78, xbp-1, ATF-4, ATF-6, MAPK) were found to be enriched in 6-OHDA + MANF treatment group(Fig. 3c、 d). HSP70 was the most significantly up-regulated gene under 6-OHDA + MANF treatment in SHSY-5Y cells. The expression of the other ER stress relative genes (SP1, IRE-1, MAPKK, SAPK, jnk-1, CHOP, PERK) was not changed under 6-OHDA + MANF treatment (Fig. 3c). To verify the differential expression of the ER stress genes in *6-OHDA* and *6-OHDA + MANF* group, qPCR was employed to measure the relative abundance of mRNA. To validate the gene expression data obtained from RNA-seq, reverse transcription-quantitative polymerase chain reaction (RT-PCR) was performed. Six changes were selected based on involvement in the ER stress pathway (HSP70, GRP78, xbp-1, ATF-4, ATF-6 and MAPK). RT-PCR confirmed the significant changes in mRNA expression that was observed by RNA-seq after 24 h of 6-OHDA + MANF treatment (Fig. 3e). Phosphorylated PERK was checked by western blot. The reaction of kinase is short, so it can be seen in 5 min after injury. At the time point of 5 mins, the samples under the treatment of 6-OHDA + MANF, phosphorylated PERK did not increase, indicating the protective effect of MANF (Fig. 3f).

MANF up-regulates HSP70 expression in SHSY-5Y cells treated with 6-OHDA

In the ER stress genes, HSP70 was the most significantly up-regulated gene. We investigated the effect of MANF on HSP70 expressions in SHSY-5Y cells treated with 6-OHDA. HSP70 expression levels did significantly decrease in cells treated with 6-OHDA compared with control cells. MANF treatment resulted in a significant increase in HSP70 expression in 6-OHDA-treated cells (*$P < 0.05$; Fig. 3d). The observed expression of log2 Ratio (MANF + 6-OHDA/6-OHDA) for HSP70 was significantly increased (fold change = 7.07) in SHSY-5Y cells of *6-OHDA + MANF* treatment group. To verify the differential expression of HSP70 in *6-OHDA* and *6-OHDA + MANF* group, qPCR was employed to measure the relative abundance of HSP70 mRNA. Compared with *6-OHDA* group, the SHSY-5Y cells in *6-OHDA + MANF* group exhibited 2.15-fold increase in HSP70 transcription, as determined by qPCR (Fig. 3e), which is consistent with the 7.07-fold increase observed by RNA-Seq analysis (Fig. 3c, d). But HSP70 expression did not significantly increase under H_2O_2 + MANF, TG + MANF and TM + MANF treatment in SHSY-5Y cells than in control cells (Fig. 4).

RNAi knockdown for HSP70 abolishes the MANF protective effect against 6-OHDA-induced apoptosis in SHSY-5Y cells

Several lines of evidence have shown that HSP70 protects cells from 6-OHDA-induced cell apoptosis. We

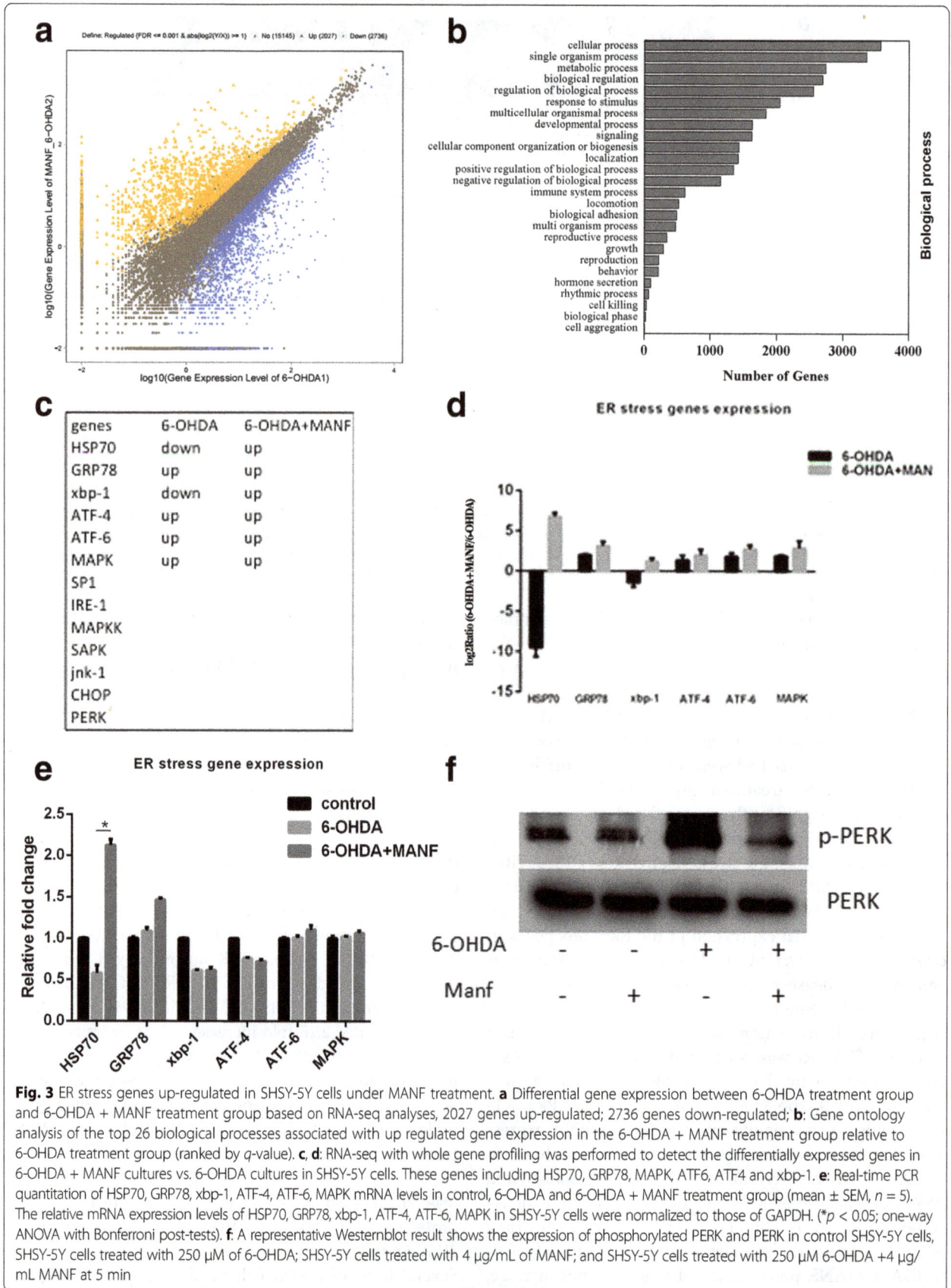

Fig. 3 ER stress genes up-regulated in SHSY-5Y cells under MANF treatment. **a** Differential gene expression between 6-OHDA treatment group and 6-OHDA + MANF treatment group based on RNA-seq analyses, 2027 genes up-regulated; 2736 genes down-regulated; **b**: Gene ontology analysis of the top 26 biological processes associated with up regulated gene expression in the 6-OHDA + MANF treatment group relative to 6-OHDA treatment group (ranked by q-value). **c, d**: RNA-seq with whole gene profiling was performed to detect the differentially expressed genes in 6-OHDA + MANF cultures vs. 6-OHDA cultures in SHSY-5Y cells. These genes including HSP70, GRP78, MAPK, ATF6, ATF4 and xbp-1. **e**: Real-time PCR quantitation of HSP70, GRP78, xbp-1, ATF-4, ATF-6, MAPK mRNA levels in control, 6-OHDA and 6-OHDA + MANF treatment group (mean ± SEM, $n = 5$). The relative mRNA expression levels of HSP70, GRP78, xbp-1, ATF-4, ATF-6, MAPK in SHSY-5Y cells were normalized to those of GAPDH. (*$p < 0.05$; one-way ANOVA with Bonferroni post-tests). **f**: A representative Westernblot result shows the expression of phosphorylated PERK and PERK in control SHSY-5Y cells, SHSY-5Y cells treated with 250 μM of 6-OHDA; SHSY-5Y cells treated with 4 μg/mL of MANF; and SHSY-5Y cells treated with 250 μM 6-OHDA +4 μg/mL MANF at 5 min

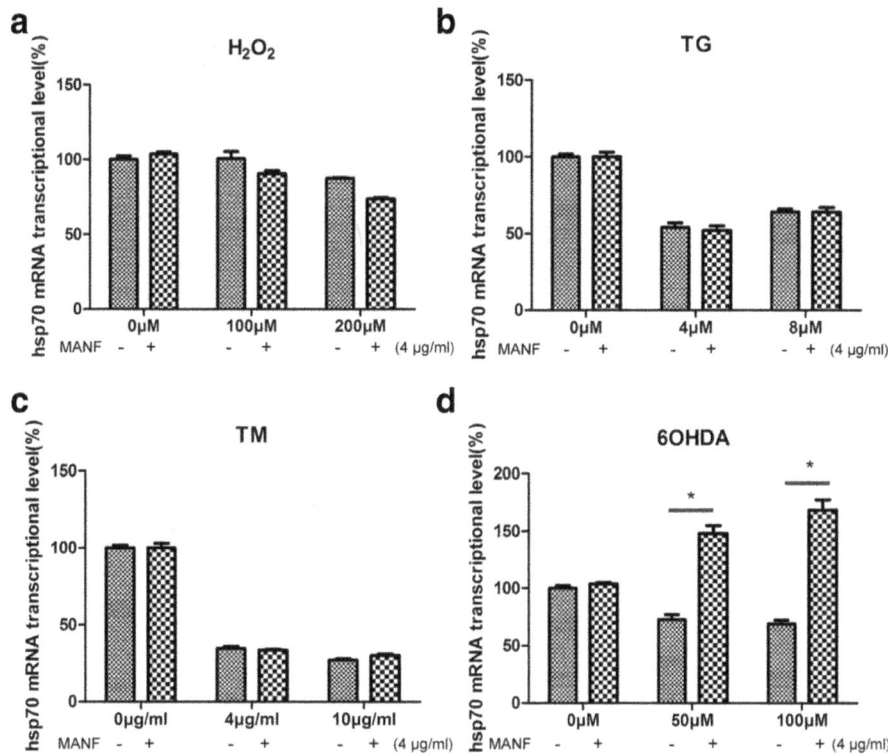

Fig. 4 MANF did not upregulate HSP70 expression levels under H_2O_2 TG and TM treatment in SHSY-5Y cells. **a** Real-time PCR quantitation of HSP70 mRNA levels in control, H_2O_2 and H_2O_2 + MANF treatment group (mean ± SEM, $n = 5$). The relative mRNA expression levels of HSP70 in SHSY-5Y cells were normalized to those of β-actin. **b** Real-time PCR quantitation of HSP70 mRNA levels in control, TG and TG + MANF treatment group (mean ± SEM, $n = 5$). **c** Real-time PCR quantitation of HSP70 mRNA levels in control, TM and TM + MANF treatment group (mean ± SEM, $n = 5$). **d** Real-time PCR quantitation of HSP70 mRNA levels in control, 6-OHDA and 6-OHDA + MANF treatment group (mean ± SEM, $n = 5$). The relative mRNA expression levels of HSP70 in SHSY-5Y cells were normalized to those of β-actin

showed that RNAi knockdown for HSP70 could block MANF-induced survival of SHSY-5Y cells. These results suggest that HSP70 inhibited 6-OHDA-induced apoptosis in SHSY-5Y cells (Fig. 5a). Similarly, TUNEL staining induced by 6-OHDA treatment did not decrease under MANF treatment in HSP70 RNAi SHSY-5Y cells (Fig. 5b, c). In parallel with this result, we found that in HSP70 RNAi SHSY-5Y cells, MANF (4 μg) treatment did not significantly inhibit the increase in cleaved caspase-3 level induced by 6-OHDA (Fig. 6c). And two independent shRNAs (shHSP70–3 and shHSP70–4) were knocked down and knocking down efficiency was 0.32 and 0.22. We found that in both shHSP70–3 and shHSP70–4 RNAi SHSY-5Y cells, the protective effect of MANF against 6-OHDA induced apoptosis disappeared. TUNEL staining induced by 6-OHDA treatment did not decrease under MANF treatment in shHSP70–3/–4 RNAi SHSY-5Y cells (Fig. 6a). In MTT assay, we did not observe that the protective effect of MANF in shHSP70–3/–4 RNAi SHSY-5Y cells (Fig. 6b).

Discussion

Recently, MANF has been recognized as an important factor that protect dopaminergic neurons in the substantia nigra from injury induced by several toxins [13]. In this study, we found that MANF inhibited 6-OHDA-induced apoptosis in SHSY-5Y cells. 6-OHDA is a neurotoxin widely used to create animal models of PD. In the experiment, the expression of TUNEL staining was observed by immunohistochemical staining to determine the number of apoptotic cells. We found that 6-OHDA increased the positive TUNEL staining, a marker of apoptosis. MANF treatment inhibited the increase of TUNEL staining induced by 6-OHDA. Our findings are consistent with recent studies, showing that MANF inhibits ER stress relative apoptosis [14]. That means, the protective effect of MANF were due to ER stress relative apoptosis suppression.

Our present understanding of the neuron protection mechanism of MANF suggests that it is involved in the regulation of ER stress and unfolded protein response (UPR) [3, 15]. In our study, expression of two ER stress marker genes, HSP70 and GRP78 were up-regulated under MANF + 6-OHDA treatment. This is in parallel with previous studies which showed that MANF reduces ER stress and inhibits ER stress-induced neuronal apoptosis [16]. We identified that MANF treatment

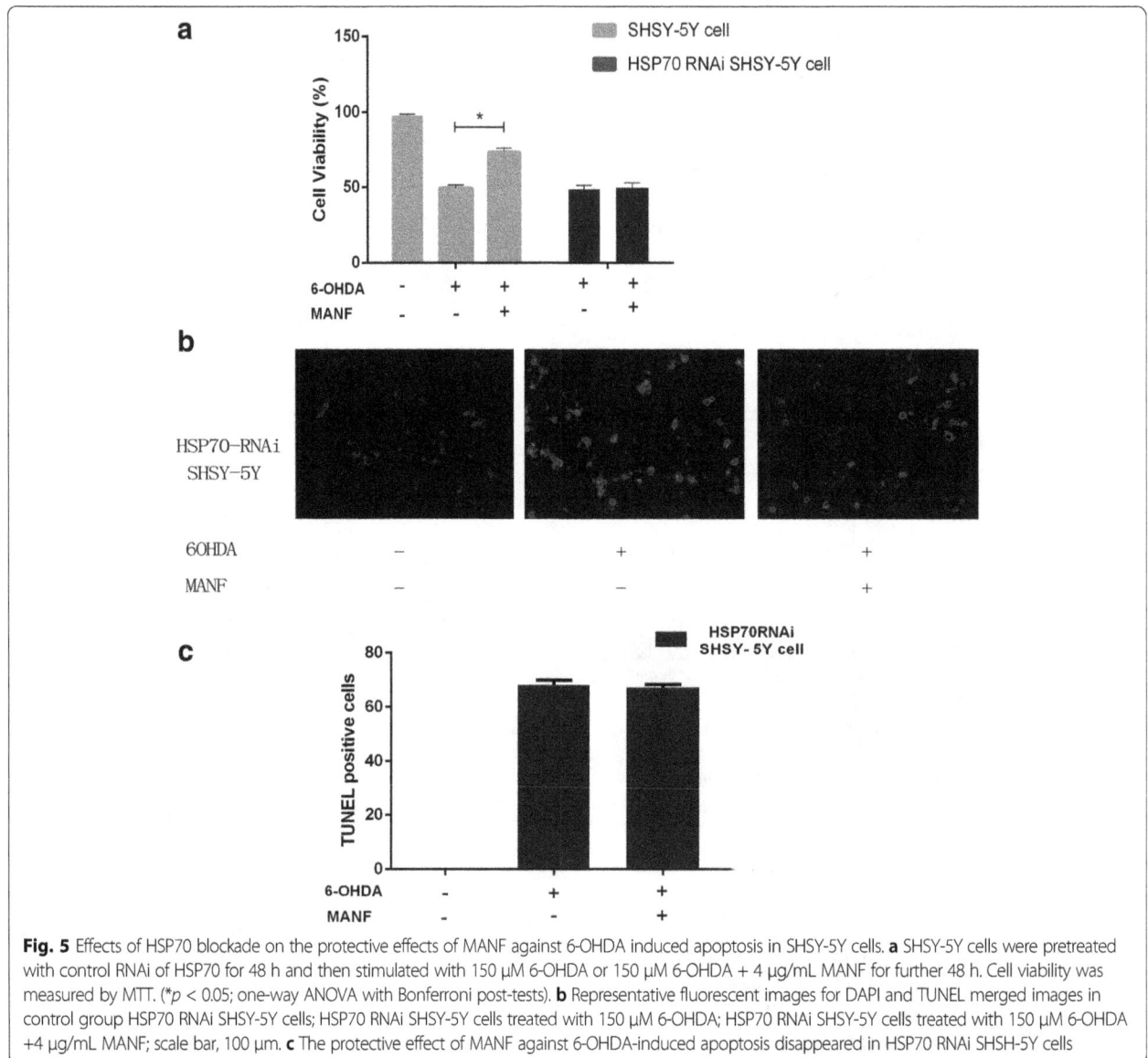

Fig. 5 Effects of HSP70 blockade on the protective effects of MANF against 6-OHDA induced apoptosis in SHSY-5Y cells. **a** SHSY-5Y cells were pretreated with control RNAi of HSP70 for 48 h and then stimulated with 150 μM 6-OHDA or 150 μM 6-OHDA + 4 μg/mL MANF for further 48 h. Cell viability was measured by MTT. (*$p < 0.05$; one-way ANOVA with Bonferroni post-tests). **b** Representative fluorescent images for DAPI and TUNEL merged images in control group HSP70 RNAi SHSY-5Y cells; HSP70 RNAi SHSY-5Y cells treated with 150 μM 6-OHDA; HSP70 RNAi SHSY-5Y cells treated with 150 μM 6-OHDA +4 μg/mL MANF; scale bar, 100 μm. **c** The protective effect of MANF against 6-OHDA-induced apoptosis disappeared in HSP70 RNAi SHSH-5Y cells

significantly up-regulated HSP70 levels in SHSY-5Y cell models, which was accompanied by a decrease in cleaved caspase-3 level, suggesting that MANF alleviates ER-induced apoptosis through HSP70 up-regulation. Lee et al. demonstrated that MANF was an ER stress-responsive gene. MANF mRNA and protein were induced on ATF6 activation in the myocardium, in vivo, consistent with the hypothesis that ER stresses, such as ischemia, which can activate ATF6, a hallmark of ER stress genes, might also induce MANF expression in the heart [17, 18]. Rescently, it has been reported that lack of MANF in vivo in mouse leads to chronic activation of UPR [3]. ER stress and chronic activation of UPR play an important role in the pathogenesis of PD [19]. Thus, MANF has significant potential as a treatment of PD.

In a whole-genome microarray and pathway analysis, the expression of genes involved in membrane transport and the ER stress was found to be altered, in the absence of MANF, in drosophilaa models [20]. In parallel with this study, our RNA-seq result revealed that many of the genes up-regulated in MANF treatment group were associated with biological processes/pathways related to stimulus response. In ER stress relative genes, HSP70 and Grp78 changed significantly. Combined with our previous work, we found they were both involved in a survival signal transduction. Jessie S et al. showed that after a transient ischemic insult, the subcellular responses to the accumulation of unfolded proteins varies between cellular compartments and are most prevalent in the cytoplasm and, to a lesser degree, in the mitochondrial matrix and ER lumen. Induction of mRNA for

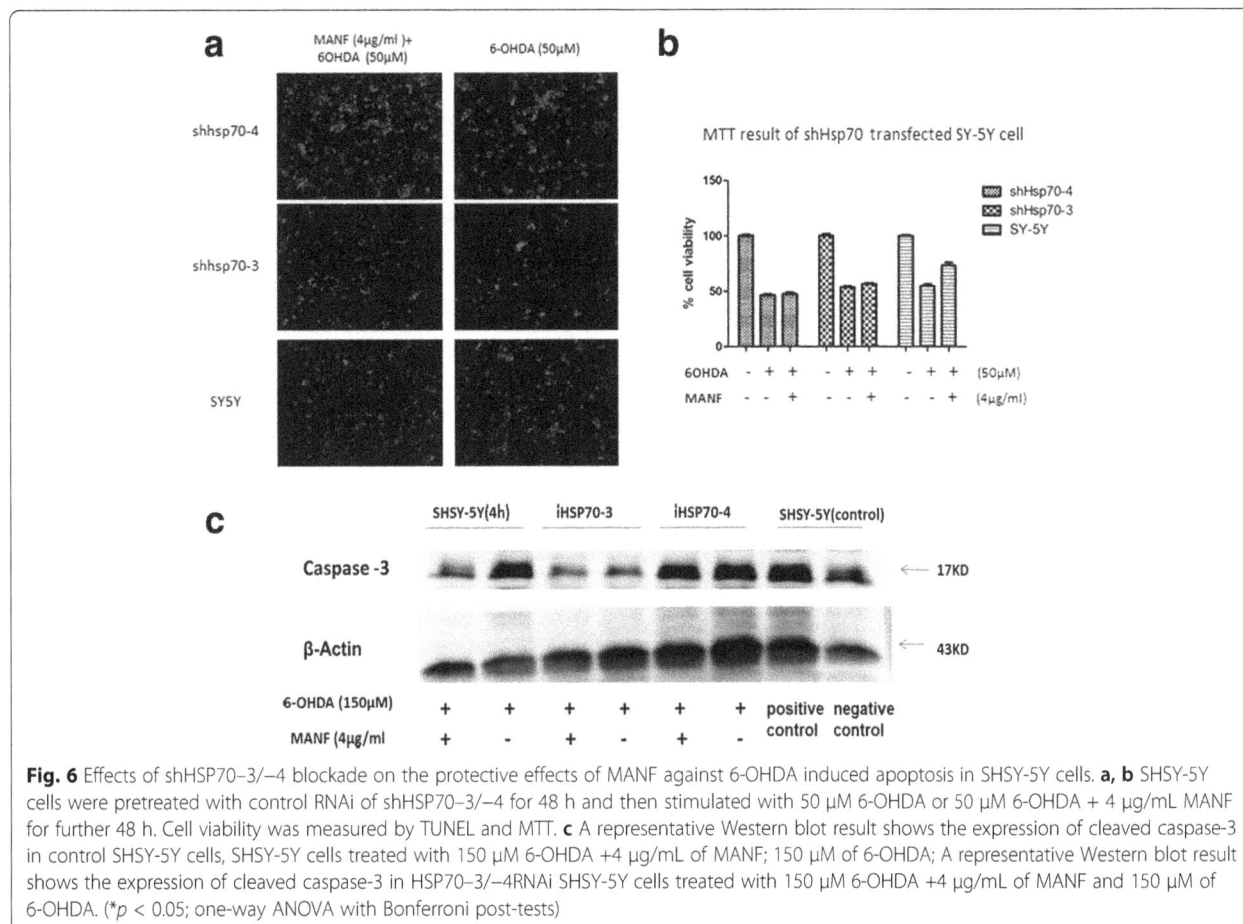

Fig. 6 Effects of shHSP70–3/–4 blockade on the protective effects of MANF against 6-OHDA induced apoptosis in SHSY-5Y cells. **a, b** SHSY-5Y cells were pretreated with control RNAi of shHSP70–3/–4 for 48 h and then stimulated with 50 μM 6-OHDA or 50 μM 6-OHDA + 4 μg/mL MANF for further 48 h. Cell viability was measured by TUNEL and MTT. **c** A representative Western blot result shows the expression of cleaved caspase-3 in control SHSY-5Y cells, SHSY-5Y cells treated with 150 μM 6-OHDA +4 μg/mL of MANF; 150 μM of 6-OHDA; A representative Western blot result shows the expression of cleaved caspase-3 in HSP70–3/–4RNAi SHSY-5Y cells treated with 150 μM 6-OHDA +4 μg/mL of MANF and 150 μM of 6-OHDA. (*$p < 0.05$; one-way ANOVA with Bonferroni post-tests)

HSP70 occurred earlier (beginning at 30 min) and more moderate (4-24 h) induction of mRNAs for ER lumen Grp78 [21]. Grp78 up-regulation is associated with HSP70-HSP90 client proteins [22]. Cellular events can trigger the unfolded protein response (UPR) and activate the expression of a number of genes involved in pro-survival pathways. Whether the HSP70 and Grp78 participate in a same signal cascade or belong to individual signaling pathways still needs to be investigated. However, aside from HSP70, no other anti-protein misfolding genes were differentially expressed in 6-OHDA + MANF treatment group, suggesting that up-regulation of HSP70 could be responsible for the protective effects of MANF in pathogenic condition of PD. Our Real time-PCR result could further show an increase in HSP70 levels in SHSY-5Y cells under MANF treatment. Similarly, in this study, we found that HSP70 knockdown inhibited the decrease in active caspase-3 levels induced by 6-OHDA, suggesting that HSP70 up-regulation may protect cells from 6-OHDA-induced apoptosis.

Various lines of evidence indicate that HSP70 siRNA transfection can further induce cell death in neuronal cells exposed to 6-OHDA [23, 24]. In our study, we showed that RNAi knockdown for HSP70 could block the protection of MANF against 6-OHDA induced apoptosis. In this research, we also observed that 6-OHDA treatment leads to suppression of HSP70 in SHSY-5Y cells. This result is on the contrary to the evidence in PC12 cells, in which 6-OHDA up-regulates the expression of HSP70. This may be due to PC12 cells and SHSY-5Y cells derived from different organs [23, 24].

HSP70 is a member of heat shock protein family, and it plays a critical function in the rescue of misfolded proteins [25–27]. HSP70-related anti-fibrillation may have contributed to the protection of dopaminergic neurons in MANF-treated cells and PD animals [28]. Earlier studies have shown that the aggregation ofα-Synuclein is linked to the pathogenesis of PD. Indeed, α-Syn is the major component of Lewy bodies. Molecular chaperones, which could modulate the pathological conversion of misfolded proteins into cytotoxic species, are recognized as key players in the avoidance of misfolding proteins [29–31]. The family of stress-inducible 70KDa heat-shock proteins (HSP70s), plays a critical function in the rescue of misfolded proteins [25–27], hence avoiding the potentially harmful effects of the aggregation of the species. Meanwhile, some studies showed that the expression of HSP70 was highly perturbed in the substantia nigra of PD patients, which was the site of neurodegeneration in this condition [32–34]. And in our H_2O_2, TG and TM system, the relationship between MANF and HSP70 was not observed. That means MANF/HSP70 was specific to 6-OHDA induced apoptosis. TM is a bacterial toxin that inhibits N-linked glycosylation of nascent proteins resulting in activation of UPR in mammalian cells [35]. TG has the ability to activate extracellular-signal regulated kinase (ERK), but tunicamycin does not [36]. It is well known that thapsigargin induces ER stress by blocking sarco-endoplasmic reticulum Ca^{2+}-ATPase [36]. H_2O_2 is a representative ROS that is generated from nearly all sources of oxidative stress and can diffuse freely in and out of tissues [37]. The cytotoxic mechanisms are different between 6-OHDA and tunicamycin. 6-OHDA increases and accumulates reactive oxygen species (ROS) to induce ER stress; however, tunicamycin blocks N-linked glycosylation, accumulating unfolded proteins that induce ER stress [38]. This may explain MANF/HSP70 was specific to 6-OHDA.

Conclusions

Our study indicates that MANF exerts a protective role against in vitro induced apoptosis in SHSY-5Y cells. This function may involve the activation of apoptosis inhibition. The regulation of HSP70 expression contributes to MANF-mediated neuroprotection. It is crucial to highlight and further characterize disease-related differences in basal and inducible gene expression levels. Further studies need to specifically define potential disease-related alterations in the reactivity to MANF and further define which molecular pathway is involved. Our results support the potential of MANF to contribute to a more protective environment for degenerating dopaminergic neurons in PD via regulation of HSP70 and cytokine secretion and therefore to be further evaluated as novel therapeutic approach for the treatment of PD.

Abbreviations
6-OHDA: 6-hydroxydopamine; ER: Endoplasmic reticulum; HSP70: Heat shock protein; MANF: Mesencephalic astrocyte-derived neurotrophic factor; PD: Parkinson's disease

Acknowledgments
Not applicable.

Funding
This study is supported by the National Major Scientific and Technological Special Project for Significant New Drugs Development (2014ZX09102043–003), National Natural Science Foundation of China (81371403), Shanghai Science and Technology Commission (13JC1401102), and Natural Science Foundation of Jiangsu Province of China (BK20140275).

Authors' contributions
HS and MJ conceived and designed the experiments; QC, JZ, YY, JG, LY and YJ performed the experiments; YL and LF analyzed the data; ZN and JF contributed discussion; HS wrote the paper; LJ contributed guidance on the manuscript. All authors read and approved the final manuscript.

Competing interests
The authors declare that they have no competing interests.

Author details
[1]Department of Neurology, Shanghai Tongji Hospital, Tongji University School of Medicine, 389 Xincun Road, Shanghai 200065, People's Republic of China. [2]School of Life Science and Technology, Tongji University, 1239 Siping Road, Shanghai 200092, People's Republic of China. [3]Biomedical Research Center, Tongji University Suzhou Institute, Building 2, 198 Jinfeng Road, Wuzhong District, Suzhou, Jiangsu 215101, China.

References
1. Petrova P, Raibekas A, Pevsner J, Vigo N, Anafi M, Moore MK, Peaire AE, Shridhar V, Smith DI, Kelly J, et al. MANF: a new mesencephalic, astrocyte-derived neurotrophic factor with selectivity for dopaminergic neurons. J Mol Neurosci. 2003;20(2):173–88.
2. Lindahl M, Saarma M, Lindholm P. Unconventional neurotrophic factors CDNF and MANF: Structure, physiological functions and therapeutic potential. Neurobiol Dis. 2017 97(Pt B):90–102.
3. Lindahl M, Danilova T, Palm E, Lindholm P, Voikar V, Hakonen E, Ustinov J, Andressoo JO, Harvey BK, Otonkoski T, et al. MANF is indispensable for the proliferation and survival of pancreatic beta cells. Cell Rep. 2014;7(2):366–75.
4. Wei SG, Yu Y, Weiss RM, Felder RB. Endoplasmic reticulum stress increases brain MAPK signaling, inflammation and renin-angiotensin system activity and sympathetic nerve activity in heart failure. Am J Physiol Heart Circ Physiol. 2016;311(4):H871–H880.
5. Jeong K, Oh Y, Kim S-J, Kim H, Park K-C, Kim SS, Ha J, Kang I, Choe W. Apelin is transcriptionally regulated by ER stress-induced ATF4 expression via a p38 MAPK-dependent pathway. Apoptosis. 2014;19(9):1399–410.
6. Cubillos-Ruiz JR, Silberman PC, Rutkowski MR, Chopra S, Perales-Puchalt A, Song M, Zhang S, Bettigole SE, Gupta D, Holcomb K, et al. ER stress sensor XBP1 controls anti-tumor immunity by disrupting Dendritic cell homeostasis. Cell. 2015;161(7):1527–38.
7. Huang J, Chen C, Gu H, Li C, Fu X, Jiang M, Sun H, Xu J, Fang J, Jin L. Mesencephalic astrocyte-derived neurotrophic factor reduces cell apoptosis via upregulating GRP78 in SH-SY5Y cells. Cell Biol Int. 2016;40(7):803–11.
8. Alani B, Salehi R, Sadeghi P, Khodagholi F, Digaleh H, Jabbarzadeh-Tabrizi S, Zare M, Korbekandi H. Silencing of Hsp70 intensifies 6-OHDA-induced apoptosis and Hsp90 Upregulation in PC12 cells. J Mol Neurosci. 2015;55(1):174–83.
9. Ortiz C, Cardemil L. Heat-shock responses in two leguminous plants: a comparative study. J Exp Bot. 2001;52(361):1711–9.
10. Lee AS. The ER chaperone and signaling regulator GRP78/BiP as a monitor of endoplasmic reticulum stress. Methods. 2005;35(4):373–81.
11. Tai KK, Pham L, Truong DD. Idebenone induces apoptotic cell death in the human dopaminergic neuroblastoma SHSY-5Y cells. Neurotox Res. 2011;20(4):321–8.
12. Trapnell C, Pachter L, Salzberg SL. TopHat: discovering splice junctions with RNA-Seq. Bioinformatics. 2009;25(9):1105–11.
13. Nuss JE, Choksi KB, DeFord JH, Papaconstantinou J. Decreased enzyme activities of chaperones PDI and BiP in aged mouse livers. Biochem Biophys Res Commun. 2008;365(2):355–61.
14. Cooper AA, Gitler AD, Cashikar A, Haynes CM, Hill KJ, Bhullar B, Liu K, Xu K, Stratheam KE, Liu R, et al. Alpha-synuclein blocks ER-Golgi traffic and Rab1 rescues neuron loss in Parkinson's models. Science. 2006;313(5785):324–8.
15. Hellman M, Arumae U, Yu LY, Lindholm P, Peranen J, Saarma M, Permi P. Mesencephalic astrocyte-derived neurotrophic factor (MANF) has a unique mechanism to rescue apoptotic neurons. J Biol Chem. 2011;286(4):2675–80.
16. Arrieta A, Blackwood EA, Stauffer WT, Pentoney AN, Thuerauf DJ, Doroudgar S, Glembotski CC. Abstract 19772: MANF, a structurally unique ER stress-inducible protein, restores ER-protein folding in ER stressed cardiac Myocytes and in the ischemic heart. Circulation. 2016;134 (Suppl_1 Suppl 1):A19772.

17. Tadimalla A, Belmont PJ, Thuerauf DJ, Glassy MS, Martindale JJ, Gude N, Sussman MA, Glembotski CC. Mesencephalic Astrocyte-derived Neurotrophic factor is an ischemia-inducible secreted endoplasmic reticulum stress response protein in the heart. Circ Res. 2008;103(11):1249–58.

18. Lee A-H, Iwakoshi NN, Glimcher LH. XBP-1 regulates a subset of endoplasmic reticulum resident chaperone genes in the unfolded protein response. Mol Cell Biol. 2003;23(21):7448–59.

19. Nuss JE, Choksi KB, DeFord JH, Papaconstantinou J. Decreased enzyme activities of chaperones PD1 and BiP in aged mouse livers. Biochem Biophys Res Commun. 2008;365(2):355–61.

20. Palgi M, Greco D, Lindstrom R, Auvinen P, Heino TI. Gene expression analysis of Drosophilaa Manf mutants reveals perturbations in membrane traffic and major metabolic changes. BMC Genomics. 2012;13:134.

21. Truettner JS, Hu B, Hu K, Liu CL, Dietrich WD. Subcellular stress response and induction of molecular chaperones and folding proteins after transient global ischemia in rats. Brain Res. 2009;1249:9–18.

22. Tan SS, Ahmad I, Bennett HL, Singh L, Nixon C, Seywright M, Barnetson RJ, Edwards J, Leung HY. GRP78 up-regulation is associated with androgen receptor status, Hsp70–Hsp90 client proteins and castrate-resistant prostate cancer. J Pathol. 2011;223(1):81–7.

23. Alani B, Salehi R, Sadeghi P, Khodagholi F, Digaleh H, Jabbarzadeh-Tabrizi S, Zare M, Korbekandi H. Silencing of Hsp70 intensifies 6-OHDA-induced apoptosis and Hsp90 upregulation in PC12 cells. J.Mol Neurosci. 2015;55(1):174–83.

24. Alani B, Salehi R, Sadeghi P, Zare M, Khodagholi F, Arefian E, Hakemi MG, Digaleh H. Silencing of Hsp90 chaperone expression protects against 6-hydroxydopamine toxicity in PC12 cells. J.Mol Neurosci. 2014;52(3):392–402.

25. Gragerov A, Nudler E, Komissarova N, Gaitanaris GA, Gottesman ME, Nikiforov V. Cooperation of GroEL/GroES and DnaK/DnaJ heat shock proteins in preventing protein misfolding in Escherichia coli. Proc Natl Acad Sci U S A. 1992;89(21):10341–4.

26. Martinez-Alonso M, Gomez-Sebastian S, Escribano JM, Saiz JC, Ferrer-Miralles N, Villaverde A. DnaK/DnaJ-assisted recombinant protein production in Trichoplusia ni larvae. Appl Microbiol Biotechnol. 2010;86(2):633–9.

27. Kedzierska S, Jezierski G, Taylor A. DnaK/DnaJ chaperone system reactivates endogenous E. coli thermostable FBP aldolase in vivo and in vitro; the effect is enhanced by GroE heat shock proteins. Cell Stress Chaperones. 2001;6(1):29–37.

28. Pastukhov YF, Plaksina DV, Lapshina KV, Guzhova IV, Ekimova IV. Exogenous protein HSP70 blocks neurodegeneration in the rat model of the clinical stage of Parkinson's disease. Dokl Biol Sci. 2014;457(1):225–7.

29. Dobson CM. Protein folding and misfolding. Nature. 2003;426(6968):884–90.

30. Young JC, Agashe VR, Siegers K, Hartl FU. Pathways of chaperone-mediated protein folding in the cytosol. Nat Rev Mol Cell Biol. 2004;5(10):781–91.

31. Balch WE, Morimoto RI, Dillin A, Kelly JW. Adapting proteostasis for disease intervention. Science. 2008;319(5865):916–9.

32. Mandel S, Grunblatt E, Maor G, Youdim MB. Early and late gene changes in MPTP mice model of Parkinson's disease employing cDNA microarray. Neurochem Res. 2002;27(10):1231–43.

33. Hauser MA, Li YJ, Xu H, Noureddine MA, Shao YS, Gullans SR, Scherzer CR, Jensen RV, McLaurin AC, Gibson JR, et al. Expression profiling of substantia nigra in Parkinson disease, progressive supranuclear palsy, and frontotemporal dementia with parkinsonism. Arch Neurol. 2005;62(6):917–21.

34. Moran LB, Duke DC, Deprez M, Dexter DT, Pearce RK, Graeber MB. Whole genome expression profiling of the medial and lateral substantia nigra in Parkinson's disease. Neurogenetics. 2006;7(1):1–11.

35. Bull VH, Thiede B. Proteome analysis of tunicamycin-induced ER stress. Electrophoresis. 2012;33(12):1814–23.

36. Kamiya T, Obara A, Hara H, Inagaki N, Adachi T. ER stress inducer, thapsigargin, decreases extracellular-superoxide dismutase through MEK/ERK signalling cascades in COS7 cells. Free Radic Res. 2011;45(6):692–8.

37. Min S-K, Lee S-K, Park J-S, Lee J, Paeng J-Y, Lee S-I, Lee H-J, Kim Y, Pae H-O, Lee S-K, et al. Endoplasmic reticulum stress is involved in hydrogen peroxide induced apoptosis in immortalized and malignant human oral keratinocytes: H2O2 induced ER stress apoptosis in oral cancer cells. J Oral Pathol Med. 2008;37(8):490–8.

38. Luo F, Wei L, Sun C, Chen X, Wang T, Li Y, Liu Z, Chen Z, Xu P. HtrA2/Omi is involved in 6-OHDA-induced endoplasmic reticulum stress in SH-SY5Y cells. J Mol Neurosci. 2012;47(1):120–7.

8

The underlying mechanism of prodromal PD: insights from the parasympathetic nervous system and the olfactory system

Shu-Ying Liu[1,2,3], Piu Chan[1,2] and A. Jon Stoessl[3*]

Abstract

Neurodegeneration of Parkinson's disease (PD) starts in an insidious manner, 30–50% of dopaminergic neurons have been lost in the substantia nigra before clinical diagnosis. Prodromal stage of the disease, during which the disease pathology has started but is insufficient to result in clinical manifestations, offers a valuable window for disease-modifying therapies. The most focused underlying mechanisms linking the pathological pattern and clinical characteristics of prodromal PD are the prion hypothesis of alpha-synuclein and the selective vulnerability of neurons. In this review, we consider the two potential portals, the vagus nerve and the olfactory bulb, through which abnormal alpha-synuclein can access the brain. We review the clinical, pathological and neuroimaging evidence of the parasympathetic nervous system and the olfactory system in the neurodegenerative process and using the two systems as models to discuss the internal homogeneity and heterogeneity of the prodromal stage of PD, including both the clustering and subtyping of symptoms and signs. Finally, we offer some suggestions on future directions for imaging studies in prodromal Parkinson's disease.

Keywords: Parkinson's disease, Prodromal, Alpha-synuclein, Parasympathetic nervous system, Olfactory system, Subtype

Background

Parkinson disease (PD), characterized by its motor symptoms (bradykinesia, resting tremor, and rigidity) [1], does not start suddenly. By the time the clinical diagnosis has been made, some 30–50% of dopaminergic neurons have been lost in the substantia nigra [2]. Symptomatic treatments are effective in most patients with PD, but currently no drugs have demonstrated convincing evidence of disease modification. One possible explanation is that the pathology of PD may be sufficiently advanced at the point of diagnosis that none of the interventions can rescue the remaining dying neurons, thus the prodromal stage of PD, during which the disease pathology has started but is insufficient to result in clinical manifestations, provides a valuable window during which disease-modifying therapies can be tested [3].

According to recent Movement Disorder Society criteria, early PD can be divided into three stages: preclinical PD (neurodegeneration has started yet without evident symptoms and signs); prodromal PD (symptoms and signs are present, but are still insufficient to define PD) and clinical PD (diagnosis of PD based on classical symptoms). The criteria are based upon probability and likelihood since it is not possible to identify prodromal PD with 100% certainty; probable prodromal PD is defined as a high likelihood (greater than 80%) and possible prodromal PD as a likelihood between 30 and 80% [4, 5]. The cardinal features of prodromal PD are non-motor and include constipation, hyposmia/anosmia, depression, REM sleep behavior disorder, orthostatic hypotension, and loss of heart rate variability [6]. Notably, many of the symptoms that emerge earlier in the disease course can be attributed to dysfunction in the peripheral nervous system or the peripheral part of the central nervous system, such as the vagus nerve (e.g. constipation),

* Correspondence: jstoessl@mail.ubc.ca
[3]Pacific Parkinson's Research Centre, Division of Neurology and Djavad Mowafaghian Centre for Brain Health, University of British Columbia and Vancouver Coastal Health, Vancouver V6T 1Z3, BC, Canada
Full list of author information is available at the end of the article

the sympathetic nervous system (e.g. orthostatic hypotension), or the olfactory bulb (hyposmia).

Neuronal aggregation of alpha-synuclein (α-syn) in Lewy bodies and Lewy neurites, the pathological signature of sporadic PD, can be found in the peripheral nervous system of PD patients [7]. It is not clear whether these structures are the original site of α-syn aggregation or whether they are subject to α-syn pathology transported from the brain. In support of the former hypothesis, truncal vagotomy has been associated with a reduced risk of PD after 20 years of follow-up (adjusted hazard ratio [HR] = 0.53; 95% CI: 0.28–0.99) [8]. Based on evidence from human studies, cell culture and animal models, the paradigm of pathological protein propagation in neurodegenerative diseases has been extended to include the concept that pathology arising from neurodegeneration-related proteins such as α-syn, amyloid-β, tau and TAR DNA-binding protein 43 (TDP43) may propagate in a prion-like fashion [9–13]. On the other hand, the prion hypothesis as selective neuronal vulnerability may be another important factor contributing to specific patterns of degeneration in human and animal brains [13]. In PD patients who underwent human fetal nigral transplantation, Lewy body-like inclusions that stained positive for α-syn were found in the grafted nigral neurons 14 years after transplantation, suggestive of cell to cell transmission [14, 15]. It is hypothesized that the propagation of α-syn in the brain starts in the dorsal motor nucleus of the glossopharyngeal and vagus nerves (DMV) and the olfactory bulb; from these two structures the α-syn pathology spreads in an ascending pattern to the pons, the midbrain, the basal forebrain and finally to the neocortex through chains of vulnerable neurons [16–18]. The so-called "Braak hypothesis" provides a mechanistic underpinning for the prodromal stage of PD, as non-motor symptoms could be explained by pathology in the peripheral nervous system and caudal brainstem that precede the onset of classic motor symptoms which do not emerge until Lewy pathology affects the substantia nigra. In this review we consider the two potential portals through which abnormal α-syn can access the brain: the vagus nerve and the olfactory bulb. We review clinical, pathological and neuroimaging evidence, and suggest future directions for studies in prodromal disease.

Constipation and the parasympathetic nervous system
Risks of PD
Constipation is a non-specific yet sensitive prodromal symptom of PD (sensitivity 79%, specificity 31% from Honolulu-Asia Aging Study) [19, 20]. At 10 years before diagnosis of PD, the incidence of constipation was already higher in those who went on to develop PD than in controls (relative risk [RR] = 2.01; 95% CI: 1.62–2.49)

while the incidence of other typical prodromal symptoms (except tremor) fails to reach significance until 5 years before diagnosis [21]. To date, eight large longitudinal cohorts confirmed the increased risk of PD in populations with chronic constipation [19, 21–27], providing sufficient evidence for the Movement Disorder Society task force to calculate a likelihood ratio (LR) for constipation in the research criteria for prodromal PD (constipation LR + = 2.2, LR– = 0.8) [5].

Underlying mechanisms and the role of α-syn
The mechanism of constipation in PD and prodromal PD is still under debate. A-syn deposition and Lewy type α-syn pathology affecting the gastrointestinal tract have been frequently reported from biopsy and postmortem studies; however, the types of antibodies, the morphological assessment of pathology and the site of biopsy varied considerably, in line with the inconsistent measures of sensitivity and specify of α-syn pathology detected between patients and healthy aged controls [28, 29]. Among the many contradictory results, one of the more consistent findings is a rostral-caudal gradient of α-syn pathology throughout the gastrointestinal canal (most dense in the lower esophagus, stomach, and upper small intestine; lowest in the colon and rectum) [7, 30], which correspond to the rostral-caudal gradient of vagal innervation [31]. The DMV is one of the earliest sites of α-syn aggregation in the central nervous system according to Braak, and more than 50% of efferent motor neurons were already lost by the time that clinical PD became manifest [32]. It is hypothesized that the accumulation of α-syn may originate in the enteric nervous system and be transported in a retrograde manner through the vagus nerve. By inducing normal α-syn to misfold in a prion-like manner, the cycle may repeat itself and lead to self-propagation and cell loss in networks of connected neurons [13].

In retrospective pathological studies of PD patients who underwent colon biopsy years before being diagnosed with PD, α-syn pathology in the gastrointestinal tract could be detected up to 20 years prior to the full manifestation of PD symptoms [33–35]. In one study of patients with REM sleep behavior disorder (RBD), which carries a high risk of future synucleinopathy, immunostaining of phosphorylated α-syn was reported in four of 17 subjects, whereas none of the 14 healthy controls was positive [36]. Even though these findings support the accumulation of α-syn in the gut as a possible peripheral mechanism for constipation, caution is required owing to inconsistency of findings and the absence of direct evidence of centripetal spread of α-syn in humans.

There is recent evidence for alterations in the gut microbiome in PD [37–39]. Whether gut microbial content is altered as a manifestation of impaired colonic motility or whether altered GI flora can result in regional neurotoxicity remains to be determined.

Evidence from medical interventions

Based on clinical and pathological evidence, further investigations were conducted into the potential neuroprotective effects of gastrointestinal interventions such as vagotomy and appendectomy. A small cohort with 34 patients who underwent appendectomy before PD onset showed that past appendectomy may be associated with more years of life without PD symptoms ($P = 0.040$) [40], however, a later population-based study of 265,758 patients with appendectomy and 1,328,790 comparison controls indicated no difference in risk of PD between subjects with or without appendectomy in mid or late life (HR = 1.00; 95% CI: 0.74–1.36) [41].. On the other hand, Svensson et al. assembled a population-based registry-linkage cohort with 14,883 patients who underwent vagotomy between 1977 and 1995 and analyzed the incidence rates and HR of PD afterwards, the overall adjusted HR between patients with truncal vagotomy was 0.85, 95% CI: 0.63–1.14; for those with follow-up of more than 20 years, adjusted HR was 0.53, 95% CI: 0.28–0.99 [8]. The study is the first evidence that by preventing vagal transport, the risk of PD decreased, supporting a possibly critical involvement of the vagus nerve in the pathogenesis of PD.

Evidence from imaging

Positron emission tomography (PET) offers a useful tool to investigate physiological dysfunction in vivo [42]. In 2014, the PET tracer 5-^{11}C-methoxydonepezil was validated for the in vivo quantification of acetylcholinesterase (AChE) density in humans and thus can serve as a biomarker for parasympathetic dysfunction. Significantly decreased ^{11}C-donepezil standard uptake values in the small intestine and pancreas were detected in twelve PD patients compared to age-matched controls (small intestine: –35%, $P = 0.003$; pancreas: –22%, $P = 0.001$); the results were similar when distribution volume was assessed (small intestine: PD 66.4 ± 15.4 control 111.9 ± 40.0, $P = 0.001$; pancreas: PD 126.2 ± 31.7 control 167 ± 64.2, $P = 0.061$) [43]. Interestingly, the rostral-caudal pattern of vagal innervation was replicated by the distribution of ^{11}C-donepezil binding: highest in the upper gastro-intestinal tract and lower in the ileum and colon. This study supports suggestions of impaired vagal activity in PD patients but there was no relationship between reduced cholinergic activity and severity of PD. However, reduced ^{11}C-donepezil uptake is not specific for decreased vagal innervation, as it might also reflect the loss of cholinergic enteric neurons.

Hyposmia and the olfactory system
Risk of PD

The other potential portal for aggregated α-syn to enter the central nervous system are the anterior olfactory structures. Olfactory loss demonstrated by objective test is the only non-motor symptom that has more than 80% specificity for the differential diagnosis of PD from other parkinsonian conditions in the MDS clinical diagnostic criteria [1]. Hyposmia is also predictive of the future development of clinical PD in both general and high-risk populations, but with lower specificity (sensitivity 79%, specificity 53% from Honolulu-Asia Aging Study; sensitivity 60%, specificity 72.6% from Prospective Validation of Risk factors for the development of Parkinson Syndromes study) [20, 44, 45]. Based on the predictive value of olfactory dysfunction and dopaminergic deficit in dopamine transporter (DAT) imaging, the nested population-based Parkinson Associated Risk Syndrome study was launched from 2008: 4999 subjects completed a 40-item University of Pennsylvania Smell Identification Test (UPSIT) in the first stage; 203 hyposmic subjects and 100 normosmic subjects underwent [123]I-ß-CIT/SPECT at the baseline of the second stage [22, 46]. The results demonstrated a significant predictive ability of hyposmia for dopaminergic dysfunction (odds ratio [OR] = 12.4, 95% CI: 1.6–96.1) at baseline and a 61% phenoconversion rate of subjects who had both hyposmia and DAT deficit (of whom there were only 23) in the 4-year follow-up [47]. For high-risk populations, Postuma et al. reported that the UPSIT scores of RBD patients who developed PD in 10 years were much lower at baseline than RBD patients who remained disease-free (HR = 2.8, 95% CI: 1.3–6.0, $P = 0.003$) [48]. Similar results were found in an RBD cohort from Spain and in a cohort of first degree relatives of PD [49–51]. The Movement Disorder Society task force determined a LR + of 4.0 and a LR– of 0.43 for olfactory dysfunction in the research criteria for prodromal PD [5].

Underlying mechanisms and the role of α-syn

Hyposmia/anosmia in PD could reflect both cortical and local pathological changes and likely involves a complex integration of central network deficits and local neural dysfunction, in which the role of α-syn may be critical. The olfactory receptor neurons are directly exposed to the external environment and thus prone to attack from viruses, toxins or other pathological particles. The axons of the olfactory neurons pass though the cribriform plate and reach the mitral or tufted cells in the olfactory bulb, whose axons project in turn to the anterior olfactory nucleus, the piriform cortex, the periamygdaloid cortex, the olfactory amygdala and entorhinal cortex [52, 53]. A-syn pathology in the olfactory mucosa of PD patients does not appear to be greater than that in healthy age-matched controls [54, 55], while in the olfactory bulb there is evidence for abnormal α-syn deposition that distinguishes PD subjects from healthy elderly controls with a sensitivity of 95% and a specificity of 91% [56]. The anterior olfactory nucleus, which receives input from the mitral and tufted cells, was the most heavily involved structure in the bulb region; the cortical nucleus of the amygdala, which receives input from the primary olfactory bulb projections, exhibited considerably more α-syn pathology and neuronal loss than other amygdaloid nuclei [53, 56]. The extent of α-syn pathology in other brain regions, including substantia nigra, amygdala, cingulate cortex and orbitofrontal cortex, was strongly correlated with pathological burden in the olfactory bulb in the brains of patients with Lewy body diseases [56, 57]. In a small cohort of PD and incidental Lewy body disease cases, α-syn pathology was found in all sub-regions of the primary olfactory cortex. Despite the fact that all the sub-regions are separated from the olfactory bulb by only a single synapse, the burden of α-syn pathology varies: highest in the frontal and temporal piriform cortex and lowest in part of anterior entorhinal cortex [58]. Together, these results support the possibility that the pathology of PD spreads along olfactory pathways but is additionally influenced by differential neural vulnerability.

Evidence from animal models showed that after injection of preformed fibrils of recombinant α-syn into the olfactory bulb, wild-type mice developed not only olfactory deficits, but also α-syn pathology in brain areas unconnected to the olfactory system after a time interval of about half a year [59]. Similar changes were seen following intranasal instillation of pro-inflammatory lipopolysaccharide [60]. Widespread propagation of α-syn pathology through connected anatomical pathways was observed in the animal study: 1 month after intranasal injection, α-syn phosphorylated on serine 129 (Pser129) was found in areas directly connected to the olfactory bulb, including piriform cortex, entorhinal cortex and cortical amygdaloid nuclei; 3 months after, the pathology had progressed to those brain areas one synapse removed from the olfactory bulb, including the hippocampus, insular cortex and frontal cortex; by 6 months Pser129-positive cells were found two synapses removed from the olfactory bulb and 12 months later Pser129 pathology was widespread in cortical associative and secondary cortical brain regions, somatosensory cortex and the anterior cingulate area [59]. The propagation model was created using preformed fibrillary assemblies of recombinant α-syn in mice, thus may provide only an indirect simulation of the behavior of α-syn in the human olfactory system.

In the aged human population, a postmortem study was performed in 164 participants who underwent olfactory testing during the longitudinal Honolulu-Asia Aging Study; incidental Lewy bodies were found in the substantia nigra or locus coeruleus in only 1.7% of subjects in the highest tertile of olfactory performance, but in 18.2% of subjects in the lowest tertile, with an age-adjusted OR of 11.0 (95% CI: 1.3–526) [61]. In another study with 320 consecutive autopsies from a general geriatric hospital, α-syn pathology restricted to the olfactory bulb was detected in 16 subjects (2% of all participants), of whom two had α-syn pathology in the anterior olfactory nucleus alone, and 14 in the peripheral olfactory bulb [62]. In accordance with the results from previous studies, the extent of α-syn pathology in the amygdala was strongly correlated with that in the olfactory bulb (Spearman correlation R [R_S] = 0.853) [56, 62]. Similar results were reported from elderly subjects with incidental Lewy body disease or Alzheimer's disease with Lewy bodies [7, 63].

Evidence from imaging
Anterior olfactory structures
Morphological analysis by structural magnetic resonance imaging (MRI) can be used to provide quantitative measurements of anatomical changes of brain structures, including volume, cortical thickness or shape. A meta-analysis of six case-control studies showed significant reduction of olfactory bulb volume in PD patients compared to heathy controls, the pooled weighted mean difference was −8.07 mm^3 (95% CI: −14.72, −1.42) for the right olfactory bulb and −10.12 mm^3 (95% CI: −16.48, −3.77) for the left olfactory bulb [64]. However, the results must be interpreted with caution as the heterogeneity between studies was quite high (I^2 = 76%). Another study compared the volume of both olfactory bulb and tracts between patients with PD and with other forms of parkinsonism including progressive supranuclear palsy (PSP), multiple system atrophy (MSA), and corticobasal degeneration (CBD) and detected the lowest volume of 198.3 ± 60.1 mm^3 in patients with PD, followed by 261.7 ± 75.5 mm^3 in PSP, 278.2 ± 77.0 mm^3 in MSA, 312.4 ± 30.2 mm^3 in CBD, and 314.6 ± 42.6 mm^3 in controls [65]. Using diffusion tensor imaging (DTI), two studies reported a significant increase of mean diffusivity, presumed to reflect axonal and myelin damage, in bilateral olfactory tracts of the PD patients. The mean diffusivity values of the olfactory tract and substantia nigra were significantly correlated with decreased 6-[^{18}F]-fluorolevodopa uptake in the putamen ($R = -0.71$, $P < 0.01$; $R = -0.52$, $P < 0.05$ respectively) [66, 67]. The findings implied that microstructural degradation of the olfactory tract and the substantia nigra parallels progression of putaminal dopaminergic dysfunction, but the time sequence of the pathological changes cannot be determined from these studies. MRI and DTI measurements of olfactory bulb/tract

degradation were associated with decreased olfactory performance [68, 69].

Network and neural transmitter systems

The process of odor identification requires short-term working memory to receive test information and long-term memory to recognize and name the odor, so a normal olfactory performance requires the integrity of both primary olfactory cortex and higher order cognitive network such as the limbic network and is modulated by varies neural transmitters [70].

Focal voxel-based morphology analysis of the olfactory sulcus showed smaller depth in the PD patients but this did not correlate with olfactory identification performance [68], while the grey matter volume in the piriform cortex was positively correlated with the olfactory performance in early PD subjects [71].

In both PD and healthy controls, olfactory stimulation activated vast brain regions in functional magnetic resonance imaging, including amygdaloid complex, hippocampal formation, lateral orbitofrontal cortex, striatum, thalamus and midbrain; compared to control subjects, the activation in amygdala and hippocampal formation was reduced in PD patients [72]. In a study using olfactory event-related potentials to identify hyposmia, further decrease of activation was found in the inferior frontal gyrus, insula and cingulate cortex as well as in amygdala and hippocampus in PD without identifiable olfactory event-related potentials [73]. Other cortical regions with decreased activation in hyposmic PD included medial frontal gyrus, middle temporal gyrus and occipital cortex [74]. In resting state, the regional homogeneity and functional connectivity within primary olfactory cortices and secondary olfactory structures were reduced in hyposmic PD; along with significantly decreased connectivity within limbic/paralimbic networks between gyrus rectus and orbital frontal cortex, parahippocampal gyrus, middle occipital gyrus, insula, temporal pole, posterior cingulate and amygdala [75]. A longitudinal ^{18}F-fluorodeoxyglucose PET study showed reduced metabolism in bilateral medial prefrontal cortex and parieto-occipito-temporal cortex in hyposmic PD at baseline and a marked metabolic reduction in the posterior regions such as posterior cingulate, precuneus, medial occipital and parieto-occipito-temporal cortex at 3-year follow-up; this pattern of reduced metabolism has some extent of similarity with the PD-related cognitive pattern reported by the Eidelberg group [76, 77]. The PD group with hyposmia had significant deteriorations in Mini-Mental State Examination score compared to normosmic PD and one standard deviation change in the olfactory score at baseline resulted in 18.7-fold increase in the risk of developing PD with dementia in 3 years [76].

The connection between olfactory impairment and cognitive decline was further revealed by PET studies: positive correlations between UPSIT scores and acetylcholinesterase (AChE) activities were found in the hippocampal formation, amygdala and neocortex ($R = 0.56$, $P < 0.0001$; $R = 0.50$, $P < 0.0001$; $R = 0.46$, $P = 0.0003$; respectively); while limbic AChE activity also correlated positively with executive cognitive ability ($r = 0.36$, $P = 0.006$) and verbal memory ($r = 0.29$, $P = 0.03$) [70]. In the same study, higher UPSIT scores were associated with better scores on cognitive measures, revealing the same underlying cholinergic mechanism behind olfactory deficits and cognitive decline. To date, the linkage between hyposmia and cognitive disorder were reported from symptomatic level, structure level, resting-state and event-related functional level, metabolic level and neurotransmitter level [45, 70, 75, 76].

Olfactory function has been reported to correlate with the integrity of other neurotransmitter systems in PD, such as binding potential of vesicular monoamine transporter type 2 in the striatum ($R = 0.30$, $P < 0.05$) and binding potential of DAT in the hippocampus, amygdala and striatum ($R_S = 0.54$, $P = 0.003$; $R_S = 0.43$, $P = 0.02$; $R_S = 0.48$, $P = 0.008$; respectively) [70, 78]. There is lack of significant correlation between binding potential of serotonin transporter in the raphe nucleus, amygdala, hippocampus, striatum or neocortex [79], which is contradictory to the results from animals [80, 81]. A summary of important imaging evidence regarding parasympathetic nervous system and olfactory system was provided in Table 1. Association with decrease of odor identification capability and striatum DAT binding were also reported in general aged populations, patients with "idiopathic" olfactory loss and high-risk populations such as leucine-rich repeat kinase 2 (LRRK2) G2019S carriers [22, 44, 49, 82, 83]. However, it is difficult to know whether this reflects a true relationship between the dopaminergic loss and olfactory dysfunction or whether both findings might simply reflect underlying prodromal PD.

The internal homogeneity and heterogeneity of prodromal mechanisms

In fact, the linkage between different prodromal symptoms and imaging signs of prodromal PD are universal. Hyposmia has been associated with constipation, depression, anxiety and mild motor symptoms [45], a combination of symptoms is more predictive of decreased DAT binding [22]. Other studies showed linkage between hyposmia, symptoms of autonomic failure and imaging evidence of sympathetic system denervation, such as lower cardiac septal: hepatic ratios of 6-^{18}F-fluorodopamine-derived radioactivity and lower cardiac ^{123}I-metaiodobenzylguanidine uptake [84–86]. In both manifest PD with RBD and idiopathic RBD patients, RBD has been linked with

Table 1 Summary of pathological and imaging evidence of parasympathetic nervous system and olfactory system involvement in PD

Structure	α-syn pathology	Structural imaging	Functional imaging	Molecular imaging
Vagus nerve	Positive	NA	NA	NA
Gastrointestinal tract	Controversy	NA	NA	Decreased ^{11}C-donepezil standard uptake values in the small intestine and pancreas following a rostral-caudal gradient [43]
Olfactory bulb	Positive	Bilateral reduction of olfactory bulb volume [64, 65, 68]	NA	NA
Olfactory tract	Positive	Bilateral increase of mean diffusivity [66, 67]	NA	NA
Olfactory cortex	Positive	Decrease of olfactory sulcus depth; decrease of piriform cortex volume [68, 71]	Reduced activation in amygdala and hippocampal formation after olfactory stimulation [72–74]; decreased regional homogeneity and functional connectivity within olfactory cortex and decreased connectivity within limbic/paralimbic networks [75]	Reduced glucose metabolism in bilateral medial prefrontal cortex and parieto-occipito-temporal cortex [76]; positive correlations between UPSIT scores and acetyl cholinesterase activities in hippo campal formation, amygdala and neocortex [70]; positive correlations between UPSIT scores and vesicular monoamine transporter type 2 binding potential in striatum [70]; positive correlations between UPSIT scores and dopamine transporter binding potential in hippocampus, amygdala and striatum [78]

hyposmia, constipation, orthostatic symptoms, hallucinations, depression and worse parkinsonian sign [87, 88]. In population-based studies, substantia nigra hyperechogenicity has been associated with constipation, hyposmia, depression and mild parkinsonian signs [89].

The cause of this clustering of motor and non-motor symptoms is unknown, although different classifications of empirical subtypes based on the clusters are proposed [90], the phenomena may simply follow the severity of pathological development of PD. Hyposmia, RBD and constipation constantly appear in different clusters, while the corresponding pathological structures are either the potential portals for α-syn aggregation (DMV and olfactory system) or are close to them (locus coeruleus/subcoeruleus complex and pedunculopotine nucleus), so it is natural that the symptoms should cluster together if α-syn propagates though the relevant structures. In support of this view, some evidence showed possible higher α-syn burden in subjects with hyposmia, RBD and reduced ^{123}I-metaiodobenzylguanidine uptake [91–93], in agreement with the Braak stage and the progression of PD. From this perspective, the homogeneity in the development of parkinsonian pathology is emphasized, and the recently described research criteria for prodromal PD assign each symptom and sign in those clusters into a combined score to predict future PD manifestation [5].

On the other hand, such a scheme may neglect important heterogeneity of mechanisms in the development of PD. Braak and colleagues have proposed a dual-hit hypothesis in which a neurotropic pathogen might enter the brain through either the gastrointestinal or the nasal route [94], either of which can result in disease progression, but potentially with different manifestations [95, 96]. Empirical nonmotor subtypes are recently proposed, which categorize patients into brainstem phenotype (brainstem route, characterized with late onset hyposmia, RBD and dysautonomia), limbic phenotype (olfactory route, characterized by anosmia, depression, fatigue and central pain) and cognitive phenotype (diffused, characterized by cognitive decline) [97, 98]. So far, no pathological evidence is available to support such subtyping and the internal axonal linkage between the olfactory bulb, olfactory cortex and basal forebrain, hypothalamus, and brainstem may introduce ambiguity in the separation of the two hypothetical routes [99, 100]. However, functional and structural network analysis based on neuroimaging may help to investigate the real propagation patterns of α-syn pathology in the brain.

Another illustration of heterogeneity in PD is based on genetic subtypes, as there is evidence of pathophysiological differences related to certain gene mutations, such as increased inflammation in LRRK2 mutation carriers [101, 102]. The lack or lesser extent of α-syn deposition in some genetic forms of PD further emphasizes these differences [103]. Compared to RBD patients, LRRK2 carriers have significantly lower prevalence of olfactory loss, cognitive decline or sleep disturbance in the prodromal stage [104–108]. Neuroimaging studies are needed to consider the functional and structural network changes in the genetic subtypes and to evaluate the differences between the sporadic subtypes and genetic subtypes in both non-manifest and manifest stages.

Even though not emphasized in this review, the sympathetic nervous system may deserve more attention in attempting to understand mechanisms of prodromal PD, as there is evidences for pre-motor involvement of peripheral noradrenergic depletion [109], while the noradrenergic nucleus locus coeruleus may be affected prior to the substantia nigra in the prodromal stage. Related biomarker such as ^{123}I-metaiodobenzylguanidine uptake and 3-methoxy-4-hydroxyphenylglycol can be potential early indicators for central neurodegeneration [110].

Conclusions

The underlying mechanism of prodromal PD includes both homogeneous and heterogeneous aspects. A-syn may proliferate in a prion-like manner and selectively cause neurodegeneration, which possibly represents as the Braak stage in pathology and lead to clusters of prodromal symptoms and signs in clinic; while the gastrointestinal tract/vagus nerve and olfactory system can be two separate routes and models of pathological progression. Further efforts are needed using neuroimaging as a tool to investigate the network changes.

Abbreviations

AChE: Acetylcholinesterase; CBD: Corticobasal degeneration; DAT: Dopamine transporter; DMV: Dorsal motor nucleus of the glossopharyngeal and vagus nerves; DTI: Diffusion tensor imaging; HR: Hazard ratio; LR: Likelihood ratio; LRRK2: Leucine-rich repeat kinase 2; MRI: Magnetic resonance imaging; MSA: Multiple system atrophy; OR: Odds ratio; PD: Parkinson's disease; PET: Positron emission tomography; Pser129: Alpha-synuclein phosphorylated on serine 129; PSP: Progressive supranuclear palsy; RBD: REM sleep behavior disorder; RR: Relative risk; TDP43: TAR DNA-binding protein 43; UPSIT: University of Pennsylvania Smell Identification Test; α-syn: Alpha-synuclein

Acknowledgements
Not applicable.

Funding
Not applicable.

Authors' contributions
SYL made substantial contributions to design and draft the manuscript; PC was involved in revising it; AJS designed, revised the manuscript; All the authors read and gave final approval of the manuscript to be published.

Competing interests
The authors declare that they have no competing interests.

Author details
[1]Department of Neurobiology, Neurology and Geriatrics, Xuanwu Hospital Capital Medical University, Beijing 100051, China. [2]Beijing Key Laboratory on Parkinson's Disease, Parkinson Disease Center of Beijing Institute for Brain Disorders, Beijing 100051, China. [3]Pacific Parkinson's Research Centre, Division of Neurology and Djavad Mowafaghian Centre for Brain Health, University of British Columbia and Vancouver Coastal Health, Vancouver V6T 1Z3, BC, Canada.

References
1. Postuma RB, Berg D, Stern M, Poewe W, Olanow CW, Oertel W, Obeso J, Marek K, Litvan I, Lang AE, et al. MDS clinical diagnostic criteria for Parkinson's disease. Mov Disord. 2015;30:1591–601.
2. Fearnley JM, Lees AJ. Ageing and Parkinson's disease: substantia nigra regional selectivity. Brain. 1991;114(Pt 5):2283–301.
3. Noyce AJ, Lees AJ, Schrag AE. The prediagnostic phase of Parkinson's disease. J Neurol Neurosurg Psychiatry. 2016;87:871–8.
4. Berg D, Postuma RB, Bloem B, Chan P, Dubois B, Gasser T, Goetz CG, Halliday GM, Hardy J, Lang AE, et al. Time to redefine PD? Introductory statement of the MDS Task Force on the definition of Parkinson's disease. Mov Disord. 2014;29:454–62.
5. Berg D, Postuma RB, Adler CH, Bloem BR, Chan P, Dubois B, Gasser T, Goetz CG, Halliday G, Joseph L, et al. MDS research criteria for prodromal Parkinson's disease. Mov Disord. 2015;30:1600–11.
6. Salat D, Noyce AJ, Schrag A, Tolosa E. Challenges of modifying disease progression in prediagnostic Parkinson's disease. Lancet Neurol. 2016;15: 637–48.
7. Beach TG, Adler CH, Sue LI, Vedders L, Lue L, White Iii CL, Akiyama H, Caviness JN, Shill HA, Sabbagh MN, et al. Multi-organ distribution of phosphorylated alpha-synuclein histopathology in subjects with Lewy body disorders. Acta Neuropathol. 2010;119:689–702.
8. Svensson E, Horvath-Puho E, Thomsen RW, Djurhuus JC, Pedersen L, Borghammer P, Sorensen HT. Vagotomy and subsequent risk of Parkinson's disease. Ann Neurol. 2015;78:522–9.
9. Goedert M. Alzheimer's and Parkinson's diseases: The prion concept in relation to assembled Abeta, tau, and alpha-synuclein. Science. 2015;349: 1255555.
10. Brettschneider J, Del Tredici K, Lee VM, Trojanowski JQ. Spreading of pathology in neurodegenerative diseases: a focus on human studies. Nat Rev Neurosci. 2015;16:109–20.
11. Jucker M, Walker LC. Self-propagation of pathogenic protein aggregates in neurodegenerative diseases. Nature. 2013;501:45–51.
12. Luk KC, Kehm V, Carroll J, Zhang B, O'Brien P, Trojanowski JQ, Lee VM. Pathological alpha-synuclein transmission initiates Parkinson-like neurodegeneration in nontransgenic mice. Science. 2012;338:949–53.
13. Walsh DM, Selkoe DJ. A critical appraisal of the pathogenic protein spread hypothesis of neurodegeneration. Nat Rev Neurosci. 2016;17:251–60.
14. Kordower JH, Chu Y, Hauser RA, Freeman TB, Olanow CW. Lewy body-like pathology in long-term embryonic nigral transplants in Parkinson's disease. Nat Med. 2008;14:504–6.
15. Li JY, Englund E, Holton JL, Soulet D, Hagell P, Lees AJ, Lashley T, Quinn NP, Rehncrona S, Bjorklund A, et al. Lewy bodies in grafted neurons in subjects with Parkinson's disease suggest host-to-graft disease propagation. Nat Med. 2008;14:501–3.
16. Braak E. Staging of brain pathology related to sporadic Parkinson's disease. Neurobiol Aging. 2003;24:197–211.
17. Kingsbury AE, Bandopadhyay R, Silveira-Moriyama L, Ayling H, Kallis C, Sterlacci W, Maeir H, Poewe W, Lees AJ. Brain stem pathology in Parkinson's disease: an evaluation of the Braak staging model. Mov Disord. 2010;25: 2508–15.
18. Dickson DW, Uchikado H, Fujishiro H, Tsuboi Y. Evidence in favor of Braak staging of Parkinson's disease. Mov Disord. 2010;25 Suppl 1:S78–82.
19. Abbott RD, Petrovitch H, White LR, Masaki KH, Tanner CM, Curb JD, Grandinetti A, Blanchette PL, Popper JS, Ross GW. Frequency of bowel movements and the future risk of Parkinson's disease. Neurology. 2001;57:456–62.
20. Ross GW, Abbott RD, Petrovitch H, Tanner CM, White LR. Pre-motor features of Parkinson's disease: the Honolulu-Asia Aging Study experience. Parkinsonism Relat Disord. 2012;18 Suppl 1:S199–202.

21. Schrag A, Horsfall L, Walters K, Noyce A, Petersen I. Prediagnostic presentations of Parkinson's disease in primary care: a case-control study. Lancet Neurol. 2015;14:57–64.

22. Jennings D, Siderowf A, Stern M, Seibyl J, Eberly S, Oakes D, Marek K. Imaging prodromal Parkinson disease: the Parkinson Associated Risk Syndrome Study. Neurology. 2014;83:1739–46.

23. Svensson E, Henderson VW, Borghammer P, Horvath-Puho E, Sorensen HT. Constipation and risk of Parkinson's disease: A Danish population-based cohort study. Parkinsonism Relat Disord. 2016;28:18–22.

24. Savica R, Carlin JM, Grossardt BR, Bower JH, Ahlskog JE, Maraganore DM, Bharucha AE, Rocca WA. Medical records documentation of constipation preceding Parkinson disease: A case-control study. Neurology. 2009;73: 1752–8.

25. Gao X, Chen H, Schwarzschild MA, Ascherio A. A prospective study of bowel movement frequency and risk of Parkinson's disease. Am J Epidemiol. 2011; 174:546–51.

26. Lin CH, Lin JW, Liu YC, Chang CH, Wu RM. Risk of Parkinson's disease following severe constipation: a nationwide population-based cohort study. Parkinsonism Relat Disord. 2014;20:1371–5.

27. Plouvier AO, Hameleers RJ, van den Heuvel EA, Bor HH, Olde Hartman TC, Bloem BR, van Weel C, Lagro-Janssen AL. Prodromal symptoms and early detection of Parkinson's disease in general practice: a nested case-control study. Fam Pract. 2014;31:373–8.

28. Ruffmann C, Parkkinen L. Gut Feelings About alpha-Synuclein in Gastrointestinal Biopsies: Biomarker in the Making? Mov Disord. 2016;31: 193–202.

29. Adler CH, Beach TG. Neuropathological basis of nonmotor manifestations of Parkinson's disease. Mov Disord. 2016;31:1114–9.

30. Gelpi E, Navarro-Otano J, Tolosa E, Gaig C, Compta Y, Rey MJ, Marti MJ, Hernandez I, Valldeoriola F, Rene R, et al. Multiple organ involvement by alpha-synuclein pathology in Lewy body disorders. Mov Disord. 2014;29: 1010–8.

31. Hopkins DA, Bieger D, deVente J, Steinbusch WM. Vagal efferent projections: viscerotopy, neurochemistry and effects of vagotomy. Prog Brain Res. 1996; 107:79–96.

32. Eadie MJ. The pathology of certain medullary nuclei in Parkinsonism. Brain. 1963;86:781–92.

33. Shannon KM, Keshavarzian A, Dodiya HB, Jakate S, Kordower JH. Is alpha-synuclein in the colon a biomarker for premotor Parkinson's disease? Evidence from 3 cases. Mov Disord. 2012;27:716–9.

34. Hilton D, Stephens M, Kirk L, Edwards P, Potter R, Zajicek J, Broughton E, Hagan H, Carroll C. Accumulation of alpha-synuclein in the bowel of patients in the pre-clinical phase of Parkinson's disease. Acta Neuropathol. 2014;127:235–41.

35. Stokholm MG, Danielsen EH, Hamilton-Dutoit SJ, Borghammer P. Pathological alpha-synuclein in gastrointestinal tissues from prodromal Parkinson disease patients. Ann Neurol. 2016;79:940–9.

36. Sprenger FS, Stefanova N, Gelpi E, Seppi K, Navarro-Otano J, Offner F, Vilas D, Valldeoriola F, Pont-Sunyer C, Aldecoa I, et al. Enteric nervous system alpha-synuclein immunoreactivity in idiopathic REM sleep behavior disorder. Neurology. 2015;85:1761–8.

37. Goldman SM, Kamel F, Ross GW, Jewell SA, Marras C, Hoppin JA, Umbach DM, Bhudhikanok GS, Meng C, Korell M, et al. Peptidoglycan recognition protein genes and risk of Parkinson's disease. Mov Disord. 2014;29:1171–80.

38. Keshavarzian A, Green SJ, Engen PA, Voigt RM, Naqib A, Forsyth CB, Mutlu E, Shannon KM. Colonic bacterial composition in Parkinson's disease. Mov Disord. 2015;30:1351–60.

39. Scheperjans F, Aho V, Pereira PA, Koskinen K, Paulin L, Pekkonen E, Haapaniemi E, Kaakkola S, Eerola-Rautio J, Pohja M, et al. Gut microbiota are related to Parkinson's disease and clinical phenotype. Mov Disord. 2015;30:350–8.

40. Mendes A, Goncalves A, Vila-Cha N, Moreira I, Fernandes J, Damasio J, Teixeira-Pinto A, Taipa R, Lima AB, Cavaco S. Appendectomy may delay Parkinson's disease Onset. Mov Disord. 2015;30:1404–7.

41. Marras C, Lang AE, Austin PC, Lau C, Urbach DR. Appendectomy in mid and later life and risk of Parkinson's disease: A population-based study. Mov Disord. 2016;31:1243–7.

42. Stoessl AJ. Neuroimaging in Parkinson's disease: from pathology to diagnosis. Parkinsonism Relat Disord. 2012;18 Suppl 1:S55–9.

43. Gjerloff T, Fedorova T, Knudsen K, Munk OL, Nahimi A, Jacobsen S, Danielsen EH, Terkelsen AJ, Hansen J, Pavese N, et al. Imaging acetylcholinesterase density in peripheral organs in Parkinson's disease with 11C-donepezil PET. Brain. 2015;138:653–63.

44. Ross GW, Petrovitch H, Abbott RD, Tanner CM, Popper J, Masaki K, Launer L, White LR. Association of olfactory dysfunction with risk for future Parkinson's disease. Ann Neurol. 2008;63:167–73.

45. Berg D, Marek K, Ross GW, Poewe W. Defining at-risk populations for Parkinson's disease: lessons from ongoing studies. Mov Disord. 2012;27:656–65.

46. Siderowf A, Jennings D, Eberly S, Oakes D, Hawkins KA, Ascherio A, Stern MB, Marek K. Impaired olfaction and other prodromal features in the Parkinson At-Risk Syndrome Study. Mov Disord. 2012;27:406–12.

47. Jennings D, Siderowf A, Stern M, Marek M. Evaluating the natural history of prodromal PD in the PARS cohort. Mov Disord. 2016;31 Suppl 2:S387.

48. Postuma RB, Gagnon JF, Vendette M, Desjardins C, Montplaisir JY. Olfaction and color vision identify impending neurodegeneration in rapid eye movement sleep behavior disorder. Ann Neurol. 2011;69:811–8.

49. Mahlknecht P, Iranzo A, Hogl B, Frauscher B, Muller C, Santamaria J, Tolosa E, Serradell M, Mitterling T, Gschliesser V, et al. Olfactory dysfunction predicts early transition to a Lewy body disease in idiopathic RBD. Neurology. 2015; 84:654–8.

50. Ponsen MM, Stoffers D, Booij J, van Eck-Smit BL, Wolters E, Berendse HW. Idiopathic hyposmia as a preclinical sign of Parkinson's disease. Ann Neurol. 2004;56:173–81.

51. Ponsen MM, Stoffers D, Twisk JW, Wolters E, Berendse HW. Hyposmia and executive dysfunction as predictors of future Parkinson's disease: a prospective study. Mov Disord. 2009;24:1060–5.

52. Benarroch EE. Olfactory system: functional organization and involvement in neurodegenerative disease. Neurology. 2010;75:1104–9.

53. Doty RL. Olfactory dysfunction in Parkinson disease. Nat Rev Neurol. 2012;8: 329–39.

54. Duda JE, Shah U, Arnold SE, Lee VM, Trojanowski JQ. The expression of alpha-, beta-, and gamma-synucleins in olfactory mucosa from patients with and without neurodegenerative diseases. Exp Neurol. 1999;160:515–22.

55. Witt M, Bormann K, Gudziol V, Pehlke K, Barth K, Minovi A, Hahner A, Reichmann H, Hummel T. Biopsies of olfactory epithelium in patients with Parkinson's disease. Mov Disord. 2009;24:906–14.

56. Beach TG, White 3rd CL, Hladik CL, Sabbagh MN, Connor DJ, Shill HA, Sue LI, Sasse J, Bachalakuri J, Henry-Watson J, et al. Olfactory bulb alpha-synucleinopathy has high specificity and sensitivity for Lewy body disorders. Acta Neuropathol. 2009;117:169–74.

57. Hubbard PS, Esiri MM, Reading M, McShane R, Nagy Z. Alpha-synuclein pathology in the olfactory pathways of dementia patients. J Anat. 2007;211: 117–24.

58. Silveira-Moriyama L, Holton JL, Kingsbury A, Ayling H, Petrie A, Sterlacci W, Poewe W, Maier H, Lees AJ, Revesz T. Regional differences in the severity of Lewy body pathology across the olfactory cortex. Neurosci Lett. 2009;453: 77–80.

59. Rey NL, Steiner JA, Maroof N, Luk KC, Madaj Z, Trojanowski JQ, Lee VM, Brundin P. Widespread transneuronal propagation of alpha-synucleinopathy triggered in olfactory bulb mimics prodromal Parkinson's disease. J Exp Med. 2016;213:1759–78.

60. He Q, Yu W, Wu J, Chen C, Lou Z, Zhang Q, Zhao J, Wang J, Xiao B. Intranasal LPS-mediated Parkinson's model challenges the pathogenesis of nasal cavity and environmental toxins. PLoS One. 2013;8:e78418.

61. Ross GW, Abbott RD, Petrovitch H, Tanner CM, Davis DG, Nelson J, Markesbery WR, Hardman J, Masaki K, Launer L, et al. Association of olfactory dysfunction with incidental Lewy bodies. Mov Disord. 2006;21:2062–7.

62. Sengoku R, Saito Y, Ikemura M, Hatsuta H, Sakiyama Y, Kanemaru K, Arai T, Sawabe M, Tanaka N, Mochizuki H, et al. Incidence and extent of Lewy body-related alpha-synucleinopathy in aging human olfactory bulb. J Neuropathol Exp Neurol. 2008;67:1072–83.

63. Beach TG, Adler CH, Lue L, Sue LI, Bachalakuri J, Henry-Watson J, Sasse J, Boyer S, Shirohi S, Brooks R, et al. Unified staging system for Lewy body disorders: correlation with nigrostriatal degeneration, cognitive impairment and motor dysfunction. Acta Neuropathol. 2009;117:613–34.

64. Li J, Gu CZ, Su JB, Zhu LH, Zhou Y, Huang HY, Liu CF. Changes in Olfactory Bulb Volume in Parkinson's Disease: A Systematic Review and Meta-Analysis. PLoS One. 2016;11:e0149286.

65. Sengoku R, Matsushima S, Bono K, Sakuta K, Yamazaki M, Miyagawa S, Komatsu T, Mitsumura H, Kono Y, Kamiyama T, et al. Olfactory function combined with morphology distinguishes Parkinson's disease. Parkinsonism Relat Disord. 2015;21:771–7.

66. Scherfler C, Schocke MF, Seppi K, Esterhammer R, Brenneis C, Jaschke W, Wenning GK, Poewe W. Voxel-wise analysis of diffusion weighted imaging reveals disruption of the olfactory tract in Parkinson's disease. Brain. 2006; 129:538–42.

67. Scherfler C, Esterhammer R, Nocker M, Mahlknecht P, Stockner H, Warwitz B, Spielberger S, Pinter B, Donnemiller E, Decristoforo C, et al. Correlation of dopaminergic terminal dysfunction and microstructural abnormalities of the basal ganglia and the olfactory tract in Parkinson's disease. Brain. 2013;136: 3028–37.

68. Wang J, You H, Liu JF, Ni DF, Zhang ZX, Guan J. Association of olfactory bulb volume and olfactory sulcus depth with olfactory function in patients with Parkinson disease. AJNR Am J Neuroradiol. 2011;32:677–81.

69. Rolheiser TM, Fulton HG, Good KP, Fisk JD, McKelvey JR, Scherfler C, Khan NM, Leslie RA, Robertson HA. Diffusion tensor imaging and olfactory identification testing in early-stage Parkinson's disease. J Neurol. 2011;258:1254–60.

70. Bohnen NI, Muller ML, Kotagal V, Koeppe RA, Kilbourn MA, Albin RL, Frey KA. Olfactory dysfunction, central cholinergic integrity and cognitive impairment in Parkinson's disease. Brain. 2010;133:1747–54.

71. Wattendorf E, Welge-Lussen A, Fiedler K, Bilecen D, Wolfensberger M, Fuhr P, Hummel T, Westermann B. Olfactory impairment predicts brain atrophy in Parkinson's disease. J Neurosci. 2009;29:15410–3.

72. Westermann B, Wattendorf E, Schwerdtfeger U, Husner A, Fuhr P, Gratzl O, Hummel T, Bilecen D, Welge-Lussen A. Functional imaging of the cerebral olfactory system in patients with Parkinson's disease. J Neurol Neurosurg Psychiatry. 2008;79:19–24.

73. Welge-Lussen A, Wattendorf E, Schwerdtfeger U, Fuhr P, Bilecen D, Hummel T, Westermann B. Olfactory-induced brain activity in Parkinson's disease relates to the expression of event-related potentials: a functional magnetic resonance imaging study. Neuroscience. 2009;162:537–43.

74. Takeda A, Saito N, Baba T, Kikuchi A, Sugeno N, Kobayashi M, Hasegawa T, Itoyama Y. Functional imaging studies of hyposmia in Parkinson's disease. J Neurol Sci. 2010;289:36–9.

75. Su M, Wang S, Fang W, Zhu Y, Li R, Sheng K, Zou D, Han Y, Wang X, Cheng O. Alterations in the limbic/paralimbic cortices of Parkinson's disease patients with hyposmia under resting-state functional MRI by regional homogeneity and functional connectivity analysis. Parkinsonism Relat Disord. 2015;21:698–703.

76. Baba T, Kikuchi A, Hirayama K, Nishio Y, Hosokai Y, Kanno S, Hasegawa T, Sugeno N, Konno M, Suzuki K, et al. Severe olfactory dysfunction is a prodromal symptom of dementia associated with Parkinson's disease: a 3 year longitudinal study. Brain. 2012;135:161–9.

77. Poston KL, Eidelberg D. Functional brain networks and abnormal connectivity in the movement disorders. Neuroimage. 2012;62:2261–70.

78. Bohnen NI, Gedela S, Herath P, Constantine GM, Moore RY. Selective hyposmia in Parkinson disease: association with hippocampal dopamine activity. Neurosci Lett. 2008;447:12–6.

79. Bohnen NI, Muller ML. In vivo neurochemical imaging of olfactory dysfunction in Parkinson's disease. J Neural Transm (Vienna). 2013;120:571–6.

80. Kapoor V, Provost AC, Agarwal P, Murthy VN. Activation of raphe nuclei triggers rapid and distinct effects on parallel olfactory bulb output channels. Nat Neurosci. 2016;19:271–82.

81. Petzold GC, Hagiwara A, Murthy VN. Serotonergic modulation of odor input to the mammalian olfactory bulb. Nat Neurosci. 2009;12:784–91.

82. Wong KK, Muller ML, Kuwabara H, Studenski SA, Bohnen NI. Olfactory loss and nigrostriatal dopaminergic denervation in the elderly. Neurosci Lett. 2010;484:163–7.

83. Sommer U, Hummel T, Cormann K, Mueller A, Frasnelli J, Kropp J, Reichmann H. Detection of presymptomatic Parkinson's disease: combining smell tests, transcranial sonography, and SPECT. Mov Disord. 2004;19:1196–202.

84. Goldstein DS, Sewell L, Holmes C. Association of anosmia with autonomic failure in Parkinson disease. Neurology. 2010;74:245–51.

85. Goldstein DS, Holmes C, Sewell L, Park MY, Sharabi Y. Sympathetic noradrenergic before striatal dopaminergic denervation: relevance to Braak staging of synucleinopathy. Clin Auton Res. 2012;22:57–61.

86. Goldstein DS, Holmes C, Bentho O, Sato T, Moak J, Sharabi Y, Imrich R, Conant S, Eldadah BA. Biomarkers to detect central dopamine deficiency and distinguish Parkinson disease from multiple system atrophy. Parkinsonism Relat Disord. 2008;14:600–7.

87. Romenets SR, Gagnon JF, Latreille V, Panniset M, Chouinard S, Montplaisir J, Postuma RB. Rapid eye movement sleep behavior disorder and subtypes of Parkinson's disease. Mov Disord. 2012;27:996–1003.

88. Postuma RB, Lang AE, Gagnon JF, Pelletier A, Montplaisir JY. How does parkinsonism start? Prodromal parkinsonism motor changes in idiopathic REM sleep behaviour disorder. Brain. 2012;135:1860–70.

89. Liepelt I, Behnke S, Schweitzer K, Wolf B, Godau J, Wollenweber F, Dillmann U, Gaenslen A, Di Santo A, Maetzler W, et al. Pre-motor signs of PD are related to SN hyperechogenicity assessed by TCS in an elderly population. Neurobiol Aging. 2011;32:1599–606.

90. Thenganatt MA, Jankovic J. Parkinson disease subtypes. JAMA Neurol. 2014; 71:499–504.

91. Ruiz-Martinez J, Gorostidi A, Goyenechea E, Alzualde A, Poza JJ, Rodriguez F, Bergareche A, Moreno F, Lopez de Munain A, Marti Masso JF. Olfactory deficits and cardiac 123I-MIBG in Parkinson's disease related to the LRRK2 R1441G and G2019S mutations. Mov Disord. 2011;26:2026–31.

92. Valldeoriola F, Gaig C, Muxi A, Navales I, Paredes P, Lomena F, De la Cerda A, Buongiorno M, Ezquerra M, Santacruz P, et al. 123I-MIBG cardiac uptake and smell identification in parkinsonian patients with LRRK2 mutations. J Neurol. 2011;258:1126–32.

93. Postuma RB, Adler CH, Dugger BN, Hentz JG, Shill HA, Driver-Dunckley E, Sabbagh MN, Jacobson SA, Belden CM, Sue LI, et al. REM sleep behavior disorder and neuropathology in Parkinson's disease. Mov Disord. 2015;30: 1413–7.

94. Hawkes CH, Del Tredici K, Braak H. Parkinson's disease: a dual-hit hypothesis. Neuropathol Appl Neurobiol. 2007;33:599–614.

95. Attems J, Walker L, Jellinger KA. Olfactory bulb involvement in neurodegenerative diseases. Acta Neuropathol. 2014;127:459–75.

96. Duda JE. Olfactory system pathology as a model of Lewy neurodegenerative disease. J Neurol Sci. 2010;289:49–54.

97. Marras C, Chaudhuri KR. Nonmotor features of Parkinson's disease subtypes. Mov Disord. 2016;31:1095–102.

98. Sauerbier A, Jenner P, Todorova A, Chaudhuri KR. Non motor subtypes and Parkinson's disease. Parkinsonism Relat Disord. 2016;22 Suppl 1:S41–6.

99. Haberly LB. Parallel-distributed processing in olfactory cortex: new insights from morphological and physiological analysis of neuronal circuitry. Chem Senses. 2001;26:551–76.

100. Carmichael ST, Clugnet MC, Price JL. Central olfactory connections in the macaque monkey. J Comp Neurol. 1994;346:403–34.

101. von Coelln R, Shulman LM. Clinical subtypes and genetic heterogeneity: of lumping and splitting in Parkinson disease. Curr Opin Neurol. 2016;29:727–34.

102. Brockmann K, Apel A, Schulte C, Schneiderhan-Marra N, Pont-Sunyer C, Vilas D, Ruiz-Martinez J, Langkamp M, Corvol JC, Cormier F, et al. Inflammatory profile in LRRK2-associated prodromal and clinical PD. J Neuroinflammation. 2016;13:122.

103. Kalia LV, Lang AE, Hazrati LN, Fujioka S, Wszolek ZK, Dickson DW, Ross OA, Van Deerlin VM, Trojanowski JQ, Hurtig HI, et al. Clinical correlations with Lewy body pathology in LRRK2-related Parkinson disease. JAMA Neurol. 2015;72:100–5.

104. Marras C, Schule B, Munhoz RP, Rogaeva E, Langston JW, Kasten M, Meaney C, Klein C, Wadia PM, Lim SY, et al. Phenotype in parkinsonian and nonparkinsonian LRRK2 G2019S mutation carriers. Neurology. 2011;77:325–33.

105. Sierra M, Sanchez-Juan P, Martinez-Rodriguez MI, Gonzalez-Aramburu I, Garcia-Gorostiaga I, Quirce MR, Palacio E, Carril JM, Berciano J, Combarros O, et al. Olfaction and imaging biomarkers in premotor LRRK2 G2019S-associated Parkinson disease. Neurology. 2013;80:621–6.

106. Mirelman A, Alcalay RN, Saunders-Pullman R, Yasinovsky K, Thaler A, Gurevich T, Mejia-Santana H, Raymond D, Gana-Weisz M, Bar-Shira A, et al. Nonmotor symptoms in healthy Ashkenazi Jewish carriers of the G2019S mutation in the LRRK2 gene. Mov Disord. 2015;30:981–6.

107. Saunders-Pullman R, Alcalay RN, Mirelman A, Wang C, Luciano MS, Ortega RA, Glickman A, Raymond D, Mejia-Santana H, Doan N, et al. REM sleep behavior disorder, as assessed by questionnaire, in G2019S LRRK2 mutation PD and carriers. Mov Disord. 2015;30:1834–9.

108. Aguirre-Mardones C, Iranzo A, Vilas D, Serradell M, Gaig C, Santamaria J, Tolosa E. Prevalence and timeline of nonmotor symptoms in idiopathic rapid eye movement sleep behavior disorder. J Neurol. 2015;262:1568–78.

109. Sakakibara R, Tateno F, Kishi M, Tsuyusaki Y, Terada H, Inaoka T. MIBG myocardial scintigraphy in pre-motor Parkinson's disease: a review. Parkinsonism Relat Disord. 2014;20:267–73.

110. Vermeiren Y, De Deyn PP. Targeting the norepinephrinergic system in Parkinson's disease and related disorders: The locus coeruleus story. Neurochem Int. 2017;102:22–32.

9

Factors predicting the instant effect of motor function after subthalamic nucleus deep brain stimulation in Parkinson's disease

Xin-Ling Su[1], Xiao-Guang Luo[1*] (iD), Hong Lv[1], Jun Wang[2], Yan Ren[1] and Zhi-Yi He[1]

Abstract

Background: Subthalamic nucleus deep brain stimulation (STN-DBS) is an effective treatment for Parkinson's disease (PD), the predictive effect of levodopa responsiveness on surgical outcomes was confirmed by some studies, however there were different conclusions about that through long- and short-term follow-ups. We aimed to investigate the factors which influence the predictive value of levodopa responsiveness, and discover more predictive factors of surgical outcomes.

Methods: Twenty-three PD patients underwent bilateral STN-DBS and completed our follow-up. Clinical evaluations were performed 1 week before and 3 months after surgery.

Results: STN-DBS significantly improved motor function of PD patients after 3 months; preoperative levodopa responsiveness and disease subtype predicted the effect of DBS on motor function; gender, disease duration and duration of motor fluctuations modified the predictive effect of levodopa responsiveness on motor improvement; the duration of motor fluctuations and severity of preoperative motor symptoms modified the predictive effect of disease subtype on motor improvement.

Conclusions: The intensity of levodopa responsiveness served as a predictor of motor improvement more accurately in female patients, patients with shorter disease duration or shorter motor fluctuations; PD patients with dominant axial symptoms benefit less from STN-DBS compared to those with limb-predominant symptoms, especially in their later disease stage.

Keywords: Parkinson's disease, Deep brain stimulation, Subthalamic nucleus, Predictive factors, Levodopa responsiveness

Background

Parkinson's disease (PD) is the second most common neurodegenerative disorder and is characterized by progressive loss of dopaminergic neurons in the substantia nigra; the cardinal clinical motor symptoms include tremor, rigidity, bradykinesia and axial symptoms [1]. Levodopa replacement therapy is the standard treatment for PD but causes motor complications as the disease progresses [1]. Subsequently, bilateral deep brain stimulation (DBS) of the subthalamic nucleus (STN) is used for patients with drug-refractory tremor or patients with intolerable motor complications. The benefits of STN-DBS are incontestable and have been proven by short-term and long-term follow-up studies [2–7].

Factors related to the outcomes of STN-DBS are a major concern to clinicians who want to predict the surgical effects in patients before the operation. P.D. Charles et al. and Jianyu Li respectively reported that patients with better preoperative levodopa responsiveness and younger age showed greater effects of surgery after 3 months [8] and after a long-term follow-up [6]; Hae

---

* Correspondence: grace_shenyang@163.com
[1]Department of Neurology, First Affiliated Hospital, China Medical University, China Medical University, 155 Nanjing North Street, Heping District, Shenyang 110001, China
Full list of author information is available at the end of the article

Yu Kim et al. [4] noted that preoperative levodopa responsiveness, gender, age and magnitude of the Hoehn and Yahr stage (H&Y stage) before surgery were predictive of surgical outcomes with more than 3 years of follow-up. However, Tsai et al. [9] discussed that preoperative levodopa responsiveness only led to consistent improvement in part III of the Unified Parkinson Disease Rating Scale (UPDRS III) 3 months after STN-DBS and this predictive effect did not exist after 18 months. They also reported that disease duration, severity or H&Y stage did not predict improvement from short- and long-term STN-DBS; this result was contrary to the findings of other studies [4, 8]. While questions remain regarding why there are differing correlations between levodopa responsiveness and surgical improvement in long-term follow-ups or compared to that of short-term follow-up, and whether there are unknown factors influencing the predictive effects of levodopa responsiveness on DBS outcomes. Additionally, no consensus exists regarding the above-mentioned predictors, and whether there are any other characteristics that can predict the effects of surgery yet to be confirmed.

In the present retrospective study, we confirmed the effects of bilateral STN-DBS with a 3-month follow-up. The 3 month was selected as a short-term follow-up because optimal surgical effects generally appear 3–6 months postoperatively [10] and most patients attained a relatively stable condition 3 months postoperatively [11]. Moreover, we aimed to identify other predictive factors for the effects of STN-DBS after 3 months, and it was worth emphasizing that we further performed stratified analyses to explore which factors modify the predictive effects of preoperative levodopa responsiveness and other analyzed predictors of postoperative motor improvement.

Methods
Patients
We studied 27 consecutive PD patients who underwent bilateral STN-DBS in the First Affiliated Hospital of China Medical University from November 2014 to November 2015, including 22 Medtronic DBS system and 5 PINS DBS system. All patients enrolled in the study have written informed consent, and the local ethics committee approved the study. The inclusion criteria for the study were as follows: 1) patients must were diagnosed as idiopathic Parkinson's disease by movement disorder neurologists based on the UK PD Brain Bank Criteria [12]; 2) disease duration > = 4 years; 3) were effective to levodopa; 4) with motor fluctuations or wearing-off phenomenon; 5) can cooperate with our follow-up. Exclusion criteria including: 1) obvious complications after surgery, such as hemorrhage, serious infection; 2) with dementia or severe psychotic symptoms; 3) marked cerebral atrophy or other abnormities on MRI.

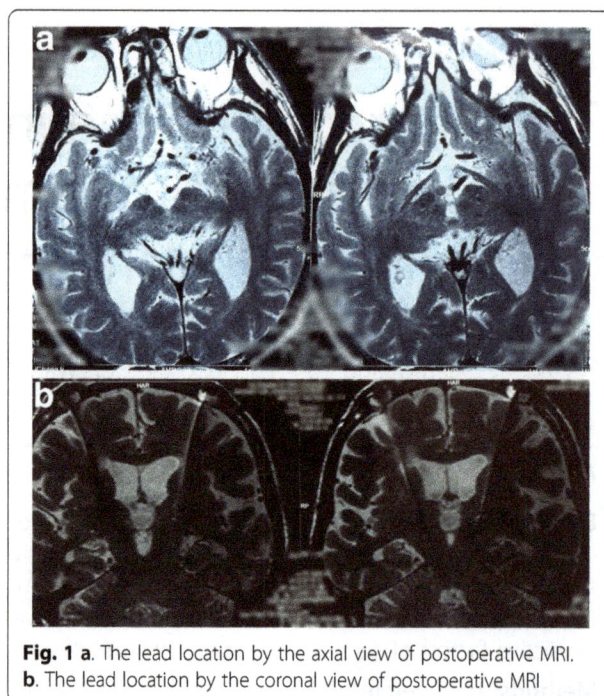

Fig. 1 a. The lead location by the axial view of postoperative MRI. **b**. The lead location by the coronal view of postoperative MRI

Surgery
We located the subthalamic nucleus by preoperative magnetic resonance imaging (MRI 3.0 T) with Leksell stereotactic frame, then compute accurate coordinates of the target by surgical-plan system, the subthalamic nuclei dorsolateral part was selected as the target; intraoperative microelectrode localization was taken use of the electrophysiological recordings, then we made a stimulation test to observe the reaction of patients to different voltages after electrode implantation, an impulse generator (IPG) was implanted subcutaneously when patients were under general anesthesia. All patients underwent MRI (1.5 T) postoperatively for the assessment of target location and surgical complications (Fig. 1). Patients followed the doctor's advices to continue to take medicine and without stimulation settings temporarily.

Programming
Approximately 1 month after surgery, we turned on the IPG when patients were totally at off-medication state (drug withdrawal more than 6 h), through repetitive tests, all the contacts were tested according to a standard protocol [13]. We set frequency at 130 Hz and pulse width at 60 us generally, the amplitude was progressively increased from 0 to 5–6 V with increments of 0.5–1.0 V or until side effects appeared. The optimal electrode contacts and voltage with the lowest threshold for inducing a beneficial results and the highest threshold for leading side effects were finally selected for chronic stimulation [7]. After setting up suitable parameters, we

adjusted the dopaminergic medication based on the patient's response to stimulation or just followed the preoperative medication plan. Then patients continued to observe at home, and accompanied with our telephone follow-up, patients came back to program when they feel uncomfortable, we adjusted the parameters on the basis of their symptoms, until up to a steady state.

Assessments

We collected the basic clinical information of all subjects before surgery. All patients with STN-DBS surgery were assessed by UPDRS III (item18–31) 1 week preoperatively and 3 months postoperatively, and to calculate the improvement of motor symptoms according to the assessment data, in other words, we measured the efficacy of STN-DBS on motor function through the change of UPDRS III scores before and after surgery (Fig. 2).

Pre-operation:

1. Acute levodopa challenge test: UPDRS III was evaluated when patients took no medicine for at least 12 h (usually overnight) which defined as "off-medication" or baseline state [14], and in the course of the maximal clinical benefit after administration of a dose of Madopar which was about 50 mg higher than the usual morning dose ("on-medication") [15], the levodopa responsiveness which refers to the percentage improvement of levodopa challenge test was equivalent to (UPDRS III score of the baseline state - UPDRS III score of best state)/UPDRS III score of baseline*100%.
2. The akinesia scores include items 23–26 of UPDRS part III; the scores of axial symptoms include dysphonia, neck rigidity, arising from a chair, gait, and postural instability (items 18, 22 along with 27–30 of UPDRS III) [16].
3. The severity of Parkinsonism was evaluated by the scores of UPDRS III and H&Y stage in off-medication condition respectively.
4. LEDD refers to levodopa equivalent daily dose which was calculated as the dose of dopamine agonist plus levodopa and MAO-B inhibitor, according to the following formula: 100 mg Madopar = 1 mg pramipexole = 100 mg piribedil = 10 mg selegiline; each dose of levodopa was 25% more effective with entacapone. [7, 17].
5. Duration of motor fluctuations refers to the time from wearing-off symptoms emerge to the time of preoperative evaluation.
6. Based on the predominant motor features in daily living activities and motor scores of UPDRS,

the disease subtype of an individual patient was classified as posture instability and gait difficulty (PIGD) [18] and limb-predominant symptoms (LPS). PIGD was defined as the scores of items 28–30, LPS was defined as the total scores of limb tremor, limb rigidity and akinesia (items 23–26). We used the ratio of the scores of LPS to the scores of PIGD to judge which subtype the patients belong to (>6 belong to LPS, <6 belong to PIGD, when the rate equal to or very close to 6, we grouped the patients according to their main complaints).

Post-operation:

Three months after STN-DBS, patients came to program the parameters, they must withdraw drugs for at least 6 h, when doctors finished the programming and patients reached to an ideal state, we assessed the score of UPDRS III at off-medication/on-stimulation condition.

The motor effects of STN-DBS was evaluated by the difference of UPDRSIII scores at off-medication state before and after operation, improvement rate was defined as follows: (preoperative UPDRS III score - postoperative UPDRS III score)/preoperative score *100%.

Statistical analysis

The effects of bilateral STN-DBS on parkinsonian motor symptoms were evaluated using Wilcoxon signed rank test (Table 2). Then we performed univariate analysis and chose the variables whose p value was less than 0.1 or with assured clinical significance, next we did multivariate analysis after adjusting the potential confounders to estimate the independent relationship between postoperative motor function improvement and each related factors. When performed further stratified analysis, we determined the cut-off point of disease duration (<10 years, > = 10 years) based on that PD patients progressed to severe disability after about 10 years of the onset [19], the dividing line of duration of motor fluctuations (<=3 years, >3 years) was determined by reference to previous studies [16, 20, 21], and we chose the mean preoperative scores of UPDRS III as cut-off point (<=50, >50) since no clear cut-off has been confirmed. A p value less than 0.05 was regarded as statistically significant. All analyses were performed using Empower (R) (www.empowerstats.com, X&Y solutions, inc. Boston MA) and R (http://www.R-project.org).

Results

Demography and baseline characteristics of the PD patients

Four of the initial 27 patients in our study were lost during the follow-up. Finally, 23 patients (11 men and

12 women, 21 Medtronic and 2 PINS) with a mean (±SD) age of 50.4 ± 8.5 years at onset, 61.7 ± 8.3 years at the time of surgery and a mean disease duration of 11.3 ± 5.8 years were remained to complete the study, their mean duration of motor fluctuations was 5.4 ± 3.9 years, and mean score of UPDRSIII in off-medication condition was 50.2 ± 18.2. The baseline characteristics of the subjects were listed as Table 1. Additionally, the parameters at 3 months postoperatively including voltage (Left, Right), pulse width and frequency was 1.904 ± 0.45 V (L), 1.821 ± 0.39 V (R), 65 ± 9.45us, 138 ± 14.83 Hz respectively, and 18 of monopolar, 1 of bipolar and 4 of double cathode stimulation.

STN-DBS significantly improved the postoperative motor function of PD patients

Patients were followed up 3 months after operation. As illustrated in Table 2 and Fig. 2, motor function including total score of UPDRS III, scores of tremor, rigidity, akinesia and axial symptoms all demonstrated a significant improvement in "off-medication/on-stimulation" state compared with preoperative baseline state. The total score of UPDRSIII improved by 56% from 50.15 ± 18.19 at baseline to 21.94 ± 11.69 at 3 months ($p < 0.001$), tremor, rigidity, akinesia, and axial symptoms were ameliorated by 83% ($p < 0.001$), 66% ($p < 0.001$), 54% ($p < 0.001$) and 40% ($p < 0.001$) respectively. The postoperative levodopa equivalent daily doses decreased 20%, from 999.32 ± 516.69 mg at baseline to 797.52 ± 414.45 mg at 3 months ($p = 0.006$) (Table 2). No patient stopped taking medication.

Preoperative levodopa responsiveness and disease subtype influenced the effect of DBS operation on motor function

During the univariate analysis (Table 3), we selected the variables which the p value less than 0.1 or variables with definite clinical significance in other studies to make further analyses, included disease subtype and preoperative levodopa responsiveness. In the multivariate analysis (Table 3), after adjusting factors of gender, disease duration, subtype, baseline UPDRS III scores, dyskinesia, age of onset, age of surgery and duration of motor fluctuations, the results showed that preoperative levodopa responsiveness tended to be positively related to the improvement of motor function in "off-medication/on-stimulation" 3 months postoperatively ($\beta = 0.9$, 95% CI 0.1, 1.7, $p = 0.055$, on the verge of 0.05), it referred to that as each increase of 1% of preoperative levodopa responsiveness, the postoperative motor function improved as the similar amplitude of 0.9%. Additionally, there was a significant difference of postoperative motor improvement between PIGD group and LPS group in multivariate analysis after adjusting levodopa responsiveness, baseline UPDRS III scores, dyskinesia and age of surgery ($\beta = -28.7$, 95% CI -49.5, -8.0, $p = 0.015$), which indicated that the motor function in PIGD group was 28.7% less improved than LPS group.

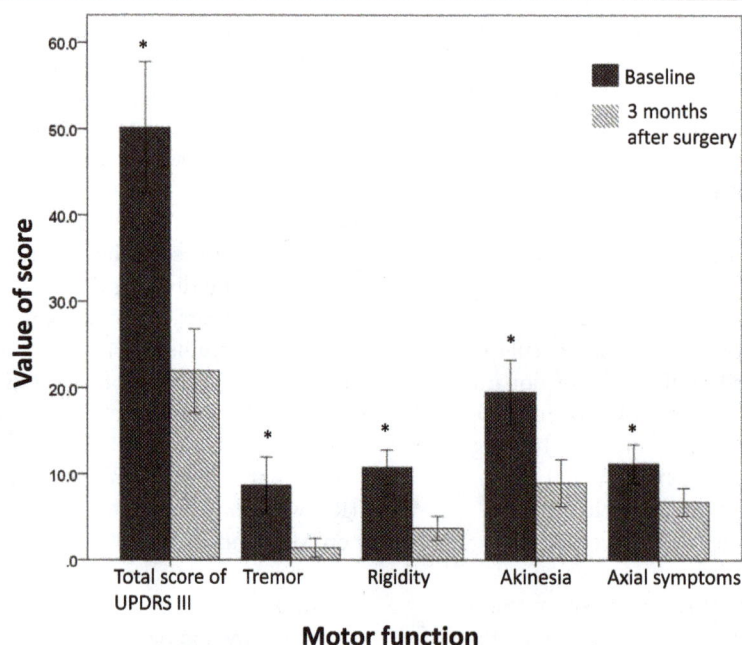

Fig. 2 The comparison of motor function between baseline and 3 months after STN-DBS. Basal and postoperative scores (mean ± SE) for of UPDRS III and tremor, rigidity, akinesia, axial symptoms were showed in the diagram. Tremor obtained the most significant improvement and axial symptoms improved least

Table 1 Demography and baseline characteristics of study subjects

Characteristics	Value
Gender(male/female)	11/12
Age of onset, y	50.4 ± 8.5
Duration, y	11.3 ± 5.8
Age of surgery, y	61.7 ± 8.3
H&Y stage (off-med)	
Mild(<3)	9 (39.1%)
Severe(≥3)	14 (60.9%)
Levodopa responsiveness, %	62.5 ± 19.3
LEDD, mg/d	999.3 ± 516.7
Dyskinesia	
No	14 (60.9%)
Yes	9 (39.1%)
Motor fluctuations duration, y	5.4 ± 3.9
Disease subtype	
LPS	12(52.2%)
PIGD	11 (47.8%)
Baseline UPDRSIII scores (off-med)	50.2 ± 18.2

Data are expressed as numbers, with percentages in parentheses, or as means ± SE. *PIGD* posture instability and gait difficulty, *LPS* Limb-predominant symptoms; Baseline refers to "off-medication" state

Gender, disease duration and duration of motor fluctuations modified the effect of preoperative levodopa responsiveness on postoperative motor improvement

In order to discover whether some factors influenced the effect of levodopa responsiveness on motor results of STN-DBS, we further did stratified analysis, here we adjusted their related covariates respectively. The results in Table 4 demonstrated that gender, duration of motor fluctuations and disease duration exerted significant influence on the preoperative levodopa responsiveness-related postoperative motor function improvement.

Each 1% increment of preoperative levodopa responsiveness led to a 1.1% increase of motor improvement in female group (β = 1.1, 95% CI 0.3,1.9, *p* = 0.0294), while there was no statistical significance in male patients (Table 4); as each increase of 1% of preoperative

levodopa responsiveness, the motor function improved 2.0% in patients with disease duration less than 10 years (β = 2.0, 95% CI 1.1,2.9, *p* = 0.0021), and no statistical significance in patients with longer disease duration (>10 years); each 1% increment of preoperative levodopa responsiveness led to a 3.1% increase of postoperative motor improvement in patients whose motor fluctuations appeared less than 3 years (β = 3.1, 95% CI 0.8,5.5, *p* = 0.0393), and no statistical significance in the others with motor fluctuations longer than 3 years (Table 4). Moreover, when stratified by factors such as age of onset, age of surgery and H&Y stage, we not found more other factors which can influenced the predicting power of Levodopa responsiveness.

The duration of motor fluctuations and severity of preoperative motor symptoms modified the effect of disease subtype on postoperative motor improvement

The results of stratified analysis in Table 4 showed that more obvious difference was existed in patients with longer motor fluctuations (> = 3 years), in other words, in those late-stage operated patients with motor fluctuation longer than 3 years, the PIGD group was 38.4% less improved than LPS group (β = −38.4, 95% CI -67.1, −9.7, *p* = 0.039); additionally, in patients with more severe motor symptoms preoperatively whose baseline UPDRSIII score > 50, the PIGD group was 41.1% less improved than LPS group (β = −41.1, 95% CI -61.8, −20.4, *p* = 0.03); we found there was no difference of surgery effect between PIGD and LPS group when stratified by other factors.

Discussion

Bilateral STN-DBS is widely used to treat PD and its distinct effects have been confirmed [2, 3, 6, 7, 11]. Compared with the "off-medication" condition prior to surgery, bilateral STN-DBS greatly improved the motor function of PD patients in "off-medication/on-stimulation" condition 3 months after surgery in our study. The total score of UPDRS III was significantly reduced by 56% of baseline. Scores of motor symptoms including tremor, rigidity, akinesia, and axial symptoms all decreased post-operatively, of these, tremor demonstrated the most

Table 2 Comparison between baseline and 3 months postoperatively

Subscale	Range of possible scores	Preoperative baseline (*N* = 23)	3 months after surgery off-medication/on-stimulation (*N* = 23)	P value
Total UPDRSIII	0–108	50.15 ± 18.19	21.94 ± 11.69; 56%	<0.001**
Tremor	0–28	8.67 ± 7.85	1.44 ± 2.65; 83%	<0.001**
Rigidity	0–20	10.76 ± 4.82	3.71 ± 3.33; 66%	<0.001**
Akinesia	0–32	19.5 ± 8.95	8.98 ± 6.48; 54%	<0.001**
Axial symptoms	0–24	11.17 ± 5.35	6.76 ± 3.84; 40%	<0.001**
LEDD, mg		999.32 ± 516.69	797.52 ± 414.45; 20%	0.006*

**p < 0.01, *p < 0.05; Akinesia refers to the sum of items 23–26 of UPDRS III; Axial symptoms was defined as the sum of the following motor scores: item 18, 22 (rigidity of the neck), items 27–30 [16]

Table 3 The correlations between various factors and postoperative improvement of motor function

Variables	Univariate analysis		Multivariate analysis	
	β	P value	β	P value
Gender (male/female)	7.1	0.451	10	0.364
Age of onset, y	−0.2	0.788	−0.3	0.719
Duration, y	−0.7	0.429	−0.3	0.852
Age of surgery, y	−0.5	0.397	−1	0.35
H&Y stage (Mild/Severe)	−6.4	0.503	5.5	0.74
Levodopa responsiveness, %	0.2	0.328	0.9	0.055
Dyskinesia(No/Yes)	−8.7	0.361	10.3	0.357
Motor fluctuations duration, y	−1	0.427	−1.7	0.495
Disease subtype (PIGD/LPS)	−17.2	0.057	−28.7	0.015*
Baseline UPDRSIII scores	0.3	0.331	0.3	0.421

*$p < 0.05$; p value which was close to 0.05 means a significant tendency; multivariate analyses of all factors adjusted the respective covariates

improvement (83%) and axial symptoms showed minimal change (40%). In addition, postoperative medication dosage showed a marked decrease compared to preoperative dosage requirements.

The marked effects of STN-DBS after both short-term and long-term follow-up are well known, however, for clinicians, it is more important to evaluate the variables that may influence the clinical outcomes of surgery to optimize the timing of an operation and to predict the therapeutic effects of surgery as accurately as possible. Preoperative levodopa responsiveness is a well-established predictor of motor improvements after STN-DBS therapy [4, 6, 10, 22]. In our study, multivariate analyses demonstrated a positive and nearly statistically significant correlation between levodopa responsiveness and postoperative motor improvement ($p = 0.055$), where the p value may be attributed to the small sample size of our study. After adjusting for potential confounds in the analyses, stratifying for gender, disease duration and duration of motor fluctuations, a significant association was found between levodopa responsiveness and postoperative motor improvement.

The strong predicting effect of levodopa responsiveness generally suggests that the resolution of PD symptoms with DBS is more related to the degeneration of the dopaminergic system; greater involvement of other neurotransmitter systems, such as acetylcholine and noradrenaline, in the disease may contribute to the less predicting effect of levodopa responsiveness. Thus, our study demonstrates the three variables that may exert influence on the predictive power of levodopa responsiveness on postoperative motor improvements. The three significant variables are female gender, shorter disease duration, and shorter duration of motor fluctuations. This result not meant a great DBS response in these people or a poor surgical response in the male patients or patients with motor fluctuation more than 3 years or disease duration longer than 10 years, our point here is to tell which subset of patients can be more accurately predicted by preoperative levodopa responsiveness rather than tell the clues for worse DBS result.

In female patients, each 1% increment of preoperative levodopa responsiveness led to a 1.1% increase of

Table 4 Factors that modify the predictive effects of levodopa responsiveness and disease subtype on motor improvement

Predictors	Stratification factors		β	95% CI	P value
Preoperative levodopa responsiveness	Gender	Female	1.1[a]	(0.3,1.9)	0.0294*
		Male	0.6[a]	(−0.4,1.6)	0.2901
	Disease duration, y	<10	2.0[a]	(1.1,2.9)	0.0021**
		>=10	−0.1[a]	(−0.9,0.8)	0.8874
	Motor fluctuations duration, y	<=3	3.1[a]	(0.8,5.5)	0.0393*
		>3	0.5[a]	(−0.4,1.3)	0.3061
Disease subtype(PIGD/LPS)	Motor fluctuations duration, y	>3	−38.4[b]	(−67.1,−9.7)	0.039*
	Disease severity	>50	−41.1[b]	(−61.8,−20.4)	0.03*

[a]refers to the value of β means that as each increase of 1% of Levodopa responsiveness, the postoperative motor function improved as a certain amplitude;
[b]refers to the value of β means the difference of motor improvement of PIGD group compared to that of LPS group; **$p < 0.01$, *$p < 0.05$; Disease severity was measured by the baseline UPDRS scores of part III

postoperative motor improvement ($p < 0.05$), these data suggest that preoperative levodopa responsiveness may be a more accurate predictor for the outcomes of motor function after STN-DBS in female PD patients. We supposed this result may be related to the greater survival of dopaminergic neurons in women owing to the protective role of estrogens against the degeneration of dopaminergic neurons which had been suggested by primate model tests [23–25] and a clinical and epidemiological study [26]; in addition, estrogens were affirmed to prevent the dopamine depletion in studies using rodent PD models induced by 6-hydroxydopamine [27] and by 1-methyl-4-phenyl-1,2,3,6-tetrahydropyridine (MPTP) [28]. Accordingly, more dopaminergic neurons survived in female PD patient suggesting less disease severity, and DBS mainly ameliorated dopaminergic-related symptoms [29], thus, better responses to levodopa preoperatively predict greater improvement in motor function after STN-DBS in female PD patients.

The other two variables that influenced the predictive potency of levodopa responsiveness on postoperative motor improvement were shorter disease duration (< 10 years) and shorter duration of motor fluctuations (< 3 years) which both imply a DBS operation in the early stages of the disease, a so-called "early stimulated" condition. Similarly, early-stimulated groups also have fewer non-dopaminergic symptoms, including freezing of gait, postural instability, falls, or cognitive disorders; thus, parkinsonian symptoms in the early stages improve with levodopa supplementation or DBS as well. The biochemical mechanism in the late stages of PD, as suggested by a longer disease duration or longer time of motor fluctuation, was not only related to the loss of nigrostriatal dopaminergic neurons but also the participation of other non-dopaminergic systems, such as loss of noradrenaline in the locus coeruleus (LC), glutamatergic hyperactivity and loss of cholinergic pedunculopontine nucleus (PPN) neurons, as described by David Devos et al. [30]. In sum, we supposed that preoperative levodopa responsiveness serves as a predictor for DBS outcomes more precisely in early-stage PD patients than late-stage patients. Generally, the PD symptoms expected to be resolved with DBS are those responsive to levodopa supplementation, which suggests that DBS mainly exerts a dopaminergic-based effect. The two variables in our study that exerted greater influence on the relationship between levodopa responsiveness and postoperative motor improvement are related to better preservation of dopamine neurons or less severity of the disease.

Another variable predicting postoperative motor improvement in our study was the subtype of disease before surgery. We observed a significant difference in motor improvement between two predominant subtypes; the PIGD group showed poorer amelioration than the LPS group ($p < 0.05$), in other words, patients with dominant symptoms of LPS preoperatively gained greater motor function improvements than those in the PIGD group. After further stratified analyses, we found this difference between the two subtypes was notable in patients with longer duration of motor fluctuations ($p < 0.05$) and in patients with severe motor symptoms before surgery ($p < 0.05$); these findings suggest that PIGD patients at a late stage of PD would benefit less from the operation than LPS patients and an early recommendation for the operation for such subtype would be desirable. Given that motor function improvement with DBS manifests primarily in dopaminergic-related symptoms, it is conceivable to understand this result since for PIGD patients, the major symptoms such as falling, balancing dysfunction and gait disorders are axial symptoms, which are not completely alleviated by levodopa but also much related to non-dopamineric neurotransmitters [29, 31] and are involved in later stages of the disease [30–32].

One major shortcoming of our study was the small sample size of 23 patients, which decreased the p value of our statistical results. Other factors related to the surgical outcomes and the predictors reported in other studies may be confirmed through the statistical analysis of a larger patient population. Another limitation of this study was that we collected UPDRS III data but not UPDRS II and IV data, so other patient aspects were not evaluated. We expect that future studies with larger patient populations will confirm these findings.

Conclusions

The intensity of preoperative levodopa responsiveness served as a predictor of motor improvement more accurately in female patients, and patients with short disease duration or shorter motor fluctuations. Patients with dominant axial symptoms as PIGD ones benefit less from STN-DBS compared to those with limb-predominant symptoms, especially in their later disease stage or with more severe motor symptoms before surgery. So it is natural and reasonable to recommend the operation to levodopa-responsive patients especially the female, patients in early stage of disease and PIGD patients at their early stage.

Acknowledgments

We are grateful for support from Professor Chang-Zhong Chen and Dr. Xing-Lin Chen who come from the United States X&Y Solutions software company, we thank they for guidance on statistical analysis by EmpowerStats.

Funding

This study was funded by the National Nature Science Foundation of China (grant.no.81371421).

Authors' contributions

XLS: study design, data collection, statistical analysis and draft the manuscript. XGL: participated in study design, analysis of results and revision of manuscript. HL: manuscript revision. JW: design and implementation of surgical procedures. YR: critical revision of the manuscript for important intellectual content. ZYH: study supervision. All authors read and approved the final manuscript.

Competing interest

The authors declare that they have no competing interests.

Author details

[1]Department of Neurology, First Affiliated Hospital, China Medical University, China Medical University, 155 Nanjing North Street, Heping District, Shenyang 110001, China. [2]Department of Neurosurgery, First Affiliated Hospital, China Medical University, China Medical University, Shenyang, China.

References

1. Lang AE, Lozano AM. Parkinson's disease. First of two parts. New Engl J Med. 1998;339:1044–53.
2. Tao Y, Liang G. Effect of subthalamic nuclei electrical stimulation in the treatment of Parkinson's disease. Cell Biochem Biophys. 2015;71(1):113–7.
3. Chiou SM, Lin YC, Huang HM. One-year outcome of bilateral Subthalamic stimulation in Parkinson disease: an eastern experience. World Neurosurg. 2015;84(5):1294–8.
4. Kim HY, Chang WS, Kang DW, Sohn YH, Lee MS, Chang JW. Factors related to outcomes of subthalamic deep brain stimulation in Parkinson's disease. J Korean Neurosurg Soc. 2013;54(2):118–24.
5. Tir M, Devos D, Blond S, Touzet G, Reyns N, Duhamel A, Cottencin O, Dujardin K, Cassim F, Destée A, Defebvre L, Krystkowiak P. Exhaustive, one-year follow-up of subthalamic nucleus deep brain stimulation in a large, single-center cohort of parkinsonian patients. Neurosurgery. 2007; 61(2):297–304.
6. Li J, Zhang Y, Li Y. Long-term follow-up of bilateral subthalamic nucleus stimulation in Chinese Parkinson's disease patients. Br J Neurosurg. 2015; 29(3):329–33.
7. Jiang LL, Liu JL, Fu XL, Xian WB, Gu J, Liu YM, Ye J, Chen J, Qian H, Xu SH, et al. Long-term efficacy of Subthalamic nucleus deep brain stimulation in Parkinson's disease: a 5-year follow-up study in China. Chin Med J. 2015; 128(18):2433–8.
8. Charles PD, Blercom NV, Krack P, Lee SL, Xie J, Besson G, Benabid A-L, Pollak P. Predictors of effective bilateral subthalamic nucleusstimulation for PD. Neurology. 2002;59:932–4.
9. Tsai ST, Lin SH, Chou YC, Pan YH, Hung HY, Li CW, Lin SZ, Chen SY. Prognostic factors of subthalamic stimulation in Parkinson's disease: a comparative study between short- and long-term effects. Stereotact Funct Neurosurg. 2009;87(4):241–8.
10. Bronstein JM, Tagliati M, Alterman RL, Lozano AM, Volkmann J, Stefani A, Horak FB, Okun MS, Foote KD, Krack P, et al. Deep brain stimulation for Parkinson disease: an expert consensus and review of key issues. Arch Neurol. 2011;68(2):165.
11. Limousin P, Krack P, Pollak P, et al. Electrical stimulation of the Subthalamic nucleus in advanced Parkinson's disease. N Engl J Med. 1998;339:1105–11.
12. Hughes AJDS, Kilford L, Lees AJ. Accuracy of clinical diagnosis of idiopathic Parkinson's disease: a clinicopathological study of 100 cases. J Neurol Neurosurg Psychiatry. 1992;55(3):181–4.
13. Volkmann J, Moro E, Pahwa R. Basic algorithms for the programming of deep brain stimulation in Parkinson's disease. Mov Disord. 2006;21(Suppl 14):S284–9.
14. Langston JW, Widner H, Goetz CG, Brooks D, Fahn S, Freeman T, Watts R. Core assessment program for intracerebral transplantations (CAPIT). Mov Disord. 1992;7(1):2–13.
15. Albanese A, Bonuccelli U, Brefel C, Chaudhuri KR, FRCP CC, Eichhorn T, Melamed E, Pollak P, Laar TV, Zappia M. Consensus statement on the role of acute dopaminergicchallenge in Parkinson s disease. Mov Disord. 2001;16:197–201.
16. Merola A, Romagnolo A, Bernardini A, Rizzi L, Artusi CA, Lanotte M, Rizzone MG, Zibetti M, Lopiano L. Earlier versus later subthalamic deep brain stimulation in Parkinson's disease. Parkinsonism Relat Disord. 2015; 21(8):972–5.
17. Tomlinson CL, Stowe R, Patel S, Rick C, Gray R, Clarke CE. Systematic review of levodopa dose equivalency reporting in Parkinson's disease. Mov Disord. 2010;25(15):2649–53.
18. Jankovic J, McDermott M, Gauthier S, Goetz C, Golbe L, Huber S, Koller W, Olanow C, Shoulson I, Stern M, et al. Variable expression of Parkinson s disease: a base-line analysis of the DATATOP cohort. Neurology. 1990;40(10):1529–34.
19. Maetzler W, Liepelt I, Berg D. Progression of Parkinson's disease in the clinical phase potential markers. Lancet Neurol. 2009;8:1158–71.
20. Mestre TA, Espay AJ, Marras C, Eckman MH, Pollak P, Lang AE. Subthalamic nucleus-deep brain stimulation for early motor complications in Parkinson's disease-the EARLYSTIM trial: early is not always better. Mov Disord. 2014; 29(14):1751–6.
21. Deuschl G, Schupbach M, Knudsen K, Pinsker MO, Cornu P, Rau J, Agid Y, Schade-Brittinger C. Stimulation of the subthalamic nucleus at an earlier disease stage of Parkinson's disease: concept and standards of the EARLYSTIM-study. Parkinsonism Relat Disord. 2013;19(1):56–61.
22. Kleiner-Fisman G, Herzog J, Fisman DN, Tamma F, Lyons KE, Pahwa R, Lang AE, Deuschl G. Subthalamic nucleus deep brain stimulation: summary and meta-analysis of outcomes. Mov Disord. 2006;21(Suppl 14):S290–304.
23. Leranth CRR, Elsworth JD, Naftolin F, Horvath TL, Redmond DE Jr. Estrogen is essential for maintaining nigrostriatal dopamine neurons in primates: implications for Parkinson's disease and memory. J Neurosci. 2000;20:8604–9.
24. Henderson VW. The neurology of menopause. Neurologist. 2006;12(3):149–59.
25. Gillies GE, Murray HE, Dexter D, McArthur S. Sex dimorphisms in the neuroprotective effects of estrogen in an animal model of Parkinson's disease. Pharmacol Biochem Behav. 2004;78(3):513–22.
26. Yadav R, Shukla G, Goyal V, Singh S, Behari M. A case control study of women with Parkinson's disease and their fertility characteristics. J Neurol Sci. 2012;319(1–2):135–8.
27. Gerlach M, Riederer P. Animal models of Parkinson's disease: an empirical comparison with the phenomenology of the disease in man. J Neural Transm. 2006;103:987–1041.
28. Dluzen DE, McDermott JL, Liu B. Estrogen alters MPTP-induced neurotoxicity in female mice: effects on striatal dopamine concentrations and release. J Neurochem. 1996;66:658–66.
29. Bejjani BP, Gervais D, Arnulf I, Papadopoulos S, Demeret S, Bonnet AM, Cornu P, Damier P, Agid Y. Axial parkinsonian symptoms can be improved: the role of levodopa and bilateral subthalamic stimulation. J Neurol Neurosurg Psychiatry. 2000;68:595–600.
30. Devos D, Defebvre L, Bordet R. Dopaminergic and non-dopaminergic pharmacological hypotheses for gait disorders in Parkinson's disease. Fundam Clin Pharmacol. 2010;24(4):407–21.
31. Fasano A, Aquino CC, Krauss JK, Honey CR, Bloem BR. Axial disability and deep brain stimulation in patients with Parkinson disease. Nat Rev Neurol. 2015;11(2):98–110.
32. Coelho M, Ferreira JJ. Late-stage Parkinson disease. Nat Rev Neurol. 2012;8(8):435–42.

10

Is ApoE ε 4 a good biomarker for amyloid pathology in late onset Alzheimer's disease?

Maowen Ba[1,2†], Min Kong[3†], Xiaofeng Li[2,4], Kok Pin Ng[2,5], Pedro Rosa-Neto[2] and Serge Gauthier[2*]

Abstract

Amyloid plaques are pathological hallmarks of Alzheimer's Disease (AD) and biomarkers such as cerebrospinal fluid (CSF) β-amyloid 1–42 (Aβ1-42) and amyloid positron emission tomographic (PET) imaging are important in diagnosing amyloid pathology in vivo. ε4 allele of the Apolipoprotein E gene (ApoE ε 4), which is a major genetic risk factor for late onset AD, is an important genetic biomarker for AD pathophysiology. It has been shown that ApoE ε 4 is involved in Aβ deposition and formation of amyloid plaques. Studies have suggested the utility of peripheral blood ApoE ε 4 in AD diagnosis and risk assessment. However it is still a matter of debate whether ApoE ε 4 status would improve prediction of amyloid pathology and represent a cost-effective alternative to amyloid PET or CSF Aβ in resource-limited settings in late onset AD. Recent research suggest that the mean prevalence of PET amyloid-positivity is 95% in ApoE ε 4-positive AD patients. This short review aims to provide an updated information on the relationship between ApoE ε 4 and amyloid biomarkers.

Keywords: Apolipoprotein E ε4, Alzheimer's disease, Amyloid

Background

Alzheimer's disease (AD) is the most common neurodegenerative dementia, which severely impacts daily living. The medical cost for AD patients is also significantly high [1]. Advance in medical research have led to the discovery of biomarkers for the diagnosis of AD pathologies, such as decreased cerebrospinal fluid (CSF) β-amyloid 1–42 (Aβ1-42), positive amyloid positron emission tomographic (PET) imaging and presence of the Apolipoprotein E ε4 allele (ApoE ε 4) for amyloid pathology [2–6]. Aβ plaque is one of the main hallmarks of AD which is related to neuronal death [1, 7, 8]. CSF-Aβ1-42 and amyloid PET imaging are able to quantify the level of Aβ pathology while amyloid PET is able to show the distribution of Aβ deposits in the brain. However, the invasive examination of lumbar puncture and expensive tests of amyloid PET have restricted their use in clinical practice for AD diagnosis and risk assessment. The search for a cost effective biomarker with good prediction for AD pathology is the goal. ApoE ε 4 is one of the major and best-established genetic risk factor for late onset AD [9–11]. It has been shown that ApoE ε 4 is involved in Aβ deposition and the formation of amyloid plaques, which accounts for its role on the pathophysiology of AD and hence a potential biomarker for diagnosing amyloid pathology. Indeed, the development in neuroimaging technology has allowed us to assess the relationship between the ApoE ε 4 and amyloid PET imaging. This review aims to summarize the current evidences regarding the relationship between the ApoE ε 4 and amyloid biomarkers.

Back to basic: the effect of ApoE ε 4 on Aβ

ApoE ε 4, which is positive in > 40% AD cases, is one of the strongest genetic risk factor for AD among the three human ApoE isoforms (ε2, ε3 and ε4 allele) [12, 13]. Histopathological studies of AD brains show that ApoE ε 4 coexist with Aβ in amyloid plaques [14], demonstrating an association between ApoE ε 4 and Aβ in the pathological structure of AD. Epitope analysis shows that the 144–148 residues in the N-terminal region of ApoE ε 4 and the 13–17 residues in Aβ as the receptor-

* Correspondence: serge.gauthier@mcgill.ca
†Equal contributors
²McGill Centre for Studies in Aging, McGill University, Douglas Institute, 6825 Lasalle Boul, Montreal, QC H4H 1R3, Canada
Full list of author information is available at the end of the article

binding domain [15], are common sites that interact with each other. ApoE ε 4 plays a key role in AD pathophysiology because it is less effective in breaking down Aβ peptide compared to other ApoE isoforms, which results in an increased risk of formation of amyloid plaques. Meanwhile, ApoE ε 4-containing lipoprotein is seldom lipidated, which reduces its stability and this leads to a lower level of ApoE ε 4/Aβ complex. The decreased level of ApoE ε 4/Aβ complex further leads to the increased Aβ aggregation. Several in vivo studies have also clearly shown that when ApoE ε 4 deficient mice crosses with APP transgenic mice, there is decreased Aβ deposition compared to human ApoE ε 2 and ApoE ε 3 [13, 16]. On the other hand, human ApoE ε 4 overexpression increases Aβ deposition [16–19]. A further detailed quantitative research of Aβ homeostasis using in vivo microdialysis in human ApoE deficient and human amyloid precursor protein crossed mice showed that Aβ clearance reduced the most in mice with by ε 4 allele, followed by ε 3 and then ε 2 alleles. [20]. These findings clearly show the significant role of ApoE ε 4 in the formation of fibrillar Aβ [16, 19] which results in cognitive impairment.

Current in clinic: the association between ApoE ε 4 and Aβ

Low CSF Aβ1-42 and high amyloid PET imaging in the brain are biomarkers which may support the diagnosis of AD. With the advancement of amyloid PET imaging and amyloid ligands development, it is now possible to visualize amyloid plaques in vivo in the brain. As mentioned above, ApoE ε 4 is a major genetic risk factor for amyloid pathology in late onset AD [9–11]. The presence of one copy of the ApoE ε 4 allele increases the risk of late onset AD by about 3.7 times while the presence of two copies increases this risk by about 12 times as compared to the ApoE ε 3 isoform [21]. More importantly when compared with non-carriers, Aβ deposition and amyloid plaque formation is greater in ApoE ε 4 carriers. In the brain of ApoE ε4/ε4 AD patient, the level of Aβ oligomers is 2.7 times higher than ApoE ε3/ε3 AD patient and this corresponds to greater total amyloid plaque burden. This suggests that ApoE ε 4 influences Aβ oligomers metabolism. ApoE increases Aβ oligomers levels in an isoform dependent manner (ε 2 < ε 3 < ε 4) [22]. A report from the Alzheimer's Disease Neuroimaging Initiative (ADNI) database shows the influence of ApoE ε 4 dose on clinical and neuroimaging biomarkers across the AD spectrum (from cognitive normal to AD patients with severe cognitive impairment. ApoE ε 4 is associated with decreased CSF beta-amyloid (Aβ$_{1-42}$) and increased cerebral Aβ deposition across the AD spectrum. ApoE ε 4 increases cerebral amyloid-β (Aβ) deposition in all the stages of AD development, and also influences Aβ-initiated cascade of downstream neurodegenerative

effects, thereby increasing the risk of AD [2]. A recent meta-analysis also shows that ApoE ε 4 carriers (either 1 or both alleles) were significantly associated with increased amyloid PET deposition, suggesting its potential effects on cortical amyloid burden [23]. The difference of amyloid plaque burden between ApoE ε 4 carriers and ApoE ε 4 non carriers patients, may be explained that Aβ deposition starts earlier and continues for a longer time in ApoE ε 4 carriers. This theory is supported by the research in neuropathology and epidemiology, which showed earlier onset of disease and higher amyloid plaque burden in younger ApoE ε 4 carriers with AD. Another possible explaination for greater plaque burden in ApoE ε 4 carrier is that there may be a higher speed of amyloid deposition in ApoE ε 4 carriers over time in the process of disease [24–27]. Further studies are needed to investigate this relationship, including subgroups analyses according to diagnosis from a more homogeneous population. In contrary, one study showed the increased amyloid deposition in the frontal cortex in ApoE ε 4 noncarriers [28]. It appears contradictory that lack of the important genetic risk factor for AD is related to increased amyloid burden. It was explained that the inconsistent outcome could be associated with confounding factors interfering with demographic characteristics, different assay protocols and even the accuracy of clinical diagnosis.

Indeed, there is a very high concordance between amyloid PET and CSF Aβ in AD patients, as demonstrated in the research on Pittsburgh compound B imaging and cerebrospinal fluid amyloid-β in a multicentre European memory clinic study published in Brain [29]. Yet, clinicians are more concerned whether the knowledge of ApoE ε 4 status would improve prediction of amyloid status and represent a cost-effective alternative to amyloid PET or CSF Aβ in resource-limited settings. One recent meta-analysis published in JAMA [30], which pooled the results of 29 cohorts worldwide to assess the prevalence of PET amyloid-positivity of different dementia syndromes as a function of age and ApoE ε 4 status. With a total sample of 1359 patients with a clinical diagnosis of probable AD, the curves of PET amyloid-positivity were formed based on age and ApoE ε 4 status. The prevalence of PET amyloid-positivity is higher in clinically diagnosed AD patients especially when ApoE ε 4-positive. The mean prevalence of PET amyloid-positivity is 95% in ApoE ε 4-positive AD patients. The prevalence of PET amyloid-positivity is always above 90% from age 50 to age 90 in clinically diagnosed ApoE ε 4-positive AD potients. The data presented good concordance between ApoE ε 4 and PET amyloid-positivity. However, in ApoE ε 4-negative AD patients, the prevalence of PET amyloid-positivity decreased with age from 86% at age 50 to 68% at age 90. The mean prevalence of PET amyloid-positivity is 77% in

ApoE ε 4-negative AD patients. Although, the prevalence of amyloid-positivity is lower in older patients with clinically diagnosed AD, especially when ApoE ε 4-negative, which instead indicate that knowledge of ApoE ε 4 status would improve the positive predictive value of amyloid PET results in older patients with clinically diagnosed AD. The weakness of the research is that ApoE ε 4 status is dichotomized as either positive or negative, without regards to the dose of ApoE ε 4 alleles. The data from solanezumab phase 3 clinical trials clearly demonstrated that the dose of ApoE ε 4 alleles correlates with amyloid burden and diagnosis of AD [31]. The prevalence of PET amyloid-positivity is 98% in ApoE ε 4/4-positive AD patients. One table adapted from the Degenhardt publication summarized the information that the dose of ApoE ε 4 alleles is a good predictor of amyloid positivity (Table 1). ApoE ε 4 status are crucial factors when ordering clinical amyloid PET scans, especially in resource-limited settings.

Although, ApoE ε 4 genotype is associated with decreased CSF $A\beta_{1-42}$ in AD patients [2, 32–34]. There were no enough available reports to assess the prevalence of concordance of ApoE ε 4 and CSF $A\beta_{1-42}$-positivity in AD patients. Future research is still required to clarify the concordance of ApoE ε 4, CSF $A\beta_{1-42}$ and amyloid PET positivity in AD patients. When the concordance is clarified, thus blood ApoE ε 4 genotype biomarker as one economic testing can be helpful in AD patients when considering amyloid evaluation in clinical practice, especially when an anti-amyloid drug would be available.

Conclusions

In summary, these basic and clinic researches support that ApoE ε 4 is highly associated with amyloid pathology in the brain. Especially, in confirmed AD patients with ApoE ε 4+, ApoE ε 4 genotype positivity almost equals brain amyloid positivity from a qualitative point of view. Future research exploring the dose-effect association between ApoE ε 4 genotypes and amyloid neuropathology of AD, or in conjunction with other markers can help to better understand the pathophysiological role of ApoE ε 4 and improve the diagnostic accuracy in AD. Considering the above relationship, blood ApoE ε 4 genotype positivity is an important referred biomarker for

amyloid pathology and should be considered for use in AD diagnosis and future pre-treatment biological testing when an anti-amyloid drug will be available.

Acknowledgements
Not applicable

Funding
MWB is supported by Yantai Yuhuangding Hospital, China.
MK is supported by Yantai Yuhuangding Hospital, China.
XFL is supported by a Fellowship Program from Chongqing Medical University
KP Ng is supported by the National Medical Research Council (NMRC) Research Training Research
SG is supported by the Canadian Institutes for Health Research

Authors' contributions
MWB and MK made equal contributions to conception and design, acquisition of data, and in drafting the manuscript. XFL and KP Ng were involved in revising it critically for important intellectual content. SG and PRN was the general supervision of the research group. All authors read and approved the final manuscript.

Competing interests
The authors declare that they have no competing interests.

Author details
[1]Department of Neurology, Yuhuangding Hospital Affiliated to Qingdao Medical University, Qingdao, Shandong 264000, People's Republic of China. [2]McGill Centre for Studies in Aging, McGill University, Douglas Institute, 6825 Lasalle Boul, Montreal, QC H4H 1R3, Canada. [3]Department of Neurology, Yantaishan Hospital, Yantai City, Shandong 264000, People's Republic of China. [4]Department of Neurology, The Second Affiliated Hospital of Chongqing Medical University, Chongqing 400010, People's Republic of China. [5]Department of Neurology, National Neuroscience Institute Singapore, Singapore, Singapore.

Table 1 Three hundred seventy Subjects with clinical diagnosis of mild to moderate AD and known ApoE ε 4 genotype (adapted from the Degenhardt publication in Psychosomatics in 2016)

	Amyloid FBP PET positive*	Amyloid FBP PET negative*	Totals	Accuracy of clinical diagnosis
ApoE ε 4(−)	107	65	172	62%
ApoE ε 4(+/−)	133	18	151	88%
ApoE ε 4(+)	46	1	47	98%

References
1. Selkoe DJ. Preventing Alzheimer's disease. Science. 2012;337(6101):1488–92.
2. Liu Y et al. Multiple Effect of APOE Genotype on Clinical and Neuroimaging Biomarkers Across Alzheimer's Disease Spectrum. Mol Neurobiol. 2015;53(7): 4539–47. [Epub ahead of print].
3. Wilson RS, et al. The apolipoprotein E epsilon 4 allele and decline in different cognitive systems during a 6-year period. Arch Neurol. 2002;59(7):1154–60.
4. Shaw LM, et al. Cerebrospinal fluid biomarker signature in Alzheimer's disease neuroimaging initiative subjects. Ann Neurol. 2009;65(4):403–13.
5. Elias-Sonnenschein LS, Bertram L, Visser PJ. Relationship between genetic risk factors and markers for Alzheimer's disease pathology. Biomark Med. 2012;6(4):477–95.
6. Klunk WE, et al. Imaging brain amyloid in Alzheimer's disease with Pittsburgh Compound-B. Ann Neurol. 2004;55(3):306–19.
7. Finder VH. Alzheimer's disease: a general introduction and pathomechanism. J Alzheimers Dis. 2010;22 Suppl 3:5–19.
8. Holtzman DM, Morris JC, Goate AM. Alzheimer's disease: the challenge of the second century. Sci Transl Med. 2011;3(77):77sr1.
9. Bu G. Apolipoprotein E, and its receptors in Alzheimer's disease: pathways, pathogenesis and therapy. Nat Rev Neurosci. 2009;10(5):333–44.

10. Yu JT, Tan L, Hardy J. Apolipoprotein E in Alzheimer's disease: an update. Annu Rev Neurosci. 2014;37:79–100.

11. Kim J, Basak JM, Holtzman DM. The role of apolipoprotein E in Alzheimer's disease. Neuron. 2009;63(3):287–303.

12. Farrer LA, et al. Effects of age, sex, and ethnicity on the association between apolipoprotein E genotype and Alzheimer disease. A meta-analysis. APOE and Alzheimer Disease Meta Analysis Consortium. JAMA. 1997;278(16):1349–56.

13. Kanekiyo T, Xu H, Bu G. ApoE and Aβ in Alzheimer's disease: accidental encounters or partners? Neuron. 2014;81(4):740–54.

14. Namba Y, et al. Apolipoprotein E immunoreactivity in cerebral amyloid deposits and neurofibrillary tangles in Alzheimer's disease and kuru plaque amyloid in Creutzfeldt-Jakob disease. Brain Res. 1991;541(1):163–6.

15. Winkler K, et al. Competition of Abeta amyloid peptide and apolipoprotein E for receptor-mediated endocytosis. J Lipid Res. 1999;40(3):447–55.

16. Irizarry MC, et al. Modulation of A beta deposition in APP transgenic mice by an apolipoprotein E null background. Ann N Y Acad Sci. 2000;920:171–8.

17. Holtzman DM, et al. Apolipoprotein E isoform-dependent amyloid deposition and neuritic degeneration in a mouse model of Alzheimer's disease. Proc Natl Acad Sci U S A. 2000;97(6):2892–7.

18. Fagan AM, et al. Human and murine ApoE markedly alters A beta metabolism before and after plaque formation in a mouse model of Alzheimer's disease. Neurobiol Dis. 2002;9(3):305–18.

19. Bales KR, et al. Lack of apolipoprotein E dramatically reduces amyloid beta-peptide deposition. Nat Genet. 1997;17(3):263–4.

20. Castellano JM, et al. Human apoE isoforms differentially regulate brain amyloid-β peptide clearance. Sci Transl Med. 2011;3(89):89ra57.

21. Corder EH, et al. Gene dose of apolipoprotein E type 4 allele and the risk of Alzheimer's disease in late onset families. Science. 1993;261(5123):921–3.

22. Hashimoto T, et al. Apolipoprotein E, especially apolipoprotein E4, increases the oligomerization of amyloid β peptide. J Neurosci. 2012;32(43):15181–92.

23. Liu Y, et al. APOE genotype and neuroimaging markers of Alzheimer's disease: systematic review and meta-analysis. J Neurol Neurosurg Psychiatry. 2015;86(2):127–34.

24. Näslund J, et al. Characterization of stable complexes involving apolipoprotein E and the amyloid beta peptide in Alzheimer's disease brain. Neuron. 1995;15(1):219–28.

25. Rebeck GW, et al. Apolipoprotein E in sporadic Alzheimer's disease: allelic variation and receptor interactions. Neuron. 1993;11(4):575–80.

26. Ashford JW. APOE genotype effects on Alzheimer's disease onset and epidemiology. J Mol Neurosci. 2004;23(3):157–65.

27. Sando SB, et al. APOE epsilon 4 lowers age at onset and is a high risk factor for Alzheimer's disease; a case control study from central Norway. BMC Neurol. 2008;8:9.

28. Ossenkoppele R, et al. Differential effect of APOE genotype on amyloid load and glucose metabolism in AD dementia. Neurology. 2013;80(4):359–65.

29. Leuzy A, et al. Pittsburgh compound B imaging and cerebrospinal fluid amyloid-β in a multicentre European memory clinic study. Brain. 2016. doi: 10.1093/brain/aww160 [Epub ahead of print].

30. Ossenkoppele R, et al. Prevalence of amyloid PET positivity in dementia syndromes: a meta-analysis. JAMA. 2015;313(19):1939–49.

31. Degenhardt EK, et al. Florbetapir F18 PET amyloid neuroimaging and characteristics in patients with mild and moderate Alzheimer dementia. Psychosomatics. 2016;57(2):208–16.

32. Tapiola T, et al. Relationship between apoE genotype and CSF beta-amyloid (1–42) and tau in patients with probable and definite Alzheimer's disease. Neurobiol Aging. 2000;21(5):735–40.

33. Yassine HN, et al. The effect of APOE genotype on the delivery of DHA to cerebrospinal fluid in Alzheimer's disease. Alzheimers Res Ther. 2016;8:25. doi:10.1186/s13195-016-0194-x.

34. Mehrabian S, et al. Cerebrospinal fluid biomarkers for Alzheimer's disease: the role of apolipoprotein E genotype, age, and sex. Neuropsychiatr Dis Treat. 2015;11:3105–10.

11

7,8-dihydroxyflavone, a small molecular TrkB agonist, is useful for treating various BDNF-implicated human disorders

Chaoyang Liu[1], Chi Bun Chan[2] and Keqiang Ye[3]*

Abstract

Brain-derived neurotrophic factor (BDNF) regulates a variety of biological processes predominantly via binding to the transmembrane receptor tyrosine kinase TrkB. It is a potential therapeutic target in numerous neurological, mental and metabolic disorders. However, the lack of efficient means to deliver BDNF into the body imposes an insurmountable hurdle to its clinical application. To address this challenge, we initiated a cell-based drug screening to search for small molecules that act as the TrkB agonist. 7,8-Dihydroxyflavone (7,8-DHF) is our first reported small molecular TrkB agonist, which has now been extensively validated in various biochemical and cellular systems. Though binding to the extracellular domain of TrkB, 7,8-DHF triggers TrkB dimerization to induce the downstream signaling. Notably, 7,8-DHF is orally bioactive that can penetrate the brain blood barrier (BBB) to exert its neurotrophic activities in the central nervous system. Numerous reports suggest 7,8-DHF processes promising therapeutic efficacy in various animal disease models that are related to deficient BDNF signaling. In this review, we summarize our current knowledge on the binding activity and specificity, structure-activity relationship, pharmacokinetic and metabolism, and the pre-clinical efficacy of 7,8-DHF against some human diseases.

Keywords: Flavonoids, Neurotrophin, BDNF, Mimetic compound, Receptor agonistic activity

Background

Neurotrophins (NT) are growth factors that regulate the development and maintenance of the peripheral and the central nervous systems [1]. It is a family of secretary proteins that includes brain-derived neurotrophic factor (BDNF), nerve growth factor (NGF), NT-3, and NT-4/NT-5 [2]. BDNF exerts its biological functions on neurons through two transmembrane receptors: the p75 neurotrophin receptor (p75NTR) and the TrkB receptor tyrosine kinase, while NGF binds to TrkA, NT-4/5 binds to TrkB, and NT-3 preferentially binds to TrkC [3, 4]. TrkB is one of the most widely distributed neurotrophic receptors (NTRs) in the brain, which is highly enriched in the neocortex, hippocampus, striatum, and brainstem [5]. Binding of BDNF to TrkB receptor triggers its dimerization through conformational changes and auto-phosphorylation of tyrosine residues in the intracellular domain, resulting in activation of signaling pathways involving mitogen-activated protein kinase (MAPK), phosphatidylinositol 3-kinase (PI3K) and phospholipase C-γ (PLC-γ).

BDNF is of particular therapeutic interest because of its neurotrophic actions on a number of neuronal populations including sensory neurons (implicated in peripheral sensory neuropathies [6]); motor neurons which are degenerated in amyotrophic lateral sclerosis (ALS) [7]; dopaminergic neurons of the substantia nigra, which are lost in Parkinson's disease (PD); and cholinergic neurons of the basal forebrain, that play a significant role in in Alzheimer's disease (AD) [8]. Moreover, BDNF protects hippocampal neurons from glutamate toxicity [9], rescues cerebellar neurons from programmed cell death [10], reduces ischemic neuronal injury [11, 12] and improves functional recovery from postinjury regeneration [13]. Thus, BDNF may represent a beneficial therapeutic agent against a variety of human disorders such as ALS, AD, PD, fetal alcohol exposure, autism and schizophrenia [14]. However, the outcomes of several clinical trials using

* Correspondence: kye@emory.edu
[3]Department of Pathology and Laboratory Medicine, Emory University School of Medicine, 615 Michael Street, Atlanta, GA 30322, USA
Full list of author information is available at the end of the article

recombinant BDNF are disappointing [15, 16], possibly because of the poor delivery and short in vivo half-life of BDNF. In addition, BDNF binds to p75NTR, a promiscuous NTR that is known to activate cell death pathways via recruitment of multiple adaptor proteins [17, 18]. To address these problems, tremendous effort has been made to generate selective agonists of TrkB including monoclonal antibodies [19] and peptide mimetics [20, 21] . Based on the fact that a monocyclic monomeric peptide resembling the a single loop of BDNF (loop 2) acts as an inhibitor of BDNF-mediated neuronal survival, O'Leary and Hughes designed bicyclic dimeric peptides that mimic a pair of solvent-exposed loops for the binding and activation of TrkB. These dimeric peptides behave as partial agonists of TrkB with respect to BDNF, which promotes the survival of embryonic chick sensory neurons in culture [20]. Recently, the tandem repeat peptide agonist approach has been employed for designing BDNF/NT-4/5 mimetics but none of these peptidyl compound exhibit satisfactory in vivo agonistic effect on TrkB [22]. Adenosine and pituitary adenylate cyclase-activating peptide (PACAP) has also been reported to transactivate TrkB in cultured hippocampal neurons, however, this G protein-coupled receptor ligand does not act as TrkB agonists as it only activates an immature form of TrkB after 1 h treatment [23–25].

To search for small molecules that mimic the biological functions of BDNF, we developed a cell-based TrkB receptor-dependent survival assay system, and used it to screen a chemical library via counter screening. The positive hits were then subjected to TrkB activation analysis in primary neurons and receptor binding assays. Finally, we identified two lead compounds: 7,8-dihydroxyflavone and deoxygedunin [26, 27], which bind to the receptor extracellular domain of TrkB, promote the receptor dimerization and autophosphorylation, and activate the downstream signaling cascades. Due to its commercial availability, and the favorable chemical and physical characteristics, 7,8-DHF is has been extensively explored in a variety of cell types and disease models since its first report in 2010 [26]. In the current review, we will summarize the main biochemical, physiological, pharmacological and functional activities of 7,8-DHF. Its therapeutic potentials against neurological and metabolic disorders will also be discussed.

Discovery of TrkB receptor agonists

In order to identify small molecules that mimic the neurotrophic activities of BDNF, we developed a cell-based survival assay using a cell permeable fluorescent dye MR(DERD)2, which produces red signal upon caspase-3 cleavage in apoptotic cells. TrkB-lacking SN56 cells (a fusion of N18TG2 neuroblastoma cells with mouse neurons from postnatal day 21- septa) and its

derived cell line T48 (which is stably transfected with TrkB) were utilized in our assay. We cultured the cells in 96-well plates and pre-incubated the cells with compounds from a library for 30 min, followed by staurosporine (STS) treatment for 9 h. MR(DEVD)2 was introduced to the cells 1 h before examination under fluorescent microscope. The apoptotic cells could be detected by the red signal, while the live cells had no signal. Using this caspase-activated fluorescent dye as a visual assay, we screened thousands of compounds from the Spectrum Collection library. Sixty-six compounds were found to selectively protect T48, but not SN56 cells, from STS-initiated apoptosis, indicating that these compounds might act either directly through TrkB receptor or its downstream signaling effectors. These positive hits were further analyzed on primary hippocampal neurons for TrkB activation and neuronal survival. 7,8-DHF is one of the positive compounds that specifically activate TrkB, but not TrkA or TrkC, at a concentration of 250 nM. It is also a bioavailable chemical that can pass through the BBB to provoke TrkB and its downstream PI3K/Akt and MAPK activation in mouse brain (cortex, hippocampus and hypothalamus) upon intraperitoneal or oral administration. In addition to cortical and hippocampal neurons, 7,8-DHF also protects other cell types including the RGC (retinal ganglion cells) and PC12 cells from excitotoxic and oxidative stress-induced apoptosis and cell death [28–30]. Fitting with these in vitro neuroprotective actions, 7,8-DHF protects the RGC cells from excitotoxic and oxidative stress-induced apoptosis in retinal glaucoma model in a TrkB-dependent manner [28]. Moreover, 7,8-DHF promotes the survival and reduces apoptosis in cortical neurons of TBI (traumatic brain injury) as administration of 7,8-DHF at 3 h post-injury reduces brain tissue damage via the PI3K/Akt pathway [31].

To demonstrate that 7,8-DHF indeed is a TrkB specific agonist, we performed in vitro filter binding assay with [3H]-labeled 7,8-DHF and purified recombinant TrkB ECD (extracellular domain) proteins. We showed that 7,8-DHF has a K_d of ~320 nM toward TrkB with a binding ratio of 1:1 (ligand versus receptor). Similarly, Biocore Surface Plasmon Resonance (SPR) and fluorescent quenching assay support the notion that 7,8-DHF directly binds to TrkB ECD with Kd about 15.4 nM. As the positive control, BDNF displays a Kd of approximately 1.7 nM. These assays also demonstrated that 7,8-DHF but not 5,7-DHF (5,7-dihydroxyflavone) interacts with TrkB but not TrkA [32]. The different binding affinities of 7,8-DHF towards TrkB obtained in these assays might be a result of distinctive binding principles and experimental conditions. Mapping assays further suggest that 7,8-DHF may directly interact with LRM/CC2 regions of TrkB ECD [26], a finding that is further supported by an subsequent molecular modeling and docking analysis [33]. Utilizing TrkB-Fc, a His-tagged fusion protein of human TrkB-ECD (C32-H430), and human IgG1 that can specifically neutralize BDNF's agonistic effect on TrkB, we demonstrated that these agents can antagonize 7,8-DHF's stimulatory effect, emphasizing that 7,8-DHF exerts its agonistic activity via binding to TrkB receptor. We tried to determine the co-crystal structure of 7,8-DHF and TrkB ECD but no satisfactory results were obtained possibly because of the highly glycosylated nature of TrkB receptor. Nevertheless, all these independent experiments strongly support that 7,8-DHF indeed preferentially interacts with TrkB but not TrkA or TrkC receptors. Since no interaction or functional studies have been performed between 7,8-DHF and the low affinity BDNF receptor p75NTR, it remains unknown if 7,8-DHF also activates p75NTR as well.

TrkB receptor internalization by 7,8-DHF

Internalization of the neurotrophin–Trk complex plays a critical role in signal transduction that initiates cell body responses to target-derived neurotrophins. The neurotrophin–Trk complex is internalized through clathrin-mediated endocytosis, leading to the formation of signaling endosomes [34, 35]. Using two independent approaches, we demonstrated that 7,8-DHF treatment triggers an internalization of activated TrkB to the early endosomes [32]. First, we analyzed TrkB receptor endocytosis in primary neurons upon BDNF or 7,8-DHF stimulation using microscopic measurement. While internalized TrkB receptors colocalized with EEA1, the early endosome marker, kinetic quantification of the co-localized TrkB/EEA1 indicates that BDNF is more potent than 7,8-DHF in stimulating TrkB internalization and early endosomes delivery in the first 10 min. At 60 min stimulation, both BDNF and 7,8-DHF substantially increase TrkB endocytosis and its early endosomal residency but 7,8-DHF seems more robust than BDNF. Second, we performed the biotinylation assay by labeling the surface protein with sulfo-NHS-SS-biotin, followed by BDNF or 7,8-DHF stimulation. Internalized biotinylated proteins were then precipitated with streptavidin, and analyzed by immunoblotting with anti-TrkB antibody against its ECD domain. Concur with the microscopic detection, both BDNF and 7,8-DHF strongly escalate TrkB internalization.

BDNF treatment elicits TrkB receptor ubiquitination and degradation [36–39]. Our recent report found that BDNF induced TrkB ubiquitination 10 min after stimulation [32]. Its ubiquitination signals tightly correlates with its Y817 phosphorylation pattern. Accordingly, the total level of TrkB is evidently reduced at 180 min, fitting with the previous findings [36–39]. 7,8-DHF treatment swiftly induces TrkB phosphorylation and the

activation sustains for more than 3 h without inducing TrkB ubiquitination or degradation; by contrast, BDNF-triggered TrkB Y817 phosphorylation with a peak signal at 10 min, decreases at 60 min and fades away at 180 min. Clearly, these findings support that 7,8-DHF and BDNF activate TrkB with different mechanisms. It remains unclear how the activated TrkB signaling induced by 7,8-DHF is turned off eventually. Conceivably, 7,8-DHF and BDNF may induce differential to dephosphorylate the phosphorylated tyrosine residues of TrkB in the signalsomes within the cytoplasms.

Structure-activity relationship (SAR) study of 7,8-DHF

Flavonoids are a large group of polyphenolic compounds containing a basic flavan nucleus with two aromatic rings (the A and the B rings) interconnected by a three-carbon-atom heterocyclic ring (the C ring). Flavonoids are divided into several big categories including flavone, flavonol, flavanone, flavanonol, flavans, anthocyanidins and isoflavonoids. 5,7-dihydroxylation is commonly found on the A ring, but 7-hydroxy ring is common in the isoflavonoids subgroups. The B ring generally has 4′-, 3′,4′- or a 3′,4′5′-hydroxylation pattern. Rare flavonoids like 7,8-DHF lack B-ring oxygenation. Flavonoids are the largest and the most diverse class of plant secondary metabolites. These compounds are naturally present in vegetables, fruits, and beverages. Bioflavonoids have been known for a long time to exert diverse biological effects. In particular, they are antioxidants and preventive agents against cancer [40]. Accumulating evidence suggests that flavonoids have the potential to improve human memory and neuro-cognitive performance via protecting the vulnerable neurons, enhancing neuronal function and stimulating neuronal regeneration [41]. Flavonoids also exert effects on LTP, one of the major mechanisms underlying learning,memory and cognitive performance through their interactions with the signaling pathways like PI 3-kinase/Akt [42], MAPK [43, 44] and PKC [45], etc.

The widespread distribution of flavonoids, their variety and their relatively low toxicity compared to other active plant compounds (e.g. alkaloids) mean that many animals, including humans, ingest significant quantities in their diet. Therefore, we tested a number of commercially available flavonoids for their TrkB agonistic activities. Our preliminary structural-activity relationship (SAR) study showed that the 7,8-dihydroxy groups are essential for the agonistic effect. We also found that the 8-hydroxy group in A ring is essential for the TrkB stimulatory effect, as 5,7-DHF, 5,6-DHF and 5,6,7-THF could not activate TrkB. The dihydroxy groups in B ring displays relatively higher TrkB agonistic activity when compared to compounds with dihydroxy groups in A ring. None of the single hydroxy flavone derivatives exhibited notable TrkB stimulatory effect and no trihydroxy flavones or dimethoxy flavones demonstrated any substantial effect [46].

The presence of 4'-position amino group enhances the agonistic effect of 7,8-DHF [46], which cannot be replaced by a hydroxy group. Interestingly, the 3' position hydroxy group escalates 7,8-DHF's agonistic activity and improves the hearing of animals thorough protecting spiral ganglion neurons from degeneration [46–48]. It is worth noting that the oxygen atom in C ring is also essential for the stimulatory activity as replacing this O atom with NH group abolishes the agonistic activity of 7,8-DHF. Together, our SAR study suggests that the catechol group (7,8-dihydroxy in A ring) might be indispensable for the agonistic activity and the 4'-hydroxy group on B ring reduces, whereas 3'-hydroxy group increases its activity.

To optimize the lead compound and conduct more comprehensive SAR studies, we synthesized dozens of 7,8-DHF derivatives via medicinal chemistry. The first generation of the optimized derivative is 4'-dimethylamino-7,8-DHF, which possesses higher agonistic effect on TrkB than the parental compound 7,8-DHF with longer in vivo activity. Because catechol group containing compounds usually possess poor pharmacokinetic profiles, as a part of our effort to optimize the lead compound 4'-dimethylamino-7,8-DHF, we synthesized numerous bioisoteres of this compound to enhance its biological or physical properties. Replacing the 7,8-dihydroxy groups with imidazole or urea ring in A-ring elevates the TrkB agonistic activity than the lead compound. Since the 4'-dimethylamino group is prone to demethylation during metabolism, we replaced the dimethylamino group with a pyrrolidino or monomethylamino group to address this potential issue. Several rounds of organic synthesis of 7,8-DHF derivatives have been performed and we have obtained a couple of synthetic benzo-imidazole derivatives displaying EC50 of about 5–10 nM in primary neurons (unpublished data). Their in vivo pharmacokinetic (PK) profiles and oral bioavailability are now under investigation.

Cytotoxicity of 7,8-DHF

7,8-DHF treatment did not induce any apparent toxicity in mice. In one of our studies, we compared the pathological changes induced by 7,8-DHF after feeding C57BL/6 mice at 5 mg/kg for 3 weeks. No adverse pathological change was detectable in the drug-treated kidney, liver, lung, muscle, spleen, cortex, hippocampus, heart, intestine and testis [46]. In addition, the complete blood count (CBC) analysis showed that there is no significant difference between drug-treated and the control saline-treated mice [49]. In another long-term feeding

experiment, female mice receiving ~ 2.4 μg 7,8-DHF/day for 20 weeks also displayed normal CBC values [49]. These data support that 7,8-DHF is not toxic to the mice during the chronic treatment. Titration experiment also reveal that 7,8-DHF does not inhibit HEK293 cell proliferation at a dose up to 50 μM [46].

Pharmacokinetics of 7,8-DHF

To study the 7,8-DHF's PK profiles, we have performed a panel of in vitro ADMET assays. We found that 7,8-DHF is stable in liver microsomal assay but labile in hepatocytes, indicating that 7,8-DHF might be readily subjected to secondary modification-conjugation. Caco-2 permeability assay, parallel artificial membrane permeability assay (PAMPA) and PAMPA-BBB assays demonstrate that 7,8-DHF possess reasonable absorption rate and is able to penetrate BBB [50]. MDR1-MDCKII permeability assay also indicates that 7,8-DHF is a weak P-glycoprotein (Pgp) substrate (unpublished data). hERG assay reveals that 7,8-DHF exhibits IC_{50} >25 μM. CYP inhibition and induction assays reveal that 7,8-DHF has no time-dependent inhibition nor induction on major CYP enzymes. Concur with this result, 12 months chronic treatment or high dose acute treatment with 7,8-DHF suggests that 7,8-DHF is non-toxic to the rodents.

In vivo PK study shows that plasma 7,8-DHF concentration peaks at 10 min with 70 ng/ml, and brain 7,8-DHF also climaxes at 10 min with concentration of 50 ng/g of brain. 7,8-DHF in plasma can still be detected after 8 h (5 ng/ml) after administration. In contrast, only 7 ng/g of 7,8-DHF can be found in brain at 4 h and it is below the quantitative limit at 6 h [50]. In vivo metabolism study shows that 7,8-DHF is subjected to glucuronidation, sulfation and methylation [33]. Among these modifications, glucuronidation and sulfation are mainly responsible for the in vivo clearance of the flavonoids. Indeed, O-methylated metabolites including 7-methoxy-8-hydroxy-flavone (7M8H-flavone) and 7-hydroxy-8-methoxy-flavone (7H8M-flavone) can be detected in both the plasma and brain samples after oral administration of 7,8-DHF. Interestingly, these monomethylated metabolites are still active in triggering TrkB activation in primary neurons and mouse brain [50].

Catechol containing compounds usually have short in vivo half-life and are prone to be cleared in the circulation system after oxidation, glucoronidation, sulfation or methylation. For instance, Apomorphine is a catechol-containing non-narcotic morphine derivative that acts as a potent dopaminergic agonist. Its metabolism occurs through several enzymatic pathways, including N-demethylation, sulfation, glucuronidation, and catechol-O-methyltransferase as well as by nonenzymatic oxidation [51]. L-DOPA is the mainstay of Parkinson's disease (PD) therapy; this drug is usually administered orally, but it is extensively metabolized in the gastrointestinal tract, so that relatively little arrives in the bloodstream as intact L-DOPA. To minimize the conversion to dopamine outside the central nervous system, L-DOPA is usually given in combination with inhibitors of amino acid decarboxylase and COMT (catechol methyltransferase) [52]. Our preliminary in vivo PK study revealed that 7,8-DHF has $t_{1/2}$ more than 2 h in mouse circulation after oral administration [50]. Conceivably, glucuronidation, sulfation and methylation pathways may explain the relative short half-life of 7,8-DHF and its synthetic derivatives.

To improve the poor PK profiles intrinsic to catechol-containing molecules, we synthesized numerous prodrugs by modifying 7,8-dihydroxy groups with esters, carbamates or phosphates to improve the oral bioavailability and brain exposure of 7,8-DHF. Currently, an optimal prodrug R7 has been found with favorable in vitro ADMET (absorption, distribution, metabolism, excretion and toxicity) characteristics. R7 exhibits approximately 18 % oral bioavailability with C_{max} of 1554.9 ng/ml, T_{max} of 0.28 h and $T_{1/2}$ for PO of 2.32 h. Noticeably, 7,8-DHF plasma concentration released from R7 (PO, 50 mg/kg) is much higher than orally administrating the same dose of parent 7,8-DHF. The oral bioavailability is increased from 4.6 % (parental 7,8-DHF) to 84.2 % (R7). Accordingly, the brain exposure for 7,8-DHF is significantly increased by R7 than the parent compound upon oral administration of comparable dosage (unpublished data). TrkB and its downstream p-Akt/p-MAPK signalings are potently activated upon oral administration of R7, which is tightly correlating with 7,8-DHF concentrations in the animal brain. R7-provoked TrkB activation also fits well with the in vivo PK data, underscoring that the released 7,8-DHF from R7 prodrug triggers a long-lasting TrkB signalings in the mouse brain. This prodrug is now under preclinical IND-enabling study for the indication of Alzheimer's disease.

7,8-DHF displays robust therapeutic efficacy toward Alzheimer's disease

There is mounting evidence that 7,8-DHF mimics the physiological activities of BDNF and exhibits promising therapeutic efficacy toward various neurological diseases including Parkinson's disease (PD) [26], Huntington's disease (HD) [27], ALS (Amyotrophic lateral sclerosis) [53, 54], Alzheimer's disease (AD) [55–58], Posttraumatic Stress Disorder (PTSD) [59], and Rett Syndrome [60]. Moreover, 7,8-DHF displays therapeutic effect toward axon regeneration [61], and spiral ganglion degeneration [48]. Noticeably, it also demonstrates therapeutic activities in mental diseases like depression [33, 56, 62, 63]. Here, we focus on discussing its effects in treating AD, the leading cause of dementia worldwide, which is characterized by the accumulation of the β-amyloid peptide (Aβ) within the brain along with deposition of hyperphosphorylated and cleaved microtubule-associated protein Tau. It is suggested that

reductions of BDNF content or TrkB inactivation may play a role in the pathogenesis of AD. Indeed, BDNF expression is reduced in the brain of AD patients and delivery of BDNF gene has been shown as a novel potential therapeutic in diverse models related to AD [64]. BDNF also displays a protective role against AD pathogenesis by increasing learning and memory of demented animals [65]. Thus, these preclinical evidence strongly supports that BDNF might be useful as a therapeutic agent for treating AD.

Reduced acetylcholine neurotransmission due to loss of neurons in the basal forebrain and depletion of choline acetyltransferase are observed in AD pathology. Currently, there are two types of medication to treat AD: cholinesterase inhibitors and NMDA antagonist. However, these drugs can only delay the inevitable symptomatic progression of the disease without eliminating the main neuropathological hallmarks of the disease (i.e. formation of senile plaques and neurofibrillary tangles) nor rescuing the neuronal loss. 7,8-DHF potently stimulates hippocampal progenitor neurogenesis. For instance, oral administration of 7,8-DHF (5 mg/kg) in wild-type C57BL/6 J mice for a few weeks strongly induces neurogenesis [46]. Intraperitoneal administration of 7,8-DHF also elicits robust neurogenesis in depressive vulnerable or non-vulnerable rat [62]. This neurotrophic effect by 7,8-DHF has also been observed in APP/PS1 AD mouse model [66]. Devi and Ohno showed that 7,8-DHF rescued memory deficits in transgenic mice that co-express five familial Alzheimer's disease mutations (5XFAD) during the spontaneous alternation Y-maze task. In addition, 7,8-DHF restores deficient TrkB signaling in 5XFAD mice without affecting endogenous BDNF levels. While 5XFAD mice exhibit elevations in the β-secretase enzyme (BACE1) that initiates amyloid-β (Aβ) generation, as observed in sporadic AD, 7,8-DHF blocks BACE1 elevations and lowers the levels of the β-secretase-cleaved C-terminal fragment of amyloid precursor protein (C99), Aβ40, and Aβ42 in the brains of these mice. Most strikingly, they demonstrated that BACE1 expression can be decreased by 7,8-DHF administration in wild-type mice, suggesting that BDNF-TrkB signaling is also important for downregulating baseline levels of BACE1. Hence, this study supports that TrkB activation with systemic 7,8-DHF administration can ameliorate AD-associated memory deficits, attributable to reductions in BACE1 expression and β-amyloidogenesis [55]. Nevertheless, the authors employed a subchronic paradigm (10 days intraperitonial injection) in aged 5X FAD mice (12–15 months old mice). Since 5X FAD mice develop amyloid plaques at 2 months old and exhibit cognitive defects at 5 months of age, we employed a different treatment strategy: feeding the mice at 2-months-old till 5-months-old and monitored the cognitive activity in

Morris Water maze. In addition, we examined the amyloid plaque deposit, synapse formation and long-term potentiation (LTP) at the end of the treatment. Our data showed that 7,8-DHF protects primary neurons from Aβ-induced cell death and promotes dendrite branching and synaptogenesis. Chronic oral administration of 7,8-DHF activates TrkB signaling and prevents Aβ deposition in 5XFAD mice [56]. In alignment with these findings, 7,8-DHF significantly increases spine density and reduces synaptic and neuronal loss in Cam/Tet-DTA, an inducible model of severe neuronal loss in hippocampus and cortex, and demonstrates substantial improvements in spatial memory in the lesioned mice [58]. These results strongly suggest that 7,8-DHF represents a novel oral bioactive therapeutic agent for treating AD.

7,8-DHF inhibits obesity through activating muscular TrkB

Obesity is a metabolic disorder with increasing prevalence worldwide. According to the World Health Organization (WHO), more than 39 % (~1.9 billion) of adults are overweight. Of these, over 600 million (~13 %) are obese in 2014. These numbers have been doubled since 1980. Therefore, developing effective pharmacotherapy to control excess body weight gain is a hot research direction nowadays.

In addition to the neurotrophic activities, BDNF/TrkB signaling also plays a critical role in food intake and body weight control. In rodents, pharmacological treatments with BDNF induce a reduction of food intake, whereas genetic models with reduced BDNF/TrkB signaling display hyperphagia and obesity [67, 68]. Recent evidence indicates that BDNF acts as an energy metabolism regulator in both CNS and peripheral organs. It has been reported that BDNF levels are low in obesity or patients with type 2 diabetes [68, 69]. BDNF is expressed in non-neurogenic tissues, including skeletal muscle, and exercise increases BDNF levels in brain, plasma and skeletal muscle. Pederson et al. reported that BDNF increased phosphorylation of AMP-activated protein kinase (AMPK) and acetyl coenzyme A carboxylase (ACC) and enhanced fatty oxidation both in vitro and *ex vivo*. These data points to the fact that BDNF is a contraction-inducible protein in skeletal muscle that is capable of enhancing lipid oxidation via activation of AMPK. Thus, BDNF appears to be an active player in both neurobiology and peripheral metabolism [70].

Because BDNF has anti-obesity activity by suppressing food intake, we thus initiated a test to see if 7,8-DHF can be used to prevent the development of obesity. We investigated the effect of 7,8-DHF (drinking the dissolved 7,8-DHF in water) on mouse body weight gain under chow diet or high-fat diet (HFD) feeding for 6 months [49]. To our surprise, 7,8-DHF consumption does not suppress food intake, which is in contrast to

BDNF administration. Nevertheless, we found that 7,8-DHF significantly decreases the body weight gain in both chow diet and HFD paradigms, with more striking effect on HFD. The white adipocyte tissue (WAT) mass is significantly decreased about 20–30 % in 7,8-DHF-treated HFD group. Indirect calorimetry study showed that 7,8-DHF treatment decreases RER (respiratory exchange ratio), favoring the usage of lipid as the main fuel. Our study also reveals the mechanism of the anti-obesity actions by 7,8-DHF. By performing experiments in animal model and cell culture (C2C12) system, we identified that 7,8-DHF mainly acts on the muscle TrkB receptors to induce uncoupling protein 1 (UCP1) expression and activates AMP-activated protein kinase (AMPK). As a result, the energy expenditure and lipid oxidation in 7,8-DHF activated muscle cells are increased, leading to the lean phenotype observed. Unexpectedly, this anti-obesity effect is predominantly associated with female mice but not male mice, presumably due to estrogen content of the animals. Mice with 7,8-DHF treatment also exhibit improved blood insulin concentration, lower blood glucose level and increased insulin sensitivity in tissues such as liver, fat and muscles, suggesting 7,8-DHF is effective in alleviating the obesity-induced diabetes as well. These exciting findings identify a new function of BDNF/TrkB signaling in the skeletal muscle that the cascade controls cellular energy expenditure, which also provides the preclinical evidence that 7,8-DHF administration is an effective means to suppress body weight gain during energy surplus.

Perspectives and future directions

7,8-DHF is a broadly validated small molecule that imitates the biological functions of BDNF via directly binding to the TrkB ECD to trigger TrkB receptor dimerization and autophosphorylation [26]. It simulates the physiological functions of BDNF like promoting neuronal survival, elevating synaptogenesis and LTP on aged hippocampal slides and enhancement of learning and memory [26, 71, 72]. More important, 7,8-DHF displays a robust therapeutic efficacy in numerous neurological and metabolic diseases. However, it should be noted that the dosage of 7,8-DHF in clinical application has to be determined carefully as over-activation of the TrkB signaling may result in devastating consequences. In transgenic mice that overexpress BDNF in the forebrain, the animals exhibit spatial learning deficits at 2–3 months of age, followed by the emergence of spontaneous seizures at ~6 months, which is possibility a result of neuronal hyperexciation [73–75]. Because BDNF acts at central synapses in pain pathways both at spinal and supraspinal levels, prolonged TrkB activation may also interfere with the nociception pathway, leading to pain hypersensitivity [76].

Further investigations on the biochemical and mechanistic natures of 7,8-DHF are also necessary to boost its applications. For instance, the precise molecular details of how 7,8-DHF induces TrkB dimerization and activation are still unclear. For instance, how could 7,8-DHF mimic so many aspects of the physiological activities of the macromolecule BDNF, given that 7,8-DHF is only 254 dalton, which is 1 % of polypeptide hormone BDNF in size? Further, the tyrosine phosphorylated residues on TrkB intracellular domain and their relative abundance are different after BDNF and 7,8-DHF stimulations [32]. What downstream effects may these molecular differences incur in view that although both PI3K/Akt and MAPK downstream pathways are activated? Clearly, further biochemical investigations into these aspects are undoubtedly needed. Additional medicinal chemistry work is also required for optimizing this promising lead compound into a nanomolar binding affinity small molecular clinical candidate, which will not only provide an innovative pharmacological intervention for treating various human disorders but also present a useful tool for dissecting the biological actions of BDNF/TrkB signalings. For example, the availability of a TrkB PET tracer, which does not exist currently, would accelerate TrkB therapeutic development and provide insight into the role of TrkB and its expression levels in neuropsychiatric and neurodegenerative diseases, as well monitoring the change of TrkB levels during antidepressant or therapeutic neuro-regeneration treatments.

Conclusions

7,8-dihydroxyflavone is a promising small molecular BDNF mimetic compound, which fully mimics the physiological actions of BDNF from neuronal survival, synpatogenesis, axonal regeneration etc. Notably, it is orally bioactive and is safe for chronic treatment. It has been extensively validated in various BDNFimplicated disease models. Hence, it acts as a good lead compound for further medicinal modification for optimizing its therapeutic efficacy toward various BDNF-mediated human disorders.

Competing interests
The authors declare no any conflict of interest.

Authors' contributions
CL prepared literature and wrote the draft; CBC and KY wrote the manuscript. All authors read and approved the final manuscript.

Acknowledgements
This work is supported by grant from National Institute of Health (NS045627) to KYe.

Author details
[1]School of Information and Safety Engineering, Zhongnan University of Economics and Law, Wuhan 430073, P.R. China. [2]Department of Physiology, University of Oklahoma Health Sciences Center, 940 Stanton L. Young Blvd., Oklahoma City, OK 73104, USA. [3]Department of Pathology and Laboratory Medicine, Emory University School of Medicine, 615 Michael Street, Atlanta, GA 30322, USA.

References
1. Lewin GR. Neurotrophins and the specification of neuronal phenotype. Philos Trans R Soc Lond B Biol Sci. 1996;351:405–11. doi:10.1098/rstb. 1996.0035.
2. Thoenen H, Zafra F, Hengerer B, Lindholm D. The synthesis of nerve growth factor and brain-derived neurotrophic factor in hippocampal and cortical neurons is regulated by specific transmitter systems. Ann N Y Acad Sci. 1991;640:86–90.
3. Kaplan DR, Miller FD. Neurotrophin signal transduction in the nervous system. Curr Opin Neurobiol. 2000;10:381–91.
4. Huang EJ, Reichardt LF. Trk receptors: roles in neuronal signal transduction. Annu Rev Biochem. 2003;72:609–42. doi:10.1146/annurev.biochem.72. 121801.161629.
5. Shelton DL, Sutherland J, Gripp J, Camerato T, Armanini MP, Phillips HS, et al. Human trks: molecular cloning, tissue distribution, and expression of extracellular domain immunoadhesins. J Neurosci Off J Soc Neurosci. 1995; 15:477–91.
6. Lindsay RM. Role of neurotrophins and trk receptors in the development and maintenance of sensory neurons: an overview. Philos Trans R Soc Lond B Biol Sci. 1996;351:365–73. doi:10.1098/rstb.1996.0030.
7. Askanas V. Neurotrophic factors and amyotrophic lateral sclerosis. Adv Neurol. 1995;68:241–4.
8. Siegel GJ, Chauhan NB. Neurotrophic factors in Alzheimer's and Parkinson's disease brain. Brain Res Brain Res Rev. 2000;33:199–227.
9. Lindholm D, Dechant G, Heisenberg CP, Thoenen H. Brain-derived neurotrophic factor is a survival factor for cultured rat cerebellar granule neurons and protects them against glutamate-induced neurotoxicity. Eur J Neurosci. 1993;5:1455–64.
10. Leeds P, Leng Y, Chalecka-Franaszek E, Chuang DM. Neurotrophins protect against cytosine arabinoside-induced apoptosis of immature rat cerebellar neurons. Neurochem Int. 2005;46:61–72. doi:10.1016/j.neuint.2004.07.001.
11. Schäbitz WR, Sommer C, Zoder W, Kiessling M, Schwaninger M, Schwab S. Intravenous brain-derived neurotrophic factor reduces infarct size and counterregulates Bax and Bcl-2 expression after temporary focal cerebral ischemia. Stroke. 2000;31:2212–7.
12. Kurozumi K, Nakamura K, Tamiya T, Kawano Y, Kobune M, Hirai S, et al. BDNF gene-modified mesenchymal stem cells promote functional recovery and reduce infarct size in the rat middle cerebral artery occlusion model. Mol Ther. 2004;9:189–97. doi:10.1016/j.ymthe.2003.10.012.
13. Koda M, Hashimoto M, Murakami M, Yoshinaga K, Ikeda O, Yamazaki M, et al. Adenovirus vector-mediated in vivo gene transfer of brain-derived neurotrophic factor (BDNF) promotes rubrospinal axonal regeneration and functional recovery after complete transection of the adult rat spinal cord. J Neurotrauma. 2004;21:329–37. doi:10.1089/089771504322972112.
14. Du X, Hill RA. 7,8-Dihydroxyflavone as a pro-neurotrophic treatment for neurodevelopmental disorders. Neurochem Int. 2015;89:170–80. doi:10.1016/j.neuint.2015.07.021.
15. Ochs G, Penn RD, York M, Giess R, Beck M, Tonn J, et al. A phase I/II trial of recombinant methionyl human brain derived neurotrophic factor administered by intrathecal infusion to patients with amyotrophic lateral sclerosis. Amyotroph Lateral Scler Other Motor Neuron Disord. 2000;1:201–6.
16. Thoenen H, Sendtner M. Neurotrophins: from enthusiastic expectations through sobering experiences to rational therapeutic approaches. Nat Neurosci. 2002;5(Suppl):1046–50. doi:10.1038/nn938.
17. Chao MV. The p75 neurotrophin receptor. J Neurobiol. 1994;25:1373–85. doi: 10.1002/neu.480251106.
18. Friedman WJ, Greene LA. Neurotrophin signaling via Trks and p75. Exp Cell Res. 1999;253:131–42. doi:10.1006/excr.1999.4705.
19. Qian MD, Zhang J, Tan XY, Wood A, Gill D, Cho S. Novel agonist monoclonal antibodies activate TrkB receptors and demonstrate potent neurotrophic activities. J Neurosci Off J Soc Neurosci. 2006;26:9394–403. doi:10.1523/jneurosci.1118-06.2006.
20. O'Leary PD, Hughes RA. Design of potent peptide mimetics of brain-derived neurotrophic factor. J Biol Chem. 2003;278:25738–44. doi:10.1074/jbc. M303209200.

21. Fletcher JM, Hughes RA. Novel monocyclic and bicyclic loop mimetics of brain-derived neurotrophic factor. J Pept Sci. 2006;12:515–24. doi:10.1002/psc.760.

22. Molina-Holgado F, Doherty P, Williams G. Tandem repeat peptide strategy for the design of neurotrophic factor mimetics. CNS Neurol Disord Drug Targets. 2008;7:110–9.

23. Lee FS, Chao MV. Activation of Trk neurotrophin receptors in the absence of neurotrophins. Proc Natl Acad Sci U S A. 2001;98:3555–60. doi:10.1073/pnas.061020198.

24. Lee FS, Rajagopal R, Kim AH, Chang PC, Chao MV. Activation of Trk neurotrophin receptor signaling by pituitary adenylate cyclase-activating polypeptides. J Biol Chem. 2002;277:9096–102. doi:10.1074/jbc.M107421200.

25. Rajagopal R, Chen ZY, Lee FS, Chao MV. Transactivation of Trk neurotrophin receptors by G-protein-coupled receptor ligands occurs on intracellular membranes. J Neurosci Off J Soc Neurosci. 2004;24: 6650–8. doi:10.1523/jneurosci.0010-04.2004.

26. Jang SW, Liu X, Yepes M, Shepherd KR, Miller GW, Liu Y, et al. A selective TrkB agonist with potent neurotrophic activities by 7,8-dihydroxyflavone. Proc Natl Acad Sci U S A. 2010;107:2687–92. doi:10.1073/pnas.0913572107.

27. Jiang M, Peng Q, Liu X, Jin J, Hou Z, Zhang J, et al. Small-molecule TrkB receptor agonists improve motor function and extend survival in a mouse model of Huntington's disease. Hum Mol Genet. 2013;22:2462–70. doi:10. 1093/hmg/ddt098.

28. Gupta VK, You Y, Li JC, Klistorner A, Graham SL. Protective effects of 7,8-dihydroxyflavone on retinal ganglion and RGC-5 cells against excitotoxic and oxidative stress. J Mol Neurosci. 2013;49:96–104. doi:10.1007/s12031-012-9899-x.

29. Han X, Zhu S, Wang B, Chen L, Li R, Yao W, et al. Antioxidant action of 7,8-dihydroxyflavone protects PC12 cells against 6-hydroxydopamine-induced cytotoxicity. Neurochem Int. 2014;64:18–23. doi:10.1016/j.neuint.2013.10.018.

30. Han XH, Cheng MN, Chen L, Fang H, Wang LJ, Li XT, et al. 7,8-dihydroxyflavone protects PC12 cells against 6-hydroxydopamine-induced cell death through modulating PI3K/Akt and JNK pathways. Neurosci Lett. 2014;581:85–8. doi:10.1016/j.neulet.2014.08.016.

31. Wu CH, Hung TH, Chen CC, Ke CH, Lee CY, Wang PY, et al. Post-injury treatment with 7,8-dihydroxyflavone, a TrkB receptor agonist, protects against experimental traumatic brain injury via PI3K/Akt signaling. PLoS One. 2014;9: e113397. doi:10.1371/journal.pone.0113397.

32. Liu X, Obianyo O, Chan CB, Huang J, Xue S, Yang JJ, et al. Biochemical and biophysical investigation of the brain-derived neurotrophic factor mimetic 7,8-dihydroxyflavone in the binding and activation of the TrkB receptor. J Biol Chem. 2014;289:27571–84. doi:10.1074/jbc.M114.562561.

33. Liu X, Chan CB, Qi Q, Xiao G, Luo HR, He X, et al. Optimization of a small tropomyosin-related kinase B (TrkB) agonist 7,8-dihydroxyflavone active in mouse models of depression. J Med Chem. 2012;55:8524–37. doi:10.1021/jm301099x.

34. Grimes ML, Zhou J, Beattie EC, Yuen EC, Hall DE, Valletta JS, et al. Endocytosis of activated TrkA: evidence that nerve growth factor induces formation of signaling endosomes. J Neurosci Off J Soc Neurosci. 1996;16: 7950–64.

35. Beattie EC, Howe CL, Wilde A, Brodsky FM, Mobley WC. NGF signals through TrkA to increase clathrin at the plasma membrane and enhance clathrin-mediated membrane trafficking. J Neurosci Off J Soc Neurosci. 2000;20:7325–33.

36. Makkerh JP, Ceni C, Auld DS, Vaillancourt F, Dorval G, Barker PA. p75 neurotrophin receptor reduces ligand-induced Trk receptor ubiquitination and delays Trk receptor internalization and degradation. EMBO Rep. 2005;6: 936–41. doi:10.1038/sj.embor.7400503.

37. Geetha T, Jiang J, Wooten MW. Lysine 63 polyubiquitination of the nerve growth factor receptor TrkA directs internalization and signaling. Mol Cell. 2005;20:301–12. doi:10.1016/j.molcel.2005.09.014.

38. Arévalo JC, Waite J, Rajagopal R, Beyna M, Chen ZY, Lee FS, et al. Cell survival through Trk neurotrophin receptors is differentially regulated by ubiquitination. Neuron. 2006;50:549–59. doi:10.1016/j.neuron.2006.03.044.

39. Jadhav T, Geetha T, Jiang J, Wooten MW. Identification of a consensus site for TRAF6/p62 polyubiquitination. Biochem Biophys Res Commun. 2008;371:521–4. doi:10.1016/j.bbrc.2008.04.138.

40. Harborne JB, Williams CA. Advances in flavonoid research since 1992. Phytochemistry. 2000;55:481–504.

41. Spencer JP. Flavonoids: modulators of brain function? Br J Nutr. 2008;99 E Suppl 1:ES60–77. doi:10.1017/s0007114508965776.

42. Vauzour D, Vafeiadou K, Rice-Evans C, Williams RJ, Spencer JP. Activation of pro-survival Akt and ERK1/2 signalling pathways underlie the anti-apoptotic effects of flavanones in cortical neurons. J Neurochem. 2007;103:1355–67. doi:10.1111/j.1471-4159.2007.04841.x.

43. Schroeter H, Bahia P, Spencer JP, Sheppard O, Rattray M, Cadenas E, et al. (−)Epicatechin stimulates ERK-dependent cyclic AMP response element activity and up-regulates GluR2 in cortical neurons. J Neurochem. 2007;101:1596–606. doi:10.1111/j.1471-4159.2006.04434.x.

44. Maher P, Akaishi T, Abe K. Flavonoid fisetin promotes ERK-dependent long-term potentiation and enhances memory. Proc Natl Acad Sci U S A. 2006;103:16568–73. doi:10.1073/pnas.0607822103.

45. Levites Y, Amit T, Youdim MB, Mandel S. Involvement of protein kinase C activation and cell survival/ cell cycle genes in green tea polyphenol (−)-epigallocatechin 3-gallate neuroprotective action. J Biol Chem. 2002;277:30574–80. doi:10.1074/jbc. M202832200.

46. Liu X, Chan CB, Jang SW, Pradoldej S, Huang J, He K, et al. A synthetic 7,8-dihydroxyflavone derivative promotes neurogenesis and exhibits potent antidepressant effect. J Med Chem. 2010;53:8274–86. doi:10.1021/jm101206p.

47. Yu Q, Chang Q, Liu X, Gong S, Ye K, Lin X. 7,8,3′-Trihydroxyflavone, a potent small molecule TrkB receptor agonist, protects spiral ganglion neurons from degeneration both in vitro and in vivo. Biochem Biophys Res Commun. 2012;422:387–92. doi:10.1016/j.bbrc.2012.04.154.

48. Yu Q, Chang Q, Liu X, Wang Y, Li H, Gong S, et al. Protection of spiral ganglion neurons from degeneration using small-molecule TrkB receptor agonists. J Neurosci Off J Soc Neurosci. 2013;33:13042–52. doi:10.1523/jneurosci.0854-13.2013.

49. Chan CB, Tse MC, Liu X, Zhang S, Schmidt R, Otten R, et al. Activation of muscular TrkB by its small molecular agonist 7,8-dihydroxyflavone sex-dependently regulates energy metabolism in diet-induced obese mice. Chem Biol. 2015;22:355–68. doi:10.1016/j.chembiol.2015.02.003.

50. Liu X, Qi Q, Xiao G, Li J, Luo HR, Ye K. O-methylated metabolite of 7,8-dihydroxyflavone activates TrkB receptor and displays antidepressant activity. Pharmacology. 2013;91:185–200. doi:10.1159/000346920.

51. LeWitt PA. Subcutaneously administered apomorphine: pharmacokinetics and metabolism. Neurology. 2004;62:S8–S11.

52. Di Stefano A, Sozio P, Cerasa LS, Iannitelli A. L-Dopa prodrugs: an overview of trends for improving Parkinson's disease treatment. Curr Pharm Des. 2011;17:3482–93.

53. Tsai T, Klausmeyer A, Conrad R, Gottschling C, Leo M, Faissner A, et al. 7,8-Dihydroxyflavone leads to survival of cultured embryonic motoneurons by activating intracellular signaling pathways. Mol Cell Neurosci. 2013;56:18–28. doi:10.1016/j.mcn.2013.02.007.

54. Korkmaz OT, Aytan N, Carreras I, Choi JK, Kowall NW, Jenkins BG, et al. 7,8-Dihydroxyflavone improves motor performance and enhances lower motor neuronal survival in a mouse model of amyotrophic lateral sclerosis. Neurosci Lett. 2014;566:286–91. doi:10.1016/j.neulet.2014.02.058.

55. Devi L, Ohno M. 7,8-dihydroxyflavone, a small-molecule TrkB agonist, reverses memory deficits and BACE1 elevation in a mouse model of Alzheimer's disease. Neuropsychopharmacology. 2012;37:434–44. doi:10.1038/npp.2011.191.

56. Zhang Z, Liu X, Schroeder JP, Chan CB, Song M, Yu SP, et al. 7,8-dihydroxyflavone prevents synaptic loss and memory deficits in a mouse model of Alzheimer's disease. Neuropsychopharmacology. 2014;39:638–50. doi:10.1038/npp.2013.243.

57. Chen C, Li XH, Zhang S, Tu Y, Wang YM, Sun HT. 7,8-dihydroxyflavone ameliorates scopolamine-induced Alzheimer-like pathologic dysfunction. Rejuvenation Res. 2014;17:249–54. doi:10.1089/rej.2013.1519.

58. Castello NA, Nguyen MH, Tran JD, Cheng D, Green KN, LaFerla FM. 7,8-Dihydroxyflavone, a small molecule TrkB agonist, improves spatial memory and increases thin spine density in a mouse model of Alzheimer disease-like neuronal loss. PLoS One. 2014;9:e91453. doi:10.1371/journal.pone.0091453.

59. Andero R, Daviu N, Escorihuela RM, Nadal R, Armario A. 7,8-dihydroxyflavone, a TrkB receptor agonist, blocks long-term spatial memory impairment caused by immobilization stress in rats. Hippocampus. 2012;22:399–408. doi:10.1002/hipo. 20906.

60. Johnson RA, Lam M, Punzo AM, Li H, Lin BR, Ye K, et al. 7,8-dihydroxyflavone exhibits therapeutic efficacy in a mouse model of Rett syndrome. J Appl Physiol. 2012;112:704–10. doi:10.1152/japplphysiol.01361.2011.

61. English AW, Liu K, Nicolini JM, Mulligan AM, Ye K. Small-molecule trkB agonists promote axon regeneration in cut peripheral nerves. Proc Natl Acad Sci U S A. 2013;110:16217–22. doi:10.1073/pnas.1303646110.

62. Blugeot A, Rivat C, Bouvier E, Molet J, Mouchard A, Zeau B, et al. Vulnerability to depression: from brain neuroplasticity to identification of biomarkers. J Neurosci Off J Soc Neurosci. 2011;31:12889–99. doi:10.1523/jneurosci.1309-11. 2011.

63. Bollen E, Vanmierlo T, Akkerman S, Wouters C, Steinbusch HM, Prickaerts J. 7,8-Dihydroxyflavone improves memory consolidation processes in rats and mice. Behav Brain Res. 2013;257:8–12. doi:10.1016/j.bbr.2013.09.029.

64. Nagahara AH, Merrill DA, Coppola G, Tsukada S, Schroeder BE, Shaked GM, et al. Neuroprotective effects of brain-derived neurotrophic factor in rodent and primate models of Alzheimer's disease. Nat Med. 2009;15:331–7. doi:10.1038/nm.1912.

65. Ando S, Kobayashi S, Waki H, Kon K, Fukui F, Tadenuma T, et al. Animal model of dementia induced by entorhinal synaptic damage and partial restoration of cognitive deficits by BDNF and carnitine. J Neurosci Res. 2002; 70:519–27. doi:10.1002/jnr.10443.

66. Hsiao YH, Hung HC, Chen SH, Gean PW. Social interaction rescues memory deficit in an animal model of Alzheimer's disease by increasing BDNF-dependent hippocampal neurogenesis. J Neurosci Off J Soc Neurosci. 2014; 34:16207–19. doi:10.1523/jneurosci.0747-14.2014.

67. Gray J, Yeo GS, Cox JJ, Morton J, Adlam AL, Keogh JM, et al. Hyperphagia, severe obesity, impaired cognitive function, and hyperactivity associated with functional loss of one copy of the brain-derived neurotrophic factor (BDNF) gene. Diabetes. 2006;55:3366–71. doi:10.2337/db06-0550.

68. Yeo GS, Connie Hung CC, Rochford J, Keogh J, Gray J, Sivaramakrishnan S, et al. A de novo mutation affecting human TrkB associated with severe obesity and developmental delay. Nat Neurosci. 2004;7:1187–9. doi:10.1038/nn1336.

69. Kernie SG, Liebl DJ, Parada LF. BDNF regulates eating behavior and locomotor activity in mice. EMBO J. 2000;19:1290–300. doi:10.1093/emboj/19.6.1290.

70. Pedersen BK, Pedersen M, Krabbe KS, Bruunsgaard H, Matthews VB, Febbraio MA. Role of exercise-induced brain-derived neurotrophic factor production in the regulation of energy homeostasis in mammals. Exp Physiol. 2009;94:1153–60. doi:10.1113/expphysiol.2009.048561.

71. Zeng Y, Liu Y, Wu M, Liu J, Hu Q. Activation of TrkB by 7,8-dihydroxyflavone prevents fear memory defects and facilitates amygdalar synaptic plasticity in aging. J Alzheimers Dis. 2012;31:765–78. doi:10.3233/jad-2012-120886.

72. Zeng Y, Lv F, Li L, Yu H, Dong M, Fu Q. 7,8-dihydroxyflavone rescues spatial memory and synaptic plasticity in cognitively impaired aged rats. J Neurochem. 2012;122:800–11. doi:10.1111/j.1471-4159.2012.07830.x.

73. Scharfman HE. Hyperexcitability in combined entorhinal/hippocampal slices of adult rat after exposure to brain-derived neurotrophic factor. J Neurophysiol. 1997;78:1082–95.

74. Isgor C, Pare C, McDole B, Coombs P, Guthrie K. Expansion of the dentate mossy fiber-CA3 projection in the brain-derived neurotrophic factor-enriched mouse hippocampus. Neuroscience. 2015;288:10–23. doi:10.1016/j.neuroscience.2014.12.036.

75. Cunha C, Angelucci A, D'Antoni A, Dobrossy MD, Dunnett SB, Berardi N, et al. Brain-derived neurotrophic factor (BDNF) overexpression in the forebrain results in learning and memory impairments. Neurobiol Dis. 2009;33:358–68. doi:10.1016/j.nbd.2008.11.004.

76. Merighi A, Salio C, Ghirri A, Lossi L, Ferrini F, Betelli C, et al. Prog Neurobiol. 2008;85:297–317. doi:10.1016/j.pneurobio.2008.04.004.

12

Environmental insults: critical triggers for amyotrophic lateral sclerosis

Bing Yu[1,2]* and Roger Pamphlett[3,4]

Abstract

Background: Amyotrophic lateral sclerosis (ALS) is a fatal neurodegenerative disease characterised by a rapid loss of lower and upper motor neurons. As a complex disease, the ageing process and complicated gene-environment interactions are involved in the majority of cases.

Main body: Significant advances have been made in unravelling the genetic susceptibility to ALS with massively parallel sequencing technologies, while environmental insults remain a suspected but largely unexplored source of risk. Several studies applying the strategy of Mendelian randomisation have strengthened the link between environmental insults and ALS, but none so far has proved conclusive. We propose a new ALS model which links the current knowledge of genetic factors, ageing and environmental insults. This model provides a mechanism as to how ALS is initiated, with environmental insults playing a critical role.

Conclusion: The available evidence has suggested that inherited defect(s) could cause mitochondrial dysfunction, which would establish the primary susceptibility to ALS. Further study of the underlying mechanism may shed light on ALS pathogenesis. Environmental insults are a critical trigger for ALS, particularly in the aged individuals with other toxicant susceptible genes. The identification of ALS triggers could lead to preventive strategies for those individuals at risk.

Keywords: Amyotrophic lateral sclerosis, Environmental risk factors, Mendelian randomisation, Mitochondrial dysfunction, Trigger, Initiation, Spread

Background

Amyotrophic lateral sclerosis (ALS) is a rapidly progressive and universally fatal neurodegenerative disease of the human motor system. It is characterised by degeneration of upper (frontal motor cortex) and lower (spinal cord and brain stem) motor neurons, leading to progressive paralysis and death, usually due to respiratory failure. Its onset peaks around the mid-60s and most patients succumb to the disease within 2–5 years of becoming symptomatic [1, 2]. ALS is classically divided into familial and sporadic forms (Table 1), though these two forms are generally clinically and pathologically indistinguishable [1, 3]. The causes of sporadic ALS remain a research challenge [4]. Recent massively parallel sequencing technologies have facilitated

disease-gene discovery, and rare variants in more than 50 genes have now been identified in association with sporadic ALS [5, 6].

The sporadic form of ALS in particular is considered to be complex disease (Table 1). A gene-time-environment model has been proposed, in which environmental risks and ageing interact with a pre-existing genetic load, followed by an unknown mechanism of self-perpetuating decline to death [1]. About 60% of the risk of sporadic ALS is genetically determined with the remaining 40% due to environmental factors [4, 7]. Advanced age and male gender are the only two established risk factors for ALS. Many environmental factors have been postulated for sporadic ALS (for comprehensive reviews see references [1, 8]), but none has been proven conclusively. Several critical issues remain unexplained, such as how sporadic ALS begins, how it spreads, and why it affects mostly motor neurons. In this article, we focus on several commonly postulated ALS-associated environmental insults that have support from Mendelian

* Correspondence: bing.yu@sydney.edu.au

[1]Sydney Medical School (Central), The University of Sydney, Camperdown, NSW 2006, Australia

[2]Department of Medical Genomics, Royal Prince Alfred Hospital and NSW Health Pathology, Camperdown, NSW 2050, Australia

Full list of author information is available at the end of the article

Table 1 Genetic characteristics of familial and sporadic ALS

	Familial ALS	Sporadic ALS
Proportion	10%	90%
Disease category	Monogenic	Complex
Inheritance	Autosomal dominant (most common) Recessive X-linked	Gene-environment interactions Gene-gene interactions Autosomal recessive variants De novo variants
Common genes (% mutations)	C9orf72 repeat expansions (24%) SOD1 (20%) TARDBP (1–5%) FUS (1–5%) Other genes (rare or unknown)	C9orf72 repeat expansions (5–10%) SOD1 (1–3%) Other genes (rare or unknown)

Abbreviations: C9orf72 chromosome 9 open reading frame 72 gene, SOD1 superoxide dismutase 1 gene, TARDBP TAR DNA binding protein gene or TDP-43, FUS fused in sarcoma gene

randomisation analyses. We also explore the consequences of gene-environment interactions, and how to further investigate the role of environmental factors in ALS. A model of ALS pathogenesis is proposed that links current knowledge of genetic factors and advancing age with the role of environmental factors (Fig. 1).

Characteristics of the motor neuron system
Motor neurons
Motor neurons, comprising the cell body, axon, dendrites and telodendria, coordinate voluntary actions and transmit signals to different muscles of the body. The axon is a long process which transmits nerve impulses over a long distance without diminution of the amplitude

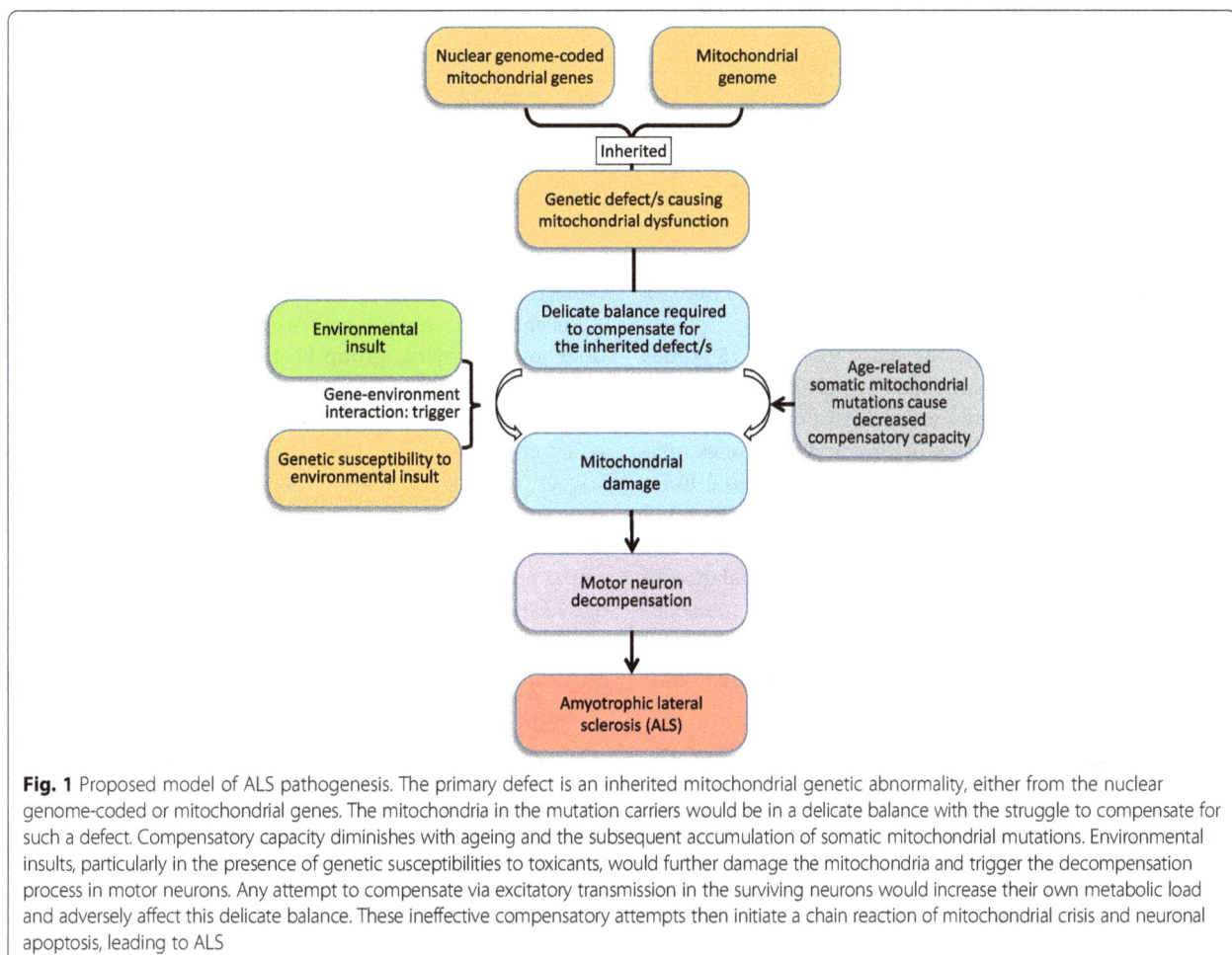

Fig. 1 Proposed model of ALS pathogenesis. The primary defect is an inherited mitochondrial genetic abnormality, either from the nuclear genome-coded or mitochondrial genes. The mitochondria in the mutation carriers would be in a delicate balance with the struggle to compensate for such a defect. Compensatory capacity diminishes with ageing and the subsequent accumulation of somatic mitochondrial mutations. Environmental insults, particularly in the presence of genetic susceptibilities to toxicants, would further damage the mitochondria and trigger the decompensation process in motor neurons. Any attempt to compensate via excitatory transmission in the surviving neurons would increase their own metabolic load and adversely affect this delicate balance. These ineffective compensatory attempts then initiate a chain reaction of mitochondrial crisis and neuronal apoptosis, leading to ALS

of the signal. For example, the motor neuron axon in the human sciatic nerve begins in the lumbar spinal cord, runs down the lower limb and reaches the foot. Dendrites form extensions that synapse with one or many other neurons and telodendria make contact with muscles at neuromuscular junctions.

Astrocytes

Astrocytes represent 20–40% of the total number of cells in mammalian brains [9]. These glial cells form a network among neurons, dendrites and axons by means of their numerous processes radiating from their cell bodies, and creating functional units [10]. They are active partners of motor neurons and integrate or modify converging information through their contacts with neuronal synapses.

Mitochondria

Mitochondria play multiple roles in calcium homeostasis, energy supply, metabolic synthesis and apoptosis [11]. There is a high density of mitochondria in motor neurons, including in the neuromuscular junction. The central nervous system consumes more energy than any other human organ, accounting for up to 20% of the body's total use [12]. Approximately 90% of cerebral ATP production occurs in the mitochondria through oxidative phosphorylation [13, 14]. ATP utilisation occurs mainly in the axon that supports various cellular functions, including phospholipid metabolism, protein synthesis, neurotransmitter cycling, and transportation of ions across cellular membranes. Sodium, calcium and potassium ions are continuously and actively passed through the membranes of cells at the expense of ATP consumption, so that neurons can recharge to fire [13, 14].

The mitochondrial genome has about a 15 times higher mutation rate than that of the nuclear genome [11]. This could be related to its high concentration of reactive oxygen species, lack of protective histones, and limited DNA repair. Importantly for mitochondrial function, there are 1158 predicted mitochondrially-targeted proteins encoded by the nuclear genome [15]. Mitochondria play a central role in the complex balance of cellular processes contributing to ageing and neurodegeneration [11, 16] (Fig. 1). Interestingly, astrocytes act as recharging stations for neurons by supplying functional mitochondria [17].

Environmental insults in ALS

It is becoming increasingly apparent that mutations in ALS-associated genes can lead to ALS. However, none of these mutations explains how the disease starts and spreads. The environmental contributions to the disease have been more challenging to uncover, in part because the lack of knowledge about disease mechanisms makes it difficult to determine which environmental insults to focus on.

Infections

Viral and bacterial infections have been implicated as risk factors for ALS in several epidemiological and clinical studies [18–20]. Enteroviral nucleic acids have been identified in the spinal cords of sporadic ALS cases more frequently than controls [21–23]. Poliovirus, a member of the enteroviral family, affects motor neurons selectively [20] and individuals who have poliomyelitis in childhood may develop a progressive motor neuron disorder up to 40 years later, termed post-polio syndrome [24]. In vitro studies suggest that enteroviral infection of human motor neurons or glial cells can become persistent [25, 26]. This could have a significant impact on the motor neuron and result in altered astrocytic glutamate transport, decreased mitochondrial activity and impaired resistance to oxidative stress [27, 28] (Fig. 1). The lack of inflammatory change in the nervous tissue of most cases makes an acute viral attack on motor neurons unlikely. A persistent viral presence in neurons, however, may result in an atypical insult that could play a role in ALS.

The poliovirus receptor is a nuclear-encoded gene specific to the primate lineage, and serves as a cellular receptor for poliovirus in the first step of poliovirus replication. Its product is a transmembrane glycoprotein belonging to the immunoglobulin superfamily. The poliovirus receptor may be involved in the differentiation of motor neurons during embryonic development. Human poliovirus receptor variants can influence the consequence of poliovirus infection and possibly result in a persistent infection that later leads to ALS [29, 30].

Recently, the neural expression of latent human endogenous retrovirus group K (HERV-K) was detected in post mortem brain tissue from patients with sporadic ALS [31]. In vitro transfection of the HERV-K genome, or its env gene alone, into cultured human neurons can trigger neurite retraction and neuronal death. Transgenic mice expressing the HERV-K env gene showed abnormalities in intrinsic cortical hyperexcitability and impaired motor function, and 50% die by 10 months of age [31].

Organophosphates

Organophosphates have been suspected as a risk factor in the pathogenesis of ALS due to their ability to damage motor neurons [32–34]. Chemicals containing organophosphates are present in fertilizers, herbicides, fungicides and insecticides and have wide agriculture and domestic usage [2, 35]. The toxicity of organophosphates is related to its acute inhibition of acetyl cholinesterase, the enzyme responsible for terminating the activity of the neurotransmitter acetylcholine. Chronic exposure to organophosphates can induce progressive brain damage by irreversibly inhibiting acetylcholinesterase, resulting in excessive simulation of cholinergic receptors and excitotoxicity [36]. Metabolites of various organophosphorus compounds [37] could also trigger neuronal damage and induce delayed neurotoxicity. Genetic susceptibility inhibiting organophosphate detoxification could be responsible for the reported association of pesticide with ALS, as will be discussed later.

An increase in ALS incidence has been reported in commercial pilots, navigators and flight attendants [33, 38]. Exposure to organophosphates has been proposed as the link in this group since engine air is supplied unfiltered to the aircraft cabin. This air can contain pyrolysed engine lubricating oils and hydraulic fluids through leaking oil seals or bearings, ruptured fluid lines, improper maintenance, or other malfunctions. Engine lubricating oils contain about 4% tricresyl phosphate [39], and hydraulic fluids contain other organophosphates, such as butyl phosphates [40].

Heavy metals

Heavy metals including lead, mercury, cadmium and selenium have been implicated in the development of ALS [32, 35, 41, 42]. It is beyond the scope of this review to cover all individual metals, but aspects of mercury and lead are of interest. Mercury exists in a wide variety of physical states, elemental, organic, and inorganic. In an aquatic environment, elemental mercury undergoes biomethylation by bacteria and algae. The organic compounds that are obtained, such as methyl-mercury and ethyl-mercury, accumulate in fish, crustaceans, and throughout the food chain to humans. Mercury intoxication in the CNS disrupts cellular metabolism and degrades several cellular constituents, eventually leading to cell death and clinical disease. The biochemical mechanisms and the clinical pictures of mercury toxicity depend on individual genetic susceptibility, the chemical forms of the metal, and the length, and concentration of exposure.

An association between ALS and occupational exposure to lead has been proposed [43, 44]. Lead from human activities includes burning fossil fuels, mining and manufacturing. Workers exposed to welding or soldering materials appear to be at risk of developing ALS [45]. The toxic effects of lead on the nervous system include lead encephalopathy (primarily in children) and a motor neuropathy (primarily in adults). The half-life of lead is 1 month in blood, about 4 years in trabecular bones (such as the patella), and about 20 years in compact bone. Skeletal muscle can also be a storage site for lead [46]. Some sources of lead have been reduced in recent years, e.g., from gasoline, paints and ceramic products, caulking, and pipe solder [47], so it will be of interest to see if the incidence of ALS decreases in the future, as

has been shown recently for Alzheimer disease in Western countries.

Physical activity

Athleticism and intense physical activity have been considered important in ALS. A 6-fold increase in ALS has been reported in Italian professional footballers, with a dose-response relationship between the duration of playing and ALS risk [48]. Excessive physical activity, repeated head injuries, and exposure to pesticides and dietary supplements or illegal substances, could underlie the risk behind these footballers. Physical stress could enhance the production of reactive oxygen species, and it has further been suggested that exercise could increase the uptake of toxicants via the neuromuscular junction into human motor neurons [42]. Intense physical activity is characteristic of agricultural work and could be cofactor for ALS with exposure to organophosphates [34].

Other environmental factors

Many other environmental factors have been investigated in relation to ALS, including organochlorines insecticides, pyrethroids, fumigants, smoking, electromagnetic fields, electric shocks, cyanotoxins and military service [8, 49]. Some persistent organic pollutants that originate from the past use of pesticides, solvents and industrial chemicals can also be risk factors for ALS. However, the available data are often conflicting. For example, organochlorines are associated with neurodegeneration in several Parkinson disease studies [50, 51], but their role in ALS is controversial. Exposure to aldrin, dieldrin, DDT (dichlorodiphenyltrichloroethane) and taxaphene tends to increase the odds ratios of ALS, but may be confounded by increasing age [49]. Smoking has been reported as a risk factor for ALS [52, 53], but the results are conflicting and lack of a clear dose-response relationship [1, 54]. The limitations of previous ALS epidemiological studies are discussed in the next section.

Military service represents a different category of risk factor since it aggregates a group of combined factors. Soldiers often received prophylactic treatment of cholinergic inhibitors to protect them against nerve gas and insect pests [55]. The deployment usually involves intensive physical activity, emotional stress and physical or psychological trauma, along with detrimental lifestyle factors such as cigarette smoking and alcohol consumption. Military personnel can also be exposed to environmental viruses, heavy metals, organophosphates, nasopharyngeal radium, exhaust from heaters or generators, high-intensity radar waves, contaminated food, explosions in the field [55, 56]. Finally, it has been suggested that exposure to diesel fuel, used extensively in the military, may underlie the increased risk of ALS in the services [56].

Challenges in ALS epidemiology

ALS could occur in number of different unique environments

Environmental risk factors for ALS have been studied for many years without any firm conclusions being drawn. Sporadic ALS is probably human-specific, since neurodegeneration affects neocortical regions and interconnections, the evolutionary consequence of *Homo sapiens*. Only higher primates have direct connections between upper and lower motor neurons, the two sets of neurons most affected by ALS. The extraordinary long motor axons with their complicated activities demand a high energy consumption. The complex natural, built and social environments that every human individual faces are unique to our species. For example, heavy metals can enter humans from breathing in particulate matter in the air, from drinking water with leached lead from pipes, or by eating accumulated mercury via the seafood chain. ALS animal models are different from humans as regards lifespan, with humans commonly living over 80 years but mice surviving only up to 3 years. An elderly human has therefore experienced vastly more cycles of mitochondrial DNA replication than an aged mouse, since the daily turnover of mitochondrial DNA is similar in mice and humans [16]. It is therefore not surprising that the use of animal models has proven less than fruitful for complex human disorders, particularly in relation to environmental risk factors.

Limitations of investigating environmental risks in ALS

Environmental factors are widely considered to play a role in ALS pathogenesis. However, none of the known environmental risk factors has been conclusively determined [1]. Criticisms have been made on epidemiological study design and selection bias. Many previous investigations of the environmental effects on ALS have small sample and effect sizes, lack population controls and are retrospective in nature. Data collection largely relies on self-reporting through questionnaires or surveys with such studies being prone to recall bias. Misclassification of exposure may be responsible, for example, for the lack of concordance between survey data and measurements of blood pollutants [33]. Most of the published studies lack data on the frequency and intensity of toxicant exposure [57]. Furthermore, interpretation of the significance of environmental risk factors can be difficult in the absence of participants' genomic information such as ALS susceptibilities.

It is difficult to assess how environmental insults initiate and influence the progression of ALS in observational studies. Even if an insult and an outcome are associated, the direction of causality can be hard to ascertain because ALS itself can obscure the intensity of an insult. For example, lead levels can be high in ALS,

but that ALS itself can reversely affect the lead levels due to the release of bone and/or muscle-stored lead during osteoporosis and muscle wasting [46]. Strategies have been proposed to overcome these limitations. Prospective studies with population controls would be ideal, but hard to execute because they involve significant investment for detailed interviews, monitoring of environmental insults, and a long period of time to recruit sufficient numbers of patients with ALS which has modest incidence.

Genetic proxies for environmental insults

The application of Mendelian randomisation can shed light on causal relationships since this uses a genetic proxy (e.g., single nucleotide variants, SNVs) as a variable to assess environmental exposure (Fig. 2) [58, 59]. The principle of Mendelian randomisation is based on Mendel's second law of independent assortment, i.e., the random assortment of genes from parents to offspring that occurs during gamete formation and conception. This implies that SNVs will not be associated with any confounding factors that may distort conventional observational studies at a population level, and such variants are unlikely to be affected by reverse causality since the genotypes are determined at conception. For a SNV to be a valid instrumental variable, it must be reliably associated with the exposure, and only be associated with the outcome through the exposure of interest (Fig. 2). Such variants should be independent of other factors affecting the outcomes [60–62]. This strategy can be used for ALS research with two related purposes: (1) to provide evidence for the existence of causal associations, and (2) to enable accurate estimation of the magnitude of the effect of lifelong exposure to an environmental insult. If environmental factors are truly a causal risk factor in ALS development, their susceptible genetic proxies would be expected to increase risk of ALS. Three examples of this strategy are given below.

1) Poliovirus is a lytic virus, but it can also establish a persistent infection like other enteroviruses [25, 30]. SNVs in the human poliovirus receptor gene can influence the consequences of the infection. For example, 56% of wild-type human neuroblastoma cells survived 28 h after poliovirus infection, but survival increased to 79% in cells with a particular SNV (rs1058402) [29]. When 110 patients with sporadic ALS and 30 with progressive muscular atrophy (PMA, the lower motor variant of ALS) were compared with 280 controls, the frequency of SNV rs1058402 was 20% in PMA cases and 12% in ALS cases, significantly higher than in controls at 7% [63]. These results support a pathogenic role of enteroviruses in ALS since affected neurons could

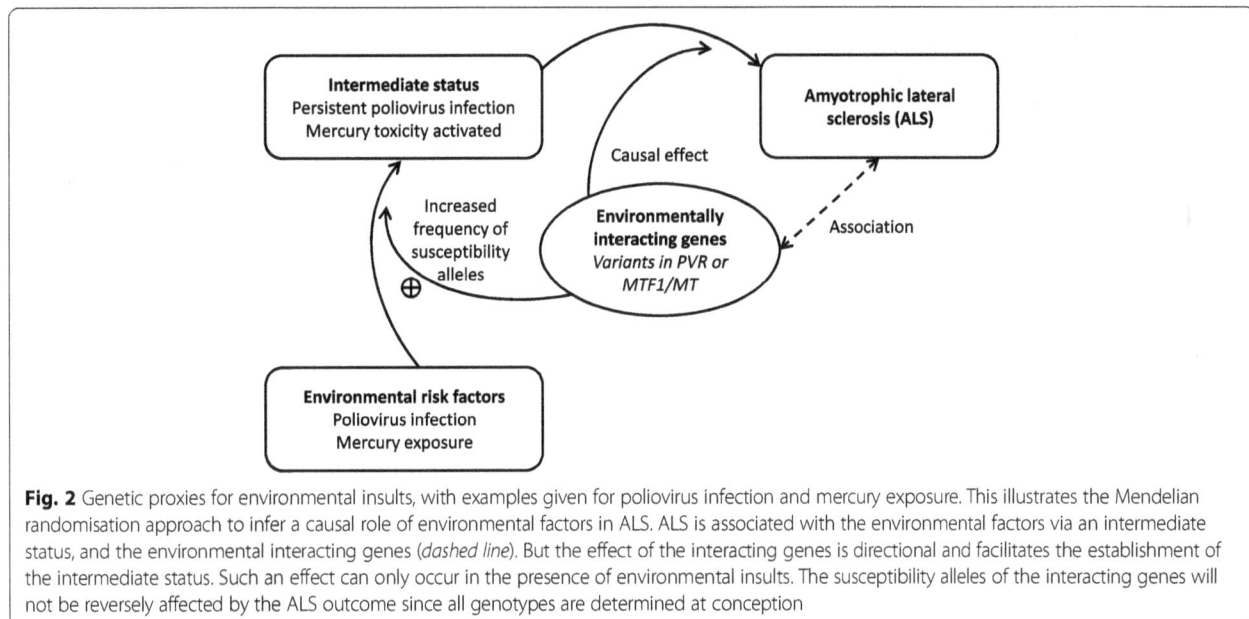

Fig. 2 Genetic proxies for environmental insults, with examples given for poliovirus infection and mercury exposure. This illustrates the Mendelian randomisation approach to infer a causal role of environmental factors in ALS. ALS is associated with the environmental factors via an intermediate status, and the environmental interacting genes (*dashed line*). But the effect of the interacting genes is directional and facilitates the establishment of the intermediate status. Such an effect can only occur in the presence of environmental insults. The susceptibility alleles of the interacting genes will not be reversely affected by the ALS outcome since all genotypes are determined at conception

survive the early cytolytic effect of poliovirus and establish the persistent infection. The expression of poliovirus receptor is weak in spinal motor neurons and strong in muscle motor endplates, suggesting that neuromuscular junctions serve as routes for viral entry into lower motor neurons [64]. A slowly accumulative cytopathic effect on spinal motor neurons along with ageing could then trigger ALS (Figs. 1 and 2). This risk factor could be target for treatment since persistent enterovirus infection can be treated with antiviral agents [65].

2) Organophosphates are activated to their reactive oxons by the cytochrome P450 system, and these oxons are hydrolysed by paraoxonase, which is encoded by *PON1*. PON1 has different levels of hydrolytic enzyme activity and such variation is genetically determined [66]. Rare *PON 1* variants or haplotypes that lead to a decrease in paraoxonase activity are associated with ALS [67, 68]. Genetic variants that reduce the ability of the body to detoxify organophosphates could therefore favour ALS development. However, the association of *PON 1* with ALS has failed to be reproduced in a large meta-analysis [69].

3) Metallothioneins (MT) are metal-binding proteins involved in the detoxification of heavy metals such as mercury. A lack of MT increases heavy metal toxicity (Fig. 2), while overexpression is protective [70]. Metal transcription factor-1 (*MTF1*) acts as a sensor and regulator for MT expression and upregulation in response to heavy metals [71] and any change in *MTF1* could disrupt the upregulation of MTs and leave motor neurons vulnerable to heavy metal damage (Fig.

2). When the relevant genetic variants in the *MT* gene family and *MTF1* were studied in 186 sporadic ALS cases and 186 controls, significant differences were found in the distribution of some SNVs in MT detoxification and *MTF1* genes between the cases and controls [72]. Less efficient metal detoxification could therefore be a risk factor for ALS.

The role of mitochondria in ALS
How is ALS initiated?
Much evidence implicates mitochondrial dysfunction in ALS. Mitochondrial shape and positioning in cells is crucial for bioenergetics [11]. Morphological changes observed in ALS mitochondria in the anterior horn of the spinal cord include smaller size, disrupted crests and edema, crystolysis and vacuolisation, indicating metabolic disturbances [73]. These changes were unlikely to be the artefacts due to ageing or post mortem process because they were significantly different from 15 age-matched control samples. Interestingly, similar changes can be found in liver and muscle cells [74, 75], supporting the concept that mitochondrial defects are inherited from either mitochondrial or nuclear genomes [74, 75] (Fig. 1).

Mitochondrial mutations are maternally inherited or result from somatic changes. These mutations can progressively increase with age through neural clonal expansion [76] (Fig. 1). High metabolic rate and ATP consumption make the human motor system particularly vulnerable to energy deficiency. Included in the 126 ALS genes in the Amyotrophic Lateral Sclerosis Online genetics Database (v6) are one mitochondrial gene (MT-ND2) and 10 nuclear genome-coded mitochondrial genes (*ATXN2, CHCHD10, GARS, MAOB, OGG1, OMA1, PARK7, SOD1*

SOD2 and *SPG7*), found when ALS genes are cross-over with MitoCarta [5, 15]. Other mitochondrial variants, particularly nuclear genome coded ones, could be misinterpreted as variants of unknown significance due to their population frequencies or less clear-cut functionality. A study of 44 ALS case-unaffected parents trios found that ALS can be transmitted in an autosomal recessive way by homozygous or compound heterozygous changes [6] (Table 1). The frequencies of ALS-related recessive alleles could therefore be higher than expected and be adversely filtered out due to the cut-off values used in the whole exome or whole genome studies.

The finding that mitochondria can be transferred from astrocytes to neurons supports the critical role of mitochondria in neurons, and the possible involvement of astrocytes in ALS pathogenesis [17, 77]. This is of interest since mercury, long suspected in the pathogenesis of ALS, first enters the CNS via uptake by perivascular astrocytes, and is found predominantly within mitochondria [78]; any transfer of mercury-laden mitochondria from astrocytes into motor neurons could result in neurotoxic damage to these neurons. Furthermore, reduced mitochondrial content with age and somatic changes in post-mitotic neurons could lead to a decline of mitochondrial function [79].

ALS-susceptible mitochondrial variants are unlikely to remain 'switched off' until mid- to late-adulthood, although they may not be sufficient to cause any overt mitochondrial disease in early life. The motor neuron system in these individuals could be in a delicate balance with a constant struggle to compensate for such a defect or defects (Fig. 1). Compensatory capacity diminishes with ageing and the compromised mitochondrial function may finally collapse. Environmental insults could further affect the mitochondria, particularly in the presence of susceptibility alleles of the interacting genes, and trigger the decompensation process in ALS susceptible individuals (Figs. 1 and 2). It is also possible that astrocytes with mitochondrial defects may be the target cells for the harmful action of some environmental insults (such as mercury, see above), while neuronal death may be a secondary event following the initial insult to astrocytes closely related with motor neurons [10, 77].

Persistent viral infection, organophosphates, heavy metals and intense physical exercise could put metabolic loads on defective mitochondria and exhaust any compensatory capacity (Fig. 1). Other mechanisms including excitotoxins, oxidative stress, or altered calcium homeostasis could participate in cell damage [77]. Disease triggers could be disguised as the root cause of ALS, and generate conflicting results in environmental studies, since these initial insults may be necessary but not sufficient for the pathogenesis of ALS. Environmental insults, even with similar intensity

and exposure time, are unlikely to have similar impacts on non-susceptible individuals.

ALS spread

Any loss of motor neurons would put extra stress on surviving motor neurons that innervate the same muscle and increase the metabolic needs to compensate for the loss. Astrocytes at this stage may fail to perform the normal maintenance to axons or neuronal cell bodies since they would divert their resources in attempts to rescue decompensating neurons. As a consequence, more neurons would enter the decompensating process. A decrease in motor unit number and an increase in cortical excitability is found before symptom onset in *SOD1* mutation carriers [80, 81]. Such excitatory compensation may not be helpful, but instead initiate a chain reaction of mitochondrial crisis and neuronal apoptosis. Excitotoxicity can increase calcium flow into the neuron, initiate oxidative stress, and result in neuronal death. A mitochondrial crisis could also influence proteasomal or autophagic protein degradation and amplify the cellular stress. Environmental risk factors such as muscle-stored heavy metals released during muscle wasting [46] could further accelerate the deterioration. Of note, a recent study has shown how human spinal interneurons, which normally inhibit motor neurons, take up heavy metals during ageing; any mercury within the mitochondria of these interneurons could lead to interneuron malfunction with subsequent excitotoxicity to motor neurons [82].

This proposed model could explain the well-known clinical and pathological pattern of ALS starting in one CNS region and 'spreading' to other adjacent region [83]. This spread may be due to a cascade of decompensating neurons. This model therefore avoids the presumption that any environmental agent travels from one neuron to another through their synapses, extracellular vesicles, or membrane contacts. The proposed model provides a unique mechanism involving a decompensation process for spreading and "gain of toxic strength" for the subsequent accelerated progression of ALS.

Association of the proposed model with known ALS features

The development of ALS has been considered as involving a six-step process [84]. Further identification of these steps could lead to novel preventive or therapeutic avenues. Our proposed model is consistent with the gene-time-environment hypothesis [1] and entails multiple steps (Fig. 1). It offers a potential single root of ALS pathogenesis, with environmental insults being a trigger for ALS initiation. The available evidence has suggested that primary inherited defect(s) could cause mitochondrial dysfunction that establishes the susceptibility of motor neurons to ALS (Fig. 1). Environmental insults then upset the delicate balance of mitochondrial function, followed by propagation and acceleration due to an ineffective compensating process. Metal homeostasis is intimately coupled to the oxidative stress response in many cell types [71]. The depletion of microtubules and neurofilaments in ALS motor neurons could result from the genetic predisposition. Consequently, it would impair normal transport and affect mitochondrial function due to lack of sufficient nutrients [85]. Environmental insults can also trigger adverse responses such as neuroinflammation that include activation of astrocytes and microglia, as well as direct motor neuron toxicity.

Persistent viral infection could be one environmental trigger of the decompensation process. It is unlikely that the relevant virus could be isolated, or any serological reaction be sufficiently generated, though microbiome studies of CNS tissue and muscle would be of interest. The model explains the paradox of the concept of virus spreading from one neuron to another with no evidence of any viral presence. Rather, the cellular stress of one neuron could be spread to activate the endogenous retrovirus in the neighbouring neurons via the expression of the env protein [31].

As suggested by Mendelian randomisation analyses, some ALS patients would have less efficient abilities to detoxify heavy metals, which could be enough to tip motor neurons beyond the point of sustained viability, resulting in the initiation of motor neuron loss and the decompensation process. Interestingly, loss of mobility and innervated nerve stimulation to muscle can accelerate the decompensation process, since more heavy metal such as lead can be released due to osteoporosis and loss of muscle bulk [46].

The proposed model emphasises gene-environment interactions, which involves multiple steps. Some crucial environmental insults might have arisen in early development, which makes them difficult to identify. For example, subclinical enterovirus or poliovirus infection, or heavy metal exposure, could occur early in life and only play a role in the initiation or acceleration stage of the disease in later life. Differently-susceptible individuals could inherit different genetic defects with different impacts on mitochondrial function and require different intensities of environmental triggers. Major inherited defects in mitochondria-related genes may only need occult or mild triggers, while other inherited variants may require a combination of environmental insults, e.g., military deployment, to evoke the onset of ALS.

Conclusion

The available evidence has suggested that inherited defect(s) could cause mitochondrial dysfunction, which would establish the primary susceptibility to ALS. Further study of the underlying mechanism may shed light on ALS pathogenesis. Environmental insults are a critical trigger for ALS, particularly in the aged individuals with other toxicant susceptible genes. The identification of ALS triggers could lead to preventive strategies for those individuals at risk.

Abbreviations

ALS: Amyotrophic lateral sclerosis; HERV-K: Human endogenous retrovirus Group K; SNV: Single nucleotide variants

Acknowledgements

We thank Dr. Marcus Hinchcliffe for discussion regarding the role of mitochondria in neurodegenerative disease.

Funding

NA.

Authors' contributions

BY conceived the topic and wrote the manuscript. RP revised the manuscript. Both authors read the final manuscript and gave approval for publication.

Competing interests

The authors declare that they have no competing interest.

Author details

[1]Sydney Medical School (Central), The University of Sydney, Camperdown, NSW 2006, Australia. [2]Department of Medical Genomics, Royal Prince Alfred Hospital and NSW Health Pathology, Camperdown, NSW 2050, Australia. [3]Discipline of Pathology, Brain and Mind Centre, The University of Sydney, 94 Mallett St, Camperdown, NSW 2050, Australia. [4]Department of Neuropathology, Royal Prince Alfred Hospital, Camperdown, NSW 2050, Australia.

References

1. Al-Chalabi A, Hardiman O. The epidemiology of ALS: a conspiracy of genes, environment and time. Nat Rev Neurol. 2013;9:617–28.
2. Bettini M, Gargiulo-Monachelli GM, Rodriguez G, Rey RC, Peralta LM, Sica RE. Epidemiology of amyotrophic lateral sclerosis patients in a centre in Buenos Aires. Arq Neuropsiquiatr. 2011;69:867–70.
3. Chio A, Traynor BJ, Lombardo F, Fimognari M, Calvo A, Ghiglione P, et al. Prevalence of SOD1 mutations in the Italian ALS population. Neurology. 2008;70:533–7.
4. McLaughlin RL, Kenna KP, Vajda A, Heverin M, Byrne S, Donaghy CG, et al. Homozygosity mapping in an Irish ALS case-control cohort describes local demographic phenomena and points towards potential recessive risk loci. Genomics. 2015;105:237–41.
5. ALSoD: Amyotrophic Lateral Sclerosis Online genetics Database http://alsod.iop.kcl.ac.uk. Accessed 29 Dec 2016.

6. Steinberg KM, Yu B, Koboldt DC, Mardis ER, Pamphlett R. Exome sequencing of case-unaffected-parents trios reveals recessive and de novo genetic variants in sporadic ALS. Sci Rep. 2015;5:9124.

7. Al-Chalabi A, Fang F, Hanby MF, Leigh PN, Shaw CE, Ye W, et al. An estimate of amyotrophic lateral sclerosis heritability using twin data. J Neurol Neurosurg Psychiatry. 2010;81:1324–6.

8. Bozzoni V, Pansarasa O, Diamanti L, Nosari G, Cereda C, Ceroni M. Amyotrophic lateral sclerosis and environmental factors. Funct Neurol. 2016;31:7–19.

9. Herculano-Houzel S. The glia/neuron ratio: how it varies uniformly across brain structures and species and what that means for brain physiology and evolution. Glia. 2014;62:1377–91.

10. Khakh BS, Sofroniew MV. Diversity of astrocyte functions and phenotypes in neural circuits. Nat Neurosci. 2015;18:942–52.

11. Osellame LD, Blacker TS, Duchen MR. Cellular and molecular mechanisms of mitochondrial function. Best Pract Res Clin Endocrinol Metab. 2012;26:711–23.

12. Swaminathan N. Why does the brain need so much power?. Scientific American MIND [Internet]. 2008; Accessed on 9 Apr 2017. Available from: https://www.scientificamerican.com/article/why-does-the-brain-need-s/.

13. Rolfe DF, Brown GC. Cellular energy utilization and molecular origin of standard metabolic rate in mammals. Physiol Rev. 1997;77:731–58.

14. Du F, Zhu XH, Zhang Y, Friedman M, Zhang N, Ugurbil K, et al. Tightly coupled brain activity and cerebral ATP metabolic rate. Proc Natl Acad Sci U S A. 2008;105:6409–14.

15. Calvo SE, Clauser KR, Mootha VK. MitoCarta2.0: an updated inventory of mammalian mitochondrial proteins. Nucleic Acids Res. 2016;44:D1251–7.

16. Payne BA, Chinnery PF. Mitochondrial dysfunction in aging: much progress but many unresolved questions. Biochim Biophys Acta. 1847;2015:1347–53.

17. Hayakawa K, Esposito E, Wang X, Terasaki Y, Liu Y, Xing C, et al. Transfer of mitochondria from astrocytes to neurons after stroke. Nature. 2016;535:551–5.

18. Vandenberghe N, Leveque N, Corcia P, Brunaud-Danel V, Salort-Campana E, Besson G, et al. Cerebrospinal fluid detection of enterovirus genome in ALS: a study of 242 patients and 354 controls. Amyotroph Lateral Scler. 2010;11:277–82.

19. Mulder DW, Rosenbaum RA, Layton DD Jr. Late progression of poliomyelitis or forme fruste amyotrophic lateral sclerosis? Mayo Clin Proc. 1972;47:756–61.

20. Salazar-Grueso EF, Roos RP. Amyotrophic lateral sclerosis and viruses. Clin Neurosci. 1995;3:360–7.

21. Woodall CJ, Riding MH, Graham DI, Clements GB. Sequences specific for enterovirus detected in spinal cord from patients with motor neurone disease. BMJ. 1994;308:1541–3.

22. Berger MM, Kopp N, Vital C, Redl B, Aymard M, Lina B. Detection and cellular localization of enterovirus RNA sequences in spinal cord of patients with ALS. Neurology. 2000;54:20–5.

23. Giraud P, Beaulieux F, Ono S, Shimizu N, Chazot G, Lina B. Detection of enteroviral sequences from frozen spinal cord samples of Japanese ALS patients. Neurology. 2001;56:1777–8.

24. Dalakas MC. The post-polio syndrome as an evolved clinical entity. Definition and clinical description. Ann N Y Acad Sci. 1995;753:68–80.

25. Destombes J, Couderc T, Thiesson D, Girard S, Wilt SG, Blondel B. Persistent poliovirus infection in mouse motoneurons. J Virol. 1997;71:1621–8.

26. Beaulieux F, Zreik Y, Deleage C, Sauvinet V, Legay V, Giraudon P, et al. Cumulative mutations in the genome of echovirus 6 during establishment of a chronic infection in precursors of glial cells. Virus Genes. 2005;30:103–12.

27. Berger MM, Jia XY, Legay V, Aymard M, Tilles JG, Lina B. Nutrition- and virus-induced stress represses the expression of manganese superoxide dismutase in vitro. Exp Biol Med (Maywood). 2004;229:843–9.

28. Legay V, Deleage C, Beaulieux F, Giraudon P, Aymard M, Lina B. Impaired glutamate uptake and EAAT2 downregulation in an enterovirus chronically infected human glial cell line. Eur J Neurosci. 2003;17:1820–8.

29. Pavio N, Couderc T, Girard S, Sgro JY, Blondel B, Colbere-Garapin F. Expression of mutated poliovirus receptors in human neuroblastoma cells persistently infected with poliovirus. Virology. 2000;274:331–42.

30. Frisk G. Mechanisms of chronic enteroviral persistence in tissue. Curr Opin Infect Dis. 2001;14:251–6.

31. Li W, Lee MH, Henderson L, Tyagi R, Bachani M, Steiner J, et al. Human endogenous retrovirus-K contributes to motor neuron disease. Sci Transl Med. 2015;7:307ra–153.

32. Sutedja NA, Veldink JH, Fischer K, Kromhout H, Heederik D, Huisman MH, et al. Exposure to chemicals and metals and risk of amyotrophic lateral sclerosis: a systematic review. Amyotroph Lateral Scler. 2009;10:302–9.

33. Su FC, Goutman SA, Chernyak S, Mukherjee B, Callaghan BC, Batterman S, et al. Association of Environmental Toxins with Amyotrophic Lateral Sclerosis. JAMA Neurol. 2016;73:803–11.

34. Das K, Nag C, Ghosh M. Familial, environmental, and occupational risk factors in development of amyotrophic lateral sclerosis. N Am J Med Sci. 2012;4:350–5.

35. Malek AM, Barchowsky A, Bowser R, Heiman-Patterson T, Lacomis D, Rana S, et al. Environmental and occupational risk factors for amyotrophic lateral sclerosis: a case-control study. Neurodegener Dis. 2014;14:31–8.

36. Chen Y. Organophosphate-induced brain damage: mechanisms, neuropsychiatric and neurological consequences, and potential therapeutic strategies. NeuroToxicology. 2012;33:391–400.

37. Kanavouras K, Tzatzarakis MN, Mastorodemos V, Plaitakis A, Tsatsakis AM. A case report of motor neuron disease in a patient showing significant level of DDTs, HCHs and organophosphate metabolites in hair as well as levels of hexane and toluene in blood. Toxicol Appl Pharmacol. 2011;256:399–404.

38. Pinkerton LE, Hein MJ, Grajewski B, Kamel F. Mortality from neurodegenerative diseases in a cohort of US flight attendants. Am J Ind Med. 2016;59:532–7.

39. Hecker H, Kincl L, McNeeley E, van Netten C, Murawski J, Vallarino JD, et al. Cabin air quality incidents project report. 2014; Accessed on 9 Apr 2017. Available from: http://www.ohrca.org/wp-content/uploads/2014/08/finalreport.pdf.

40. Solbu K, Daae HL, Thorud S, Ellingsen DG, Lundanes E, Molander P. Exposure to airborne organophosphates originating from hydraulic and turbine oils among aviation technicians and loaders. J Environ Monit. 2010;12:2259–68.

41. Callaghan B, Feldman D, Gruis K, Feldman E. The association of exposure to lead, mercury, and selenium and the development of amyotrophic lateral sclerosis and the epigenetic implications. Neurodegener Dis. 2011;8:1–8.

42. Pamphlett R, Kum JS. Heavy metals in locus ceruleus and motor neurons in motor neuron disease. Acta Neuropathol Commun. 2013;1:81.

43. Gresham LS, Molgaard CA, Golbeck AL, Smith R. Lead exposure and ALS. Neurology. 1992;42:2228–9.

44. Kamel F, Umbach DM, Munsat TL, Shefner JM, Hu H, Sandler DP. Lead exposure and amyotrophic lateral sclerosis. Epidemiology. 2002;13:311–9.

45. Strickland D, Smith SA, Dolliff G, Goldman L, Roelofs RI. Amyotrophic lateral sclerosis and occupational history. A pilot case-control study. Arch Neurol. 1996;53:730–3.

46. Conradi S, Ronnevi LO, Vesterberg O. Lead concentration in skeletal muscle in amyotrophic lateral sclerosis patients and control subjects. J Neurol Neurosurg Psychiatry. 1978;41:1001–4.

47. Patrick L. Lead toxicity, a review of the literature. Part 1: exposure, evaluation, and treatment. Altern Med Rev. 2006;11:2–22.

48. Chio A, Benzi G, Dossena M, Mutani R, Mora G. Severely increased risk of amyotrophic lateral sclerosis among Italian professional football players. Brain. 2005;128:472–6.

49. Kamel F, Umbach DM, Bedlack RS, Richards M, Watson M, Alavanja MC, et al. Pesticide exposure and amyotrophic lateral sclerosis. NeuroToxicology. 2012; 33:457–62.

50. Elbaz A, Clavel J, Rathouz PJ, Moisan F, Galanaud JP, Delemotte B, et al. Professional exposure to pesticides and Parkinson disease. Ann Neurol. 2009;66:494–504.

51. Hernandez AF, Gonzalez-Alzaga B, Lopez-Flores I, Lacasana M. Systematic reviews on neurodevelopmental and neurodegenerative disorders linked to pesticide exposure: methodological features and impact on risk assessment. Environ Int. 2016;92-93:657–79.

52. Armon C. Smoking may be considered an established risk factor for sporadic ALS. Neurology. 2009;73:1693–8.

53. Alonso A, Logroscino G, Jick SS, Hernan MA. Association of smoking with amyotrophic lateral sclerosis risk and survival in men and women: a prospective study. BMC Neurol. 2010;10:6.

54. Wang H, O'Reilly EJ, Weisskopf MG, Logroscino G, McCullough ML, Thun MJ, et al. Smoking and risk of amyotrophic lateral sclerosis: a pooled analysis of 5 prospective cohorts. Arch Neurol. 2011;68:207–13.

55. Beard JD, Engel LS, Richardson DB, Gammon MD, Baird C, Umbach DM, et al. Military service, deployments, and exposures in relation to amyotrophic lateral sclerosis etiology. Environ Int. 2016;91:104–15.

56. Pamphlett R, Rikard-Bell A. Different occupations associated with amyotrophic lateral sclerosis: is diesel exhaust the link? Plos One. 2013;8:e80993.

57. Flegal KM, Brownie C, Haas JD. The effects of exposure misclassification on estimates of relative risk. Am J Epidemiol. 1986;123:736–51.

58. Smith GD, Ebrahim S. 'Mendelian randomization': can genetic epidemiology contribute to understanding environmental determinants of disease? Int J Epidemiol. 2003;32:1–22.

59. Munafo MR, Araya R. Cigarette smoking and depression: a question of causation. Br J Psychiatry. 2010;196:425–6.

60. Angrist JD, Imbens GW, Rubin DB. Identification of causal effects using instrumental variables. J Am Stat Assoc. 1996;91:444–55.

61. Clarke PS, Windmeijer F. Instrumental variable estimators for binary outcomes. J Am Stat Assoc. 2012;107:1638–52.

62. Wehby GL, Ohsfeldt RL, Murray JC. 'Mendelian randomization' equals instrumental variable analysis with genetic instruments. Stat Med. 2008;27:2745–9.

63. Saunderson R, Yu B, Trent RJ, Pamphlett R. A polymorphism in the poliovirus receptor gene differs in motor neuron disease. NeuroReport. 2004;15:383–6.

64. Leon-Monzon ME, Illa I, Dalakas MC. Expression of poliovirus receptor in human spinal cord and muscle. Ann N Y Acad Sci. 1995;753:48–57.

65. Alidjinou EK, Sane F, Bertin A, Caloone D, Hober D. Persistent infection of human pancreatic cells with Coxsackievirus B4 is cured by fluoxetine. Antivir Res. 2015;116:51–4.

66. Costa LG, Giordano G, Cole TB, Marsillach J, Furlong CE. Paraoxonase 1 (PON1) as a genetic determinant of susceptibility to organophosphate toxicity. Toxicology. 2013;307:115–22.

67. Morahan JM, Yu B, Trent RJ, Pamphlett R. A gene-environment study of the paraoxonase 1 gene and pesticides in amyotrophic lateral sclerosis. NeuroToxicology. 2007;28:532–40.

68. Ticozzi N, LeClerc AL, Keagle PJ, Glass JD, Wills AM, van Blitterswijk M, et al. Paraoxonase gene mutations in amyotrophic lateral sclerosis. Ann Neurol. 2010;68:102–7.

69. Wills AM, Cronin S, Slowik A, Kasperaviciute D, Van Es MA, Morahan JM, et al. A large-scale international meta-analysis of paraoxonase gene polymorphisms in sporadic ALS. Neurology. 2009;73:16–24.

70. Miles AT, Hawksworth GM, Beattie JH, Rodilla V. Induction, regulation, degradation, and biological significance of mammalian metallothioneins. Crit Rev Biochem Mol Biol. 2000;35:35–70.

71. Giedroc DP, Chen X, Apuy JL. Metal response element (MRE)-binding transcription factor-1 (MTF-1): structure, function, and regulation. Antioxid Redox Signal. 2001;3:577–96.

72. Morahan JM, Yu B, Trent RJ, Pamphlett R. Genetic susceptibility to environmental toxicants in ALS. Am J Med Genet B Neuropsychiatr Genet. 2007;144B:885–90.

73. Sasaki S, Iwata M. Mitochondrial alterations in the spinal cord of patients with sporadic amyotrophic lateral sclerosis. J Neuropathol Exp Neurol. 2007; 66:10–6.

74. Nakano Y, Hirayama K, Terao K. Hepatic ultrastructural changes and liver dysfunction in amyotrophic lateral sclerosis. Arch Neurol. 1987;44:103–6.

75. Vielhaber S, Kunz D, Winkler K, Wiedemann FR, Kirches E, Feistner H, et al. Mitochondrial DNA abnormalities in skeletal muscle of patients with sporadic amyotrophic lateral sclerosis. Brain. 2000;123(Pt 7):1339–48.

76. Payne BA, Wilson IJ, Yu-Wai-Man P, Coxhead J, Deehan D, Horvath R, et al. Universal heteroplasmy of human mitochondrial DNA. Hum Mol Genet. 2013;22:384–90.

77. Sica RE, Nicola AF, Gonzalez Deniselle MC, Rodriguez G, Monachelli GM, Peralta LM, et al. Sporadic amyotrophic lateral sclerosis: new hypothesis regarding its etiology and pathogenesis suggests that astrocytes might be the primary target hosting a still unknown external agent. Arq Neuropsiquiatr. 2011;69:699–706.

78. Chang LW, Hartmann HA. Electron microscopic histochemical study on the localization and distribution of mercury in the nervous system after mercury intoxication. Exp Neurol. 1972;35:122–37.

79. Linnane AW, Marzuki S, Ozawa T, Tanaka M. Mitochondrial DNA mutations as an important contributor to ageing and degenerative diseases. Lancet. 1989;1:642–5.

80. Aggarwal A, Nicholson G. Detection of preclinical motor neurone loss in SOD1 mutation carriers using motor unit number estimation. J Neurol Neurosurg Psychiatry. 2002;73:199–201.

81. Vucic S, Nicholson GA, Kiernan MC. Cortical hyperexcitability may precede the onset of familial amyotrophic lateral sclerosis. Brain. 2008;131:1540–50.

82. Pamphlett R, Kum JS. Age-related uptake of heavy metals in human spinal Interneurons. Plos One. 2016;11:e0162260.

83. Ravits J. Focality, stochasticity and neuroanatomic propagation in ALS pathogenesis. Exp Neurol. 2014;262 Pt B:121-126.

84. Al-Chalabi A, Calvo A, Chio A, Colville S, Ellis CM, Hardiman O, et al. Analysis of amyotrophic lateral sclerosis as a multistep process: a population-based modelling study. Lancet Neurol. 2014;13:1108–13.

85. Ilieva EV, Ayala V, Jove M, Dalfo E, Cacabelos D, Povedano M, et al. Oxidative and endoplasmic reticulum stress interplay in sporadic amyotrophic lateral sclerosis. Brain. 2007;130:3111–23.

13

Salidroside reduces tau hyperphosphorylation via up-regulating GSK-3β phosphorylation in a tau transgenic *Drosophila* model of Alzheimer's disease

Bei Zhang[1,2†], Qiongqiong Li[1†], Xingkun Chu[2], Suya Sun[1*] and Shengdi Chen[1,2*]

Abstract

Background: Alzheimer's disease (AD) is an age-related and progressive neurodegenerative disease that causes substantial public health care burdens. Intensive efforts have been made to find effective and safe treatment against AD. Salidroside (Sal) is the main effective component of *Rhodiola rosea L.*, which has several pharmacological activities.

The objective of this study was to investigate the efficacy of Sal in the treatment of AD transgenic *Drosophila* and the associated mechanisms.

Methods: We used tau transgenic *Drosophila* line (TAU) in which tau protein is expressed in the central nervous system and eyes by the Gal4/UAS system. After feeding flies with Sal, the lifespan and locomotor activity were recorded. We further examined the appearance of vacuoles in the mushroom body using immunohistochemistry, and detected the levels of total glycogen synthase kinase 3β (t-GSK-3β), phosphorylated GSK-3β (p-GSK-3β), t-tau and p-tau in the brain by western blot analysis.

Results: Our results showed that the longevity was improved in salidroside-fed *Drosophila* groups as well as the locomotor activity. We also observed less vacuoles in the mushroom body, upregulated level of p-GSK-3β and downregulated p-tau following Sal treatment.

Conclusion: Our data presented the evidence that Sal was capable of reducing the neurodegeneration in tau transgenic *Drosophila* and inhibiting neuronal loss. The neuroprotective effects of Sal were associated with its up-regulation of the p-GSK-3β and down-regulation of the p-tau.

Keywords: Alzheimer's disease, Salidroside, *Drosophila*, Glycogen synthase kinase 3β, Tau

Background

Alzheimer's disease (AD) is a progressive and fatal brain disorder, and affects approximately 36 million people worldwide. This number is expected to double during the next 20 years [1]. Neuropathologically, it is characterized by accumulation of extracellular senile plaques consisting of deposits of beta-amyloid (Aβ) and intracellular neurofibrillary tangles consisting of hyperphosphorylated

tau protein, which ultimately lead to neuronal loss and brain atrophy [2, 3].

In fact, the tau hypothesis suggests that neurofibrillary tangles in the brain represent a major component of the pathophysiology of Alzheimer's disease [4], which is attributable to an abnormal phosphorylation of tau protein in the brains of AD patients. Under normal circumstances, tau protein is a neuronal microtubule-associated protein that has a crucial role in assemblage and stabilization of microtubules on neuronal axons and the inhibition of apoptosis [5, 6]. However, when tau is abnormally hyperphosphorylated, it destabilizes microtubules by decreasing the binding affinity of tau, and consequently

---

* Correspondence: sunsuya@shsmu.edu.cn; chen_sd@medmail.com.cn
†Equal contributors
[1]Department of Neurology and Institute of Neurology, Ruijin Hospital, Shanghai Jiao Tong University School of Medicine, 197 Ruijin Er Road, Shanghai 200025, China
Full list of author information is available at the end of the article

leads to microtubule destabilization, disruption of the axonal transport system, and ultimately, the formation of intracellular neurofibrillary tangles (NFTs). NFT formation spreads to various brain areas during AD progression, ultimately causing neuronal death [7–13]. Previous studies have shown that increasing tau phosphorylation occurs early in the development of AD [14, 15], and that Aβ associated clinical cognitive decline is identified only following such elevated tau phosphorylation [14, 16]. It is expected that intervening the formation of these toxic assemblies would attenuate the appearance and development of the symptoms of AD. Although many researches have discovered a great deal of pharmaceutical treatments for AD, no effective compound has been found so far for this debilitating neurodegenerative disease.

Over the past decades, drug therapies for AD primarily aim at slowing down the cognitive decline and ameliorating the behavioral symptoms, but the pharmacological effects of these drugs remain unsatisfactory. Salidroside (Sal), as one of the active ingredients extracted from the root of Rhodiola rosea L, which is extensively used in traditional folk medicine in Asian and European countries and has been reported to exhibit various strong pharmacological activities. The main effects of Sal are described as anti-oxidative, anti-apoptosis, anti-inflammatory, anti-cancer, and anti-fatigue effects [17–23]. Additional studies have shown that Sal exerts a neuroprotective effect. For example, Sal is able to protect neurons from apoptosis induced by various factors [24–26]. It remains undemonstrated whether Sal exerts neuroprotection against tau-induced toxicity in AD.

In the present study, we investigated the therapeutic potential of Sal in tau transgenic AD model. We found that Sal treatment could improve locomotor functions and prolong lifespan of AD transgenic Drosophila. Moreover, we demonstrated that Sal could protect neurons against tau-induced toxicity, which might be associated with regulation of GSK-3β.

Methods

Reagents

Salidroside (Sal, Purity > 99.7%) was obtained from the Green Valley Pharmaceutical Corporation (Shanghai, China). It was dissolved in PBS to a stock concentration of 100 mM and stored at −20 °C. Donepezil was supplied by Eisai Pharmaceutical Co., Ltd. (Tokyo, Japan).

The following antibodies were used: Phospho-GSK-3β antibody, GSK-3β antibody, Mouse monoclonal Phospho-tau (ser396) antibody and tau (Cell Signaling Technology), Mouse monoclonal anti-β-actin antibody (Sigma–Aldrich, Clone AC-15), HRP-conjugated goat anti-mouse IgG (Jackson Immuno Research Laboratories, PA, USA). All chemicals were purchased from Sigma-Aldrich except those noted otherwise.

Drosophila stocks

All Drosophila stocks were maintained at 25 °C under a 12:12 h light: dark cycle at constant 65% humidity as previously described [27]. The flies were raised in 50 ml plastic vials containing standard Drosophila medium. Transgenic upstream activating sequence (UAS) carrying human tau was obtained from Drosophila Stock Center (Institute of Biochemistry and Cell Biology, Shanghai).

Longevity assay

New flies were collected within 24 h after eclosion for the experiment. At least 100 flies of each genotype were collected and divided into fresh food vials of 20 flies. Food vials were changed every 2–3 days, and the number of dead flies was counted at that time. The survival times described were given as median standard error of the median. Survival curves were analyzed using Kaplan-Meier estimation and log-rank statistical analysis.

Climbing assay

Locomotor function of Drosophila was measured according to the climbing assay as previously reported [28]. Briefly, 10 male flies per 25 ml tube ($n = 30$ for each group) were placed at the bottom, and given 30 min to recover. After 10 s of climbing, the numbers of Drosophila between the 0, 5, 10, 15, 20 and 25 ml scale marks were recorded with a video camera. The experiment was performed three times. The results for each group were calculated by the formula below:

$$
\begin{aligned}
\text{Climbing Index} =\ & (\text{flies above 20 ml scale mark}) \times 1 \\
& + (\text{flies between 15 and 20 ml scale marks}) \times 0.8 \\
& + (\text{flies between 10 and 15 ml scale marks}) \times 0.6 \\
& + (\text{flies between 5 and 10 ml scale marks}) \times 0.4 \\
& + (\text{flies below 5 ml scale mark}) \times 0.2.
\end{aligned}
$$

Histological analysis

For immunostaining analysis, flies ($n = 10$ for each group) were fixed in freshly prepared 4% paraformaldehyde, processed to embed in paraffin blocks, and sectioned at a thickness of 5 μm. Sections were placed on slides, stained with hematoxylin and eosin, and examined by bright field illumination using a Leica DM 2500 microscope at the magnification of 60×. The areas of the vacuoles in the cell body or neuropil regions were captured.

Western blot analysis

After treatment, fly heads ($n = 50$ for each group) were homogenized in lysis buffer (50 mM Tris–HCl pH 8.0, 150 mM NaCl, 1% NP-40, 0.5% sodium deoxycholate,

0.1% SDS) with protease inhibitor cocktail (Roche, Basle, Switzerland) and 1 mM phenylmethyl sulfonyl-fluoride (PMSF) for 30 min on ice. Total extracts were centrifuged at 14,000 × g for 30 min and boiled in 4× SDS loading buffer for 5 min. The samples were subjected to SDS polyacrylamide gel electrophoresis (SDS-PAGE) and transferred to a polyvinylidene fluoride membrane (Millipore, Bedford, MA, USA). The membranes were blocked using 5% skim milk in TBST for 1 h then incubated at 4 °C overnight with respective primary antibodies to t-GSK-3β(1:1000), p-GSK-3β(1:1000), t-tau (1:1000), p-tau (1:1000) and β-actin (1:5000). After being washed three times with TBST, the membranes were incubated with horseradish peroxidase (HRP)-conjugated goat anti-rabbit/mouse antibody (1:10000) for 2 h at room temperature. Visualized with the indicated antibodies using Immobilon Western Chemiluminescent HRP Substrate (Millipore) and analyzed by ImageJ (National Institutes of Health) software. All the experiments were performed at least three times and the most representative results were shown.

Statistical analysis

All statistical analysis was performed using SPSS software 19.0(SPSS Inc., Chicago, IL). The Kaplan–Meier test was used to assess the difference in the lifespan curves. Two-group comparisons were analyzed using Student t-test. A comparison of three or more groups was performed using one-way ANOVA followed by Tukey's test. All experiments were carried out in triplicate ($n = 3$) and results were expressed as the mean ± standard error of the mean (SEM). Calculated comparisons were at confidence interval (CI) 95%. A P-value < 0.05 was considered statistically significant.

Results

Sal prolonged the lifespan of AD transgenic flies

Drosophila AD models were generated by expressing human tau, which have been assisted in the identification of novel targets for therapy [29]. These models show intracellular neurofibrillary tangles consisting of hyperphosphorylated tau protein and ultimately significant reduction in longevity [29, 30]. To assess the effect of Sal in living organisms, we firstly fed human tau transgenic flies with Sal in various concentrations (2 μM, 6 μM and 20 μM) or Donepezil (10 μM, the clinically approved drug for the treatment of AD) as positive control and measured their survival duration. We found that the lifespan of Sal-treated flies was more prolonged compared to that of the untreated flies. Sal treatment increased both the survival rate and the median survival time of flies, which is comparable to the improving effect of Donepezil (Fig. 1).

Sal treatment improved locomotor activity in AD flies

Locomotor assay is a behavioral paradigm to assess the neural functional abnormalities based on the negative geotaxis against gravity. We fed tau flies with Sal or Donepezil at different time points (10, 20, 30, and 40 days), and we found Sal treatment improved the climbing ability of these AD transgenic flies significantly in a dose dependent manner after 30 days compared to the control (the ctrl group) (Fig. 2). However, no obvious difference was observed between the treated and non-treated groups at time points of 10 and 20 days (Fig. 2).

Effects of Sal on neuronal loss in AD flies

The tau flies were able to replicate the features of human in progressive neurodegeneration with some extent as previously reported [31]. The appearance of vacuoles in the brain is thought as a hallmark of neurodegeneration in Drosophila, which represents the neuronal loss of brain [27]. As seen in Fig. 3, the transgenic AD fly model showed numerous vacuoles and exhibited loosely packed neurons all over the mushroom body at postnatal 30 days. Sal treatment in the dose of 6 μM was able to prevent these histological abnormalities in vacuoles and neuronal

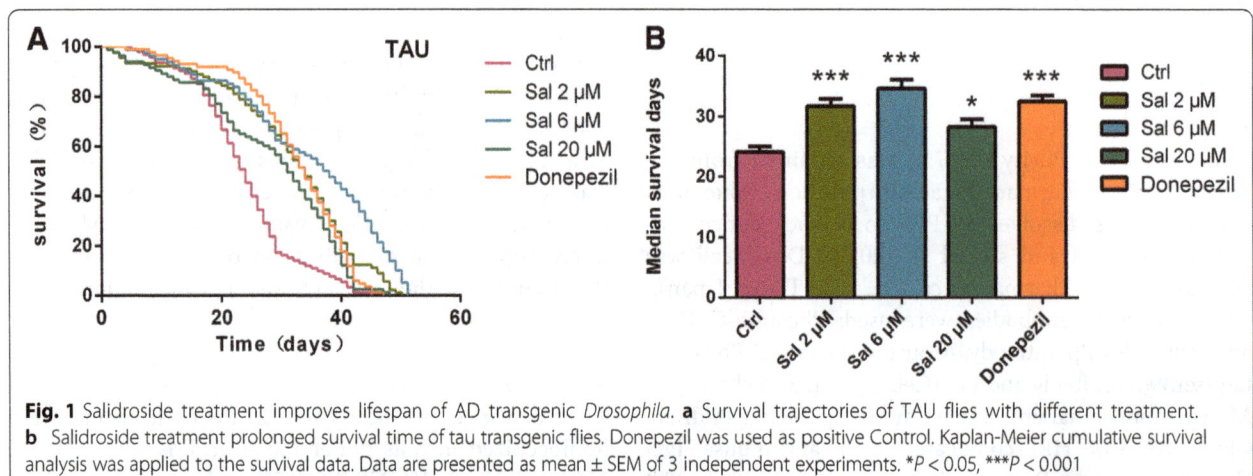

Fig. 1 Salidroside treatment improves lifespan of AD transgenic Drosophila. **a** Survival trajectories of TAU flies with different treatment. **b** Salidroside treatment prolonged survival time of tau transgenic flies. Donepezil was used as positive Control. Kaplan-Meier cumulative survival analysis was applied to the survival data. Data are presented as mean ± SEM of 3 independent experiments. *P < 0.05, ***P < 0.001

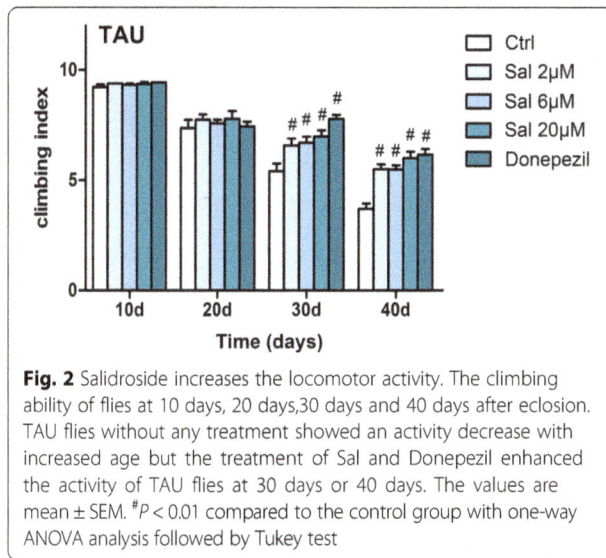

Fig. 2 Salidroside increases the locomotor activity. The climbing ability of flies at 10 days, 20 days,30 days and 40 days after eclosion. TAU flies without any treatment showed an activity decrease with increased age but the treatment of Sal and Donepezil enhanced the activity of TAU flies at 30 days or 40 days. The values are mean ± SEM. #$P < 0.01$ compared to the control group with one-way ANOVA analysis followed by Tukey test

packing phenotype, which appeared a better therapeutic effect than that in Donepezil- treated group.

Sal regulated GSK-3β phosphorylation

To explore the signaling pathways that may be involved in Sal effects, we next assessed whether Sal affected GSK-3β phosphorylation and tau phosphorylation in flies, as GSK-3β signal pathway exerts a crucial role in promoting neuronal survival under a variety of circumstances, while tau hyperphosphorylation and microtubule destabilization is widely acknowledged in AD [32–34]. We detected GSK-3β protein expression in *Drosophila* brain after Sal or Donepezil treatment, and found that Sal increased the level of p-GSK-3β effectively while decreased the level of p-tau, a downstream target of GSK-3β (Fig. 4). This result indicates that the neuroprotective

effects of Sal in the tau transgenic AD flies might be associated with the regulation of GSK-3β.

Discussion

During the last decade, *Drosophila* has emerged and been recognized as a powerful model to study human neurodegenerative diseases including AD. Although this model can not detect memory and cognitive function, the short generation time and short lifespan make it particularly amenable to study such age-related disorders [30, 35–37]. In the present study, we showed that Sal treatment prolonged the lifespan and improved locomotor abilities in a tau-expressing transgenic *Drosophila* model. Furthermore, we demonstrated that Sal could dramatically attenuate the neuronal loss in the brains. As far as we know, this is the first evidence for Sal play an important protective role in neurons through up-regulatingGSK-3β phosphorylation in transgenic flies. As Sal was reported with property of non-toxic and mitigated neurotoxicity [38], our study provides a potential promising drug candidate for AD therapy.

In the last two decades, drug discovery and development efforts for AD have been dominated by the "amyloid cascade hypothesis," focusing on targets defined by this hypothesis and proposing amyloid as the main cause of neural death and dementia. Unfortunately, several clinical trials with anti-Aβ agents failed, thus challenging the hypothesis that Aβ accumulation is the initiating event in the pathological cascade of AD, so we need to explore some novel therapeutic approaches and targets [39]. In recent years, tau-based treatments for AD have become a point of increasing focus and future investigational therapies [40]. Inhibition of the toxicity of tau in the brain may offer significant promise for the treatment of this disease. Our experiments in tau-expressing transgenic *Drosophila* showed that Sal attenuated tau-induced cytotoxicity

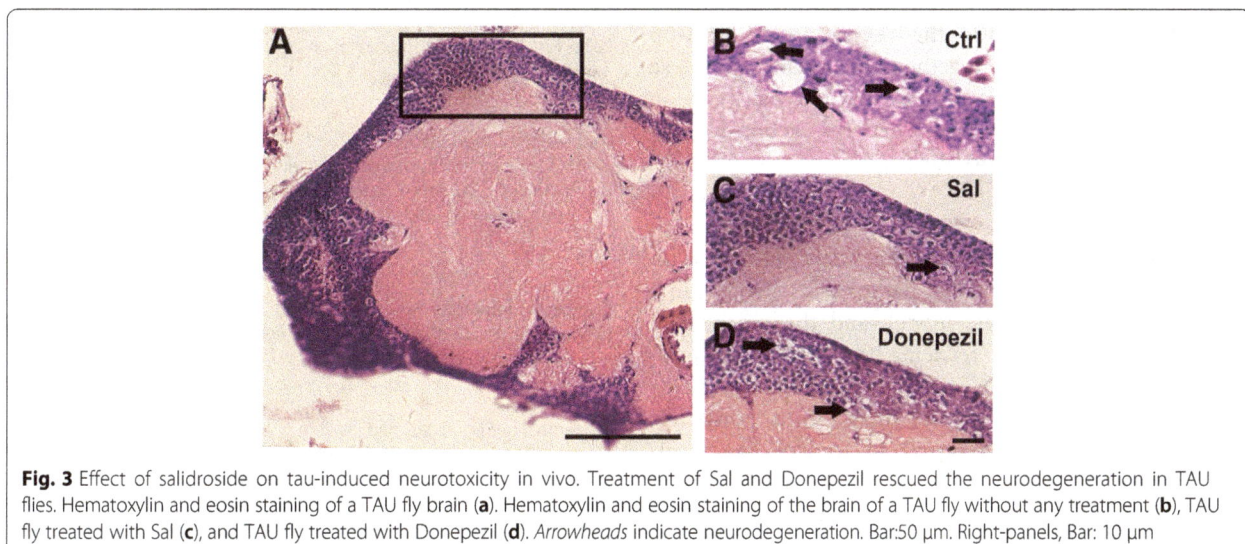

Fig. 3 Effect of salidroside on tau-induced neurotoxicity in vivo. Treatment of Sal and Donepezil rescued the neurodegeneration in TAU flies. Hematoxylin and eosin staining of a TAU fly brain (**a**). Hematoxylin and eosin staining of the brain of a TAU fly without any treatment (**b**), TAU fly treated with Sal (**c**), and TAU fly treated with Donepezil (**d**). *Arrowheads* indicate neurodegeneration. Bar:50 μm. Right-panels, Bar: 10 μm

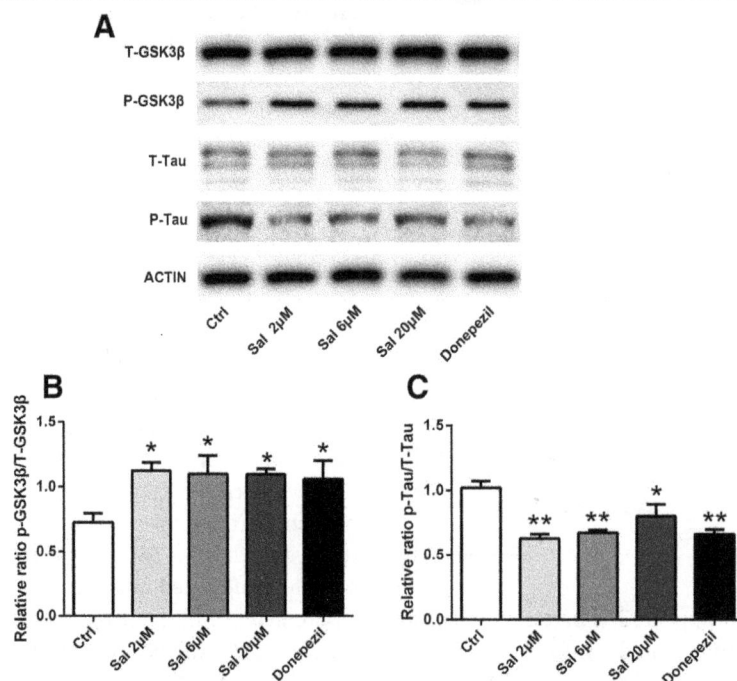

Fig. 4 Salidroside inhibits tau-induced neurotoxicity by activating the GSK-3β in vivo. **a** Tau-expressing transgenic flies were treated with Sal or Donepezil for 30 days. The levels of total GSK-3β, total tau, phosphorylated GSK-3β and phosphorylated tau were detected and compared with the control group. **b** The expression levels of GSK-3β, tau and their phosphorylated form were detected. All data are presented as mean ± SEM.*$p < 0.05$, **$p < 0.01$ (one-way ANOVA and Tukey's test)

effectively, suggesting a novel effect of Sal through inhibiting the tau phosphorylation in AD brain.

GSK-3β is a ubiquitously expressed serine/threonine kinase that plays a key role in the pathogenesis of AD. GSK-3β phosphorylates tau in most serine and threonine residues hyperphosphorylated in paired helical filaments [41]. The effect of Sal in the flies increased GSK-3β phosphorylation significantly, while inhibiting tau phosphorylation simultaneously. These results suggest a possible causal relationship for Sal effect between tau hyperphosphorylation and the regulation of GSK-3β phosphorylation. Taken together, the findings of these experiments support the proposition that Sal plays an important role in providing the neuroprotection for AD by regulating tau phosphorylation.

Conclusion

In summary, we demonstrated that the treatment with Sal relieved the behavioral and pathological changes in a tau transgenic Drosophila model, and the mechanism was associated with its reducing tau hyperphosphorylation via up-regulating GSK-3β phosphorylation. These findings suggest that the Sal may protect neurons from degeneration in brains of AD models, and provide a potential approach in prevention and treatment of AD models. Although Sal has been prescribed to patients with cardiovascular disease and exhibited

various pharmacological activities, further multiple studies should be carried out to evaluate the efficacies of Sal against AD.

Acknowledgements
We thank Dr. Nan-Jie Xu for helpful comments on the manuscript, and Dr. Gang Pei for providing transgenic Drosophila.

Funding
This work was supported by grants from the National Natural Science Fund (91332107, 81430022, 81371407). All founding were used for the design, collection, analysis and interpretation of data and in writing in the manuscript.

Authors' contributions
All authors read and approved the final manuscript. BZ summarized the background. QL, XC and BZ performed the experiment. BZ and QL conceived, designed, and performed the paper. SC and SS revised the paper.

Competing interests
The authors declare that they have no competing interest.

Author details
[1]Department of Neurology and Institute of Neurology, Ruijin Hospital, Shanghai Jiao Tong University School of Medicine, 197 Ruijin Er Road, Shanghai 200025, China. [2]Laboratory of Neurodegenerative Diseases, Institute of Health Sciences, Shanghai Institutes for Biological Sciences (SIBS), Chinese Academy of Sciences (CAS) & Shanghai Jiao Tong University School of Medicine (SJTUSM), Shanghai 200025, China.

References

1. Wimo A, et al. The worldwide economic impact of dementia 2010. Alzheimers Dement. 2013;9(1):1–11. e3.

2. Querfurth HW, LaFerla FM. Alzheimer's disease. N Engl J Med. 2010; 362(4):329–44.

3. Hardy J, Selkoe DJ. The amyloid hypothesis of Alzheimer's disease: progress and problems on the road to therapeutics. Science. 2002;297(5580):353–6.

4. Hutton M, Hardy J. The presenilins and Alzheimer's disease. Hum Mol Genet. 1997;6(10):1639–46.

5. Scholz T, Mandelkow E. Transport and diffusion of Tau protein in neurons. Cell Mol Life Sci. 2014;71(16):3139–50.

6. Ballatore C, et al. Microtubule stabilizing agents as potential treatment for Alzheimer's disease and related neurodegenerative tauopathies. J Med Chem. 2012;55(21):8979–96.

7. Brunden KR, et al. Brain-penetrant microtubule-stabilizing compounds as potential therapeutic agents for tauopathies. Biochem Soc Trans. 2012; 40(4):661–6.

8. Duan Y, et al. Advances in the pathogenesis of Alzheimer's disease: focusing on tau-mediated neurodegeneration. Transl Neurodegener. 2012;1(1):24.

9. Grundke-Iqbal I, et al. Abnormal phosphorylation of the microtubule-associated protein tau (tau) in Alzheimer cytoskeletal pathology. Proc Natl Acad Sci U S A. 1986;83(13):4913–7.

10. Grundke-Iqbal I, et al. Microtubule-associated protein tau. A component of Alzheimer paired helical filaments. J Biol Chem. 1986;261(13):6084–9.

11. Iqbal K, et al. Defective brain microtubule assembly in Alzheimer's disease. Lancet. 1986;2(8504):421–6.

12. Kosik KS, Joachim CL, Selkoe DJ. Microtubule-associated protein tau (tau) is a major antigenic component of paired helical filaments in Alzheimer disease. Proc Natl Acad Sci U S A. 1986;83(11):4044–8.

13. Gomez-Isla T, et al. Neuronal loss correlates with but exceeds neurofibrillary tangles in Alzheimer's disease. Ann Neurol. 1997;41(1):17–24.

14. Desikan RS, et al. Amyloid-beta–associated clinical decline occurs only in the presence of elevated P-tau. Arch Neurol. 2012;69(6):709–13.

15. Obulesu M, Venu R, Somashekhar R. Tau mediated neurodegeneration: an insight into Alzheimer's disease pathology. Neurochem Res. 2011;36(8):1329–35.

16. Desikan RS, et al. Amyloid-beta associated volume loss occurs only in the presence of phospho-tau. Ann Neurol. 2011;70(4):657–61.

17. Zhu Y, et al. Salidroside protects against hydrogen peroxide-induced injury in cardiac H9c2 cells via PI3K-Akt dependent pathway. DNA Cell Biol. 2011;30(10):809–19.

18. Shi K, et al. Salidroside protects retinal endothelial cells against hydrogen peroxide-induced injury via modulating oxidative status and apoptosis. Biosci Biotechnol Biochem. 2015;79(9):1406–13.

19. Jin H, et al. Therapeutic intervention of learning and memory decays by salidroside stimulation of neurogenesis in aging. Mol Neurobiol. 2016;53(2):851–66.

20. Feng Y, et al. Optimization on Preparation Conditions of Salidroside Liposome and Its Immunological Activity on PCV-2 in Mice. Evid Based Complement Alternat Med. 2015;2015:178128.

21. Liu S, et al. Salidroside rescued mice from experimental sepsis through anti-inflammatory and anti-apoptosis effects. J Surg Res. 2015;195(1): 277–83.

22. Zhao G, et al. Salidroside inhibits the growth of human breast cancer in vitro and in vivo. Oncol Rep. 2015;33(5):2553–60.

23. Li X, et al. Effect of Tongxinluo on nerve regeneration in mice with diabetic peripheral neuropathy. Cell Mol Biol (Noisy-le-Grand). 2015;61(5):103–7.

24. Xian H, et al. MADP, a salidroside analog, protects hippocampal neurons from glutamate induced apoptosis. Life Sci. 2014;103(1):34–40.

25. Zhang B, et al. Neuroprotective effects of salidroside through PI3K/Akt pathway activation in Alzheimer's disease models. Drug Des Devel Ther. 2016;10:1335–43.

26. Xiao L, et al. Salidroside protects Caenorhabditis elegans neurons from polyglutamine-mediated toxicity by reducing oxidative stress. Molecules. 2014;19(6):7757–69.

27. Wang Y, et al. The combination of aricept with a traditional Chinese medicine formula, smart soup, may be a novel way to treat Alzheimer's disease. J Alzheimers Dis. 2015;45(4):1185–95.

28. Lee FK, et al. The role of ubiquitin linkages on alpha-synuclein induced-toxicity in a Drosophila model of Parkinson's disease. J Neurochem. 2009;110(1):208–19.

29. Mudher A, et al. GSK-3beta inhibition reverses axonal transport defects and behavioural phenotypes in Drosophila. Mol Psychiatry. 2004;9(5):522–30.

30. Folwell J, et al. Abeta exacerbates the neuronal dysfunction caused by human tau expression in a Drosophila model of Alzheimer's disease. Exp Neurol. 2010;223(2):401–9.

31. Greeve I, et al. Age-dependent neurodegeneration and Alzheimer-amyloid plaque formation in transgenic Drosophila. J Neurosci. 2004;24(16):3899–906.

32. Rapoport M, et al. Tau is essential to beta -amyloid-induced neurotoxicity. Proc Natl Acad Sci U S A. 2002;99(9):6364–9.

33. Mohamed NV, et al. Spreading of tau pathology in Alzheimer's disease by cell-to-cell transmission. Eur J Neurosci. 2013;37(12):1939–48.

34. Iqbal K, Gong CX, Liu F. Microtubule-associated protein tau as a therapeutic target in Alzheimer's disease. Expert Opin Ther Targets. 2014;18(3):307–18.

35. Tan Y, Ji YB, Zhao J. Research progress of transgenic Drosophila model of Alzheimer disease. Yao Xue Xue Bao. 2013;48(3):333–6.

36. Caesar I, et al. Curcumin promotes A-beta fibrillation and reduces neurotoxicity in transgenic Drosophila. PLoS One. 2012;7(2):e31424.

37. Iijima K, Gatt A, Iijima-Ando K. Tau Ser262 phosphorylation is critical for Abeta42-induced tau toxicity in a transgenic Drosophila model of Alzheimer's disease. Hum Mol Genet. 2010;19(15):2947–57.

38. Gao J, et al. Salidroside ameliorates cognitive impairment in a d-galactose-induced rat model of Alzheimer's disease. Behav Brain Res. 2015;293:27–33.

39. Panza F, et al. Tau-Centric Targets and Drugs in Clinical Development for the Treatment of Alzheimer's Disease. Biomed Res Int. 2016;2016:3245935.

40. Harrington CR, et al. Cellular Models of Aggregation-dependent Template-directed Proteolysis to Characterize Tau Aggregation Inhibitors for Treatment of Alzheimer Disease. J Biol Chem. 2015;290(17):10862–75.

41. Ma T. GSK3 in Alzheimer's disease: mind the isoforms. J Alzheimers Dis. 2014;39(4):707–10.

14

Meta-analysis of risk factors for Parkinson's disease dementia

Yaqian Xu, Jing Yang and Huifang Shang*

Abstract

Background: Parkinson's disease (PD) is a common heterogeneous neurodegenerative disorder in elder population. Parkinson's disease dementia (PDD) is one of the most common non-motor manifestations in PD patients. No comprehensive review has been conducted to assess risk factors for PDD.

Methods: A systemic search for studies on PDD risk factors was performed. Cohort and case–control studies that clearly defined PDD and presented relevant data were included. The data were analyzed to generate a pooled effect size and 95 % confidence interval (CI). Publication bias was assessed using the Egger's test and the Begg's test.

Results: A systematic search was conducted and yielded 5195 articles. After screening, 25 studies were included in the current analysis. Development of PDD was positively associated with age (odds ratio [OR] 1.07, 95 % CI 1.03-1.13), male (OR 1.33, 95 % CI 1.08-1.64), higher Unified Parkinson's Disease Rating Scale (UPDRS) part III scores (relative risk [RR] 1.04, 95 % CI 1.01-1.07), hallucination (OR 2.47, 95 % CI 1.36-4.47), REM sleep behavior disorder (RBD) (OR 8.38, 95 % CI 3.87-18.08), smoking (ever vs. never) (RR 1.93, 95 % CI 1.15-3.26) and hypertension (OR 1.57, 95 % CI 1.11-2.22). An inverse association was found between education (RR 0.94, 95 % CI 0.91-0.98) and PDD. Other reported factors, including age of onset, disease duration of PD, Hoehn and Yahr stage and diabetes mellitus were not significantly associated with PDD.

Conclusions: Advanced age, male, higher UPDRS III scores, hallucination, RBD, smoking and hypertension increase the risk of PDD, whereas higher education is a protective factor for PDD.

Keywords: Parkinson's disease, Dementia, Risk factors, Predictors

Background

Parkinson's disease (PD), a heterogeneous neurodegenerative disorder in elder population, is characterized by cardinal motor symptoms including bradykinesia, rigidity, tremor and postural instability [1]. Recently, increasing evidence shows that PD is a disease with many non-motor symptoms (NMS) including dementia, sleep disorders, mood disorders, urinary dysfunction, and olfactory disorders [2]. Among NMS, Parkinson disease dementia (PDD) is one of the most common symptoms with a mean prevalence of 31.3 % in PD patients [3]. Among general population, PDD incidence rate is approximately 38.7 to 112.5 per 1000 person-year among several cohort studies conducted in different regions [3, 4]. It has been suggested

that PD patients who developed dementia tend to have increased health care burden, declined quality of life and increased mortality [5–7]. However, effective treatment for PDD is currently unclear [8]. Being able to predict PDD development accurately would provide opportunities for intervention as well as novel treatments and might prolong survival [9].

Several demographic, motor and non-motor features have been identified as predictors for PDD. Advanced age is the most common risk factor for dementia and for later diagnosis of PDD in PD patients [10]. More advanced disease stage as well as specific Parkinson subtype, the akinetic-rigid subtype, was found to be associated with increased risk for PDD, whereas the evaluation scales are not coherent [11, 12]. Some studies suggested that REM sleep behavior disorder (RBD), hallucination, mood disorders and olfactory dysfunction are strong predictors for

* Correspondence: hfshang2002@163.com
Department of Neurology, West China Hospital, Sichuan University, 610041 Chengdu, Sichuan, China

PDD, but the results were not consistent across studies [13–15]. Up to date, no comprehensive meta-analysis on clinical risk factors for PDD has been conducted. A 2014 review on the predictors of PDD by Moore et al. summarized major study results on different risk factors, including clinical predictors, biological predictors, neuroimaging predictors and genetic predictors [9]. In that previous review, the authors presented all possible influences of those factors on PDD, but did not provide quantitative evaluation of the predictors. In order to quantitatively evaluate the effects of different factors on PDD, we conducted this systematic review and meta-analysis via an extensive search of observational studies and a meta-analysis on multiple factors.

Methods

Search strategy

We conducted the search according to the Preferred Reporting Items for Systematic Review and Meta-analysis (PRISMA 2009) guideline. We searched MEDLINE and EMBASE database for studies reporting predictors for later diagnosis of PDD. No language restrictions were used. The keywords we selected were: "Parkinson Disease" AND "Dementia" AND "Risk" OR "Predict" OR "Age" OR "Age of Onset" OR "Education" OR "Family history" OR "Hallucination" OR "Sleep Disorders" OR "Constipation" OR "Olfactory Disorders" OR "Color Vision" OR "Depression" OR "Anxiety" OR "Mood Disorders" OR "Erectile Dysfunction" OR "Urinary Dysfunction" OR "Hypertension" OR "Coronary Artery Disease" OR "Head Injury" OR "Diabetes Mellitus" OR "Smoking" OR "Alcohols" OR "Coffee" OR "Pesticides". We also hand searched the reference lists of relevant reviews and articles with required data for missed references. The final search was carried out on December 1, 2015.

Inclusion criteria

We included articles that met the predefined criteria: 1) cohort or case–control studies assessed at least one risk factor preceding a later diagnosis of PDD; 2) compared PDD patients with PD patients who did not develop dementia; 3) clearly stated diagnostic criteria for PD and PDD, and carried out by an experienced clinician; 4) reported odds ratio (OR), relative risk (RR) or equivalent values representing risks of developing dementia or case–control studies with cases defined as diagnosed PDD; and 5) reported data that could be easily obtained via questionnaires.

Exclusion criteria

Reviews, editorials, case reports, commentaries, letters that reported no new data, meta-analysis, handouts, and abstracts were excluded from the study. We excluded studies that: 1) reported on treatment or management of PDD; 2) reported a diseases other than PDD or PD; 3) studied only young onset PD; 4) did not use a PD nondemented group as comparable group to PDD group or did not provide adequate data on the comparable group; 5) were twin studies; 6) reported one predictor repeatedly in one study population (if >1 paper reported on one study population, we chose the larger one, and where population is equal, we chose the most recent one); 7) reported on predictors that were not easily available in most clinical settings (i.e. questionnaires designed for a certain population or country); 8) reported only uncommon genetic risk factors; 9) reported measures other than OR, RR or equivalent values, or from which an OR could not be calculated. Two authors (X.Y. and J.Y.) independently evaluated the eligibility of all studies, and if there was disagreement between authors, the articles were further evaluated by a third author (H.S.) and discussed in detail until an agreement has been reached.

Data extraction and quality assessment

Study characteristics, PDD diagnostic criteria, a risk estimate of the main study finding, and secondary findings were extracted using a unified form. We did not include studies that reported dementia before or within one year to the onset of PD, since these cases did not fulfill the diagnostic criteria for PDD and were more likely cases of dementia with Lewy bodies (DLB). If studies did not report OR, RR or equivalent measures, raw data were screened to determine whether ORs could be calculated. When the studies reported both the crude OR/RRs and the adjusted OR/RRs, the adjusted figures were extracted. We calculated a quality score to assess the quality of the studies according to the Newcastle-Ottawa Scale (NOS). Length of time that any predictor precedes the diagnosis of PDD was not analyzed in the study due to inconsistent reporting.

Statistical analysis

We combined the reported risks first separately for case–control and cohort studies, and second for all studies together, in cases where two or more studies reported on the same factor. The data were analyzed to generate a pooled effect size and 95 % confidence interval (CI). We examined the heterogeneity across studies using the I^2 statistic [16, 17]. Where statistically significant heterogeneity was found ($p < 0.05$), we used randomized effects model to combine results. We assessed publication bias using the Egger's test and the Begg's test, and constructed funnel plot in order to visualize any possible asymmetry [18]. Two-tailed P values less than 0.05 were considered statistically significant. All analyses were performed using Stata version 12.0 (StataCorp, College Station, TX).

Results

The electronic search yielded 5195 articles, all of which were reviewed by titles and abstracts. Full text of 278 articles were reviewed, of which 23 articles met the inclusion criteria. We also hand searched the references of the articles, 2 of which were included into the analysis. Finally, a total of 25 articles were included in the meta-analysis. Full details of the studies included were provided (Additional files 1 and 2). The selection process is shown in a flow diagram (Fig. 1).

We found age (OR 1.07, 95 % CI 1.03-1.13), gender (Male) (OR 1.33, 95 % CI 1.08-1.64) and hypertension (OR 1.57, 95 % CI 1.11-2.22), to be significantly associated with later diagnosis of PDD (Fig. 2), whereas age of onset (AOO) (RR 1.03, 95 % CI 0.97-1.09), disease duration of PD (RR 1.00, 95 % CI 0.96-1.03), and type 2 diabetes mellitus (OR 1.16, 95 % CI 0.58-2.42) were not associated with risk of PDD (Fig. 3). Although education was only reported in three cohort studies, it was the only factor we found to decrease PDD risk (RR 0.94, 95 % CI 0.91-0.98) (Fig. 3). Lifestyle related risk factors were poorly reported. Previous and current smokers were reported to have increased risk of developing PDD (RR 1.88, 95 % CI 1.06-3.34) comparing with non-smoking PD population. However, alcohol consumption (RR 1.1, 95 % CI 0.6-2.2) and coffee consumption (RR 0.9, 95 % CI 0.5-1.8), reported in one study population, was not a significant risk factor for PDD [19].

Two general scales evaluating PD patient's motor features were included in this study. Our result showed that higher score in Unified Parkinson's Disease Rating Scale (UPDRS) part III (RR 1.04, 95 % CI 1.01-1.07) increased the risk of PDD, but higher Hoehn and Yahr stage (RR 1.24, 95 % CI 0.92-1.66) was not associated with the development PDD. Studies analyzing the association between PD motor subtypes and PDD were not included in the present meta-analysis because of limited data. Two common non-motor symptoms of PD patients, hallucination (OR 2.47, 95 % CI 1.36-4.47) and RBD (OR 8.38, 95 % CI 3.87-18.08), were both strong predictors of PDD. Single studies also reported positive association between PDD and family history of dementia (first-degree relatives), urinary dysfunction, impaired color vision or orthostatic blood pressure drop and no significant association between family history of PD (first-degree relatives), exposure to pesticides, occupational exposure to chemicals and PDD [13, 15, 20]. Details of factors not included in the meta-analysis were provided (Additional file 3).

Assessment of publication bias

The funnel plot for each included factors were individually examined visually. The shape was presented essentially symmetrical in age, AOO, gender, smoking, disease duration, education, UPDRS III, hallucination, RBD, hypertension, diabetes mellitus and Hoehn and Yahr stage, which was proved by Begg's and Egger's test.

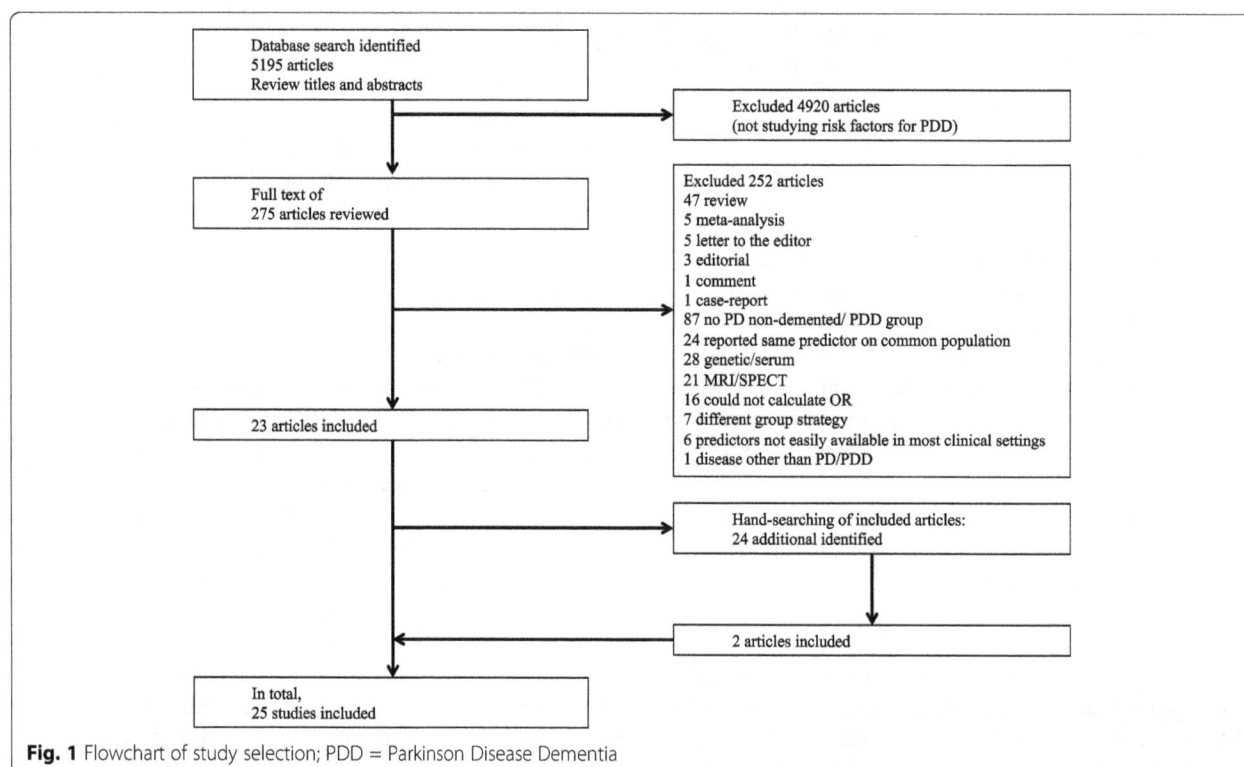

Fig. 1 Flowchart of study selection; PDD = Parkinson Disease Dementia

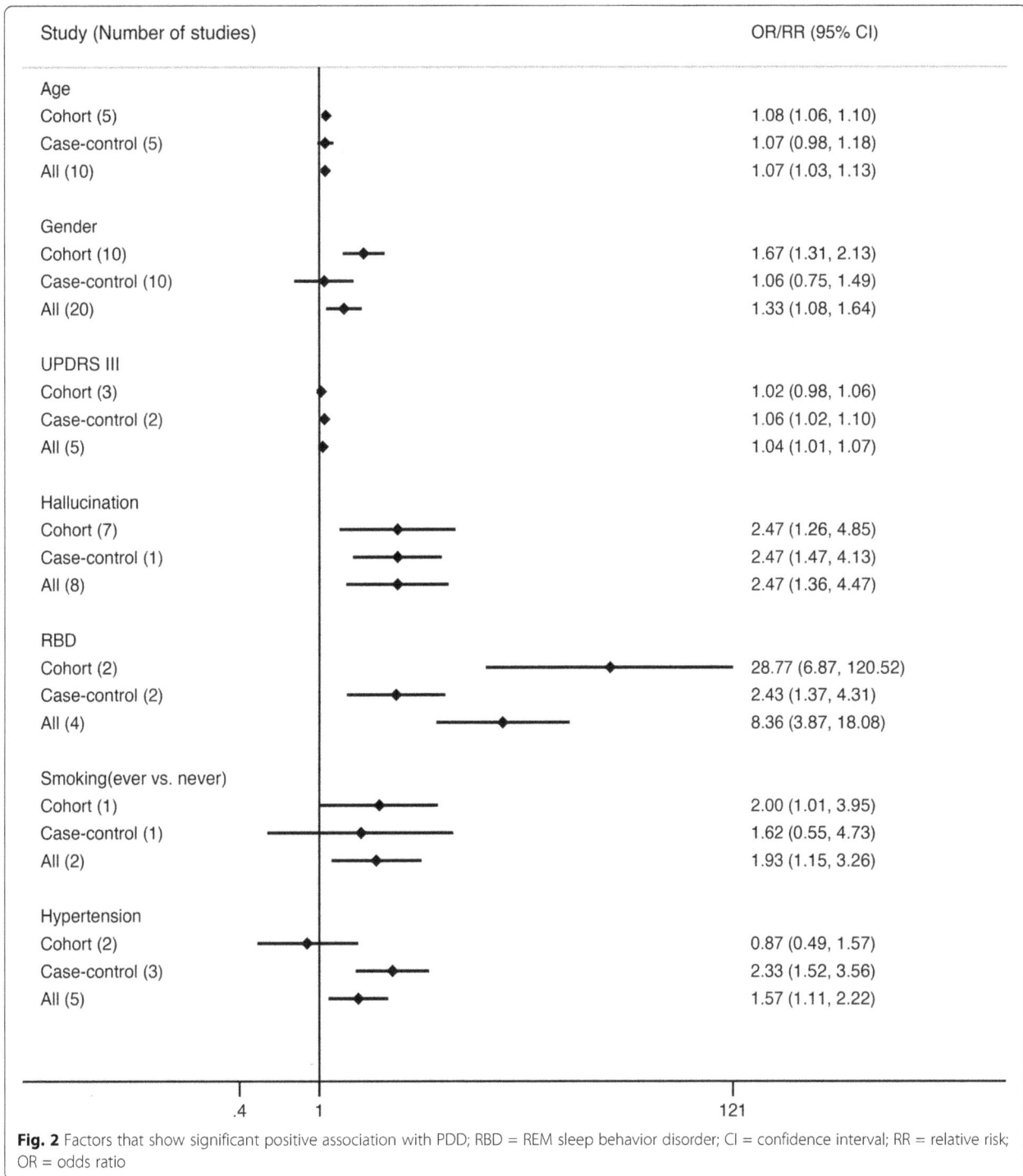

Fig. 2 Factors that show significant positive association with PDD; RBD = REM sleep behavior disorder; CI = confidence interval; RR = relative risk; OR = odds ratio

Discussion

This study identified 12 individual predictors that have potential value in screening for PDD. The identified risk factors include demographic characteristics, lifestyle factors, non-motor features of PD, and widely accepted scales evaluating PD. Some of the factors may present pathogenic importance while others could represent the relationship between symptoms and cognitive decline.

Together, these factors tend to be markers preceding diagnosis of PDD in PD patients. Of the identified factors, 7 factors were significant predictors for subsequent diagnosis of PDD, the understanding of which may contribute to higher quality of care and improve quality of life in PD patients.

Age, AOO and disease duration were all common risk factors for PDD. However, since these three factors are

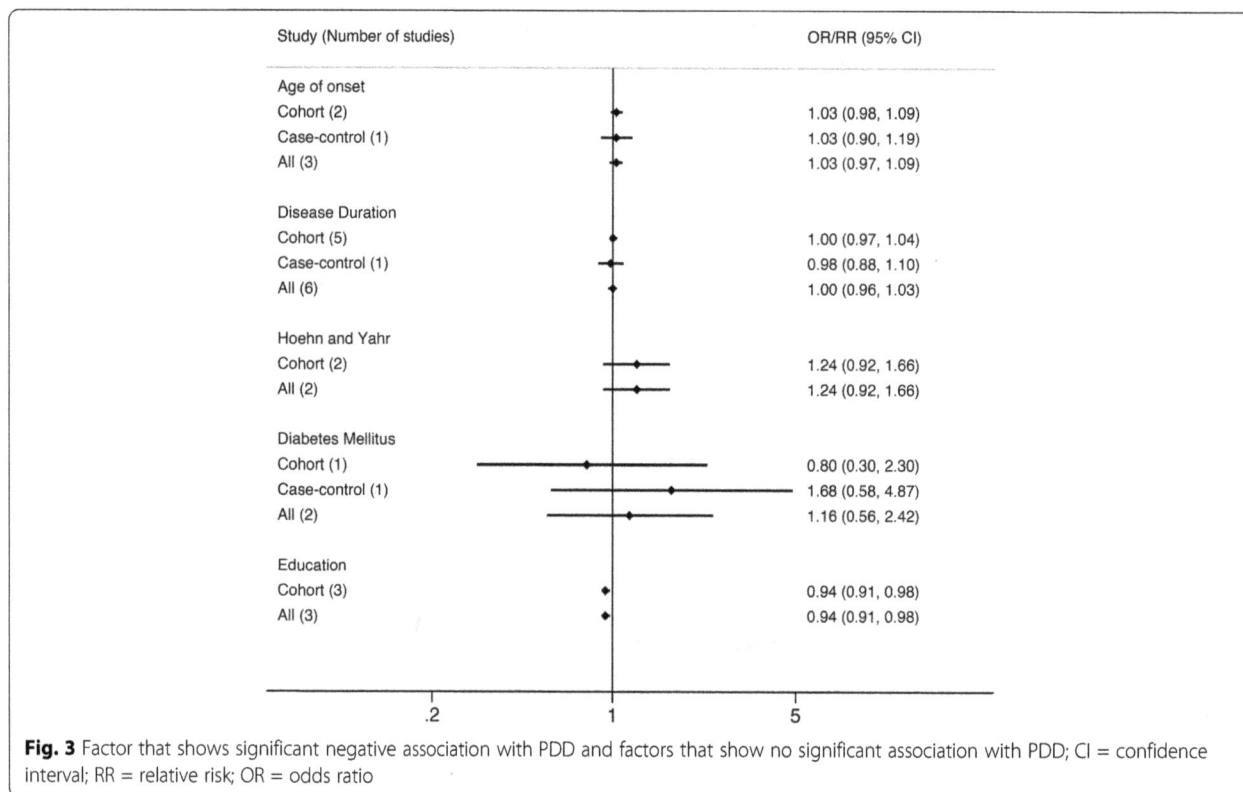

Fig. 3 Factor that shows significant negative association with PDD and factors that show no significant association with PDD; CI = confidence interval; RR = relative risk; OR = odds ratio

interdependent, their individual effect on PDD is under debate. One study comparing early and late onset PD patients suggested that late onset PD group presents with more severe impaired sensory abilities, sleep disorders and dementia [21]. Another study adjusted cofounding found that among the three factors, only age remained an independent risk factor for PDD [22]. Similarly, we found that older age had a significant influence on later diagnosis of PDD, while AOO and disease duration was not associated with PDD. Our study suggested that advanced age as a risk factor for PDD may be independent from PD related time factors, like AOO or disease duration. Many neuropathological studies have provided evidences on the effect of aging. Recent studies with α-synuclein immunostaining found a strong association between the age-related increase of Lewy bodies in cortical areas and the development of PDD [23, 24]. Another study found that cortical amyloid-β deposition and aging together might be associated with PDD [25]. Few other studies revealed that MAPT genotype, related with tau transcription, has a strong influence on the risk of PDD [26, 27]. Goris et al. found that, among MAPT haplotypes, PD patients with H1 homozygotes had an increased rate of cognitive decline, which was dependent on age [28, 29]. These age-related pathological processes together may increase the risk of PDD with aging.

We also found male to be a risk factor for PDD. However, some studies suggested that there might be no relationship between gender and PDD if potential confounding factors, including age, history of dementia, smoking and number of siblings, were adjusted [20, 22]. In the present meta-analysis, all data included for the factor gender were unadjusted data. Therefore, our study illustrated that male, before adjustment, is a positive predictor for PDD, but provided no evidence on the results after confounding factors were adjusted. The only protective factor we found in the current meta-analysis is higher education. Similar with our results, one study found that when compared with elementary school level, PDD patients with university level education were at lower risk of developing dementia [30]. One possible explanation is that education might modify the risk of cognitive decline by greater functional brain reserve in PD patients [31]. However, in a recent systematic review looking into education and dementia in Alzheimer's disease (AD), the authors suggested that although lower education is associated with greater risk of dementia, the findings varied by region, age, gender and ethnicity [32]. The association between education and dementia in PD also need further studying with confounding adjusted.

A recent meta-analysis on risk factors for PD suggested that smoking, alcohol and coffee consumption decreases the risk of PD [33]. In the current meta-analysis we found that a history of smoking increased the risk of dementia in PD by almost two fold. On the other hand, alcohol and coffee consumption has been reported to have no significant association with PDD [19]. Smoking, different from alcohol and coffee consumption, stand as an independent risk factor for PDD. One possible mechanism is related with vascular factors. We found that hypertension was associated with PDD while diabetes was not significantly associated with PDD. Because smoking is also a risk factor for hypertension and that hypertension is related with AD-type pathologies in dementia, it is possible that smoking affect dementia in PD via vascular route [34, 35]. However, after adjustment for the possibility of confounding vascular factors in one included study, smoking still exists as an increased risk for PDD [19]. Biologically, greater depletion of cholinergic cells in the nucleus basalis of Meynert has been observed in PDD [36], yet the up-regulation of central nicotine acetylcholine receptors by nicotine contrasts the mechanism [37, 38]. Another published meta-analysis found that smoking was also a cause of cognitive decline in AD patients as well as in patients with other dementia, in which the authors suggested that non-smokers have lower inflammation or oxidative stress that may lead to a reduction in cognitive decline [39, 40].

We found that higher UPDRS III score was positively related with later diagnosis of PDD, whereas Hoehn and Yahr stage was not significantly associated with PDD. This result suggests that severe motor dysfunction is associated with PDD risk, and that the risk is more likely associated with individual motor dysfunctions. In a study that discovered no significant association between UPDRS III and PDD, researchers found that within the UPDRS III section, gait dysfunction was strongly associated with eventual development of dementia [13]. Gait dysfunction is important for the classification of the postural instability and gait difficulties (PIGD) subtype, and several longitudinal studies have discovered that 25 % to 64.9 % of PIGD PD patients would be diagnosed with PDD by the end of follow-up [11, 12]. Also, researchers have found that increased loss of cholinergic nuclei may relate with both cognitive decline and motor features including rigidity, gait, and balance [12, 41]. However, only two studies were evaluated regarding Hoehn and Yahr stage, the result should be interpreted with caution.

We discovered RBD and hallucination are strongly associated with later diagnosis of PDD. Several studies suggested that patients with RBD had a higher rate of MCI at baseline and a shorter duration towards diagnosis of dementia [42–44]. Cholinergic deficit due to degeneration of ascending pathway that took place in both RBD and dementia with Lewy bodies might be the cause [45]. Visual hallucinations were also discovered to have positive association with cognitive impairment in early PD [46]. In terms of mechanism, pathological studies in PD indicated that visual hallucination might share common limbic pathology with cognitive decline and dementia [14]. In functional MRI assessment, preceding image recognition, patients with visual hallucinations have reduced activation in ventral/lateral visual associated cortices [47]. However, a reverse relation was found in previous study suggesting that cognitive impairment at baseline precedes later development of hallucination [48]. Both RBD and hallucination were also associated with MCI, an important predictor for PDD [49, 50], in early Parkinson disease [42, 46]. None of the studies included in our meta-analysis adjusted RBD or hallucination for baseline cognitive impairment, therefore the causal relation is unclear from the present study.

Limitations

We only selected factors that were easily obtained in primary care environment. Variables that used less common inventories, like color vision and olfactory dysfunction, were not included in the analysis. Also, genetic tests have been excluded from the analysis for similar reasons. Mild cognitive impairment, an important risk factor of incidence dementia in PD [50, 51], was not included in the meta-analysis because most studies on mild cognitive impairment used a different group strategy by separating the participants into PD-normal cognition, PD-mild cognitive impairment and PDD group, which differs from most of other PDD risk factor studies. Motor subtypes were not analyzed in this meta-analysis also because of differences in group strategy.

Not all studies adjusted risk factors for confounders, and those adjusted were mostly adjusted for different confounders. We included both factors unadjusted and factors adjusted where possible, which may have increased the degree of significance for some risk factors. Few factors were reported in studies to be positively associated or not associated with later diagnosis of PDD but without specified OR or RR to be extracted. Though we have calculated OR or RR where possible, there may still be data neglected.

Statistically significant heterogeneity was found in 8 of the meta-analyses performed in our study. Two risk factors, age and AOO, were found to have high heterogeneity ($I^2 > 75$ %). Gender, education, hallucination, UPDRS III, RBD and hypertension were found to have moderate heterogeneity (50 % $< I^2 <$ 75 %). The presence of heterogeneity was as expected because of the differences in the characteristics of studies, the length of follow-up, study population scale, population characteristics, diagnostic criteria used and whether factors were crude or adjusted. The follow-up period in the cohort studies and the diagnostic criteria for PDD in both cohort and case–control studies varied, we did not adjust these factors in this meta-analysis due to limited number of included studies. Thus, the results of this analysis should be interpreted cautiously, especially for those factors that were reported in less than three studies and that were with high heterogeneities.

In the present meta-analysis, we included studies with NOS score higher than 5, which ensured study quality. Also, we performed sub-group analysis by different study design in order to minimize heterogeneity. We combined analytical results according to the heterogeneity analysis, and did not find significant publication bias. Therefore, our results were considered to be robust.

Conclusions

This is the first systematic review and meta-analysis on widely evaluated risk factors of PDD. This study found advanced age, male, high UPDRS III scores, presence of hallucination, presence of RBD, ever smoking and history of hypertension are positive predictors to later diagnosis of PDD, whereas education is a protective factor of PDD. This study laid the foundation to future comparative assessment on risk factors for PDD, and lead to a better understanding of PDD risks.

Additional files

Additional file 1: Details of studies included in the meta-analysis. This file included details of all studies included in this meta-analysis, categorized by risk factors. Details including first author, year of publication, country, study design, number of participants and NOS scores. (DOCX 119 kb)

Additional file 2: Details of the study results. This file provided detailed results of meta-analysis of each risk factor. (DOCX 159 kb)

Additional file 3: Details of factors not included in the meta-analysis. This file provided data of risk factors for Parkinson's disease dementia that were mentioned in literature, but were not included in the meta-analysis due to limited number of studies or differences in study design. (DOCX 93 kb)

Abbreviations

AD, Alzheimer's disease; AOO, age of onset; CI, confidence interval; DLB, dementia with lewy bodies; NOS, Newcastle-Ottawa scale; OR, odds ratio; PD, Parkinson's disease; PDD, Parkinson's disease dementia; PIGD, postural instability and gait difficulties; PRISMA, preferred reporting items for systematic review and meta-analysis; RBD, REM sleep behavior disorder; RR, relative risk; UPDRS, Unified Parkinson's Disease Rating Scale.

Acknowledgement

We would like to thank all authors of the original research studies included in this meta-analysis. We thank Ms. Cong Li for statistical assistance and thank Ms. Hong Xie for proofreading of this meta-analysis.

Funding

No funding considering this study.

Authors' contributions

YX and HS conceived and designed the study. YX, JY and HS reviewed the literature. YX undertook the statistical analysis. YX and HS wrote the manuscript. YX, JY and HS contribute in discussions and reviewed the manuscript. All authors read and approved the final manuscript.

Authors' information

Huifang Shang, corresponding author, professor and vice director of Department of Neurology, West China Hospital of Sichuan University, Chengdu, 610041, China.

Competing Interests

The authors declare that they have no competing interests.

References

1. de Lau LM, Giesbergen PC, de Rijk MC, Hofman A, Koudstaal PJ, Breteler MM. Incidence of parkinsonism and Parkinson disease in a general population: the Rotterdam Study. Neurology. 2004;63:1240–4.
2. Schapira AH. The measurement and importance of non-motor symptoms in Parkinson disease. Eur J Neurol. 2015;22:2–3.
3. Aarsland D, Kurz MW. The epidemiology of dementia associated with Parkinson's disease. Brain Pathol (Zurich, Switzerland). 2010;20:633–9.
4. Hobson P, Meara J. Risk and incidence of dementia in a cohort of older subjects with Parkinson's disease in the United Kingdom. Mov Disord. 2004; 19:1043–9.
5. Hely MA, Reid WG, Adena MA, Halliday GM, Morris JG. The Sydney multicenter study of Parkinson's disease: the inevitability of dementia at 20 years. Mov Disord. 2008;23:837–44.
6. Leroi I, McDonald K, Pantula H, Harbishettar V. Cognitive impairment in Parkinson disease: impact on quality of life, disability, and caregiver burden. J Geriatr Psychiatry Neurol. 2012;25:208–14.
7. Emre M, Aarsland D, Brown R, Burn DJ, Duyckaerts C, Mizuno Y, et al. Clinical diagnostic criteria for dementia associated with Parkinson's disease. Mov Disord. 2007;22:1689–707. quiz 837.
8. Marder K, Tang MX, Alfaro B, Mejia H, Cote L, Jacobs D, et al. Postmenopausal estrogen use and Parkinson's disease with and without dementia. Neurology. 1998;50:1141–3.
9. Moore SF, Barker RA. Predictors of Parkinson's disease dementia: towards targeted therapies for a heterogeneous disease. Parkinsonism Relat Disord. 2014;20 Suppl 1:S104–7.
10. Aarsland D, Kvaloy JT, Andersen K, Larsen JP, Tang MX, Lolk A, et al. The effect of age of onset of PD on risk of dementia. J Neurol. 2007;254:38–45.
11. Alves G, Larsen JP, Emre M, Wentzel-Larsen T, Aarsland D. Changes in motor subtype and risk for incident dementia in Parkinson's disease. Mov Disord. 2006;21:1123–30.
12. Burn DJ, Rowan EN, Allan LM, Molloy S, O'Brien JT, McKeith IG. Motor subtype and cognitive decline in Parkinson's disease, Parkinson's disease with dementia, and dementia with Lewy bodies. J Neurol Neurosurg Psychiatry. 2006;77:585–9.
13. Anang JB, Gagnon JF, Bertrand JA, Romenets SR, Latreille V, Panisset M, et al. Predictors of dementia in Parkinson disease: A prospective cohort study. Neurology. 2014;83:1253–60.
14. Zhu K, van Hilten JJ, Putter H, Marinus J. Risk factors for hallucinations in Parkinson's disease: results from a large prospective cohort study. Mov Disord. 2013;28:755–62.
15. Baba T, Kikuchi A, Hirayama K, Nishio Y, Hosokai Y, Kanno S, et al. Severe olfactory dysfunction is a prodromal symptom of dementia associated with Parkinson's disease: a 3 year longitudinal study. Brain. 2012;135:161–9.
16. Higgins JP, Thompson SG, Deeks JJ, Altman DG. Measuring inconsistency in meta-analyses. BMJ (Clinical research ed). 2003;327:557–60.
17. DerSimonian R, Laird N. Meta-analysis in clinical trials. Control Clin Trials. 1986;7:177–88.
18. Egger M, Smith GD, Phillips AN. Meta-analysis: principles and procedures. BMJ (Clinical research ed). 1997;315:1533–7.
19. Levy G, Tang MX, Cote LJ, Louis ED, Alfaro B, Mejia H, et al. Do risk factors for Alzheimer's disease predict dementia in Parkinson's disease? An exploratory study. Mov Disord. 2002;17:250–7.
20. Marder K, Flood P, Cote L, Mayeux R. A pilot study of risk factors for dementia in Parkinson's disease. Mov Disord. 1990;5:156–61.
21. Zhou MZ, Gan J, Wei YR, Ren XY, Chen W, Liu ZG. The association between non-motor symptoms in Parkinson's disease and age at onset. Clin Neurol Neurosurg. 2013;115:2103–7.

22. Hughes TA, Ross HF, Musa S, Bhattacherjee S, Nathan RN, Mindham RH, et al. A 10-year study of the incidence of and factors predicting dementia in Parkinson's disease. Neurology. 2000;54:1596–602.

23. Mattila PM, Rinne JO, Helenius H, Dickson DW, Roytta M. Alpha-synuclein-immunoreactive cortical Lewy bodies are associated with cognitive impairment in Parkinson's disease. Acta Neuropathol. 2000;100:285–90.

24. Hurtig HI, Trojanowski JQ, Galvin J, Ewbank D, Schmidt ML, Lee VM, et al. Alpha-synuclein cortical Lewy bodies correlate with dementia in Parkinson's disease. Neurology. 2000;54:1916–21.

25. Compta Y, Parkkinen L, O'Sullivan SS, Vandrovcova J, Holton JL, Collins C, et al. Lewy- and Alzheimer-type pathologies in Parkinson's disease dementia: which is more important? Brain. 2011;134:1493–505.

26. Seto-Salvia N, Clarimon J, Pagonabarraga J, Pascual-Sedano B, Campolongo A, Combarros O, et al. Dementia risk in Parkinson disease: disentangling the role of MAPT haplotypes. Arch Neurol. 2011;68:359–64.

27. Williams-Gray CH, Mason SL, Evans JR, Foltynie T, Brayne C, Robbins TW, et al. The CamPaIGN study of Parkinson's disease: 10-year outlook in an incident population-based cohort. J Neurol Neurosurg Psychiatry. 2013;84:1258–64.

28. Winder-Rhodes SE, Hampshire A, Rowe JB, Peelle JE, Robbins TW, Owen AM, et al. Association between MAPT haplotype and memory function in patients with Parkinson's disease and healthy aging individuals. Neurobiol Aging. 2015;36:1519–28.

29. Goris A, Williams-Gray CH, Clark GR, Foltynie T, Lewis SJ, Brown J, et al. Tau and alpha-synuclein in susceptibility to, and dementia in. Parkinson's Disease Ann Neurol. 2007;62:145–53.

30. Zoccolella S, dell'Aquila C, Abruzzese G, Antonini A, Bonuccelli U, Canesi M, et al. Hyperhomocysteinemia in levodopa-treated patients with Parkinson's disease dementia. Mov Disord. 2009;24:1028–33.

31. Glatt SL, Hubble JP, Lyons K, Paolo A, Troster AI, Hassanein RE, et al. Risk factors for dementia in Parkinson's disease: effect of education. Neuroepidemiology. 1996;15:20–5.

32. Sharp ES, Gatz M. Relationship between education and dementia: an updated systematic review. Alzheimer Dis Assoc Disord. 2011;25:289–304.

33. Noyce AJ, Bestwick JP, Silveira-Moriyama L, Hawkes CH, Giovannoni G, Lees AJ, et al. Meta-analysis of early nonmotor features and risk factors for Parkinson disease. Ann Neurol. 2012;72:893–901.

34. Virdis A, Giannarelli C, Neves MF, Taddei S, Ghiadoni L. Cigarette smoking and hypertension. Curr Pharm Des. 2010;16:2518–25.

35. Iadecola C. Hypertension and dementia. Hypertension. 2014;64:3–5.

36. Jellinger KA. Morphological substrates of dementia in parkinsonism. A critical update. J Neural Transm Suppl. 1997;51:57–82.

37. Grenhoff J, Svensson TH. Pharmacology of nicotine. Br J Addict. 1989;84:477–92.

38. Levin ED. Nicotinic systems and cognitive function. Psychopharmacology. 1992;108:417–31.

39. Anstey KJ, von Sanden C, Salim A, O'Kearney R. Smoking as a risk factor for dementia and cognitive decline: a meta-analysis of prospective studies. Am J Epidemiol. 2007;166:367–78.

40. Bruno RS, Traber MG. Vitamin E biokinetics, oxidative stress and cigarette smoking. Pathophysiology. 2006;13:143–9.

41. Bohnen NI, Kaufer DI, Ivanco LS, Lopresti B, Koeppe RA, Davis JG, et al. Cortical cholinergic function is more severely affected in parkinsonian dementia than in Alzheimer disease: an in vivo positron emission tomographic study. Arch Neurol. 2003;60:1745–8.

42. Postuma RB, Bertrand JA, Montplaisir J, Desjardins C, Vendette M, Rios Romenets S, et al. Rapid eye movement sleep behavior disorder and risk of dementia in Parkinson's disease: a prospective study. Mov Disord. 2012;27:720–6.

43. Marion MH, Qurashi M, Marshall G, Foster O. Is REM sleep behaviour disorder (RBD) a risk factor of dementia in idiopathic Parkinson's disease? J Neurol. 2008;255:192–6.

44. Nomura T, Inoue Y, Kagimura T, Nakashima K. Clinical significance of REM sleep behavior disorder in Parkinson's disease. Sleep Med. 2013;14:131–5.

45. Emre M. Dementia in Parkinson's disease: cause and treatment. Curr Opin Neurol. 2004;17:399–404.

46. Uc EY, McDermott MP, Marder KS, Anderson SW, Litvan I, Como PG, et al. Incidence of and risk factors for cognitive impairment in an early Parkinson disease clinical trial cohort. Neurology. 2009;73:1469–77.

47. Meppelink AM, de Jong BM, Renken R, Leenders KL, Cornelissen FW, van Laar T. Impaired visual processing preceding image recognition in Parkinson's disease patients with visual hallucinations. Brain. 2009;132:2980–93.

48. van Rooden SM, Heiser WJ, Kok JN, Verbaan D, van Hilten JJ, Marinus J. The identification of Parkinson's disease subtypes using cluster analysis: a systematic review. Mov Disord. 2010;25:969–78.

49. Pedersen KF, Larsen JP, Tysnes OB, Alves G. Prognosis of mild cognitive impairment in early Parkinson disease: the Norwegian ParkWest study. JAMA Neurol. 2013;70:580–6.

50. Litvan I, Aarsland D, Adler CH, Goldman JG, Kulisevsky J, Mollenhauer B, et al. MDS Task Force on mild cognitive impairment in Parkinson's disease: critical review of PD-MCI. Mov Disord. 2011;26:1814–24.

51. Janvin CC, Larsen JP, Aarsland D, Hugdahl K. Subtypes of mild cognitive impairment in Parkinson's disease: progression to dementia. Mov Disord. 2006;21:1343–9.

15

Clinical features and genotype-phenotype correlation analysis in patients with *ATL1* mutations: A literature reanalysis

Guo-hua Zhao[1,2] and Xiao-min Liu[3*]

Abstract

Background: The hereditary spastic paraplegias (HSPs) are a group of clinically and genetically heterogeneous disorders. Approximately 10% of the autosomal dominant (AD) HSPs (ADHSPs) have the spastic paraplegia 3A (SPG3A) genotype which is caused by *ATL1* gene mutations. Currently there are more than 60 reported *ATL1* gene mutations and the genotype-phenotype correlation remains unclear. The study aims to investigate the genotype-phenotype correlation in SPG3A patients.

Methods: We performed a reanalysis of the clinical features and genotype-phenotype correlations in 51 reported studies exhibiting an *ATL1* gene mutation.

Results: Most HSPs-SPG3A patients exhibited an early age at onset (AAO) of <10 years old, and showed an autosomal dominant pure spastic paraplegia. We found that 14% of the HSPs-SPG3A patients presented complicated phenotypes, with distal atrophy being the most common complicated symptom. The AAO of each mutation group was not statistically significant ($P > 0.05$). The mutational spectrum associated with *ATL1* gene mutation is wide, and most mutations are missense mutations, but do not involve the functional motif of *ATL1* gene encoded atlastin-1 protein.

Conclusions: Our findings indicate that there is no clear genotype-phenotype correlation in HSPs-SPG3A patients. We also find that exons 4, 7, 8 and 12 are mutation hotspots in *ATL1* gene.

Keywords: Hereditary spastic paraplegia, SPG3A, Age at onset, *ATL1*, Mutation, Genotype-phenotype correlation

Background

The hereditary spastic paraplegias (HSPs) are a group of clinically heterogeneous neurological disorders, which are classified into "pure" or "complicated" HSP according to the clinical features. The pure HSP is defined by progressive spasticity and weakness limited to the lower limbs, while the complicated HSP may include other neurological manifestations such as optic atrophy, retinal pigmentation, seizures, deafness, neuropathy and mental retardation. In the clinic, HSPs can also be classified into early onset (mainly 1st decade of life) and late onset (between the 2nd and 4th decade) type. The main

pathological changes of HSP include the axonal degeneration of the corticospinal tracts and back column [1, 2].

Genetic mutations are the main cause of HSPs and there are currently over 72 spastic paraplegia genes or genetic loci (designated SPG1-SPG72 genetic type in order of their discovery) in which mutations can occur [3]. HSPs can be inherited as autosomal dominant (AD), autosomal recessive (AR) or X-linked trait or a spastic paraplegia syndrome. Among identified mutations, approximately 40% of definite autosomal dominant pure HSP mutations are in the spastic paraplegia 4 (*SPG4/ SPAST*) gene which encodes the spastin protein [4, 5].

SPG3A is the second most common type of HSP which accounts for approximately 10% of autosomal dominant HSP [6] and is caused by mutations in the atlastin-1 (*ATL1*) gene. The atlastin-1 protein is a member of the dynamin family of large guanosine

* Correspondence: greenfield008@sina.com
[3]Department of Neurology, Qianfoshan Hospital, Shandong University, Jinan 16766, China
Full list of author information is available at the end of the article

triphosphatases (GTPases) which contains three conserved motif-P loops (74GAFRKGKS81), RD (217RD) and DxxG (146DTQG) which are characteristic regions for guanylate binding/GTPase active sites [6]. HSPs-SPG3A phenotype (HSPs with *ATL1* gene mutations) was generally a pure HSP with age at onset (AAO) less than 10 years old [6]. Patients characterize progressive bilateral and mostly symmetric lower extremity weakness and spasticity.

Currently there are more than 60 different *ATL1* gene mutations described, including numerous missense, small deletion, small insertion and splice site mutations, as well as whole exon deletions [6–56]. However, the genotype-phenotype correlation remains unclear [13]. In this study, we perform a reanalysis of all published studies ($n = 51$) to identify the clinical features and then genotype-phenotype correlations in HSPs caused by *ATL1* gene mutations.

Methods

We conducted a literature search using databases from PubMed (http://ncbi.nlm.nih.gov/pubmed) and the China National Knowledge Infrastructure (CNKI) (http://cnki.net) with the keyword "SPG3A" or "*ATL1*", which resulted in 51 articles describing *ATL1* gene mutations [6–56]. We collected information related to the age at onset (AAO), age at examination, pure or complicated form, involvement of upper and lower limbs, Babinski signs, urinary urgency and other symptoms or signs for individually affected patients directly from relevant papers. Asymptomatic individuals were also included, but excluded from the analysis of AAO and pure or complicated form. Patients with elderly sensory neuropathy caused by *ATL1* gene mutations were excluded in this study [57, 58]. We reanalysed the clinical and genetic data in *ATL1* gene mutant patients and performed a correlation analysis of AAO with mutational class in *ATL1* gene. Comparisons of data were performed using two-way ANOVA. Tests were considered statistically significant for $P < 0.05$.

Results

The patients' clinical information and the *ATL1* gene mutation of 51 reports are summarized in Additional file 1: Table S1. The published studies contain data for 142 families with known *ATL1* gene mutations. These 142 families included 130 (91.54%) autosomal dominant HSP (ADHSP) families, 10 (7.04%) sporadic families, one (0.70%) ARHSP family, and one (0.70%) family with unknown inheritance mode. Gender information was available in 151 patients, including 88 male patients and 63 female patients (ratio is 1.40:1). The main clinical features included lower spasticity (99.68%, 313/314), upper spasticity (10.03%, 30/299), Babinski sign (87.83%, 231/263) and urinary urgency (16.37%, 38/232). AAO data were available in 355 subjects from infancy to the seventh decade, in which 301 (84.79%) patients had AAO < 10 years old, whereas 54 (15.21%) patients had AAO >10 years old. Patient information for pure or complicated type was available in 440 patients, including 378 (85.90%) pure HSP and 62 (14.10%) complicated HSP patients. Distal atrophy or neuropathy is the most common symptom in patients with complicated *SPG3A* gene mutations (69.35%, 43/62). In addition, 15/142 families (10.56%) showed incomplete penetrance.

In total, there were 61 different types of mutations reported, which were divided into five broad groups: 130 (91.54%) families had missense mutations (54 types), six (4.23%) had small insertions (4 types), four had (2.82%) small deletions (2 types), one (0.70%) had presumed splice site mutation (1 type), and one (0.70%) had whole exon deletion (1 type). The mutations were located in exon 3 (0.70%, $n = 1$), exon 4 (11.26%, $n = 16$), exon 5 (1.41%, $n = 2$), exon 6 (0.70%, $n = 1$), exon 7 (24.65%, $n = 35$), exon 8 (12.68%, $n = 18$), exon 9 (1.41%, $n = 2$), exon 10 (5.63%, $n = 8$), exon 11 (1.41%, $n = 2$), exon 12 (38.73%, $n = 55$), exon 13 (0.70%, $n = 1$), and intron 1 (0.70%, $n = 1$). A total of 124 (87.32%) mutations were found in exons 4, 7, 8 and 12. No mutations were detected in exons 1, 2 and 14. Figure 1 shows the locations of *ATL1* gene mutations and the number of mutations found in the families. Most mutations did not involve in the functional motif of atlastin-1, except R217Q, c.35-3C > T and exon 4 deletion [7, 13, 40]. The most commonly reported mutations were R239C ($n = 31$) and R495W ($n = 14$). All the published mutations are listed in Ensemble database (ensemble.org).

The AAOs of each mutation group are summarized in Table 1. The patients with missense mutations had a slightly lower AAO, however this difference is not statistically significant ($F = 1.273$, $P = 0.282$). The patients with splice site mutation and exon deletion were not included in the statistics because there was only one patient in each group.

Discussion

HSPs-SPG3A patients account for approximately 10% of ADHSP. Although several large cohorts of patients with mutant *ATL1* gene were reported [17, 21, 27, 29, 32, 36, 45, 50, 54, 56], a genotype-phenotype correlation still remains unclear. Here, we reanalysed the observations on 142 families and confirmed three previously reported observations. First, we find that most HSPs-SPG3A patients exhibiting early AAO and autosomal dominant pure spastic paraplegia there have a wide mutational spectrum associated with *ATL1* gene mutations. Second, we find that most mutations are missense but do not involve the functional motifs of atlastin-1. Third, we note

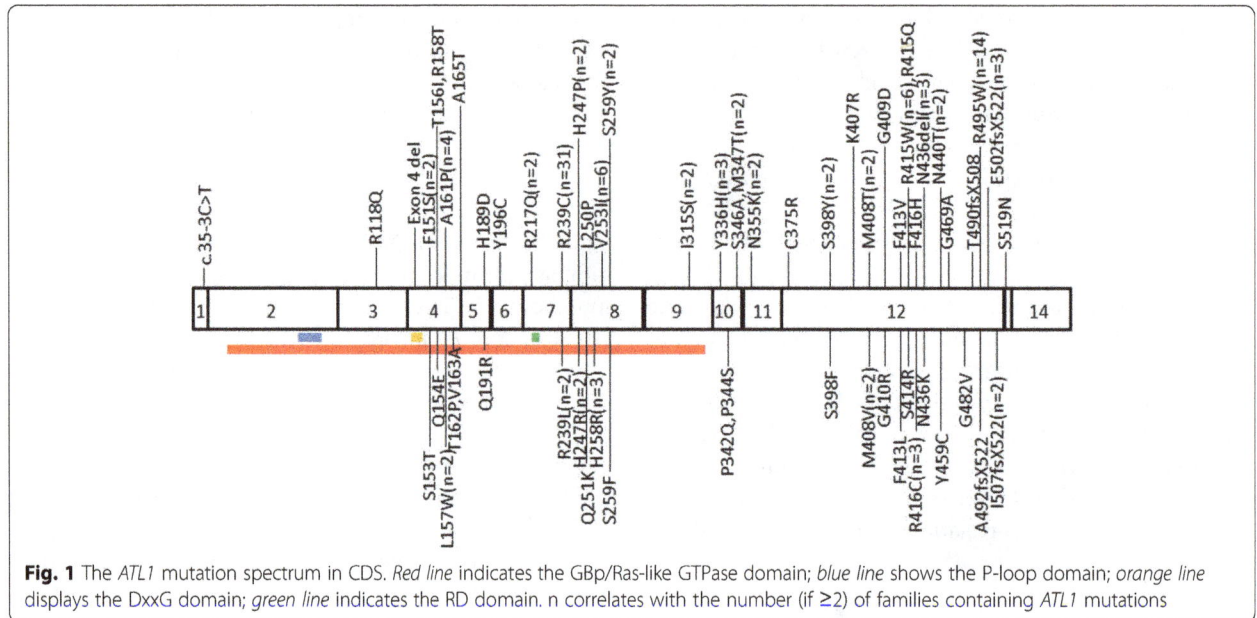

Fig. 1 The *ATL1* mutation spectrum in CDS. *Red line* indicates the GBp/Ras-like GTPase domain; *blue line* shows the P-loop domain; *orange line* displays the DxxG domain; *green line* indicates the RD domain. n correlates with the number (if ≥2) of families containing *ATL1* mutations

that exon 4, 7, 8 and 12 might be mutation hotspots. Additionally, we found that the complicated type was prevalent in HSPs-SPG3A patients, and that distal atrophy or neuropathy is the most common complicated symptoms.

ATL1 gene mutations are thought to be the most common cause of hereditary spastic paraplegia with an AAO < 10 years [17]. Our re-analysis of the 51 reported studies showed that 84.79% patients exhibited early AAO (<10 years), but we found that 15.21% patients had a later AAO (>10 years). Therefore, *ATL1* gene mutation analysis should not be limited to early onset HSP [11, 34].

Our re-analysis also showed no correlation between AAO and mutational classes. More studies with larger sample sizes may be required to resolve this issue because of the limited number of small insertion, small deletion, splice site mutation and exon deletion. In addition, there was variability of AAOs between families with the same mutation, even within the same family. Some members in different families exhibiting the same

mutation had different AAOs. For example, the AAOs for the A161P *ATL1* gene mutation could be childhood or age 45–55 in different families [11]. We found that both childhood-onset HSP and late onset HSP (after age 40 years) occurred in the same family with A161P mutation [21]. Furthermore, intrafamilial variability in AAO varied from eight to 28 years in a family with R495W mutation [21]. One family member with complicated HSP showed AAOs >30 years, whereas another family member with pure HSP presented AAO at puberty, but both members had a R416C mutation in the *ATL1* gene, suggesting a clear intrafamilial variability. Hedera et al. reported a family in which patients had a variable AAO from five to 39 years, and two subjects were functionally asymptomatic despite abnormalities in neurological examinations [15]. Patients in an ADHSP family carrying the *ATL1* R416C mutation were found to have variable clinical characteristics, both the pure phenotype with early onset and the complicated phenotype with later onset [41]. Differences of AAO and clinical features between families with the same mutation or in the same family might be due to variability in expression of this mutation or maybe to related to other genetic or epigenetic factors [11, 18, 34]. Overall, the comparison of the clinical data for all *ATL1* gene mutation families failed to reveal any genotype-phenotype correlation as demonstrated in other types of ADHSP [13].

ATL1 gene was commonly thought to be associated with pure spastic paraplegia manifesting as lower limb spasticity, decreased vibration sense in the lower limbs, and sphincter disturbances. Information for pure or complicated HSPs were available in 440 patients, including 378 (85.90%) pure patients and 62 (14.10%)

Table 1 The comparison of AAOs between different kinds of mutations

Mutation type	No. of families	No. of subjects	Mean age at onset (years)
Missense	109	271	7.47 ± 11.97
Small insertion	6	10	13.60 ± 12.39
Small deletion	4	12	8.25 ± 11.87
Splice site	1	1	44
Exon deletion	1	1	Not available

$F = 1.273$, $P = 0.282$. No.: number

complicated patients. Our re-analysis suggests that most *ATL1* gene mutations usually display a pure phenotype, but *ATL1* gene mutation can also been found in patients with complicated phenotype of HSPs. The complicated symptoms of HSPs-SPG3A patients included seizure, optic atrophy, sensory impairment, mental retardation, ataxia, distal atrophy and peripheral axonal neuropathy (Additional file 1: Table S1). Additionally, we found that distal atrophy is the most common symptom in complicated HSPs-SPG3A patients (69.35%, 43/62).

The early-onset and relatively non-progressive nature of lower extremity spasticity in HSPs-SPG3A patients closely resembles symptoms of patients with spastic diplegic cerebral palsy. Because of this, many HSPs-SPG3A cases have been misdiagnosed as cerebral palsy even when there is no antecedent of a perinatal sentinel event and no lesions detected on brain imaging [10, 28, 31, 47]. However, reaching a HSP diagnosis in paediatric cases is challenging, especially in the absence of a positive family history. However, the occurrence of a de novo *ALT1* gene mutation must be considered in patients with spastic diplegic cerebral palsy, when other causes can not be identified.

Disease severity in HSPs-SPG3A patients is most commonly mild, although the severity of spasticity increases with disease duration. In general, the onset of disease symptoms in children has a long phase of relatively slow progression. In many cases, symptoms remain unchanged up to old age. Additionally, there are some asymptomic cases that contain the *ATL1* gene mutations. Incomplete penetrance has been previously reported in 10.56% HSPs families [8, 12, 15, 24, 27, 45]. The scarce penetrance of the mutations favours a modulator gene or strong epigenetic factor hypothesis, which may influence the phenotype. However, previous reports have shown the existence of some severe symptoms in HSPs-SPG3A patient. For example, Haberlova et al. reported a HSPs-SPG3A patient with a severe and early complicated phenotype, which was caused by the M408T mutation in *ATL1* gene [25]. Furthermore, a de novo G409D mutation in the *ATL1* gene exhibited an extremely severe spastic paraplegia combined with general hypertonia and hypokinesia since the neonatal period in one patient [47].

Linkage analysis suggests that mutations in the *ATL1* gene account for approximately 10% of ADHSP. The reported frequency of *ATL1* gene mutations varied from 2.9 to 38.7% though most studies reported a frequency of less than 15%. For example, we found that there were eight studies which reported a frequency of *ATL1* gene mutations less than 15%: 2.9% [27] in ADHSP families, 3.7% in ADSHP probands [45], 4.2% in HSP families [36], 8.3% in unrelated early onset pure ADHSP families [9], 6.6% in a heterogeneous population including both pure and complicated HSP phenotypes [21], 8.6% in ADHSP families [29], 11.3% in the ADHSP families [32], and 11.7% in ADHSP probands [44]. We also found four studies which reported a higher frequency of *ATL1* gene mutations: 20.0% in pure HSP [55], 20.0% (3/15) in early onset autosomal dominant HSP [13], 38.5% in SPG4-negative pure ADHSP families [11], and 38.7% in pure ADHSP families [15]. We also found that there was a difference in the frequency of *ATL1* gene mutations reported with different AAOs. For example, Namekawa et al. reported that the frequency of *ATL1* gene mutation in ADHSP was 6.6%, whereas the frequency was 13.5% in ADHSP families with onset before age 20, and it increased to 31.8% in ADHSP families with onset before age 10 [17]. The frequency variation may be caused by the differences in ethical criteria, number of patients and inclusion criteria, such as pure and complicated phenotypes of the patients, AAOs and *SPAST* mutations.

This study found that most *ATL1* gene mutations were located at exons 4, 7, 8 and 12, which is consistent with a previous study [29], which suggests that these exons should be given priority when performing molecular diagnosis. In addition, R239C ($n = 31$) [6, 9, 11, 13, 15, 17, 21, 22, 27–29, 31, 32, 36, 39, 45, 51, 53, 54, 56] and R495W ($n = 14$) [15–17, 21, 32, 36, 43, 50, 52, 54] mutations were the most commonly reported mutations in all studied families. Zhao et al. reported that the three families with R239C mutations were not apparently related and haplotype analysis did not exclude a distant founder effect [6]. Namekawa et al. reported that the R495W mutation could occur by independent mutational events [59]. Genetic testing should be performed in HSPs patients with very early-onset pure spastic paraplegia.

It is still not understood how the atlastin-1 protein functions and it is also unclear how autosomal dominant mutations in *ATL1* gene lead to the degeneration of upper motor neurons. In our analysis of the literature we found that all *ATL1* gene mutations except 3 (R217Q, c.35-3C < T, and exon 4 deletion) fell outside the GTPase-related motifs or the conserved motifs identified in the *ATL1* gene sequence which are thought to alter the structure of atlastin-1 and its interaction with other proteins [6, 11, 13, 16]. We find that most mutations are missense which suggests a gain-of-function pathogenic mechanism that is dependent on the position of the mutation, gene modifier and environmental factors [32]. This is supported by studies using yeast two-hybrid assay and co-immunoprecipitation of wild-type and p.del436N atlastin proteins which show that the p.del436N mutant protein can still oligomerize with wild-type atlastin, supporting a loss-of-function disease mechanism [23]. Atlastin-1 interacts with spastin (*SPG4*), suggesting that they may be a part of a common biological cascade whose disruption can result in motor neuron death [60].

Conclusions

Our reanalysis demonstrates that most HSPs-SPG3A patients exhibited a pure autosomal dominant HSP with early AAO. The causal *ATL1* gene mutations are missense mutations and exons 4, 7, 8 and 12 should be prioritized for genetic testing. We find that there is no clear genotype-phenotype correlation.

Abbreviations

AAO: Age at onset; AD: Autosomal dominant; ADHSP: Autosomal dominant HSP; AR: Autosomal recessive; GTPases: Guanosine triphosphatases; HSP: Hereditary spastic paraplegias; SPG3A: Spastic paraplegia 3A

Acknowledgements

Not applicable.

Funding

This study was supported by the National Scientific Foundations of China (81000484), Natural Scientific Fundation of Zhejiang Province (LY17H090002), the Research Fundation of Zhejiang Health (2008QN017, 2016144072), the Natural Science Foundation of Shandong Province (ZR2013HQ016), and the Key Research and Development Project of Shandong Province (2015GGH318011).

Authors' contributions

All authors read and approved the final manuscript. GZ and XL conceived, designed and performed the paper. GZ revised the paper.

Competing interests

The authors declare that they have no competing interest.

Author details

[1]Department of Neurology, Second Affiliated Hospital, School of Medicine, Zhejiang University, Hangzhou 310009, China. [2]Department of Neurology, Fourth Affiliated Hospital, School of Medicine, Zhejiang University, Yiwu 322000, China. [3]Department of Neurology, Qianfoshan Hospital, Shandong University, Jinan 16766, China.

References

1. Harding AE. Classification of the hereditary ataxia and paraplegias. Lancet. 1983;1(8334):1151–5.
2. Mc Dermott CJ, et al. Hereditary spastic paraparesis: a review of new developments. J Neurol Neurosurg Psychiatry. 2000;69(2):150–60.
3. Gan-Or Z, et al. Mutations in CAPN1 cause autosomal- recessive hereditary spastic paraplegia. Am J Hum Genet. 2016;98(5):1038–46.
4. Hazan J, et al. Spastin, a new AAA protein, is altered in the most frequent form of autosomal dominant spastic paraplegia. Nat Genet. 1999;23(3):296–303.
5. Tallaksen CM, Durr A, Brice A. Recent advances in hereditary spastic paraplegia. Current Opinion Neurol. 2001;14:457–63.
6. Zhao X, et al. Mutations in a newly identified GTPase gene cause autosomal dominant hereditary spastic paraplegia. Nat Genet. 2001;29(3):326–31.
7. Muglia M, Magariello A, Nicoletti G. Further evidence that SPG3A gene mutations cause autosomal dominant hereditary spastic paraplegia. Ann Neurol. 2002;51(6):794–5.
8. Tessa A, Casali C, Damiano M. SPG3A: An additional family carrying a new atlastin mutation. Neurology. 2002;59(12):2002–5.
9. Wilkinson PA, et al. SPG3A mutation screening in English families with early onset autosomal dominant hereditary spastic paraplegia. J Neurol Sci. 2003; 216(1):43–5.
10. Sartori E, et al. Infancy onset hereditary spastic paraplegia associated with a novel atlastin mutation. Neurology. 2003;61(4):580–1.
11. Sauter SM, et al. Novel mutations in the Atlastin gene (SPG3A) in families with autosomal dominant hereditary spastic paraplegia and evidence for late onset forms of HSP linked to the SPG3A locus. Hum Mutat. 2004; 23(1):98.
12. D'Amico A, et al. Incomplete penetrance in an SPG3A-linked family with a new mutation in the atlastin gene. Neurology. 2004;62(11):2138–9.
13. Abel A, et al. Early onset autosomal dominant spastic paraplegia caused by novel mutations in SPG3A. Neurogenetics. 2004;5(4):239–43.
14. Hedera P, et al. Novel mutation in the SPG3A gene in an African American family with an early onset of hereditary spastic paraplegia. Arch Neurol. 2004;61(10):1600–3.
15. Dürr A, et al. Atlastin1 mutations are frequent in young-onset autosomal dominant spastic paraplegia. Arch Neurol. 2004;61(12):1867–72.
16. Scarano V, et al. The R495W mutation in SPG3A causes spastic paraplegia associated with axonal neuropathy. J Neurol. 2005;252(8):901–3.
17. Namekawa M, et al. SPG3A is the most frequent cause of hereditary spastic paraplegia with onset before age 10 years. Neurology. 2006;66(1):112–4.
18. Rainier S, et al. De novo occurrence of novel SPG3A/atlastin mutation presenting as cerebral palsy. Arch Neurol. 2005;63(3):445–7.
19. Chen SQ, et al. Severe hereditary spastic paraplegia caused by a de novo SPG3A mutation. Sci China. 2005;51(15):1854–6. In Chinese.
20. Matsui M, et al. A novel mutation in the SPG3A gene (atlastin) in hereditary spastic paraplegia. J Neurol. 2007;54(7):972–4.
21. Ivanova N, et al. Hereditary spastic paraplegia 3A associated with axonal neuropathy. Arch Neurol. 2007;64(5):706–13.
22. Li XH, et al. A SPG3A mutation with a novel foot phenotype of hereditary spastic paraplegia in a Chinese Han family. Chin Med J (Engl). 2007;120(9):834–7.
23. Meijer IA, et al. Characterization of a novel SPG3A deletion in a French-Canadian family. Ann Neurol. 2007;61(6):599–603.
24. Ming L. SPG3A-hereditary spastin paraplegia with genetic anticipation and incomplete penetrance. Zhonghua Yi Xue Yi Chuan Xue Za Zhi. 2007;24(1):15–8. In Chinese.
25. Haberlová J, et al. Extending the clinical spectrum of SPG3A mutations to a very severe and very early complicated phenotype. J Neurol. 2008;255(6):927–8.
26. Loureiro JL, et al. Novel SPG3A and SPG4 mutations in dominant spastic paraplegia families. Acta Neurol Scand. 2009;119(2):113–8.
27. Svenstrup K, et al. Sequence variants in SPAST, SPG3A and HSPD1 in hereditary spastic paraplegia. J Neurol Sci. 2009;284(1–2):90–5.
28. Chan KY, et al. Hereditary spastic paraplegia: identification of an SPG3A gene mutation in a Chinese family. Hong Kong Med J. 2009;15(4):304–7.
29. Smith BN, et al. Four novel SPG3A/atlastin mutations identified in autosomal dominant hereditary spastic paraplegia kindreds with intra-familial variability in age of onset and complex phenotype. Clin Genet. 2009;75(5):485–9.
30. Fusco C, et al. Hereditary spastic paraplegia and axonal motor neuropathy caused by a novel SPG3A de novo mutation. Brain Dev. 2010;32(7):592–4.
31. Kwon MJ, et al. Clinical and genetic analysis of a Korean family with hereditary spastic paraplegia type 3. Ann Clin Lab Sci. 2010;40(4):375–9.
32. Alvarez V, et al. Mutational spectrum of the SPG4 (SPAST) and SPG3A (ATL1) genes in Spanish patients with hereditary spastic paraplegia. BMC Neurol. 2010;10:89.
33. de Leva MF, et al. Complex phenotype in an Italian family with a novel mutation in SPG3A. J Neurol. 2010;257(3):328–31.

34. Orlacchio A, et al. Late-onset hereditary spastic paraplegia with thin corpus callosum caused by a new SPG3A mutation. J Neurol. 2011;258(7): 1361–3.

35. Al-Maawali A, et al. Hereditary spastic paraplegia associated with axonal neuropathy: a novel mutation of SPG3A in a large family. J Clin Neuromuscul Dis. 2011;12(3):143–6.

36. McCorquodale III DS, et al. Mutation screening of spastin, atlastin, and REEP1 in hereditary spastic paraplegia. Clin Genet. 2011;79(6):523–30.

37. Magariello A, et al. The p.Arg416Cys mutation in SPG3a gene associated with a pure form of spastic paraplegia. Muscle Nerve. 2012;45(6):919–20.

38. Fusco C, et al. Very early onset and severe complicated phenotype caused by a new spastic paraplegia 3A gene mutation. J Child Neurol. 2012;27(10): 1348–50.

39. Sulek A, et al. Screening for the hereditary spastic paraplaegias SPG4 and SPG3A with the multiplex ligation-dependent probe amplification technique in a large population of affected individuals. Neurol Sci. 2012; 34(2):239–42.

40. Terada T, et al. SPG3A-linked hereditary spastic paraplegia associated with cerebral glucose hypometabolism. Ann Nucl Med. 2013;27(3):303–8.

41. de Bot ST, et al. ATL1 and REEP1 mutations in hereditary and sporadic upper motor neuron syndromes. J Neurol. 2013;260(3):869–75.

42. Varga RE, et al. Do not trust the pedigree: reduced and sex-dependent penetrance at a novel mutation hotspot in ATL1 blurs autosomal dominant inheritance of spastic paraplegia. Hum Mutat. 2013;34(6):860–3.

43. Loureiro JL, et al. Autosomal dominant spastic paraplegias: a review of 89 families resulting from a portuguese survey. JAMA Neurol. 2013;70(4): 481–7.

44. Lu X, et al. Genetic analysis of SPG4 and SPG3A genes in a cohort of Chinese patients with hereditary spastic paraplegia. J Neurol Sci. 2014; 347(1–2):368–71.

45. Luo Y, et al. Mutation and clinical characteristics of autosomal-dominant hereditary spastic paraplegias in China. Neurodegener Dis. 2014;14(4): 176–83.

46. Shin JW, et al. Novel mutation in the ATL1 with autosomal dominant hereditary spastic paraplegia presented as dysautonomia. Auton Neurosci. 2014;185:141–3.

47. Yonekawa T, et al. Extremely severe complicated spastic paraplegia 3A with neonatal onset. Pediatr Neurol. 2014;51(5):726–9.

48. Khan TN, et al. Evidence for autosomal recessive inheritance in SPG3A caused by homozygosity for a novel ATL1 missense mutation. Eur J Hum Genet. 2014;22(10):1180–4.

49. Klein CJ, et al. Application of whole exome sequencing in undiagnosed inherited polyneuropathies. J Neurol Neurosurg Psychiatry. 2014;85(11): 1265–72.

50. Ishiura H, et al. Molecular epidemiology and clinical spectrum of hereditary spastic paraplegia in the Japanese population based on comprehensive mutational analyses. J Hum Genet. 2014;59(3):163–72.

51. Leonardi L, et al. De novo mutations in SPG3A: a challenge in differential diagnosis and genetic counselling. Neurol Sci. 2015;36(6):1063–4.

52. Park H, et al. Mutational spectrum of the SPAST and ATL1 genes in Korean patients with hereditary spastic paraplegia. J Neurol Sci. 2015;357(1–2): 167–72.

53. Zhao N, et al. Mutation analysis of four Chinese families with pure hereditary spastic paraplegia: pseudo-X-linked dominant inheritance and male lethality due to a novel ATL1 mutation. Genet Mol Res. 2015;14(4): 14690–7.

54. Elert-Dobkowska E, et al. Molecular spectrum of the SPAST, ATL1 and REEP1 gene mutations associated with the most common hereditary spastic paraplegias in a group of Polish patients. J Neurol Sci. 2015;359(1–2):35–9.

55. Polymeris AA, et al. A series of Greek children with pure hereditary spastic paraplegia: clinical features and genetic findings. J Neurol. 2016;263(8): 1604–11.

56. Balicza P, et al. Genetic background of the hereditary spastic paraplegia phenotypes in Hungary-An analysis of 58 probands. J Neurol Sci. 2016; 364(1):116–21.

57. Guelly C, et al. Targeted high-throughput sequencing identifies mutations in atlastin-1 as a cause of hereditary sensory neuropathy type I. Am J Hum Genet. 2011;88(1):99–105.

58. Leonardis L, et al. The N355K atlastin 1 mutation is associated with hereditary sensory neuropathy and pyramidal tract features. Eur J Neurol. 2012;19(7):992–8.

59. Namekawa M, et al. A founder effect and mutational hotpots may contribute to the most frequent mutations in the SPG3A gene. Neurogenetics. 2016;7(2):131–2.

60. Sanderson CM, et al. Spastin and atlastin, two proteins mutated in autosomal-dominant hereditary spastic paraplegia, are binding partners. Hum Mol Genet. 2006;15(2):307–18.

16

Utility of susceptibility-weighted imaging in Parkinson's disease and atypical Parkinsonian disorders

Zhibin Wang[1], Xiao-Guang Luo[1*] and Chao Gao[2]

Abstract

In the clinic, the diagnosis of Parkinson's disease (PD) largely depends on clinicians' experience. When the diagnosis is made, approximately 80% of dopaminergic cells in the substantia nigra (SN) have been lost. Additionally, it is rather challenging to differentiate PD from atypical parkinsonian disorders (APD). Clinially-available 3T conventional MRI contributes little to solve these problems. The pathologic alterations of parkinsonism show abnormal brain iron deposition, and therefore susceptibility-weighted imaging (SWI), which is sensitive to iron concentration, has been applied to find iron-related lesions for the diagnosis and differentiation of PD in recent decades. Until now, the majority of research has revealed that in SWI the signal intensity changes in deep brain nuclei, such as the SN, the putamen (PUT), the globus pallidus (GP), the thalamus (TH), the red nucleus (RN) and the caudate nucleus (CN), thereby raising the possibility of early diagnosis and differentiation. Furthermore, the signal changes in SN, PUT and TH sub-regions may settle the issues with higher accuracy. In this article, we review the brain iron deposition of PD, MSA-P and PSP in SWI in the hope of exhibiting a profile of SWI features in PD, MSA and PSP and its clinical values.

Keywords: Parkinson's disease, Multiple system atrophy Parkinsonian predominant type, Progressive supranuclear palsy, Susceptibility-weighted imaging, Iron deposition, Biomarker

Background

Parkinson's disease (PD) is characterized by resting tremor, rigidity, bradykinesia and postural instability accompanied by non-motor symptoms [1]. The criteria for PD diagnosis largely relay on clinicians' experience, and an accurate diagnosis often needs 3 to 5 years of follow-up. When PD is diagnosed, approximately 80% of dopaminergic cells in the substantia nigra pars compacta (SNc) have been lost [2]. Researches miss the opportunity for unraveling the mechanism of PD in the early stage to develop disease-modifying therapy which is deemed to prevent the disease progression or complications, though no such therapy exists at present [3]. On the other hand, atypical parkinsonian disorders (APD) are a group of heterogeneous neurodegenerative diseases including multiple system atrophy parkinsonian predominant type (MSA-P), progressive supranuclear palsy (PSP), and others. However, in the early stage of parkinsonism, PD and APD often show similar symptoms that are extremely difficult to distinguish, even for experienced neurologists [4]. Thus, it is critical to find the biomarkers for the diagnosis and differentiation of PD in the early stage. In the clinic, the biomarkers detected by positron emission tomography (PET) and single photon emission computed tomography (SPECT) can directly visualize the loss of dopaminergic cells [5, 6]. However, MRI is less expensive, non-invasive and avoids the radiation of radiotracers compared with PET and SPECT. During the past decades, a number of imaging signs were found by conventional MRI such as the "swallow tail sign", the pontine atrophy, the "hummingbird sign", etc. Although the specificities of these signs are high, the sensitivities are highly magnetic-intensity dependent [7–9]. The ultra-high field MRI is not wildly accepted in clinic as

* Correspondence: grace_shenyang@163.com
[1]Neurology Department, The First Affiliated Hospital of China Medical University, 155# Nanjing Bei Street Heping District, Shenyang 110001, People's Republic of China
Full list of author information is available at the end of the article

the results of the high expense and potential security problems.

The most ideal biomarkers must be involved in the pathologic changes of PD and APD such that the potential biomarkers can indicate the underlying pathologic processes. The abnormal iron deposition in the deep brain nuclei in parkinsonism was first described by Lhermitte et al. in 1924 [10]. Most studies have discovered that iron increases consistently in SN of PD, and the iron content is associated with disease severity [11]. Recently, abnormal iron deposition was also found in APD such as MSA-P, PSP and others [12–15]. Interestingly, the regions that are rich in iron among neurodegenerative diseases vary from each other [15, 16]. Iron may play a key role in the neuropathology of neurodegenerative diseases [12]. Therefore, the iron concentration and iron distribution in deep brain nuclei may work as promising biomarkers in PD and APD. Also, iron can change the magnetic susceptibility of tissues where it deposits. Susceptibility-weighted imaging (SWI), a novel MRI technique, is sensitive to magnetic susceptibility of tissue, and thus can detect the iron-related information of neurodegenerative parkinsonism working as a promising detecting tool in PD and APD [16, 17]. Here we review about brain iron deposition of PD, MSA-P and PSP in SWI in the hope of exhibiting a profile of SWI feature in PD, MSA and PSP and its clinical values.

Susceptibility-weighted imaging

SWI exploits the differences in magnetic susceptibility of tissues, which describes the magnetic response of tissues placed in an external magnetic field, to develop an enhanced image contrast for conventional MRI [18–20]. By applying a gradient-recalled echo (GRE) sequence with relatively long echo time (TE), a SW image combines a phase image with a magnitude image under high-intensity magnetic field such as 3T and 7T, to add the magnetic susceptibility information to the structure of the brain in situ (as shown in Fig. 1) [19]. The high-intensity field ensures a high spatial resolution and contrast-to-noise

ratio for the further study of detailed structures in the brain [21]. Image phase variations reflect the static magnetic field inhomogeneities, which are influenced by a macroscopic effect and a microscopic effect [19, 22]. The macroscopic effect, also called the geometry effect, is that the configuration of tissues, such as white matter tract, capillary beds, the interstitial space and others, distorts the homogeneity of the local field [19, 22, 23]. The microscopic effect is described as the homogeneity of the local field being distorted by substances with different magnetic susceptibility [18, 19, 22, 24]. Thus, the variances in the magnetic susceptibility of tissues are derived from both the geometry of the tissue and the substances' reaction to the applied field.

According to the reaction to the applied field, the substances can be classified into paramagnetic and diamagnetic. The paramagnetic substances mainly include ferritin containing ferric iron, deoxygenated hemoglobin, and ceruloplasmin, while the diamagnetic ones include myelin, calcium, and oxygenated hemoglobin [23]. Generally, the grey matter is paramagnetic because of the iron, and the white matter is diamagnetic due to the myelin [25, 26]. In comparison, iron has the highest concentration in the deep grey nuclei, while the other substances are relatively minimal [12]. Abnormal iron deposition patterns were found in the brain of patients with parkinsonism. Excess iron can cause damage to neuron through free radical production [13, 27, 28]. Therefore, iron is thought to play a key role in the pathogenesis of neurodegenerative parkinsonism [12, 13, 28, 29]. The abnormal iron deposition results in changed iron distribution and concentration in the brain, and thereby changing the susceptibility of tissue. SWI is able to identify the susceptibility alteration through recording the phase changes caused by the iron deposition through the multiplication of phase image with magnitude image for several times, which enables the increasing of phase contrast and indirect evaluation of iron content in parkinsonism [30–33]. What's more, the sensitivity of SWI is higher and the error under the same signal-to-noise ratio is lower compare

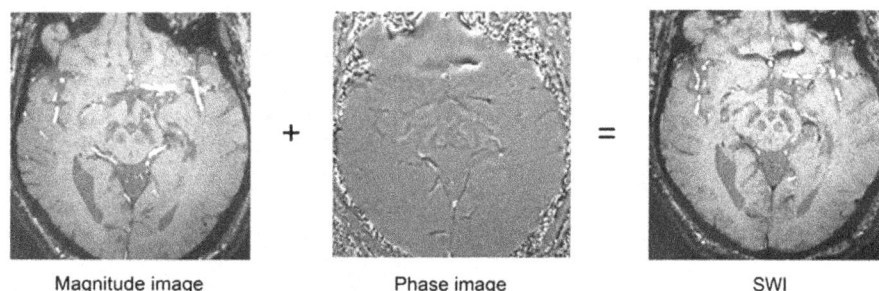

Magnitude image   Phase image   SWI

Fig 1 A SW image is developed from the combination of a magnitude image and a phase image

with T2*-weighted imaging, often considered the gold standard for the evaluation of brain iron content [34–38]. Thus, SWI is reliable for the clinical usage of evaluating the iron content of deep brain nuclei. However, SWI has drawbacks as well. The phase is not a local physical property, because the phase of a certain region is affected not only by the susceptibility of this region, but also by that of the surrounding areas [23, 26, 39]. It means that the phase image reflects comprehensive information about susceptibility changes. Moreover, a process called convolution in the formation of phase image makes it very difficult to distinguish paramagnetic iron from diamagnetic calcium [23]. Furthermore, the reproducibility is low, because the phase can be affected by the orientation of structures relative to the applied field [40].

To solve the problems of SWI, quantitative susceptibility mapping (QSM) is designed to quantify the iron content through measuring the susceptibility of certain areas directly [23, 39–43]. QSM is developed from SWI by solving the ill-posed inverse effect-to-source problem. Because the susceptibility is an intrinsic property of tissue, QSM can produce more precise image avoiding the non-locality of phase, and can differentiate iron from calcium [23]. Moreover, QSM can avoid the effect of the orientation relative to the applied field, due to the susceptibility value in QSM is isotropic [26]. What's more, QSM shows a higher reproducibility compared with R2* mapping to measure iron content [40]. Although this technique may be useful for assessing iron in deep structure with high iron content, the diamagnetic myelin level in white matter may impact the measurement. Little research has been conducted about the application of QSM for the diagnosis and differentiation of parkinsonism [42–44]. Therefore, QSM has a very promising future to study the parkinsonism-related iron deposition [36].

Brain iron deposition
Brain iron accumulation in the physiologic state
The brain iron distribution is uneven
The iron levels of basal ganglia are high [34, 45, 46]. Histological studies have shown that normally the caudate nucleus (CN), the putamen (PUT), the globus palidus (GP), the red nucleus (RN), and the substantia nigra (SN) are rich in iron, while the iron content of cortex is relatively low [45, 46]. In the cortex, the motor cortex (MC) is richest in iron, while the prefrontal and temporal cortices are the poorest [45]. Although the exact order of the iron level of deep nuclei does not reach a consensus between postmortem studies, those studies imply the heterogeneous distribution of brain iron in normal aging [45, 46].

Even within the same deep brain nuclei, the iron distribution is uneven. Histological studies reveal that the SN pars reticulata (SNr) in the ventral SN is rich

in iron, while the SNc in the dorsol SN is poor [47, 48]. Zecca et al. reported that the neuromelanin is the major iron-stored place in the SN neurons [49]. According to these facts, it is concluded that physiologically, iron deposition is heterogeneous, even in the same deep brain nuclei like SN.

The speed of brain iron deposition is uneven
A bunch of studies have approved that the speed of iron deposition across the brain is not even. In SN and GP, the iron concentration grows quickly in the early 20 years of life, then more gradually, and stops after 30 years of age [45, 49]. For CN and PUT, the maximal speed of iron accumulation was during the first 50 to 60 years old of life [45]. In some areas of the brain, iron deposition occurs through the whole life span. Interestingly, the iron content of the medulla oblongata is low and does not increase with advancing of age [45, 46].

The function of the brain iron
Iron functioning in the brain mainly exists in the forms of hemoglobin, iron-containing enzyme and non-haemin iron [13, 28, 45]. The iron involved in normal aging and neurodegenerative parkinsonism belongs to the non-haemin which is a cofactor of several enzymes that are associated with myelin formation and neurotransmitter production [13, 27–29, 45, 50, 51]. The period of the fastest iron deposition coincides with when the myelin of the brain forms the fastest in the early stage of life [12, 29, 45]. There is other evidence that iron deficiency can impair neural development, behavioral and cognitive function probably via damage to the myelin formation and neurotransmitter production [28].

Brain iron deposition in neurodegenerative parkinsonism
Brain iron accumulation in PD
Pathological and MRI studies indicate that the SN is the most relevant area of the brain in PD [17, 49, 52–55]. The iron concentration of the SN on the affected side of PD is approximately 80% more than that in healthy controls (HC), while overall iron contents in the brain between PD and HC are close [2, 31]. The reason for this phenomenon is unclear, but the elevated iron level of SN may relate to the localized pathogenesis such as permeability changes of the blood brain barrier (BBB), inflammation state, gene mutation-induced abnormal protein function in iron storage and transport, etc. [56–58] Furthermore, excess iron can cause cell death through reactive oxygen species derived from Fenton's reaction by which iron catalyzes hydrogen peroxide [11–13, 27, 29]. Notably, an insight into the relationship between the ferric (III) or ferrous (II) state of iron and alpha-synuclein enables a better understanding of the pathogenesis of PD. Fe (II) takes part in the Fenton reaction producing

hydrogen peroxide, and then Fe (II) is oxidized to Fe (III). Levin et al. reported that alpha-synuclein aggregation is independent of oxidizing agents, while is highly correlated with the amount of Fe (III) [59]. This is in line with the fact that the Fe2+/Fe3+ ratio shift to the Fe3+ in PD [59, 60]. Iron chelators can protect neurons from death in vitro, and PD patients may benefit from the decrease in iron level [12, 61, 62]. Some researchers believe that a localized, elevated iron level is caused by the iron-chelated neuromelanin that is released from dead neurones injured by aggregation of alpha-synuclein [54]. In this case, the increased extracellular neuromelanin is the cause of elevated iron level. In contrary, others suggested that the iron level increased primarily, and then neuromelanin increased as a compensatory factor to chelate redundant iron [11]. It is still debatable whether abnormal iron deposition is the primary cause of neuropathology or just an epiphenomenon [12, 13].

Brain iron accumulation in APD

MSA and PSP are the most common APD and clinically the most important differential diagnosis for PD [48]. Autopsy research suggested that brownish discoloration of deep brain nuclei relates to iron deposition [48, 63]. In MSA, discoloration and atrophy of posteriolateral PUT was remarkable compared with PD and PSP in autopsy [48, 63, 64]. However, neither discoloration nor atrophy of RN, dendate nucleus (DN) and subthalamic nucleus (STN) were found in MSA [48, 63, 64]. In PSP, remarkable atrophy and discoloration were revealed in cerebellar WM and STN [65–68]. Both MSA and PSP showed various degrees of the atrophy of SN, GP, TH and CN [48, 63–66, 68]. More researches are needed to further specify the spatial distribution of iron deposition in APD.

SWI in Parkinson's disease and atypical parkinsonian disorders

SWI in the diagnosis of Parkinson's disease

The majority of research approved that SWI was feasible to indirectly quantify the iron content of different regions of brain through comparing the phase values in SWI which was highly correlated with the iron content [17, 19, 22, 24]. Thus, the comparison of iron content in SWI is conducted by comparing the phase value indirectly rather than by comparing the iron content directly like QSM. There are various forms of iron deposition patterns of PD imaged by SWI among the researches. Some researches supported that iron deposition patterns in SWI can distinguish PD from HC. Jiuquan Zhang et al. reported that the iron concentration was elevated significantly only in the SN of PD compared with HC in SWI [17]. The iron contents of the SNc, CN and RN in PD were significantly higher than those in HC in a SWI study by Wei Zhang et al. [33]. Also, Wu et al.

demonstrated the iron accumulation in the SN, RN, CN, PUT, and GP of PD was more remarkable than that of HC [69]. An elevated iron level of the SN was common in PD among SWI research, because the SN is the most pathologically relevant site of PD and become atrophy and brownish discoloration in autopsy [48, 67, 70]. Notably, Dashtipour et al. did not find remarkably increased iron content of SN in PD, and it may be explained by the small sample size [31]. However, the discrepancy of iron accumulation in other nuclei, such as RN, CN, PUT, and GP, in SWI is unclear. One possible reason is that deep brain nuclei are pathologically involved simultaneously with different degrees of iron accumulation [70]. In addition, different iron deposition patterns may relate to disease progression [31]. Furthermore, research has demonstrated that the iron content of the SN is inversely correlated with the severity of PD as measured by UPDRS-motor score and H-Y stage [17, 30, 48], while no correlations were found between the iron content of the SN and the duration, progression, prognosis and levodopa response of PD [17, 31, 33, 69, 71, 72]. Even though with the heterogeneity of iron deposition speed and distribution in the whole disease process, SWI still fails to characterize specific clinical features of PD. For instance, SWI cannot detect the difference between earlier-onset and later-onset PD patients [17]. Neither could SWI show difference between the early and intermediate/advanced stages of PD [69]. Mechanisms, such as gene mutation, alteration of the BBB, and inflammation, may underlie the speed, onset and spatial distribution of iron deposition [12, 29, 50]. Further studies are needed to figure out whether there are correlations between iron content of SN and specific clinical features.

In recent years, a novel imaging biomarker called nigrosome 1, which is the sub-region of the SN, has been extensively studied by researchers. According to the immuno-staining of calbindin that can bind to calcium, the SNc is subdivided into nigrosome (caldbindin-poor) and nigral matrix (caldbindin-rich). Nigrosome 1 is the largest nigrosome containing the biggest group of dopaminergic cells and is affected in almost every PD patient [73]. It was reported that 7T MRI could visualize the three-layered structure of SN and could distinguish patients with PD from HC with both high sensitivity and specificity [14, 74, 75]. In 3T SWI, nigrosome 1 also shows dorsolateral hyperintensity of SN in HC, and disappears in PD with 100% sensitivity and high specificity (shown in Fig. 2) [47, 73]. These evidences suggested that 3T SWI is a reliable tool for the visualization of nigrosome 1 and the diagnosis of PD. However, in some studies nigrosome 1 hyperintensity also disappears in MSA-P and PSP in SWI [14, 53]. Therefore, nigrosome 1 is a safe biomarker for neurodegenerative parkinsonism rather than PD.

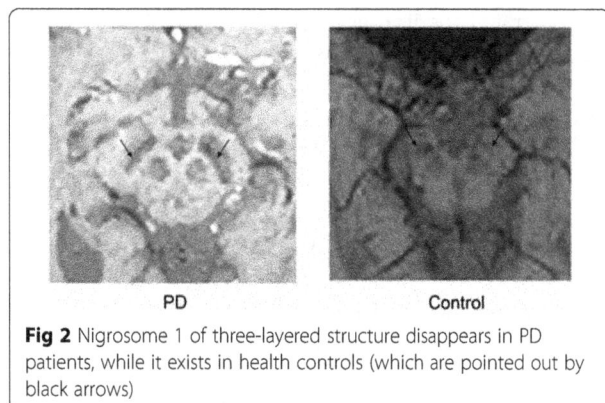

Fig 2 Nigrosome 1 of three-layered structure disappears in PD patients, while it exists in health controls (which are pointed out by black arrows)

SWI in the differentiation of PD from APD

The iron deposition patterns of MSA-P imaged by SWI

At present, the most promising signs in SWI that characterize MSA-P focus on signal changes in PUT due to its remarkably high iron level demonstrated by autopsy [32, 48, 63, 76]. As the mechanism of SWI, the signal intensity of certain region is decreased when paramagnetic iron accumulates. Researchers designed a visual scale of the PUT hypointensity for visual differentiation [71, 76, 77]. The visual scales contain a set of standard images of putaminal hypointensity graded from 0 to 3. The higher the grade reaches, the lower the signal intensity is [71, 76, 77]. Grade 3 hypointensity of the posterior PUT was reported to discriminate MSA-P from PD [77]. This finding was consistent with the iron deposition pattern of MSA-P in autopsy that the iron content of posterior PUT in MSA-P was remarkably higher than that in PD [48, 63, 64]. Some researchers even suggested more detailed criteria for differentiation. For example, Wang et al. reported that when the PUT was sub-divided into 4 regions (lower inner, lower outer, upper inner and upper outer), the lower inner part of the PUT performed the best on receiver operating characteristic curve to distinguish MSA-P from PD [72]. Except for the studies about the iron levels in the local areas of PUT, Han et al. found that the topography of iron deposition of the PUT showing posteriolateral-to-anteriomedial ascending signal intensity, was highly specific for MSA-P patients, even in the early stage without obvious clinical symptoms [32]. Although the aforementioned biomarkers are still controversial and need further validation, they are still by far the most promising biomarkers and are clinically available. It was even suggested by Yoon et al. that SWI was potentially able to replace PET in the diagnosis of MSA-P because in PUT there was positive correlation between a low metabolism rate in PET and the low signal intensity in SWI [16]. However, Kwon et al. found no correlation between the metabolism rate in PET and the signal intensity in SWI [78]. The potential that SWI indicates the dysfunction of dopaminergic neurons imaged by PET needs further studies.

Other deep nuclei, such as the CN and pulvinar TH (PT), were also studied. Meijer et al. reported that the iron content of the CN on the affected side of MSA-P was remarkably higher than that of PD in SWI [77]. By contrast, Wang et al. demonstrated that the iron content of the CN cannot distinguish MSA-P from PD in SWI [72]. On autopsy, neuronal loss of the CN correlated with iron deposition is common and severe in MSA-P but unusual and mild in PD [12, 48]. The discrepancies between different studies may come from the variety of inclusion criteria, with patients at different MSA-P stages. Only a few study investigated about PT. Wang et al. found that the higher iron content of the PT in MSA-P, but failed to show statistical significance between groups [72]. For CN and PT, more researches are warranted to validate their potentials as biomarkers.

The iron deposition patterns of PSP imaged by SWI

There are different iron deposition patterns of PSP in SWI because of various forms of neuropathological processes [65]. Meijer et al. reported that elevated iron levels of the RN and dentate nucleus (DN) on the affected side could distinguish PSP from PD [77]. These findings are consistent with the pathological results of Dickson that only the RN and DN were damaged consistently and severely in PSP, but were spared in PD and MSA [48]. Gupta et al. found that increased iron content of the RN and the PUT was able to differentiate PSP from MSA-P and PD [71]. Notably, the iron level of the PUT is suggested to be the biomarker for the diagnosis of MSA-P in many studies [32, 48, 63, 76]. One possible speculation for this controversy is that local iron content and specific deposition patterns such as dense iron deposition in lower outer part of PUT, are more specific than overall content in MSA-P, while the overall iron content of PUT is a characteristic feature for PSP [71, 76, 77]. In addition, Han et al. demonstrated that elevated iron contents of GP and TH were the most valuable biomarkers in SWI to differentiate PSP from MSA-P and PD [32]. From neuropathological studies, neuronal loss of GP and TH is more severe in PSP than in MSA, but spared in PD [48, 63, 66]. However, due to the diverse results, consensus regarding the features of SWI imaging for PSP is hard to reach and further studies aiming at finding SWI biomarkers should consider the disease stage and combine the SWI results with iron-related neuropathology.

The drawbacks among SWI research

SWI is a promising biomarker that provides more information for early and differential diagnosis of parkinsonism, however present studies have several drawbacks that need to be addressed in the future. (1) Few research combined the SWI results of parkinsonism with pathological investigations [32, 71]. (2) Most of patients involved in studies have received levodopa replacement therapy, which may change the iron deposition pattern in SWI [17]. (3) Most of the studies are retrospective [72], and the follow-up of a few prospective studies are relatively short [8]. (4) The difference in scan parameters of SWI such as slice thickness, matrix size, etc., should be considered to interpret the discrepancy of results [17, 69]. Also, standardization for regions of interest drawn by hand and uniformed image analysis should be applied [33].

Conclusion

SWI characterizes brain iron deposition patterns of PD to illustrate the iron-related pathologic alterations in vivo and compensates for some drawbacks of routine MRI. Many researches have confirmed that SWI is a promising tool for the diagnosis and differential diagnosis of PD through discovering iron-related biomarkers, and more accessible in the clinic. Further studies should take the stages of neurodegenerative parkinsonism into consideration to acquire better correlations between SWI findings and neuropathologic results. With the underling pathological procedures illustrated by SWI, it will be possible to diagnose PD in the early stage and differentiate PD from APD.

Abbreviations

APD: Atypical parkinsonian disorders; BBB: Blood brain barrier; CN: Caudate nucleus; DN: Dentate nucleus; GM: Grey matter; GP: Globus pallidus; HC: Healthy controls; LC: Locus coeruleus; MC: Motor cortex; MSA-P: Multiple system atrophy parkinsonian predominant type; PD: Parkinson's disease; PSP: Progressive supranuclear palsy; PT: Pulvinar thalamus; PUT: Putamen; RN: Red nucleus; SN: Substantia nigra; SNc: SN pars compacta; SNr: SN pars reticulate; STN: Subthalamic nucleus; SWI: Susceptibility-weighted imaging; TH: Thalamus; WM: White matter

Acknowledgements

Not applicable.

Funding

This work was funded by China National Nature Science Fund (No. 81371421). The role of this funding body was in writing the manuscript.

Authors' contributions

ZBW: draft the manuscript. XGL: raised the idea of this review and revised the manuscript. CG: revised the manuscript. All authors read and approved the final manuscript.

Competing interests

The authors declare that they have no competing interests.

Author details

[1]Neurology Department, The First Affiliated Hospital of China Medical University, 155# Nanjing Bei Street Heping District, Shenyang 110001, People's Republic of China. [2]Neurology Department, Ruijin Hospital, Shanghai Jiaotong University School of Medicine, Ruijin 2nd Road 197, Shanghai 200025, People's Republic of China.

References

1. Reichmann H. Clinical criteria for the diagnosis of Parkinson's disease. Neurodegener Dis. 2010;7:284–90.
2. Pavese N, Brooks DJ. Imaging neurodegeneration in Parkinson's disease. Biochim Biophys Acta. 2009;1792:722–9.
3. Salat D, Noyce AJ, Schrag A, Tolosa E. Challenges of modifying disease progression in prediagnostic Parkinson's disease. Lancet Neurol. 2016;15:637–48.
4. David R, Williams M, Litvan I. Parkinsonian Syndromes. Continuum. 2013;19:1189–212.
5. S. Thobois S, Guillouet S, Broussolle E. Contributions of PET and SPECT to the understanding of the pathophysiology of Parkinson's disease. Neurophysiol Clin. 2001;31:321–40.
6. Catafau AM, Tolosa E, DaTSCAN Clinically Uncertain Parkinsonian Syndromes Study Group. Impact of dopamine transporter SPECT using 123I-Ioflupane on diagnosis and management of patients with clinically uncertain Parkinsonian syndromes. Mov Disord. 2004;19:1175–82.
7. Morelli M, Arabia G, Salsone M, Novellino F, Giofre L, Paletta R, et al. Accuracy of magnetic resonance parkinsonism index for differentiation of progressive supranuclear palsy from probable or possible Parkinson disease. Mov Disord. 2011;26:527–33.
8. Meijer FJ, Aerts MB, Abdo WF, Prokop M, Borm GF, Esselink RA, et al. Contribution of routine brain MRI to the differential diagnosis of parkinsonism: a 3-year prospective follow-up study. J Neurol. 2012;259:929–35.
9. Schrag A, Kingsley D, Phatouros C, Mathias CJ, Lees AJ, Daniel SE, Quinn NP. Clinical usefulness of magnetic resonance imaging in multiple system atrophy. J Neurol Neurosurg Psychiatry. 1998;65:65–71.
10. Lhermitte J, Kraus WM, McAlpine D. On the occurrence of abnormal deposits of iron in the brain in parkinsonism with special referene to its localisation. J Neurol Psychopathol. 1924;5:195–208.
11. Zucca FA, Segura-Aguilar J, Ferrari E, Munoz P, Paris I, Sulzer D, et al. Interactions of iron, dopamine and neuromelanin pathways in brain aging and Parkinson's disease. Prog Neurobiol. 2015. doi:10.1016/j.pneurobio.2015.09.012.
12. Ward RJ, Zucca FA, Duyn JH, Crichton RR, Zecca L. The role of iron in brain ageing and neurodegenerative disorders. Lancet Neurol. 2014;13:1045–60.
13. Li K, Reichmann H. Role of iron in neurodegenerative diseases. J Neural Transm. 2016;123:389–99.
14. Kim JM, Jeong HJ, Bae YJ, Park SY, Kim E, Kang SY, et al. Loss of substantia nigra hyperintensity on 7 Tesla MRI of Parkinson's disease, multiple system atrophy, and progressive supranuclear palsy. Parkinsonism Relat Disord. 2016;26:47–54.
15. Boelmans K, Holst B, Hackius M, Finsterbusch J, Gerloff C, Fiehler J, et al. Brain iron deposition fingerprints in Parkinson's disease and progressive supranuclear palsy. Mov Disord. 2012;27:421–7.
16. Yoon RG, Kim SJ, Kim HS, Choi CG, Kim JS, Oh J, et al. The utility of susceptibility-weighted imaging for differentiating Parkinsonism-predominant multiple system atrophy from Parkinson's disease: correlation with 18F-flurodeoxyglucose positron-emission tomography. Neurosci Lett. 2015;584:296–301.
17. Zhang J, Zhang Y, Wang J, Cai P, Luo C, Qian Z, et al. Characterizing iron deposition in Parkinson's disease using susceptibility-weighted imaging: an in vivo MR study. Brain Res. 2010;1330:124–30.
18. Haacke EM, Xu Y, Cheng Y-CN, Reichenbach Jr R. Susceptibility weighted imaging (SWI). Magn Reson Med. 2004;52:612–8.
19. Tuite PJ, Mangia S, Michaeli S. Magnetic Resonance Imaging (MRI) in Parkinson's Disease. J Alzheimer's Dis Parkinsonism. 2013;Suppl 1:001.

20. Vertinsky AT, Coenen VA, Lang DJ, Kolind S, Honey CR, Li D, et al. Localization of the subthalamic nucleus: optimization with susceptibility-weighted phase MR imaging. AJNR Am J Neuroradiol. 2009;30:1717–24.

21. Cosottini M, Frosini D, Pesaresi I, Donatelli G, Cecchi P, Costagli M, et al. Comparison of 3T and 7T susceptibility-weighted angiography of the substantia nigra in diagnosing Parkinson disease. AJNR Am J Neuroradiol. 2015;36:461–6.

22. Haacke EM, Mittal S, Wu Z, Neelavalli J, Cheng YCN. Susceptibility-weighted imaging: technical aspects and clinical applications, part 1. AJNR Am J Neuroradiol. 2008;30:19–30.

23. Liu C, Li W, Tong KA, Yeom KW, Kuzminski S. Susceptibility-weighted imaging and quantitative susceptibility mapping in the brain. J Magn Reson Imaging. 2015;42:23–41.

24. Mittal S, Wu Z, Neelavalli J, Haacke EM. Susceptibility-weighted imaging: technical aspects and clinical applications, part 2. AJNR Am J Neuroradiol. 2009;30:232–52.

25. Shmueli K, de Zwart JA, van Gelderen P, Li TQ, Dodd SJ, Duyn JH. Magnetic susceptibility mapping of brain tissue in vivo using MRI phase data. Magn Reson Med. 2009;62:1510–22.

26. Schweser F, Deistung A, Lehr BW, Reichenbach JR. Quantitative imaging of intrinsic magnetic tissue properties using MRI signal phase: an approach to in vivo brain iron metabolism? Neuroimage. 2011;54:2789–807.

27. Dusek P, Roos PM, Litwin T, Schneider SA, Flaten TP, Aaseth J. The neurotoxicity of iron, copper and manganese in Parkinson's and Wilson's diseases. J Trace Elem Med Biol. 2015;31:193–203.

28. Hagemeier J, Geurts JJ, Zivadinov R. Brain iron accumulation in aging and neurodegenerative disorders. Expert Rev Neurother. 2012;12:1467–80.

29. Kruer MC. The neuropathology of neurodegeneration with brain iron accumulation. Int Rev Neurobiol. 2013;110:165–94.

30. Dabrowska M, Schinwelski M, Sitek EJ, Muraszko-Klaudel A, Brockhuis B, Jamrozik Z, et al. The role of neuroimaging in the diagnosis of the atypical parkinsonian syndromes in clinical practice. Neurol Neurochir Pol. 2015;49:421–31.

31. Dashtipour K, Liu M, Kani C, Dalaie P, Obenaus A, Simmons D, et al. Iron accumulation is not homogenous among patients with Parkinson's disease. Parkinson's Dis. 2015;2015:324843.

32. Han YH, Lee JH, Kang BM, Mun CW, Baik SK, Shin YI, et al. Topographical differences of brain iron deposition between progressive supranuclear palsy and parkinsonian variant multiple system atrophy. J Neurol Sci. 2013;325:29–35.

33. Zhang W, Sun SG, Jiang YH, Qiao X, Sun X, Wu Y. Determination of brain iron content in patients with Parkinson's disease using magnetic susceptibility imaging. Neurosci Bull. 2009;25:353–60.

34. Haacke EM, Ayaz M, Khan A, Manova ES, Krishnamurthy B, Gollapalli L, Ciulla C, Kim I, Petersen F, Kirsch W. Establishing a baseline phase behavior in magnetic resonance imaging to determine normal vs. abnormal iron content in the brain. J Magn Reson Imaging. 2007;26:256–64.

35. Pirpamer L, Hofer E, Gesierich B, De Guio F, Freudenberger P, Seiler S, et al. Determinants of iron accumulation in the normal aging brain. Neurobiol Aging. 2016;43:149–55.

36. Barbosa JH, Santos AC, Tumas V, Liu M, Zheng W, Haacke EM, et al. Quantifying brain iron deposition in patients with Parkinson's disease using quantitative susceptibility mapping, R2 and R2. Magn Reson Imaging. 2015;33:559–65.

37. Ning N, Zhang L, Gao J, Zhang Y, Ren Z, Niu G, et al. Assessment of iron deposition and white matter maturation in infant brains by using enhanced T2 star weighted angiography (ESWAN): R2* versus phase values. PLoS One. 2014;9:e89888.

38. Wang C, Fan G, Xu K, Wang S. Quantitative assessment of iron deposition in the midbrain using 3D-enhanced T2 star weighted angiography (ESWAN): a preliminary cross-sectional study of 20 Parkinson's disease patients. Magn Reson Imaging. 2013;31:1068–73.

39. Reichenbach JR, Schweser F, Serres B, Deistung A. Quantitative susceptibility mapping: concepts and applications. Clin Neuroradiol. 2015;25 Suppl 2:225–30.

40. Santin MD, Didier M, Valabregue R, Yahia Cherif L, Garcia-Lorenzo D, Loureiro de Sousa P, et al. Reproducibility of R2 * and quantitative susceptibility mapping (QSM) reconstruction methods in the basal ganglia of healthy subjects. NMR Biomed. 2016. doi:10.1002/nbm.3491.

41. Deistung A, Schweser F, Reichenbach JR. Overview of quantitative susceptibility mapping. NMR Biomed. 2016. doi:10.1002/nbm.3569.

42. Du G, Liu T, Lewis MM, Kong L, Wang Y, Connor J, et al. Quantitative susceptibility mapping of the midbrain in Parkinson's disease. Mov Disord. 2016;31:317–24.

43. Guan X, Xuan M, Gu Q, Huang P, Liu C, Wang N, et al. Regionally progressive accumulation of iron in Parkinson's disease as measured by quantitative susceptibility mapping. NMR Biomed. 2016. doi:10.1002/nbm.3489.

44. Azuma M, Hirai T, Yamada K, Yamashita S, Ando Y, Tateishi M, et al. Lateral asymmetry and spatial difference of iron deposition in the substantia nigra of patients with Parkinson disease measured with quantitative susceptibility mapping. AJNR Am J Neuroradiol. 2016;37:782–8.

45. Hallgren B, Sourander P. The effect of age on the non-haemin iron in the human brain. J Neurochem. 1958;3:41–51.

46. Ramos P, Santos A, Pinto NR, Mendes R, Magalhães T, Almeida A. Iron levels in the human brain: A post-mortem study of anatomical region differences and age-related changes. J Trace Elem Med Biol. 2014;28:13–7.

47. Blazejewska AI, Schwarz ST, Pitiot A, Stephenson MC, Lowe J, et al. Visualization of nigrosome 1 and its loss in PD. Neurology. 2013;81:534–40.

48. Dickson DW. Parkinson's disease and Parkinsonism: Neuropathology. Cold Spring Harb Perspect Med. 2012. doi:10.1101/cshperspect.a009258.

49. Zecca L, Gallorini M, Schünemann V, Trautwein AX, Gerlach M, Riederer P, Vezzoni P, Tampellini D. Iron, neuromelanin and ferritin content in the substantia nigra of normal subjects at different ages: consequences for iron storage and neurodegenerative processes. J Neurochem. 2001;76:1766–73.

50. Thomas M, Jankovic J. Neurodegenerative disease and iron storage in the brain. Curr Opin Neurol. 2004;17:437–42.

51. Heidari M, Gerami SH, Bassett B, Graham RM, Chua AC, Aryal R, et al. Pathological relationships involving iron and myelin may constitute a shared mechanism linking various rare and common brain diseases. Rare Dis. 2016;4:e1198458.

52. Jin L, Wang J, Jin H, Fei G, Zhang Y, Chen W, et al. Nigral iron deposition occurs across motor phenotypes of Parkinson's disease. Eur J Neurol. 2012;19:969–76.

53. Reiter E, Mueller C, Pinter B, Krismer F, Scherfler C, Esterhammer R, et al. Dorsolateral nigral hyperintensity on 3.0T susceptibility-weighted imaging in neurodegenerative Parkinsonism. Mov Disord. 2015;30:1068–76.

54. Kitao S, Matsusue E, Fujii S, Miyoshi F, Kaminou T, Kato S, et al. Correlation between pathology and neuromelanin MR imaging in Parkinson's disease and dementia with Lewy bodies. Neuroradiology. 2013;55:947–53.

55. Zeccaa L, Fariello R, Riederer P, Sulzer D, Gatti A, Tampellini D. The absolute concentration of nigral neuromelanin, assayed by a new sensitive method, increases throughout the life and is dramatically decreased in Parkinson's disease. FEBS Lett. 2002;510:216–20.

56. Schneider SA, Dusek P, Hardy J, Westenberger A, Jankovic J, Bhatia KP. Genetics and Pathophysiology of Neurodegeneration with Brain Iron Accumulation (NBIA). Curr Neuropharmacol. 2013;11:59–79.

57. Duck KA, Connor JR. Iron uptake and transport across physiological barriers. Biometals. 2016;29:573–91.

58. Hu Y, Yu SY, Zuo LJ, Piao YS, Cao CJ, Wang F, et al. Investigation on abnormal iron metabolism and related inflammation in Parkinson disease patients with probable RBD. PLoS One. 2015;10:e0138997.

59. Levin J, Hogen T, Hillmer AS, Bader B, Schmidt F, Kamp F, et al. Generation of ferric iron links oxidative stress to alpha-synuclein oligomer formation. J Parkinson's Dis. 2011;1:205–16.

60. Peng Y, Wang C, Xu HH, Liu YN, Zhou F. Binding of alpha-synuclein with Fe(III) and with Fe(II) and biological implications of the resultant complexes. J Inorg Biochem. 2010;104:365–70.

61. Dusek P, Schneider SA, Aaseth J. Iron chelation in the treatment of neurodegenerative diseases. J Trace Elem Med Biol. 2016. doi:10.1016/j.jtemb.2016.03.010.

62. Aguirre P, Mena NP, Carrasco CM, Munoz Y, Perez-Henriquez P, Morales RA, et al. Iron Chelators and Antioxidants Regenerate Neuritic Tree and Nigrostriatal Fibers of MPP+/MPTP-Lesioned Dopaminergic Neurons. PLoS One. 2015;10:e0144848.

63. Jellinger KA. Neuropathology of multiple system atrophy: new thoughts about pathogenesis. Mov Disord. 2014;29:1720–41.

64. Benarroch EE. New findings on the neuropathology of multiple system atrophy. Auton Neurosci. 2002;96:59–62.

65. Wakabayashi K, Takahashi H. Pathological heterogeneity in progressive supranuclear palsy and corticobasal degeneration. Neuropathology. 2004;24:79–86.

66. Dickson DW, Rademakers R, Hutton ML. Progressive supranuclear palsy: pathology and genetics. Brain Pathol. 2007;17:74–82.

67. Ferrer I, Martinez A, Blanco R, Dalfo E, Carmona M. Neuropathology of sporadic Parkinson disease before the appearance of parkinsonism: preclinical Parkinson disease. J Neural Transm. 2011;118:821–39.

68. Collins SJ, Ahlsog JE, Parisi JE, Maraganore DM. Progressive supranuclear palsy: neuropathologically based diagnostic clinical criteria. J Neurol Neurosurg Psychiatry. 1995;58:167–73.

69. Wu SF, Zhu ZF, Kong Y, Zhang HP, Zhou GQ, Jiang QT, Meng XP. Assessment of cerebral iron content in patients with Parkinson's disease by the susceptibility-weighted MRI. Eur Rev Med Pharmacol Sci. 2014;18:2605–8.

70. Braak H, Del Tredici K, Rüb U, de Vos RA, Jansen Steur EN, Braak E. Staging of brain pathology related to sporadic Parkinson's disease. Neurobiol Aging. 2003;24:197–211.

71. Gupta D, Saini J, Kesavadas C, Sarma PS, Kishore A. Utility of susceptibility-weighted MRI in differentiating Parkinson's disease and atypical parkinsonism. Neuroradiology. 2010;52:1087–94.

72. Wang Y, Butros SR, Shuai X, Dai Y, Chen C, Liu M, et al. Different iron-deposition patterns of multiple system atrophy with predominant parkinsonism and idiopathetic Parkinson diseases demonstrated by phase-corrected susceptibility-weighted imaging. AJNR Am J Neuroradiol. 2012;33:266–73.

73. Schwarz ST, Afzal M, Morgan PS, Bajaj N, Gowland PA, Auer DP. The 'Swallow Tail' Appearance of the Healthy Nigrosome – A New Accurate Test of Parkinson's Disease: A Case-control and Retrospective Cross-Sectional MRI Study at 3T. PLoS One. 2014;9:e93814.

74. Lehericy S, Bardinet E, Poupon C, Vidailhet M, Francois C. 7 Tesla magnetic resonance imaging: a closer look at substantia nigra anatomy in Parkinson's disease. Mov Disord. 2014;29:1574–81.

75. Mirco Cosottini M, Daniela Frosini M, Ilaria Pesaresi M, Mauro Costagli P, Laura Biagi P, Roberto Ceravolo M, et al. MR Imaging of the Substantia Nigra at 7 T Enables Diagnosis of Parkinson Disease. Radiology. 2014;271:831–8.

76. Leea J-H, Baikb S-K. Putaminal Hypointensity in the Parkinsonian Variant of Multiple System Atrophy: Simple Visual Assessment Using Susceptibility-Weighted Imaging. J Mov Disord. 2011;4:60–3.

77. Meijer FJ, van Rumund A, Fasen BA, Titulaer I, Aerts M, Esselink R, et al. Susceptibility-weighted imaging improves the diagnostic accuracy of 3T brain MRI in the work-up of parkinsonism. AJNR Am J Neuroradiol. 2015;36:454–60.

78. Kwon GH, Jang J, Choi HS, Hwang EJ, Jung SL, Ahn KJ, Kim BS, Yoo IR, Kim SH, Haacke EM. The phase value of putamen measured by susceptibility weighted images in Parkinson's disease and in other forms of Parkinsonism: a correlation study with F18 FP-CIT PET. Acta Radiol. 2015. doi:10.1177/0284185115604515.

17

Role of BACE1 in Alzheimer's synaptic function

Brati Das and Riqiang Yan*⊙

Abstract

Alzheimer's disease (AD) is the most common age-dependent disease of dementia, and there is currently no cure available. This hallmark pathologies of AD are the presence of amyloid plaques and neurofibrillary tangles. Although the exact etiology of AD remains a mystery, studies over the past 30 have shown that abnormal generation or accumulation of β-amyloid peptides (Aβ) is likely to be a predominant early event in AD pathological development. Aβ is generated from amyloid precursor protein (APP) via proteolytic cleavage by β-site APP cleaving enzyme 1 (BACE1). Chemical inhibition of BACE1 has been shown to reduce Aβ in animal studies and in human trials. While BACE1 inhibitors are currently being tested in clinical trials to treat AD patients, it is highly important to understand whether BACE1 inhibition will significantly impact cognitive functions in AD patients. This review summarizes the recent studies on BACE1 synaptic functions. This knowledge will help to guide the proper use of BACE1 inhibitors in AD therapy.

Keywords: Amyloid deposition, β-amyloid peptide, BACE1, Secretase, BACE1 substrates, Synaptic functions

Background

Alzheimer's disease (AD) is an age-dependent chronic neurodegenerative disease that is characterized by the presence of amyloid deposition, neurofibrillary tangles, synaptic dysfunction, and neuronal cell death [1, 2]. The common effector of this neurodegenerative process is the excessive production or accumulation of β-amyloid (Aβ), which has several deleterious effects on synaptic activity [3, 4]. For over 30 years, amyloid precursor protein (APP) has been a main target for investigating the progression of AD. Aβ is generated from APP through proteolysis in a two-step process: β-secretase, known as β-site APP cleaving enzyme 1 (BACE1), initiates the cleavage of APP to release the membrane-anchored C-terminal fragment, and then γ-secretase subsequently cleaves this fragment to excise Aβ in 40–43 amino acid sequences [5]. These sequences form hydrophobic aggregates, which constitute the senile plaques in AD. Risk factors associated with development of AD pathology involve genetic predisposition (familial early-onset forms), allele forms of apolipoprotein E (i.e, ApoE-4 has the strongest impact), age, lifestyle, and converging evidence

which suggests that many newly identified mutations are linked to altered APP processing leading to amyloidogenic pathogenesis [6, 7].

BACE1 has been an important target for therapeutic intervention because of its indispensable role in the generation of Aβ [8–12]. However, BACE1 also functions as a housekeeping enzyme and is involved in the processing of many other proteins that are responsible for proper functioning of neuronal tissue [Fig. 1]. Hence, complete removal of BACE1 enzymatic activity could potentially cause unwanted side effects. The most relevant of these is the effect of BACE1 on synaptic functions, which are related to AD pathology. To this end, this review aims to summarize our knowledge associated with the beneficial and detrimental effects of BACE1 in synaptic functions so that we can have a clearer understanding of the synaptic regulation by BACE1. This understanding will ultimately be beneficial for finding an optimally effective strategy to provide BACE1 drugs to AD patients.

Pathophysiology of AD and synaptic deficiencies

AD, along with stroke, is the third most common disease affecting the US population, afflicting ~7% of individuals ages 65–74, 53% at ages 75–84, and 40% at ages 85 and older, respectively [13]. Worldwide, it affects nearly 44

* Correspondence: yanr@ccf.org

Department of Neurosciences, Lerner Research Institute, Cleveland Clinic, 9500 Euclid Avenue/NC30, Cleveland, OH 44195, USA

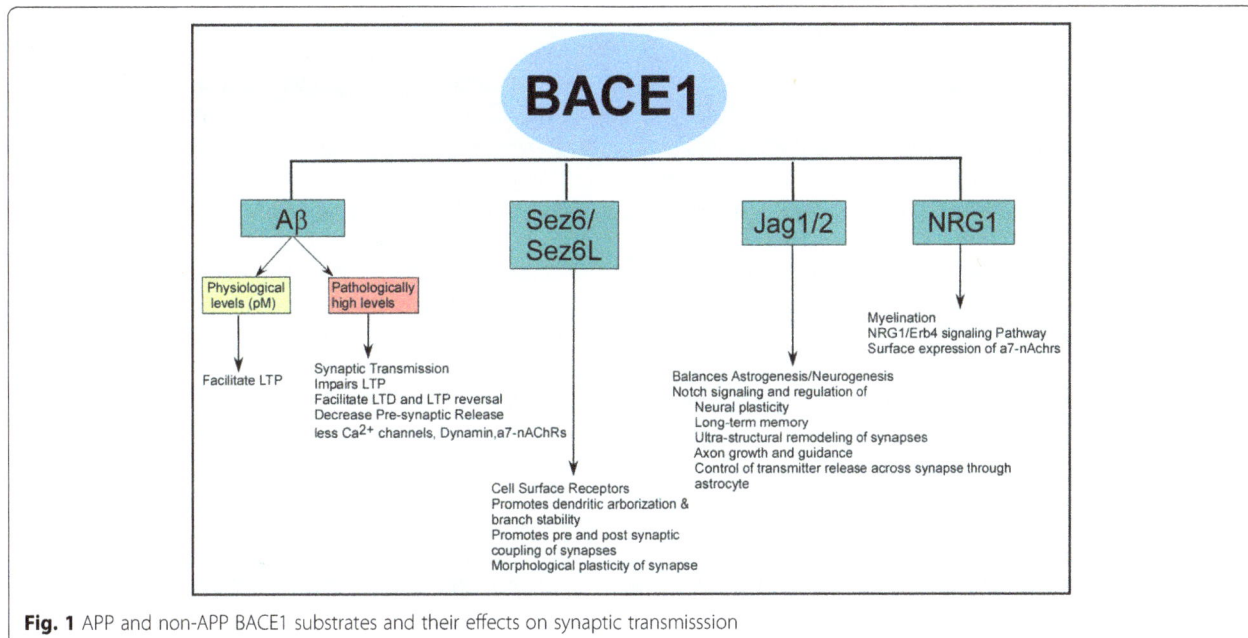

Fig. 1 APP and non-APP BACE1 substrates and their effects on synaptic transmisssion

million people and is one of major causes of age-dependent disability [14]. With no definitive cure or treatment course in sight, the global cost of Alzheimer's and dementia is estimated to be $605 billion. The pathological characteristics of AD present as cortical atrophy, neuro-inflammation, neuronal cell death, loss of synaptic connections, and the accumulation of neurofibrillary tangles and senile plaques [15].

The exact cause of AD is still unknown; however, genetic mutations in APP, presenilin 1 (PS1), or presenilin 2 (PS2) have been shown to promote the formation of amyloid plaques, which are a hallmark of AD pathology [16, 17]. The apolipoprotein E (ApoE) gene encodes three isoforms: ApoE2, ApoE3, and ApoE4. The ApoE4 isoform is identified as a genetic risk factor for late-onset AD because of its impact on the clearance of Aβ and amyloid deposition [18–21]. ApoE can also impact Aβ accumulation through its receptor, as ApoE receptor knockout mice have shown to increase Aß accumulation due to reduced clearance [22].

On the other hand, some AD risk genes are also involved in synaptic plasticity; loss of synaptic function in AD is evident long before any substantial loss of neurons [23]. PS1 is a component in the synaptic junction [24] and has been shown to regulate calcium homeostasis and the release of certain neurotransmitters [25–28]. An AD mouse model with a PS1 mutation also exhibits disruption in homeostatic scaling, a mechanism for preventing groups of neurons from altering their firing patterns too drastically in response to changes in the environment [29]. ApoE may also regulate synaptic functions through its receptor, ApoE receptor 2 (ApoER2), which is known to promote synaptic plasticity and memory formation in

mice [30]. Toxic soluble Aß can also be directly cleared from the synapse via ApoE receptors [31]. In mouse models, ApoER2 increases the number of dendritic spines and synapses and stabilizes them by regulating the assembly of a complex of proteins involved in synaptic terminals across neurons, a process which is important for learning and memory [32]. In spite of the association of these proteins with synaptic functions, the effect of these genetic mutations on AD cognitive dysfunction remains to be fully established.

Growing numbers of studies suggest that Aβ is likely to be the early effector molecule in AD cognitive dysfunction [see reviews [4, 33, 34]. Although the precise biochemical mechanisms underlying how variously assembled forms of Aβ cause synaptic dysfunction remain to be determined, biochemical and morphological studies have shown accumulation of Aβ at the synaptic terminals [35, 36]. This local accumulation is likely attributable to the fact that BACE1 initiates the generation of Aβ at the synaptic terminals [37]. Elevated levels of BCE1 have been directly correlated with Aβ-induced pathology in AD brains [38–40]. Increased amyloidogenic processing at the expense of nonamyloidogenic processing promotes Aβ accumulation at synapses in AD.

On the other hand, many scaffolding proteins like mGluR proteins, Shank, Homer, and postsynaptic density 95 (PSD95) are known to form complexes at synaptic terminals, and Aβ accumulation at synaptic terminals leads to disruption of these scaffolding protein interactions, resulting in morphological and physiological alterations such as thinning of the synaptic terminals, alteration in the molecular composition of the PSD, and disruption of synaptic signaling pathways [41–45]. Hence, abnormal accumulation of Aβ is largely considered to be toxic to synaptic functions at multiple levels.

Effects of BACE1 on synaptic functions

BACE1 is indispensable for the generation of Aβ, as germline deletion of the BACE1 gene abolishes the generation of Aβ [46–48]. BACE1 is therefore a molecule that is directly linked to synaptic functions, at least through its effects on Aβ accumulation in cells and synapses. BACE1 is predominantly expressed in brain and is richly expressed by neurons [37, 49, 50]. Accumulation of BACE1 is observed in normal and dystrophic presynaptic terminals surrounding amyloid plaques in brains of AD mouse models and patients, likely causing a vicious cycle by increasing Aβ production near synapses. Because of this, inhibition of BACE1 is logically viewed to reduce Aβ-mediated synaptic dysfunctions and to be potentially beneficial to AD patients. Hence, BACE1 inhibitors are being developed and tested for treating AD patients [51, 52].

However, whether BACE1 inhibition causes any unwanted effects on synaptic function has also attracted significant attention. This knowledge is critical for understanding the efficacy of BACE1 inhibitors in AD patients. It has been shown that BACE1 is normally expressed in broad brain regions, with rich expression by hippocampal granule cells. BACE1 has been shown to play a critical role in synaptic development and plasticity through cleavage of its various substrates [51, 53, 54]. The effects of BACE1 on synaptic functions are likely to be through multiple mechanisms, as discussed below.

1. BACE1 deficiency alters synaptic plasticity in relation to APP cleavage: Long-term changes in the strength of synaptic transmission are the basis of memory formation. Any correlated activity in the pre- and postsynaptic compartments of a synapse in a repeated pattern either strengthens synaptic connections (long term potentiation; LTP) or conversely weakens them (long term depression; LTD) [55]. High levels of Aβ disturbs the balance of reactive oxygen species (ROS) in synaptic boutons and can interfere with pre- and postsynaptic function, presumably by affecting NMDARs, presynaptic P/Q type Ca^{2+} channels, and/ or α7-nAChRs, and thus interrupting subsequent Ca^{2+} signaling and leading to altered synaptic function [56]. Mice lacking the BACE1 gene show no β-secretase activity and thus have nearly abolished Aβ (Aβ40 and Aβ42) production in the brain compared to wild-type controls. A deletion of the BACE1 gene in mouse models of AD was able to rescue hippocampal-dependent memory deficits resulting from Aβ accumulation [49] and to ameliorate impaired hippocampal cholinergic regulation of

neuronal excitability [57]. Alternatively, BACE1 cleavage of APP will also produce a 99-amino acid C-terminal fragment, referred to as βAPPc or APP-C99. This βAPPc has been shown to impair synaptic functions [58]. BACE1 deficiency benefits AD patients likely through reducing this toxic fragment. These findings implicate that BACE1 may be a good therapeutic target for treating AD [59, 60]. However, recent research progress may suggest otherwise. Since BACE1 has normal physiological functions in synaptic transmission and plasticity in CA1 region of hippocampus, BACE1-null mice displays deficits in both synaptic transmission and plasticity at the hippocampal Schaffer collateral to CA1 synapses [49, 61]. There is a significant increase in the pair pulse ratio (PPF) in BACE1-null mice when compared to wild-type [49]. Because changes in PPF ratio have been attributed to alterations in presynaptic release probability [62], the increased PPF ratio seen in BACE1-null mice may indicate a deficit in presynaptic release [49]. Consistently, BACE1-null mice display altered synaptic plasticity in CA1 and CA3 regions [49, 63]. In addition to presynaptic alterations, changes in PPF ratio can also be attributed to postsynaptic modifications, such as in the subunit composition of AMPA receptors (AMPARs) [64]. Physiological concentrations of Aβ (in pM range) have been shown to facilitate synaptic plasticity [65] and BACE1 deficiency will cause a remarkable reduction in Aβ. Such a loss of physiological levels of Aβ may also lead to synaptic deficits.

2. BACE1 deficiency alters synaptic plasticity in relation to neuregulin-1 cleavage: An alternative possibility is that the synaptic dysfunctions in BACE1-null mice may arise from abnormal processing of substrates other than APP, i.e., neuregulin-1 (Nrg1) [66–68]. Nrg1 has a plethora of functions in the central and peripheral nervous systems, which include regulation of myelination, radial and tangential neuronal migration of glutamatergic and GABAergic neurons, and synaptic plasticity [69]. To exert these functions, Nrg1 is required to be cleaved by membrane-anchored proteases, and BACE1 is one such protease. BACE1 deficiency reduces Nrg1 signaling activity and causes defects in these functions as manifested in BACE1-null mice [70, 71].
Many behaviors in animals with Nrg1 mutations exhibit a close resemblance to putative characteristics of schizophrenia, such as impaired pre-pulse inhibition, and spontaneous hyperactivity, which can be reversed by clozapine [72]. Nrg1 and its signaling receptor, the ErbB4 receptor, have been

identified as leading candidates for schizophrenia susceptibility genes [73]. It has also been shown that Nrg1-ErbB4 signaling enhances excitatory synapse formation on interneurons and inhibitory synapse formation on pyramidal neurons [74, 75]. Specifically, deletion of ErbB4 from fast-spiking interneurons, such as chandelier and basket cells, has been shown to cause relatively subtle but consistent synaptic defects [74]. Deletion of ErbB4 in interneurons increases miniature excitatory postsynaptic current (mEPSC) frequency and amplitude, but increases miniature inhibitory postsynaptic current frequency in pyramidal neurons [75, 76]. In addition, Nrg1 increases both the number and size of PSD-95 puncta, indicating that Nrg1 stimulates the formation of new synapses and strengthens existing synapses. Nrg1 could also stimulate the stability of PSD-95 in a manner that requires tyrosine kinase activity of ErbB4 [77]. Together, these results suggest that Nrg1 plays a significant role in excitatory synapse development, possibly via stabilizing PSD-95 [76]. By abolishing Nrg1 cleavage to reduce Nrg1-ErbB4 signaling in synapses, BACE1 deficiency likely contributes to synaptic dysfunctions as reported in BACE1-null mice discussed above.

3. BACE1 deficiency alters synaptic plasticity in relation to Sez6 cleavage: Another family of proteins, the seizure-related gene 6 (Sez6) and its family member Sez6L, were identified as BACE1 substrates through an unbiased proteomic approach and were recently validated as strong substrates of BACE1 [78]. Sez6 and Sez6-like (Sez6L) are nearly exclusively cleaved by BACE1 and not by other proteases in the brain and are guided by their sub-cellular location and their function. They share an NPxY motif and a phosphotyrosine-binding domain (PTB) with another BACE1 substrate, amyloid precursor protein (APP). In BACE1-null and BACE1/2-double-null mice, a marked reduction in the shedding of Sez6 and Sez6L proteins has been confirmed. Their levels in BACE1-null cerebrospinal fluid (CSF) are significantly reduced to ~10% of the wild-type condition. Although the exact molecular functions of Sez6 and Sez6L are not yet fully understood, homology in their protein-binding domains to other cell surface receptors suggests that they may act as receptors at the cell surface [79], as they were originally identified as membrane proteins with five copies of short consensus repeat with a complement C3b/C4b binding site and were seen to be elevated after bursts of neuronal activity [80]. The interaction domains suggest adhesive and/or receptor trafficking functions of these proteins; however, their binding partners are

not yet known. Sez-6 is required for normal dendritic arborization of cortical neurons, which is critical for neuronal transfer of information. Its localization along developing and mature dendritic branches and in dendritic spines modulates branch stability. In the absence of Sez-6, mice exhibit short dendrites while cultured cortical neurons display excessive neurite branching. Despite the noticeable effect on branching of dendrites, no obvious effect on an overall growth of the dendritic arbor is reported [81]. Excessive dendritic branching does not always mean a better condition for synapse formation, as studies have found that postsynaptic specializations on these branches (labeled with PSD-95) were dramatically reduced [82]. In the absence of Sez-6, spine numbers are reduced, with reduced excitatory synaptic connectivity between layers II/III and layer V pyramidal neurons in Sez-6-null mice. As spontaneous miniature EPSCs (mEPSCs) or EPSCs with minimal stimulation were not altered, the reduction might be because of uncoupling of pre- and postsynaptic ends of synapses due to altered branching patterns. There is also evidence for reduced synaptic density, punctate staining of PSD-95, and LTP in the frontal cortex of Sez6-null mice. Sez-6 proteins are therefore important for specifying proper dendritic arborization and for development of excitatory synapses on cortical neurons [81]. There is an activity-driven up-regulation of Sez-6 expression after 2 h post-high frequency stimulation [83]. Sez-6 expression levels are highly enriched in brain regions associated with ongoing morphological plasticity, such as the hippocampus and cerebellum in postnatal brain. In Sez-6 deficiency, animals exhibit poor motor coordination and balance, suppressed activity in the open field, reduced anxiety, as well as cognitive deficits. Thus Sez6 protein signaling is critical for excitatory synapse development and function [81] and synaptic circuit refinement [84]. Besides synapse formation and maintenance, Sez6 family members are also expressed and cleaved in lungs and pancreas [79, 85]. Since Sez6 and Sez6L are exclusive substrates of BACE1, they can be used as a direct readout for BACE1 activity in CSF and as a control condition where BACE1 inhibitors can be developed in a substrate-specific manner (for APP) without hampering the physiological actions of BACE1 on other essential proteins like Sez6 that are critical for proper synchronous synaptic transmission.

4. BACE1 deficiency alters synaptic plasticity in relation to jagged cleavage: Jagged-1 (Jag1) has been identified as a BACE1 substrate [86] and is known to play important roles in neural development and

synaptic functions. Jag1 regulates astrogenesis/neurogenesis via the Notch signaling pathway [87–89]. Because of abrogated Jag1 cleavage, BACE1-null mice exhibit increased astrogenesis and reduced neurogenesis due to increased Jag1-Notch interactions [87]. This is consistent with a prior report that astrocytes negatively regulate neurogenesis through the Notch pathway [90]. Although Notch and its ligands are expressed at low levels in the adult brain [91, 92], they are needed for long-term memory, which is dependent on ultra-structural remodeling of synapses. Hence Notch has an important role in the neural plasticity underlying consolidated memory. Loss of Notch function produces memory deficits in *Drosophila melanogaster* [93] and impairs proper morphology of dendritic spines [91] in the mouse hippocampus. Thus Jag, as a Notch regulator, is important for synaptic plasticity that contributes to memory formation.

On the other hand, a shift in the balance between neurogenesis and astrogenesis in BACE1-null mice likely contributes to aberrant synaptic transmission. Astrocytes regulate synaptic function and plasticity in close association with synapses [94]. They are involved in synaptogenesis as well as synapse function and elimination. This tight structural and functional partnership between the perisynaptic astrocytic process and the neuronal pre- and postsynaptic structures constitutes the "tripartite synapse" [95]. Astrocyte processes enclose synapses and define functional domains by ensheathing neuronal somas, axons, dendrites, and synapses occupying non overlapping territories, and thus establish gradually independent domains which are also developmentally regulated [96, 97]. This process of segregation, also known as astrocyte tiling, is thought to be regulated by "contact inhibition" between neighboring astrocytes and is crucial for normal functions of the nervous system because, in disease and post-injury conditions, astrocytes lose their tiling ability and display intermingled process morphology [98]. Astrocytes have also been known to regulate glutamatergic postsynaptic strength by increasing the number and stabilizing of AMPAR and NMDAR at the postsynaptic end of synapses [99]. Hence, BACE1 inhibition may impact synaptic functions due to an imbalance in total astrocytes and neurons.

Conclusion

Since BACE1 is the rate-limiting enzyme in the amyloid cascade, it is considered to be one of the promising targets for AD therapy. A rare human mutation at the BACE1 cleavage site of APP has been identified, which results in a 40% decrease in Aβ production in vitro, a reduced propensity of Aβ to aggregate, a five- to seven-fold reduced risk of developing AD, and improved cognitive function in elderly subjects without AD [100–102]. Hence, BACE1 inhibition is likely to be beneficial to AD patients. However, caution should also be taken considering the role of BACE1 in synaptic plasticity. For example, the BACE1 inhibitor verubecestat (MK-8931) showed great promise in early human and animal trials [103], but a recent announcement that Merck was stopping one of its trials suggested cause for concern. By better understanding the physiological and pathological functions of BACE1, anticipation and possible circumvention of mechanism-based side effects that may arise due to BACE1 inhibition can be accomplished. Decoding molecular mechanisms that underlie AD pathogenesis will help us to develop efficient therapeutic approaches to combat disease progression.

Acknowledgements
Due to space limitations, not all related studies regarding BACE1 substrates in synaptic functions are cited, but many of these studies were discussed in reviews cited in this article.

Funding
R Yan is supported by grants (MH103942, NS074256 and AG046929) from the National Institutes of Health.

Authors' contributions
Both BD and RY wrote this review. Both authors read and approved the final manuscript.

Competing interests
The authors declare that they have no competing interests.

References
1. Musiek ES, Holtzman DM. Three dimensions of the amyloid hypothesis: time, space and 'wingmen'. Nat Neurosci. 2015;18(6):800–6. doi:10.1038/nn.4018
2. Selkoe DJ, Hardy J. The amyloid hypothesis of Alzheimer's disease at 25 years. EMBO Mol Med. 2016;8(6):595–608. doi:10.15252/emmm.201606210
3. Malenka RC, Malinow R. Alzheimer's disease: recollection of lost memories. Nature. 2011;469(7328):44–5. doi:10.1038/469044a
4. Yan R, Fan Q, Zhou J, Vassar R. Inhibiting BACE1 to reverse synaptic dysfunctions in Alzheimer's disease. Neurosci Biobehav Rev. 2016;65:326–40. doi:10.1016/j.neubiorev.2016.03.025
5. Haass C. Take five–BACE and the gamma-secretase quartet conduct Alzheimer's amyloid beta-peptide generation. EMBO J. 2004;23(3):483–8. doi:10.1038/sj.emboj.7600061
6. Karch CM, Cruchaga C, Goate AM. Alzheimer's disease genetics: from the bench to the clinic. Neuron. 2014;83(1):11–26. doi:10.1016/j.neuron.2014.05.041
7. Tanzi RE. The genetics of Alzheimer disease. Cold Spring Harb Perspect Med. 2012;2(10) doi:10.1101/cshperspect.a006296

8. Hussain I, Powell D, Howlett DR, Tew DG, Meek TD, Chapman C, et al. Identification of a novel aspartic protease (asp 2) as beta-secretase. Mol Cell Neurosci. 1999;14(6):419–27. doi:10.1006/mcne.1999.0811

9. Lin X, Koelsch G, Wu S, Downs D, Dashti A, Tang J. Human aspartic protease memapsin 2 cleaves the beta-secretase site of beta-amyloid precursor protein. Proc Natl Acad Sci U S A. 2000;97(4):1456–60.

10. Sinha S, Anderson JP, Barbour R, Basi GS, Caccavello R, Davis D, et al. Purification and cloning of amyloid precursor protein beta-secretase from human brain. Nature. 1999;402(6761):537–40. doi:10.1038/990114

11. Vassar R, Bennett BD, Babu-Khan S, Kahn S, Mendiaz EA, Denis P, et al. Beta-secretase cleavage of Alzheimer's amyloid precursor protein by the transmembrane aspartic protease BACE. Science. 1999;286(5440):735–41.

12. Yan R, Bienkowski MJ, Shuck ME, Miao H, Tory MC, Pauley AM, et al. Membrane-anchored aspartyl protease with Alzheimer's disease beta-secretase activity. Nature. 1999;402(6761):533–7. doi:10.1038/990107

13. Hebert LE, Scherr PA, Bienias JL, Bennett DA, Evans DA. Alzheimer disease in the US population: prevalence estimates using the 2000 census. Arch Neurol. 2003;60(8):1119–22. doi:10.1001/archneur.60.8.1119

14. Alzheimer's A. 2016 Alzheimer's disease facts and figures. Alzheimers Dement. 2016;12(4):459–509

15. Holtzman DM, Morris JC, Goate AM. Alzheimer's disease: the challenge of the second century. Sci Transl Med. 2011;3(77):77sr71. doi:10.1126/scitranslmed.3002369

16. De Strooper B, Iwatsubo T, Wolfe MS. Presenilins and gamma-secretase: structure, function, and role in Alzheimer disease. Cold Spring Harb Perspect Med. 2012;2(1):a006304. doi:10.1101/cshperspect.a006304

17. Li Y, Bohm C, Dodd R, Chen F, Qamar S, Schmitt-Ulms G, et al. Structural biology of presenilin 1 complexes. Mol Neurodegener. 2014;9:59. doi:10.1186/1750-1326-9-59

18. Liu CC, Liu CC, Kanekiyo T, Xu H, Bu G. Apolipoprotein E and Alzheimer disease: risk, mechanisms and therapy. Nat Rev Neurol. 2013;9(2):106–18. doi:10.1038/nrneurol.2012.263

19. Saunders AM, Schmader K, Breitner JC, Benson MD, Brown WT, Goldfarb L, et al. Apolipoprotein E epsilon 4 allele distributions in late-onset Alzheimer's disease and in other amyloid-forming diseases. Lancet. 1993;342(8873):710–1.

20. Strittmatter WJ, Saunders AM, Schmechel D, Pericak-Vance M, Enghild J, Salvesen GS, Roses AD. Apolipoprotein E: high-avidity binding to beta-amyloid and increased frequency of type 4 allele in late-onset familial Alzheimer disease. Proc Natl Acad Sci U S A. 1993;90(5):1977–81.

21. Holtzman DM, Herz J, Bu G. Apolipoprotein E and apolipoprotein E receptors: normal biology and roles in Alzheimer disease. Cold Spring Harb Perspect Med. 2012;2(3):a006312. doi:10.1101/cshperspect.a006312

22. Shibata M, Yamada S, Kumar SR, Calero M, Bading J, Frangione B, et al. Clearance of Alzheimer's amyloid-ss(1-40) peptide from brain by LDL receptor-related protein-1 at the blood-brain barrier. J Clin Invest. 2000;106(12):1489–99. doi:10.1172/JCI10498

23. Selkoe DJ. Alzheimer's disease is a synaptic failure. Science. 2002;298(5594):789–91. doi:10.1126/science.1074069

24. Georgakopoulos A, Marambaud P, Efthimiopoulos S, Shioi J, Cui W, Li HC, et al. Presenilin-1 forms complexes with the cadherin/catenin cell-cell adhesion system and is recruited to intercellular and synaptic contacts. Mol Cell. 1999;4(6):893–902.

25. Bezprozvanny I, Hiesinger PR. The synaptic maintenance problem: membrane recycling, Ca2+ homeostasis and late onset degeneration. Mol Neurodegener. 2013;8:23. doi:10.1186/1750-1326-8-23

26. Ho A, Shen J. Presenilins in synaptic function and disease. Trends Mol Med. 2011;17(11):617–24. doi:10.1016/j.molmed.2011.06.002

27. Mattson MP. ER calcium and Alzheimer's disease: in a state of flux. Sci Signal. 2010;3(114):pe10. doi:10.1126/scisignal.3114pe10

28. Kazim SF, Iqbal K. Neurotrophic factor small-molecule mimetics mediated neuroregeneration and synaptic repair: emerging therapeutic modality for Alzheimer's disease. Mol Neurodegener. 2016;11(1):50. doi:10.1186/s13024-016-0119-y

29. Pratt KG, Zimmerman EC, Cook DG, Sullivan JM. Presenilin 1 regulates homeostatic synaptic scaling through Akt signaling. Nat Neurosci. 2011;14(9):1112–4. doi:10.1038/nn.2893

30. Wasser CR, Masiulis I, Durakoglugil MS, Lane-Donovan C, Xian X, Beffert U, et al. Differential splicing and glycosylation of Apoer2 alters synaptic plasticity and fear learning. Sci Signal. 2014;7(353):ra113. doi:10.1126/scisignal.2005438

31. Gylys KH, Fein JA, Tan AM, Cole GM. Apolipoprotein E enhances uptake of soluble but not aggregated amyloid-beta protein into synaptic terminals. J Neurochem. 2003;84(6):1442–51.

32. Dumanis SB, Cha HJ, Song JM, Trotter JH, Spitzer M, Lee JY, et al. ApoE receptor 2 regulates synapse and dendritic spine formation. PLoS One. 2011;6(2):e17203. doi:10.1371/journal.pone.0017203

33. Forner S, Baglietto-Vargas D, Martini AC, Trujillo-Estrada L, LaFerla FM. Synaptic impairment in Alzheimer's disease: a Dysregulated symphony. Trends Neurosci. 2017;40(6):347–57. doi:10.1016/j.tins.2017.04.002

34. Tu S, Okamoto S, Lipton SA, Xu H. Oligomeric Abeta-induced synaptic dysfunction in Alzheimer's disease. Mol Neurodegener. 2014;9:48. doi:10.1186/1750-1326-9-48

35. Audrain M, Fol R, Dutar P, Potier B, Billard JM, Flament J, et al. Alzheimer's disease-like APP processing in wild-type mice identifies synaptic defects as initial steps of disease progression. Mol Neurodegener. 2016;11:5. doi:10.1186/s13024-016-0070-y

36. Coleman P, Federoff H, Kurlan R. A focus on the synapse for neuroprotection in Alzheimer disease and other dementias. Neurology. 2004;63(7):1155–62.

37. Kandalepas PC, Sadleir KR, Eimer WA, Zhao J, Nicholson DA, Vassar R. The Alzheimer's beta-secretase BACE1 localizes to normal presynaptic terminals and to dystrophic presynaptic terminals surrounding amyloid plaques. Acta Neuropathol. 2013;126(3):329–52. doi:10.1007/s00401-013-1152-3

38. Fukumoto H, Cheung BS, Hyman BT, Irizarry MC. Beta-secretase protein and activity are increased in the neocortex in Alzheimer disease. Arch Neurol. 2002;59(9):1381–9.

39. Holsinger RM, McLean CA, Beyreuther K, Masters CL, Evin G. Increased expression of the amyloid precursor beta-secretase in Alzheimer's disease. Ann Neurol. 2002;51(6):783–6. doi:10.1002/ana.10208

40. Yang LB, Lindholm K, Yan R, Citron M, Xia W, Yang XL, et al. Elevated beta-secretase expression and enzymatic activity detected in sporadic Alzheimer disease. Nat Med. 2003;9(1):3–4. doi:10.1038/nm0103-3

41. Almeida CG, Tampellini D, Takahashi RH, Greengard P, Lin MT, Snyder EM, Gouras GK. Beta-amyloid accumulation in APP mutant neurons reduces PSD-95 and GluR1 in synapses. Neurobiol Dis. 2005;20(2):187–98. doi:10.1016/j.nbd.2005.02.008

42. Roselli F, Hutzler P, Wegerich Y, Livrea P, Almeida OF. Disassembly of shank and homer synaptic clusters is driven by soluble beta-amyloid(1-40) through divergent NMDAR-dependent signalling pathways. PLoS One. 2009;4(6):e6011. doi:10.1371/journal.pone.0006011

43. Roselli F, Tirard M, Lu J, Hutzler P, Lamberti P, Livrea P, et al. Soluble beta-amyloid1-40 induces NMDA-dependent degradation of postsynaptic density-95 at glutamatergic synapses. J Neurosci. 2005;25(48):11061–70. doi:10.1523/JNEUROSCI.3034-05.2005

44. Wang LW, Berry-Kravis E, Hagerman RJ. Fragile X: leading the way for targeted treatments in autism. Neurotherapeutics. 2010;7(3):264–74. doi:10.1016/j.nurt.2010.05.005

45. Golovyashkina N, Penazzi L, Ballatore C, Smith AB 3rd, Bakota L, Brandt R. Region-specific dendritic simplification induced by Abeta, mediated by tau via dysregulation of microtubule dynamics: a mechanistic distinct event from other neurodegenerative processes. Mol Neurodegener. 2015;10:60. doi:10.1186/s13024-015-0049-0

46. Cai H, Wang Y, McCarthy D, Wen H, Borchelt DR, Price DL, Wong PC. BACE1 is the major beta-secretase for generation of Abeta peptides by neurons. Nat Neurosci. 2001;4(3):233–4. doi:10.1038/85064

47. Luo Y, Bolon B, Kahn S, Bennett BD, Babu-Khan S, Denis P, et al. Mice deficient in BACE1, the Alzheimer's beta-secretase, have normal phenotype and abolished beta-amyloid generation. Nat Neurosci. 2001;4(3):231–2. doi:10.1038/85059

48. Roberds SL, Anderson J, Basi G, Bienkowski MJ, Branstetter DG, Chen KS, McConlogue L. BACE knockout mice are healthy despite lacking the primary beta-secretase activity in brain: implications for Alzheimer's disease therapeutics. Hum Mol Genet. 2001;10(12):1317–1324.

49. Laird FM, Cai H, Savonenko AV, Farah MH, He K, Melnikova T, et al. BACE1, a major determinant of selective vulnerability of the brain to amyloid-beta amyloidogenesis, is essential for cognitive, emotional, and synaptic functions. J Neurosci. 2005;25(50):11693–709. doi:10.1523/JNEUROSCI.2766-05.2005

50. Zhao J, Fu Y, Yasvoina M, Shao P, Hitt B, O'Connor T, et al. Beta-site amyloid precursor protein cleaving enzyme 1 levels become elevated in neurons around amyloid plaques: implications for Alzheimer's disease pathogenesis. J Neurosci. 2007;27(14):3639–49. doi:10.1523/JNEUROSCI.4396-06.2007

51. Vassar R, Kuhn PH, Haass C, Kennedy ME, Rajendran L, Wong PC, Lichtenthaler SF. Function, therapeutic potential and cell biology of BACE proteases: current status and future prospects. J Neurochem. 2014;130(1):4–28. doi:10.1111/jnc.12715

52. Yan R. Stepping closer to treating Alzheimer's disease patients with BACE1 inhibitor drugs. Transl Neurodegener. 2016;5:13. doi:10.1186/s40035-016-0061-5

53. Yan R. Physiological functions of the beta-site Amyloid precursor protein cleaving enzyme 1 and 2. Front Mol Neurosci. 2017;10:97. doi:10.3389/fnmol.2017.00097

54. Yan R, Vassar R. Targeting the beta secretase BACE1 for Alzheimer's disease therapy. Lancet Neurol. 2014;13(3):319–29. doi:10.1016/S1474-4422(13)70276-X

55. Morris RG. D.O. Hebb: the Organization of Behavior, Wiley: New York; 1949. Brain Res Bull. 1999;50(5–6):437.

56. Wang H, Megill A, Wong PC, Kirkwood A, Lee HK. Postsynaptic target specific synaptic dysfunctions in the CA3 area of BACE1 knockout mice. PLoS One. 2014;9(3):e92279. doi:10.1371/journal.pone.0092279

57. Ohno M, Sametsky EA, Younkin LH, Oakley H, Younkin SG, Citron M, et al. BACE1 deficiency rescues memory deficits and cholinergic dysfunction in a mouse model of Alzheimer's disease. Neuron. 2004;41(1):27–33.

58. Tamayev R, Matsuda S, Arancio O, D'Adamio L. Beta- but not gamma-secretase proteolysis of APP causes synaptic and memory deficits in a mouse model of dementia. EMBO Mol Med. 2012;4(3):171–9. doi:10.1002/emmm.201100195

59. Citron M. Strategies for disease modification in Alzheimer's disease. Nat Rev Neurosci. 2004;5(9):677–85. doi:10.1038/nrn1495

60. Vassar R. Beta-secretase (BACE) as a drug target for Alzheimer's disease. Adv Drug Deliv Rev. 2002;54(12):1589–602.

61. Dominguez D, Tournoy J, Hartmann D, Huth T, Cryns K, Deforce S, et al. Phenotypic and biochemical analyses of BACE1- and BACE2-deficient mice. J Biol Chem. 2005;280(35):30797–806. doi:10.1074/jbc.M505249200

62. Manabe T, Wyllie DJ, Perkel DJ, Nicoll RA. Modulation of synaptic transmission and long-term potentiation: effects on paired pulse facilitation and EPSC variance in the CA1 region of the hippocampus. J Neurophysiol. 1993;70(4):1451–9.

63. Wang H, Song L, Laird F, Wong PC, Lee HK. BACE1 knock-outs display deficits in activity-dependent potentiation of synaptic transmission at mossy fiber to CA3 synapses in the hippocampus. J Neurosci. 2008;28(35):8677–81. doi:10.1523/JNEUROSCI.2440-08.2008

64. Rozov A, Zilberter Y, Wollmuth LP, Burnashev N. Facilitation of currents through rat Ca2+–permeable AMPA receptor channels by activity-dependent relief from polyamine block. J Physiol. 1998;511(Pt 2):361–77.

65. Puzzo D, Privitera L, Leznik E, Fa M, Staniszewski A, Palmeri A, Arancio O. Picomolar amyloid-beta positively modulates synaptic plasticity and memory in hippocampus. J Neurosci. 2008;28(53):14537–45. doi:10.1523/JNEUROSCI.2692-08.2008

66. Hu X, Fan Q, Hou H, Yan R. Neurological dysfunctions associated with altered BACE1-dependent Neuregulin-1 signaling. J Neurochem. 2016;136(2):234–49. doi:10.1111/jnc.13395

67. Fleck D, Garratt AN, Haass C, Willem M. BACE1 dependent neuregulin processing: review. Curr Alzheimer Res. 2012;9(2):178–83.

68. Savonenko AV, Melnikova T, Laird FM, Stewart KA, Price DL, Wong PC. Alteration of BACE1-dependent NRG1/ErbB4 signaling and schizophrenia-like phenotypes in BACE1-null mice. Proc Natl Acad Sci U S A. 2008;105(14):5585–90. doi:10.1073/pnas.0710373105

69. Mei L, Nave KA. Neuregulin-ERBB signaling in the nervous system and neuropsychiatric diseases. Neuron. 2014;83(1):27–49. doi:10.1016/j.neuron.2014.06.007

70. Hu X, Hicks CW, He W, Wong P, Macklin WB, Trapp BD, Yan R. Bace1 modulates myelination in the central and peripheral nervous system. Nat Neurosci. 2006;9(12):1520–5. doi:10.1038/nn1797

71. Fleck D, van Bebber F, Colombo A, Galante C, Schwenk BM, Rabe L, et al. Dual cleavage of neuregulin 1 type III by BACE1 and ADAM17 liberates its EGF-like domain and allows paracrine signaling. J Neurosci. 2013;33(18):7856–69. doi:10.1523/JNEUROSCI.3372-12.2013

72. Stefansson H, Sigurdsson E, Steinthorsdottir V, Bjornsdottir S, Sigmundsson T, Ghosh S, et al. Neuregulin 1 and susceptibility to schizophrenia. Am J Hum Genet. 2002;71(4):877–92. doi:10.1086/342734

73. Harrison PJ, Law AJ. Neuregulin 1 and schizophrenia: genetics, gene expression, and neurobiology. Biol Psychiatry. 2006;60(2):132–40. doi:10.1016/j.biopsych.2005.11.002

74. Del Pino I, Garcia-Frigola C, Dehorter N, Brotons-Mas JR, Alvarez-Salvado E, Martinez de Lagran M, et al. Erbb4 deletion from fast-spiking interneurons causes schizophrenia-like phenotypes. Neuron. 2013;79(6):1152–68. doi:10.1016/j.neuron.2013.07.010

75. Fazzari P, Paternain AV, Valiente M, Pla R, Lujan R, Lloyd K, et al. Control of cortical GABA circuitry development by Nrg1 and ErbB4 signalling. Nature. 2010;464(7293):1376–80. doi:10.1038/nature08928

76. Ting AK, Chen Y, Wen L, Yin DM, Shen C, Tao Y, et al. Neuregulin 1 promotes excitatory synapse development and function in GABAergic interneurons. J Neurosci. 2011;31(1):15–25. doi:10.1523/JNEUROSCI.2538-10.2011

77. Munro KM, Nash A, Pigoni M, Lichtenthaler SF, Gunnersen JM. Functions of the Alzheimer's disease protease BACE1 at the synapse in the central nervous system. J Mol Neurosci. 2016;60(3):305–15. doi:10.1007/s12031-016-0800-1

78. Kuhn PH, Koroniak K, Hogl S, Colombo A, Zeitschel U, Willem M, et al. Secretome protein enrichment identifies physiological BACE1 protease substrates in neurons. EMBO J. 2012;31(14):3157–68. doi:10.1038/emboj.2012.173

79. Pigoni M, Wanngren J, Kuhn PH, Munro KM, Gunnersen JM, Takeshima H, et al. Seizure protein 6 and its homolog seizure 6-like protein are physiological substrates of BACE1 in neurons. Mol Neurodegener. 2016;11(1):67. doi:10.1186/s13024-016-0134-z

80. Shimizu-Nishikawa K, Kajiwara K, Kimura M, Katsuki M, Sugaya E. Cloning and expression of SEZ-6, a brain-specific and seizure-related cDNA. Brain Res Mol Brain Res. 1995;28(2):201–10.

81. Gunnersen JM, Kim MH, Fuller SJ, De Silva M, Britto JM, Hammond VE, et al. Sez-6 proteins affect dendritic arborization patterns and excitability of cortical pyramidal neurons. Neuron. 2007;56(4):621–39. doi:10.1016/j.neuron.2007.09.018

82. Quitsch A, Berhorster K, Liew CW, Richter D, Kreienkamp HJ. Postsynaptic shank antagonizes dendrite branching induced by the leucine-rich repeat protein Densin-180. J Neurosci. 2005;25(2):479–87. doi:10.1523/JNEUROSCI.2699-04.2005

83. Havik B, Rokke H, Dagyte G, Stavrum AK, Bramham CR, Steen VM. Synaptic activity-induced global gene expression patterns in the dentate gyrus of adult behaving rats: induction of immunity-linked genes. Neuroscience. 2007;148(4):925–36. doi:10.1016/j.neuroscience.2007.07.024

84. Miyazaki T, Hashimoto K, Uda A, Sakagami H, Nakamura Y, Saito SY, Takeshima H. Disturbance of cerebellar synaptic maturation in mutant mice lacking BSRPs, a novel brain-specific receptor-like protein family. FEBS Lett. 2006;580(17):4057–4064. doi:10.1016/j.febslet.2006.06.043.

85. Stutzer I, Selevsek N, Esterhazy D, Schmidt A, Aebersold R, & Stoffel M. Systematic proteomic analysis identifies beta-site amyloid precursor protein cleaving enzyme 2 and 1 (BACE2 and BACE1) substrates in pancreatic beta-cells. J Biol Chem. 2013;288(15):10536–10547. doi:10.1074/jbc.M112.444703.

86. He W, Hu J, Xia Y, & Yan R. Beta-site amyloid precursor protein cleaving enzyme 1 (BACE1) regulates Notch signaling by controlling the cleavage of Jagged 1 (Jag1) and Jagged 2 (Jag2) proteins. J Biol Chem. 2014;289(30):20630–20637. doi:10.1074/jbc.M114.579862.

87. Hu X, He W, Luo X, Tsubota KE, Yan R. BACE1 regulates hippocampal astrogenesis via the Jagged1-notch pathway. Cell Rep. 2013;4(1):40–9. doi:10.1016/j.celrep.2013.06.005

88. Gaiano N, Fishell G. The role of notch in promoting glial and neural stem cell fates. Annu Rev Neurosci. 2002;25:471–90. doi:10.1146/annurev.neuro.25.030702.130823

89. Morrison SJ, Perez SE, Qiao Z, Verdi JM, Hicks C, Weinmaster G, & Anderson DJ. Transient Notch activation initiates an irreversible switch from neurogenesis to gliogenesis by neural crest stem cells. Cell. 2000;101(5):499–510.

90. Wilhelmsson U, Faiz M, de Pablo Y, Sjoqvist M, Andersson D, Widestrand A, et al. Astrocytes negatively regulate neurogenesis through the Jagged1-mediated notch pathway. Stem Cells. 2012;30(10):2320–9. doi:10.1002/stem.1196

91. Alberi L, Liu S, Wang Y, Badie R, Smith-Hicks C, Wu J, et al. Activity-induced notch signaling in neurons requires arc/Arg3.1 and is essential for synaptic plasticity in hippocampal networks. Neuron. 2011;69(3):437–44. doi:10.1016/j.neuron.2011.01.004

92. Stump G, Durrer A, Klein AL, Lutolf S, Suter U, Taylor V. Notch1 and its ligands Delta-like and jagged are expressed and active in distinct cell populations in the postnatal mouse brain. Mech Dev. 2002;114(1–2):153–9.

93. Presente A, Boyles RS, Serway CN, de Belle JS, Andres AJ. Notch is required for long-term memory in drosophila. Proc Natl Acad Sci U S A. 2004;101(6):1764–8. doi:10.1073/pnas.0308259100

94. Clarke LE, Barres BA. Emerging roles of astrocytes in neural circuit development. Nat Rev Neurosci. 2013;14(5):311–21. doi:10.1038/nrn3484

95. Araque A, Parpura V, Sanzgiri RP, Haydon PG. Tripartite synapses: glia, the unacknowledged partner. Trends Neurosci. 1999;22(5):208–15.

96. Bushong EA, Martone ME, Jones YZ, Ellisman MH. Protoplasmic astrocytes in CA1 stratum radiatum occupy separate anatomical domains. J Neurosci. 2002;22(1):183–92.

97. Halassa MM, Fellin T, Takano H, Dong JH, Haydon PG. Synaptic islands defined by the territory of a single astrocyte. J Neurosci. 2007;27(24):6473–7. doi:10.1523/JNEUROSCI.1419-07.2007

98. Oberheim NA, Takano T, Han X, He W, Lin JH, Wang F, et al. Uniquely hominid features of adult human astrocytes. J Neurosci. 2009;29(10):3276–87. doi:10.1523/JNEUROSCI.4707-08.2009

99. Beattie EC, Stellwagen D, Morishita W, Bresnahan JC, Ha BK, Von Zastrow M, et al. Control of synaptic strength by glial TNFalpha. Science. 2002; 295(5563):2282–5. doi:10.1126/science.1067859

100. Benilova I, Gallardo R, Ungureanu AA, Castillo Cano V, Snellinx A, Ramakers M, et al. The Alzheimer disease protective mutation A2T modulates kinetic and thermodynamic properties of amyloid-beta (Abeta) aggregation. J Biol Chem. 2014;289(45):30977–89. doi:10.1074/jbc.M114.599027

101. Jonsson T, Atwal JK, Steinberg S, Snaedal J, Jonsson PV, Bjornsson S, et al. A mutation in APP protects against Alzheimer's disease and age-related cognitive decline. Nature. 2012;488(7409):96–9. doi:10.1038/nature11283

102. Maloney JA, Bainbridge T, Gustafson A, Zhang S, Kyauk R, Steiner P, et al. Molecular mechanisms of Alzheimer disease protection by the A673T allele of amyloid precursor protein. J Biol Chem. 2014;289(45):30990–1000. doi:10.1074/jbc.M114.589069

103. Kennedy ME, Stamford AW, Chen X, Cox K, Cumming JN, Dockendorf MF, et al. The BACE1 inhibitor verubecestat (MK-8931) reduces CNS beta-amyloid in animal models and in Alzheimer's disease patients. Sci Transl Med. 2016; 8(363):363ra150. doi:10.1126/scitranslmed.aad9704

18

Bis(9)-(−)-Meptazinol, a novel dual-binding AChE inhibitor, rescues cognitive deficits and pathological changes in APP/PS1 transgenic mice

Yuhuan Shi[1†], Wanying Huang[1†], Yu Wang[1], Rui Zhang[1], Lina Hou[1], Jianrong Xu[1], Zhuibai Qiu[2], Qiong Xie[2], Hongzhuan Chen[1], Yongfang Zhang[1*] and Hao Wang[1*]

Abstract

Background: Alzheimer's disease (AD) is a progressive and irreversible neurodegenerative brain disorder, which is the most common form of dementia. Intensive efforts have been made to find effective and safe treatment against AD. Acetylcholinesterase inhibitors (AChEIs) have been widely used for the treatment of mild to moderate AD. In this study, we investigated the effect of Bis(9)-(−)-Meptazinol (B9M), a novel potential dual-binding acetylcholinesterase (AChE) inhibitor, on learning and memory abilities, as well as the underlying mechanism in the APP/PS1 mouse model of AD.

Methods: B9M (0.1 μg/kg, 0.3 μg/kg, and 1 μg/kg) was administered by subcutaneous injection into eight-month-old APP/PS1 transgenic mice for four weeks. Morris water maze, nest-building and novel object recognition were used to examine learning and memory ability. Aβ levels and Aβ plaque were evaluated by ELISA and immunochemistry.

Results: Our results showed that chronic treatment with B9M significantly improved the cognitive function of APP/PS1 transgenic mice in the Morris water maze test, nest-building test and novel object recognition test. Moreover, B9M improved cognitive deficits in APP/PS1 mice by a mechanism that may be associated with its inhibition of the AChE activity, Aβ plaque burden, levels of Aβ and the consequent activation of astrocytes and microglia in the brain of APP/PS1 transgenic mice. Most of important, the most effective dose of B9M in the present study is 1 μg/kg, which is one thousand of the dosage of Donepezil acted as the control treatment. Furthermore, B9M reduced Aβ plaque burden better than Donepezil.

Conclusion: These results indicate that B9M appears to have potential as an effective AChE inhibitor for the treatment of AD with symptom-relieving and disease-modifying properties.

Keywords: Bis(9)-(−)-Meptazinol, AChE inhibitor, Alzheimer's disease

Background

Alzheimer's disease (AD) is a typical neurodegenerative brain disorder, which is the most common form of dementia. However, the molecular etiology of AD remains unclear [1]. The characteristic changes of AD in the brain are characterized by precipitated amyloid plaques (Aβ) [2], tau-protein aggregation [3], neuroinflammation [4], and decreased levels of acetylcholine (ACh) [5]. Multiple evidences have suggested that Aβ accumulation in the brain is the principal factor inducing other pathological features including the formation of neurofibrillary tangles (NFTs), the progressive loss or death of cholinergic neurons and the activation of immune system [6].

Acetylcholinesterase inhibitors (AChEIs), which ameliorate the cognitive and behavioral defects of the patients by enhancing central cholinergic neurotransmission,

---

* Correspondence: zhangyongfang1@yahoo.com;
angela_wanghao@hotmail.com
†Yuhuan Shi and Wanying Huang contributed equally to this work.
[1]Department of Pharmacology and Chemical Biology, Institute of Medical Sciences, Shanghai JiaoTong University School of Medicine, Shanghai 200025, People's Republic of China
Full list of author information is available at the end of the article

have been widely used for the treatment of mild to moderate AD [7]. However, high dosage of AChEIs could lead to side effects, such as gastrointestinal reactions, bradycardia and muscle spasm. And AChEIs can't directly interact with Aβ to slow down or reverse the progression of AD. Therefore, the clinical effectiveness of AChEIs has still been questioned.

Given the complex and multifactorial etiology of AD, it is generally accepted that a multi-target therapeutic approach is very necessary for AD treatment [8]. Thus, multi-target directed-ligands (MTDLs) design has been proposed to be an advanced strategy to develop novel disease-modifying drugs for AD [9, 10]. It is therefore not surprising that Aβ, other than AChE, becomes a significant therapeutic target for the design of MTDLs to ameliorate symptoms and progression of AD simultaneously [11].

In recent years, a great number of studies have shown that the peripheral anionic site (PAS) of AChE greatly accelerates Aβ deposition and promotes the assembly of Aβ into fibrils [12, 13]. Blocking PAS is efficacious for the prevention of Aβ deposition by reducing insoluble Aβ and consequently facilitating Aβ clearance. Therefore, dual-binding AChEIs, which are able to bind to both the catalytic active site (CAS) and PAS simultaneously, are of particular interest in AD therapy. According to this strategy, Bis(9)-(-)-Meptazinol (B9M) was designed and synthesized by connecting two (-)-Meptazinols with nonamethylene by our group, in an effort to identify novel drug candidate for AD. Molecular docking has revealed that B9M bound to CAS and PAS via hydrophobic interactions with Trp86 and Trp286 of AChE respectively and two "water bridges" situated at the two wings of B9M stabilized this interaction [14]. In vitro studies showed that B9M could evidently inhibit AChE activity in a reversible and selective mode and prevent AChE-induced Aβ aggregation.

However, whether B9M could rescue cognitive impairment in the animal models of AD remains unknown. APP/PS1 transgenic mice, which overexpress the Swedish mutation of human amyloid precursor protein (APP) together with human presenilin-1 (PS1) deleted in exon 9, have shown cognitive deficits, Aβ deposits and cholinergic nerve degeneration mimicking AD pathology [15]. Therefore, in the present study, eight-month-old APP/PS1 mice were utilized to assess whether B9M could alleviate the learning and memory deficits and Aβ aggregation of AD with the aim of evaluating the potential of B9M for the treatment of AD.

Methods

Chemicals

B9M was synthesized by School of Pharmacy, Fudan University (Shanghai, China). Donepezil was from Sigma

Aldrich (St Louis, MO, USA). Aβ monoclonal antibody (6E10) was purchased from Covance (Emeryville, CA, USA). Monoclonal antibody of glial fibrillary acidic protein (GFAP), an astrocyte-specific protein, was obtained from Millipore (Temecula, CA, USA). Polyclonal antibody of ionized calcium-binding adapter molecule 1 (IBA-1), a microglia-specific protein, was from Arigo biolaboratories (Taiwan, China). Amplex Red Acetylcholine/Acetylcholinesterase assay kit and $A\beta_{40}$, $A\beta_{42}$ ELISA kits were purchased from Invitrogen (Carlsbad, CA, USA). Pierce BCA protein assay kit was from Thermo Fisher Scientific (Rockford, IL, USA). All other reagents were obtained from commercial sources.

Animals and treatments

APP/PS1 transgenic mice and their wild-type littermates were obtained from the Model Animal Research Center of Nanjing University. All the mice were housed in a temperature-controlled room (22–24 °C) with a 12 h light/dark circle, and allowed free access to food and water. Animals were treated in accordance with the Guide for the Care and Use of Laboratory Animal. The experiments were carried out under the approval of the Institutional Animal Care and Use Committee of Shanghai Jiaotong University School of Medicine.

Eight-month-old APP/PS1 mice were randomly assigned into five groups ($n = 9$–11/group). Three B9M-treated groups were injected subcutaneously with B9M at the dose of 0.1, 0.3, 1 µg/kg into APP/PS1 mice for four weeks. Donepezil-treated group (1000 µg/kg) was administered by gavage. APP/PS1 and wild-type littermates mice were subcutaneously injected with equal volumes of 0.9% normal saline daily. After the treatment of four weeks, behavioral tests were carried out according to the experimental time schedule in Fig. 1.

Behavioral tests

Morris water maze test (MWM)

The test was performed in a circular water tank (120 cm in diameter) containing opaque water (22 ± 1 °C) at a depth of 25 cm and dividing into four quadrants. A hidden escape platform (9 cm in diameter) was placed in the center of one quadrant, with its surface 1 cm below the water. The mice were subjected to acquisition trial four times a day for five consecutive days. During each trial, the mice were placed in water at one of the four starting positions and the starting position was randomly selected. The latency to reach the platform was measured using a computer-controlled video tracking system (Morris water maze video analysis system, Shanghai Yishu Software Technology Co., Shanghai, China). Each mouse was allowed to swim for 60 s. Mice that failed to find the hidden platform within 60 s were placed on it for 30 s. The same platform location was used for all

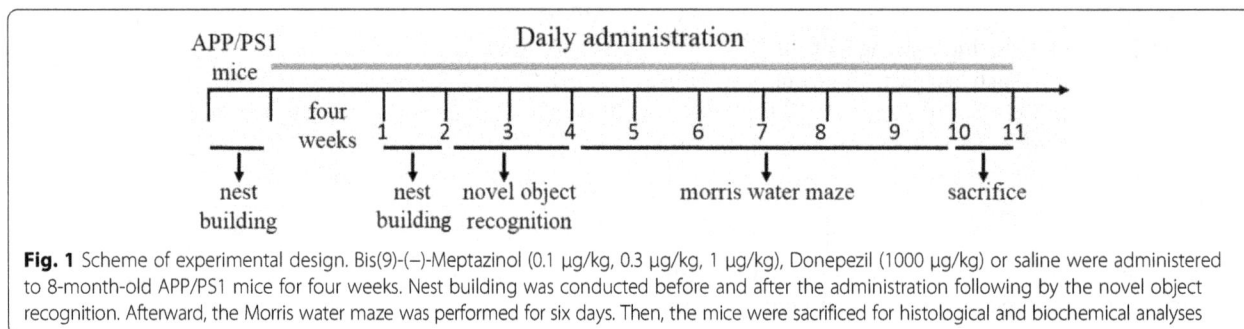

Fig. 1 Scheme of experimental design. Bis(9)-(−)-Meptazinol (0.1 µg/kg, 0.3 µg/kg, 1 µg/kg), Donepezil (1000 µg/kg) or saline were administered to 8-month-old APP/PS1 mice for four weeks. Nest building was conducted before and after the administration following by the novel object recognition. Afterward, the Morris water maze was performed for six days. Then, the mice were sacrificed for histological and biochemical analyses

mice. The platform was removed on the sixth day, and the mice were subjected to the spatial probe trial test for 60 s. The time and distance spent in the target quadrant were recorded.

Nest-building test

Mouse was placed into an individual cage for 3 days. A nestlet (5 cm × 5 cm) was placed in the middle of the cage lined with fresh bedding 1 h before the night phase, ad libitum access to food and fresh water. No further environmental enrichment items were provided. After 24 h, the nests were assessed on a 5-point scale [16, 17]: 1 = less than 10% torn up, 2 = 10–50% torn up, 3 = less than 50% intact nestlet, 4 = recognizable but flat nest, 5 = a nearly doughnut-like nest.

Novel object recognition test

The apparatus consisted of a square open field (30 cm × 30 cm × 30 cm). The objects used in the experiments were 50 ml plastic centrifuge tube (2.8 cm × 2.8 cm × 11.4 cm) and LEGO blocks (3 cm × 3 cm × 11 cm). All objects were of sufficient weight such that they could not be moved by the animals. The procedure of three 10-min trials was adopted from a previously publication with slight modification [18]. In the first trial (habituation), each mouse was placed individually into the empty chamber for 10 min. Twenty-four hours later, in the second trial (learning trial), two identical objects were placed into the open field 5 cm from the wall and let the mouse explore 10 min in the chamber. After 3 h (testing trial), one of the objects was replaced with a novel object and the mouse was put back into the chamber for 10 min. Objects and their placement in the open field were varied for each mouse to avoid positional biases. To control possible odor cues, the chamber and objects were cleaned with 75% ethanol at the end of each trial. Exploration was defined as direct contact of the nose or front paws with the object. The recognition index (RI) is defined as explorative time for the new object divided by the total explorative time for the both objects.

Brain tissue preparation

After the behavioral tests, mice were randomly selected, anesthetized with 5% chloral hydrate and perfused transcardially with 0.9% saline. The brains of the mice were rapidly removed and immediately placed in 4% paraformaldehyde for fixation, embedded in paraffin, and then cut into sections (3 µm thick), which were placed at 4 °C for immunohistochemical analysis. Cerebral cortex and hippocampus of the remaining mice were harvested and dissected on an ice plate and then immediately stored in a − 80°Crefrigerator for further biochemical measurements.

Immunohistochemistry examination

After being deparaffinized and rehydrated, the sections were treated with citric acid (pH 6.0) for 30 min followed by 20 min incubation with 0.3% peroxide. Subsequently, the sections were blocked with 10% normal horse serum and 1% BSA in TBS for 1 h, followed by incubation with primary antibodies overnight at 4 °C. The antigens of secondary antibodies were detected by standard ABC-DAB methods. Anti-6E10, anti-GFAP and anti-IBA1 antibodies were used to stain Aβ plaques, astrocytes, and microglia respectively. Then the slides were counterstained with hematoxylin and visualized using Leica Qwin software. Aβ plaques were also stained with 1% Thioflavin S (ThS) for 5 min in dark, and then washed with 70% ethanol once and distilled water twice (3 min each time). The images were captured using a fluorescence microscope and quantified with Image-Pro Plus 6.0 software.

AChE activity assay

The cortex and hippocampus were homogenized in 9-fold (w/v) of 0.9% saline. The homogenate was centrifuged at 4000 g for 10 min at 4 °C. The supernatant was gathered for protein analysis. The BCA kit was used to quantify the concentration of extracted protein. The activity of AChE in cortex and hippocampus was determined using the Amplex Red Acetylcholine/Acetylcholinesterase assay kit. All procedures complied with the manufacturer's instructions.

Determination of Aβ levels

The cortex and hippocampus were homogenized with 3-fold (w/v) of RIPA lysis buffer, containing 1% proteinase inhibitor phenylmethylsulfonyl fluoride (PMSF). After incubation for 20 min on ice, the homogenized brain tissues were centrifuged at 14000 g for 1 h at 4 °C. The supernatant (soluble fraction) of brain lysates was collected to quantify soluble $A\beta_{40}$ and $A\beta_{42}$. The acquired pellet was incubated with guanidine buffer (6.25 M guanidine-HCl, 50 mM Tris-HCl, pH 8.0) containing 1% PMSF for 2 h at room temperature, and then centrifuged at 14000 g for 1 h at 4 °C [19]. The resultant supernatant was collected to quantify insoluble $A\beta_{40}$ and $A\beta_{42}$. The concentration of soluble Aβ and insoluble Aβ was determined using $A\beta_{40}$ and $A\beta_{42}$ ELISA kits according to the manufacturer's instructions.

Statistical analysis

Data were expressed as mean ± standard error of mean (SEM). The statistics were carried out by one-way or two-way analysis of variance (ANOVA) followed by the LSD test. The difference between two groups was assessed using Student's t-tests. Statistical analysis was conducted by SPSS 13.0 software (Chicago, IL, USA) and $p < 0.05$ was considered statistically significant.

Results

Behavioral tests

B9M reversed the spatial learning and memory ability of APP/PS1 mice

To evaluate the spatial learning and memory ability of mice, Morris water maze test was performed including acquisition trial and probe trial, which primarily depends on the hippocampus. Wild type mice treated with vehicle and APP/PS1 mice treated with vehicle, B9M or Donepezil were assessed. The latency to the target platform for all groups during the 5 days of training is shown in Fig. 2a. As previously demonstrated, APP/PS1 mice exhibited a higher latency to locate the platform in the Morris water maze test than WT mice because of synaptic dysfunction and long-term potentiation (LTP) deficits in these animals [20]. Interestingly, we found that B9M administration for 4 weeks in 8 month-old APP/PS1 mice significantly reduced their latency to locate the platform, and the improvement in the spatial learning tasks occurred on fourth or fifth day (1 μg/kg on day 4: $p < 0.05$, 1 μg/kg on day 5: $p < 0.01$, vs APP/PS1 mice). On the sixth day, the platform in the pool was removed for the probe trail. As shown in Fig. 2c and d, the B9M-treated APP/PS1 mice stayed in the target quadrant for a longer time (0.3 μg/kg: $p < 0.05$, 1 μg/kg: $p < 0.01$, vs APP/PS1 mice), and swam shorter distance in the platform location (0.3 μg/kg, 1 μg/kg: $p < 0.05$, vs APP/PS1 mice). In addition, no significant difference

was detected between Donepezil-treated APP/PS1 mice (1000 μg/kg) and B9M-treated APP/PS1 mice (1 μg/kg) ($p > 0.05$), indicating that B9M possessed higher potency than Donepezil. These findings were supported by representative images of routes of travel during the probe trail (Fig. 2b), which demonstrated that the mice treated with B9M swam closer to the previous hidden platform position than the APP/PS1 mice. No differences in swimming speed were present among all groups, which indicated that the observed differences in escape latencies and swimming time or distance were not due to the differences in locomotor ability (Fig. 2e).

B9M improved hippocampal-mediated nesting behavior in APP/PS1 mice

Nesting test, quantifying the ability of the mice to build a nest from a nestlet, was used as a reliable measure of hippocampal-mediated cognitive ability [21]. As shown in Fig. 3a, a significant decrease in nesting was observed in APP/PS1 mice before treatment ($p < 0.001$ vs wild type mice). Four weeks administration of B9M significantly reversed the nesting deficiency of APP/PS1 mice (0.1 μg/kg, 0.3 μg/kg, 1 μg/kg: $p < 0.01$, vs APP/PS1 mice) (Fig. 3b). And no significant difference was observed between the treatment with B9M at the dose of 1 μg/kg and that with Donepezil at the dose of 1000 μg/kg ($p > 0.05$), suggesting that the dosage of B9M to improve cognitive deficits is much less compared with Donepezil.

B9M enhanced novel object recognition in APP/PS1 mice

The advantages of novel object recognition task are that there is no explicit need for food or water restriction and several behavioral endpoints can be rapidly obtained, including general activity, reactivity to novelty, and learning and memory [22]. As shown in Fig. 4a, after four weeks treatment of B9M, no significant differences were found in the time exploring two identical objects during the learning phase, which indicated that the mice had no preference for the position of the objects and surroundings. Three hours later, in the testing phase with two different objects (one novel, the other familiar), the recognition index (RI) had significant difference between APP/PS1 mice and wild type mice, suggesting that APP/PS1 mice failed to discriminate between novel and familiar objects (Fig. 4b). However, drug-treated groups preferred to explore the novel object. Compared with vehicle-treated APP/PS1 mice, 1 μg/kg B9M dramatically increased the RIs from 45.62 to 67.74% ($p < 0.001$), and 1000 μg/kg Donepezil increased the RIs from 47.15 to 70.46% ($p < 0.001$). These results suggest that B9M has an advantage in dosage than Donepezil enhance novel object recognition in APP/PS1 mice.

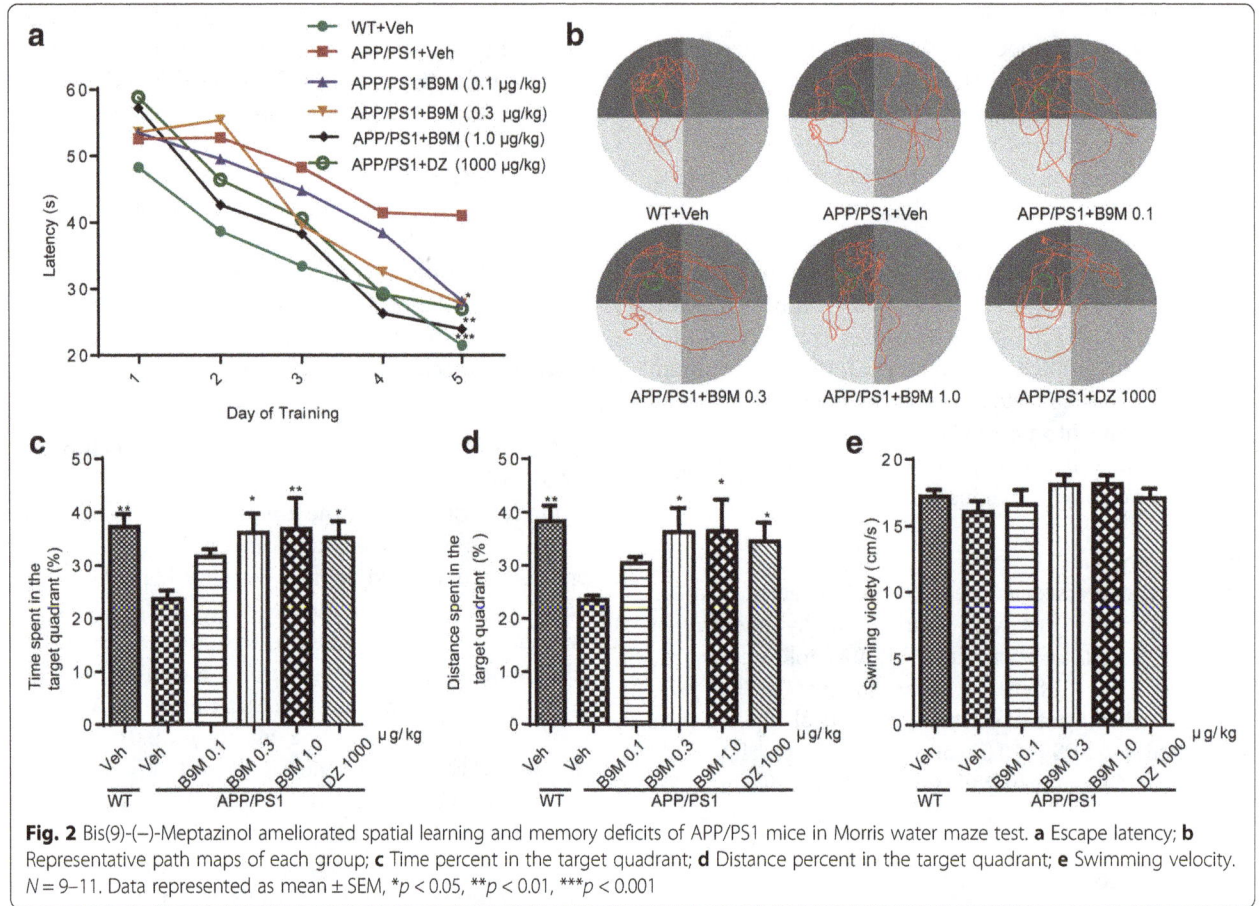

Fig. 2 Bis(9)-(−)-Meptazinol ameliorated spatial learning and memory deficits of APP/PS1 mice in Morris water maze test. **a** Escape latency; **b** Representative path maps of each group; **c** Time percent in the target quadrant; **d** Distance percent in the target quadrant; **e** Swimming velocity. $N = 9$–11. Data represented as mean ± SEM, $*p < 0.05$, $**p < 0.01$, $***p < 0.001$

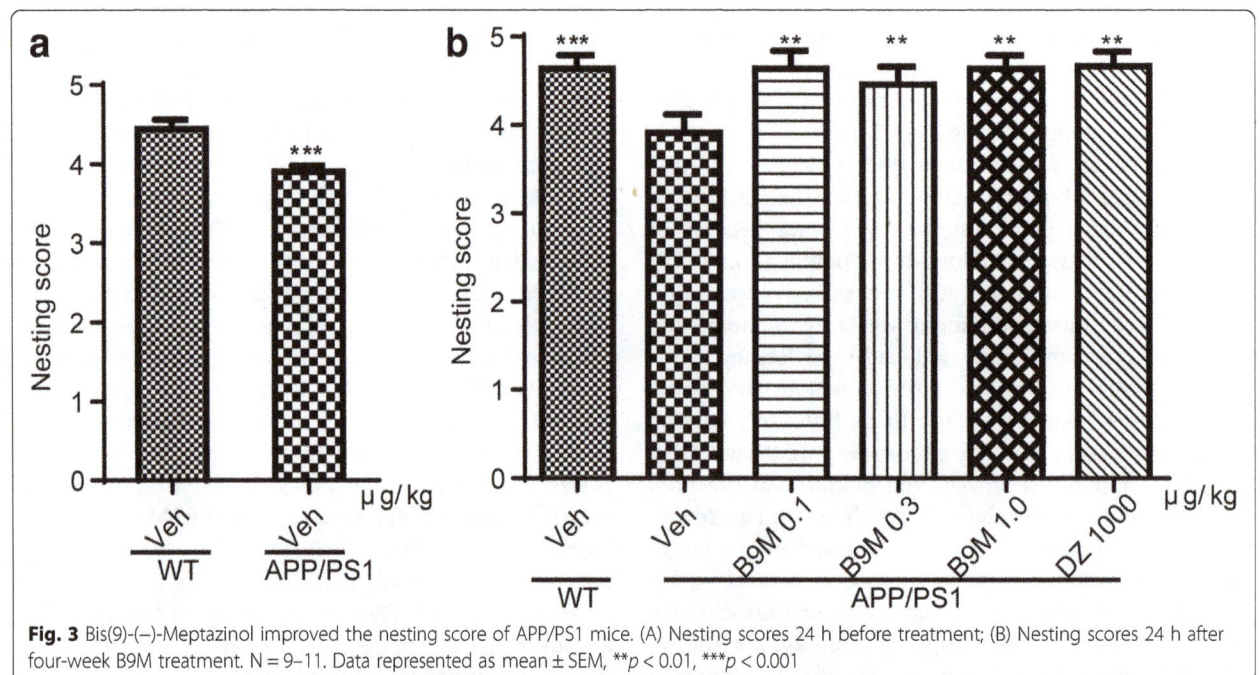

Fig. 3 Bis(9)-(−)-Meptazinol improved the nesting score of APP/PS1 mice. (A) Nesting scores 24 h before treatment; (B) Nesting scores 24 h after four-week B9M treatment. N = 9–11. Data represented as mean ± SEM, $**p < 0.01$, $***p < 0.001$

B9M inhibited AChE activity in APP/PS1 mice

It has been proved that cholinergic deficits generally lead to the memory and cognitive impairment in AD. It is generally known that AChE is the primary enzyme degrading ACh [23]. As shown in Fig. 5a and b, consistent with previous study, we found that AChE activity in the cortex and hippocampus of APP/PS1 mice was significantly elevated compared with wild type mice ($p < 0.001$ and $p < 0.01$ respectively). And compared with APP/PS1 mice, B9M administration for 4 weeks significantly reduced AChE activity in the cortex (0.1 µg/kg, 0.3 µg/kg, 1 µg/kg: $p < 0.05$, vs APP/PS1 mice) and hippocampus (0.1 µg/kg, 0.3 µg/kg: $p < 0.05$, 1 µg/kg: $p < 0.01$, vs APP/PS1 mice), which showed an obvious inhibitory effect of B9M on AChE activity. Most of all, the AChE activity in B9M-treated APP/PS1 mice at the dose of 1 µg/kg was remarkably inhibited to 77.80% in cortex ($p < 0.05$) and 60.06% in hippocampus ($p < 0.01$), similar to the inhibitory effect of Donepezil at the dose of 1000 µg/kg ($p > 0.05$), indicating that B9M could reverse the increased AChE activity in APP/PS1 mice.

B9M decreased Aβ in APP/PS1 mice

To determine whether B9M could alter Aβ levels in the brain of APP/PS1 mice, the immunohistological and biochemical assays were performed. As shown in Fig. 6a and b, the nine-month-old APP/PS1 mice displayed strong Aβ immunoreactivity, a neuropathological manifestation of AD, compared with the wild type mice. Statistic results showed that the Aβ deposition in the B9M-treated mice was significantly reduced in the cortex (1 µg/kg: $p < 0.05$, vs APP/PS1 mice) and hippocampus (1 µg/kg: $p < 0.05$, vs APP/PS1 mice) compared with APP/PS1 mice, confirming the robustness of these results (Fig. 6c and d). In the meantime, Donepezil at the dose of 1000 µg/kg also inhibited Aβ deposition in APP/PS1 mice, but there was no significant difference compared with model group. In addition, these findings were clearly supported by an obvious decrease in the levels of the thioflavin S-positive senile plaques in the group treated with B9M at the dose of 1 µg/kg, which were significantly lower than those in the vehicle-treated APP/PS1 mice ($p < 0.05$) (Fig. 6e and f).

High levels of soluble and insoluble Aβ$_{40}$ and Aβ$_{42}$ were detected in the cortex and hippocampus of APP/PS1 mice by Sandwich ELISA assays, confirming our above observation. We detected a remarkable reduction in the soluble Aβ$_{40}$ (0.3 µg/kg: $p < 0.01$, 1 µg/kg: $p < 0.05$, vs APP/PS1 mice) and insoluble Aβ$_{42}$ (0.1 µg/kg: $p < 0.05$, 1 µg/kg: $p < 0.01$, vs APP/PS1 mice) levels in the cortex of B9M-treated APP/PS1 mice (Fig. 7a and d). Simultaneously, the insoluble Aβ$_{40}$ and insoluble Aβ$_{42}$ levels of the hippocampus with the treatment of B9M were significantly decreased in a dose-dependent manner (Fig. 8b and d). Together, these data showed that Aβ burden was significantly decreased by the administration of B9M in APP/PS1 mice.

B9M reduced the activation of astrocytes and microglia in APP/PS1 mice

Astrocyte activation is characterized by the appearance of a hypertrophic soma and processes and is

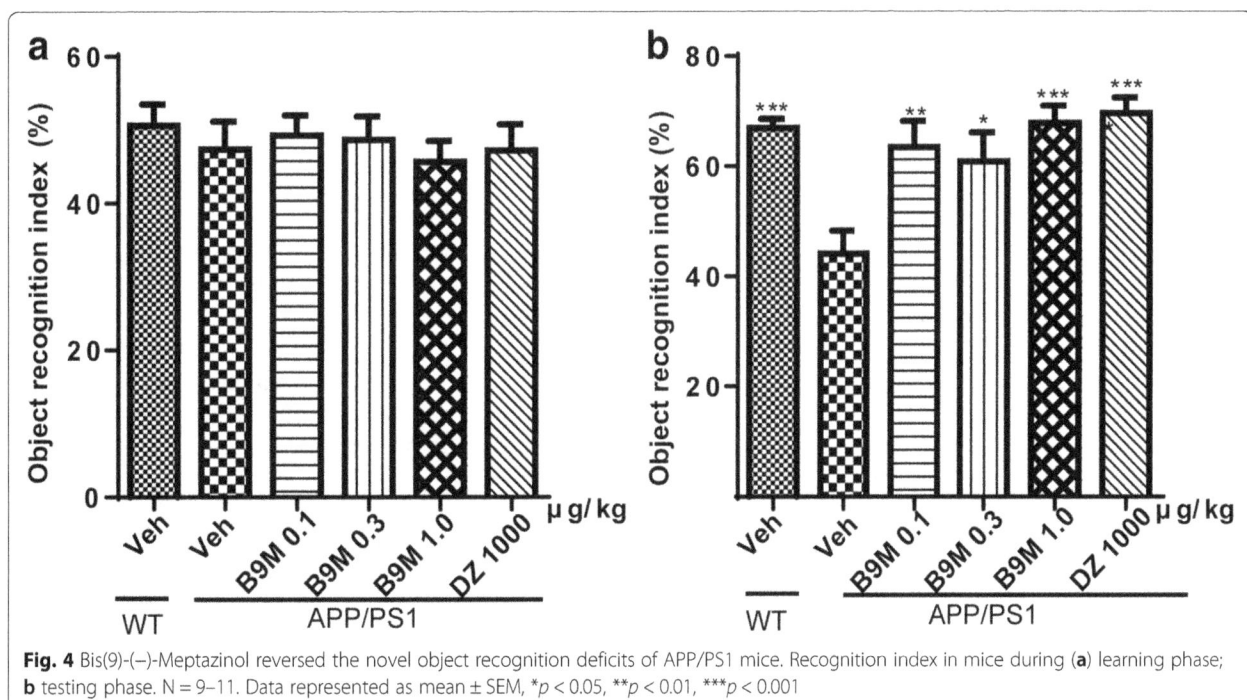

Fig. 4 Bis(9)-(−)-Meptazinol reversed the novel object recognition deficits of APP/PS1 mice. Recognition index in mice during (**a**) learning phase; **b** testing phase. N = 9–11. Data represented as mean ± SEM, *$p < 0.05$, **$p < 0.01$, ***$p < 0.001$

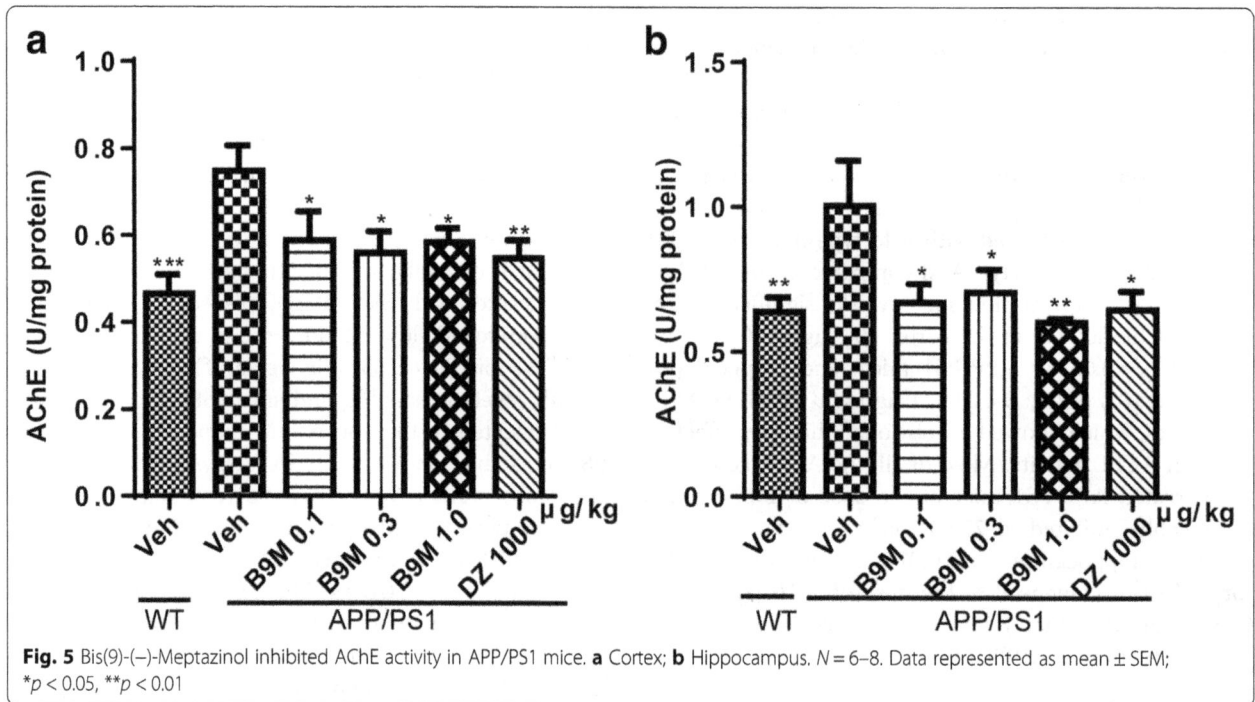

Fig. 5 Bis(9)-(–)-Meptazinol inhibited AChE activity in APP/PS1 mice. **a** Cortex; **b** Hippocampus. $N = 6$–8. Data represented as mean ± SEM; *$p < 0.05$, **$p < 0.01$

often accompanied by an increase in the expression of GFAP, a major intermediate filament protein specific to astrocytes [24]. In the meantime, microglial activation is associated with the distribution of Aβ plaques and neurofibrillary tangles, which has been related to neurodegeneration, dementia progression and AD severity [25]. To identify whether B9M has an inhibitory effect on the activation of astrocytes and microglia cells, we evaluated GFAP and IBA1 immunoreactivity respectively (Fig. 9a and b). Consistent with previous results [26], our data revealed a significant increase in GFAP staining in APP/PS1 mice in contrast to wild type mice (Fig. 9c). However, B9M treatment decreased GFAP immunoreactivity in hippocampal in a dose-dependent manner (0.3 μg/kg: $p < 0.01$, 1 μg/kg: $p < 0.01$, vs APP/PS1 mice). In addition, we found that IBA1-positive microglia cells were significantly increased in APP/PS1 mice ($p < 0.0001$ vs wild type mice), which was remarkably decreased by B9M treatment (1 μg/kg, $p < 0.05$, vs APP/PS1 mice) (Fig. 9d). These results indicated that B9M evidently inhibited the activation of astrocytes and microglia in APP/PS1 mice.

Discussion

Our study provided a property of B9M as a therapeutic compound that ameliorated the histopathological hallmarks of AD and reversed the associated cognitive and learning deficits in APP/PS1 mice. B9M treatment correlated to alleviating brain levels of Aβ as well as the soluble or insoluble Aβ40/Aβ42, inhibited the AChE activation and ameliorated astroglial and microglial

reactivity in the hippocampus. In addition, treatment of APP/PS1 mice with B9M effectively improved cognitive ability and memory dysfunction compared to treatment of these mice with vehicle. Above all, 1 μg/kg is the optimal concentration to improve the learning and memory function and reverse the process of AD. Furthermore, the capability of B9M directly decreasing Aβ aggregation is stronger than that of Donepezil at the dose of 1000 μg/kg. The results indicate that B9M possesses a promising therapeutic effect in AD by improving the symptoms as well as modifying the disease.

Our previous studies showed B9M banded simultaneously on the CAS and PAS of AChE and exhibited high potent AChE inhibitory activity ($IC_{50} = 3.9$ nM). B9M also inhibited AChE induced Aβ aggregation, indicating its potential for AD treatment [14]. Furthermore, B9M showed memory ameliorating effects at the dose of 1 μg/kg in scopolamine-induced mice model [27]. Thus, based on our previous results, three doses of B9M (0.1, 0.3, 1 μg/kg) were administered to APP/PS1 mice and three behavioral tests were conducted to evaluate learning and memory ability in the present study. Interestingly, the results of Morris water maze suggested that B9M influenced the time and distance percent in the target quadrant in a dose-dependent manner and 1 μg/kg was the optimal dose with the effect in accord with 1000 μg/kg Donepezil. Three doses of B9M showed similar cognitive improvement in novel object test and nest-building test possibly due to the different sensitivity of the behavior tests which are regulated by different regions of brain. For example, medial preoptic area and

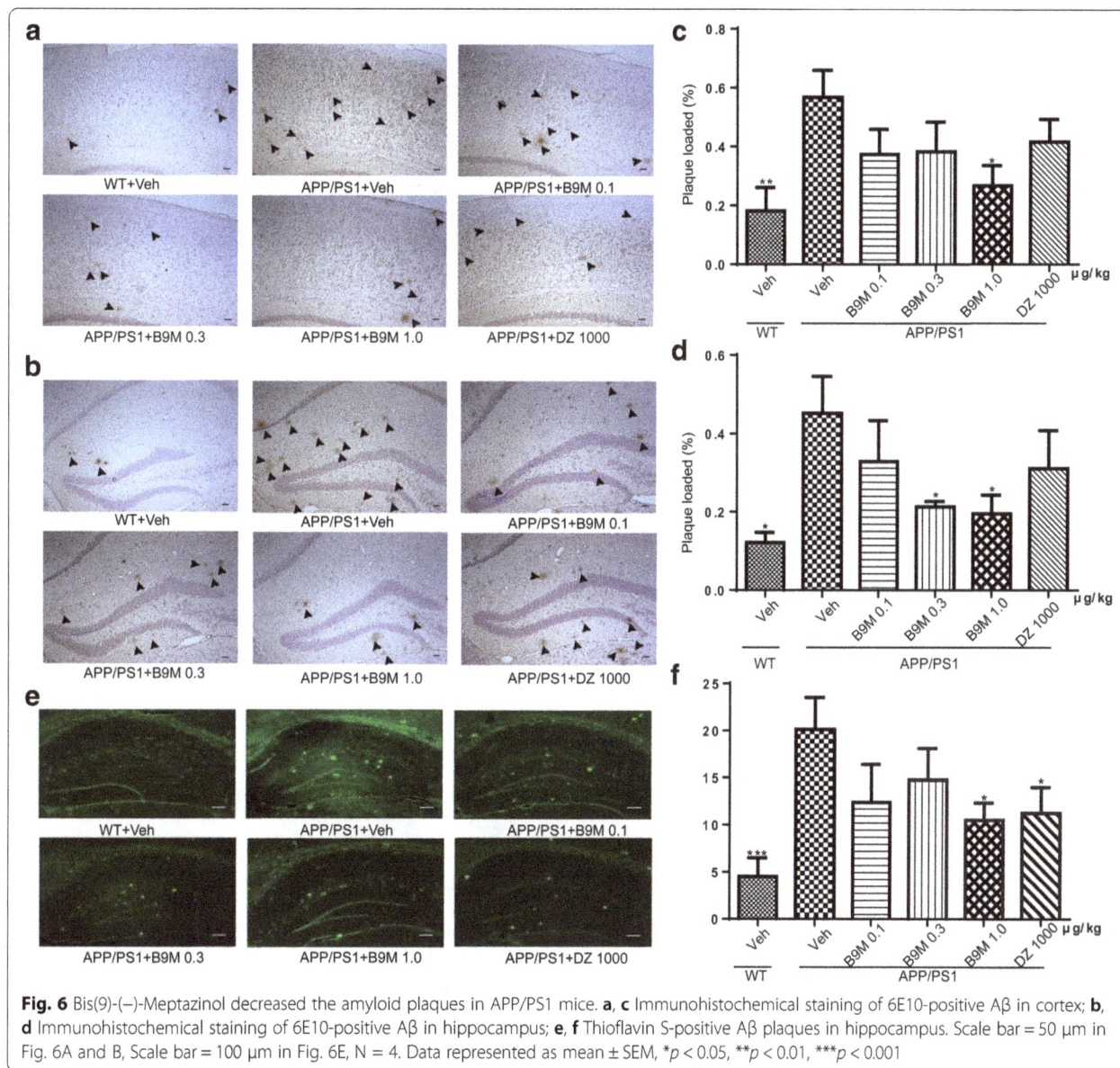

Fig. 6 Bis(9)-(−)-Meptazinol decreased the amyloid plaques in APP/PS1 mice. **a, c** Immunohistochemical staining of 6E10-positive Aβ in cortex; **b, d** Immunohistochemical staining of 6E10-positive Aβ in hippocampus; **e, f** Thioflavin S-positive Aβ plaques in hippocampus. Scale bar = 50 μm in Fig. 6A and B, Scale bar = 100 μm in Fig. 6E, N = 4. Data represented as mean ± SEM, $*p < 0.05$, $**p < 0.01$, $***p < 0.001$

hippocampus are different to the treatment of B9M [28]. Therefore, it can be inferred that 1 μg/kg B9M could strongly rescue learning and memory deficits of AD mice, comparable with the effect of control drug Donpezil at the dose of 1000 μg/kg.

Our previous studies in vitro have confirmed that B9M, acted as dual-binding AChEI, not only had a high affinity with CAS to inhibit AChE activity, but also exerted preferential affinity with PAS, which led to strong inhibitory effect on AChE and AChE-induced Aβ accumulation. Thus, we tested the AChE activity as well as the accumulation of Aβ in these transgenic mice. Our findings suggested that B9M effectively decreased the AChE activity in cortex and hippocampus of APP/PS1 mice, which is consistent with the aforementioned studies [16]. Moreover, 1 μg/kg B9M and the 1000 μg/kg

Donepezil have similar inhibitory effects on AChE activity.

Histopathological and biochemical analysis were applied to further explore the effect of B9M on plaque burdens and Aβ levels. The Aβ deposition was markedly decreased in B9M-treated group at the dose of 1 μg/kg compared with vehicle-treated transgenic mice. Meanwhile, B9M significantly reduced soluble and insoluble Aβ levels, which was confirmed by ELISA analysis. The optimum dose of B9M (1 μg/kg) was much lower than that of Donepezil (1000 μg/kg). Thus, it can be inferred that B9M directly or indirectly leads to fewer Aβ plaques via the combination with CAS and PAS of AChE.

The most commonly used anti-AD drug at present is AChEI, but it does not halt the pathological progression

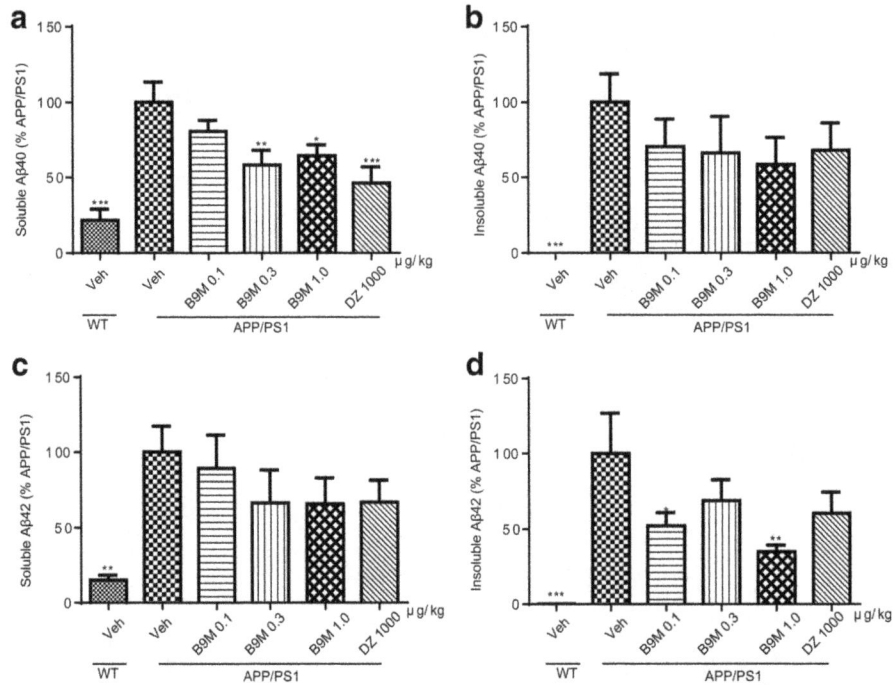

Fig. 7 Bis(9)-(−)-Meptazinol treatment reduced Aβ levels in the cortex of APP/PS1 mice. **a** Soluble Aβ$_{40}$; **b** Insoluble Aβ$_{40}$; **c** Soluble Aβ$_{42}$; **d** Insoluble Aβ$_{42}$. N = 6–8. Data represented as mean ± SEM, *$p < 0.05$, **$p < 0.01$, ***$p < 0.001$

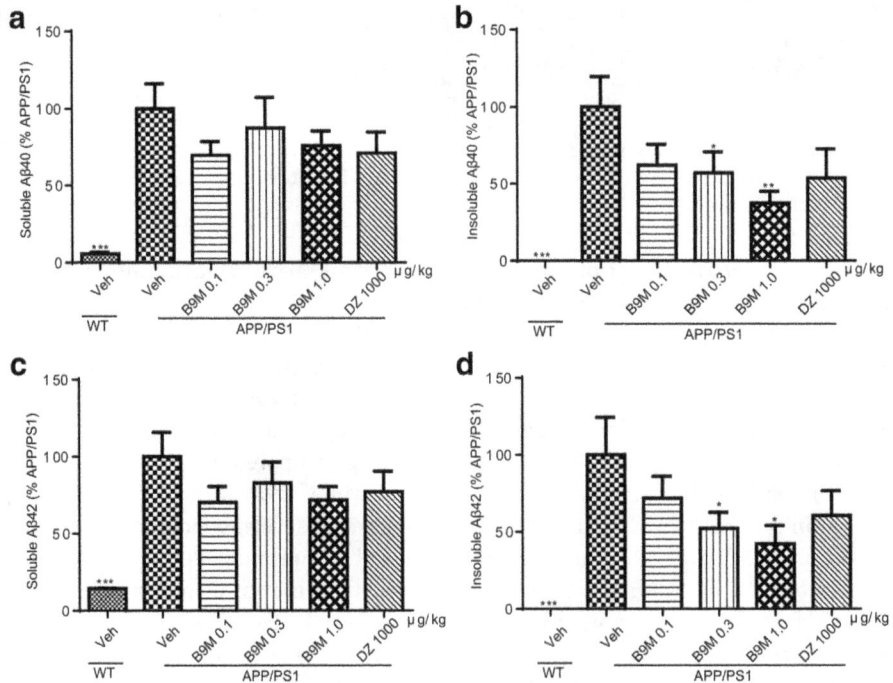

Fig. 8 Bis(9)-(−)-Meptazinol treatment reduced Aβ levels in the hippocampus of APP/PS1 mice. **a** Soluble Aβ$_{40}$; **b** Insoluble Aβ$_{40}$; **c** Soluble Aβ$_{42}$; **d** Insoluble Aβ$_{42}$. N = 6–8. Data represented as mean ± SEM, *$p < 0.05$, **$p < 0.01$, ***$p < 0.001$

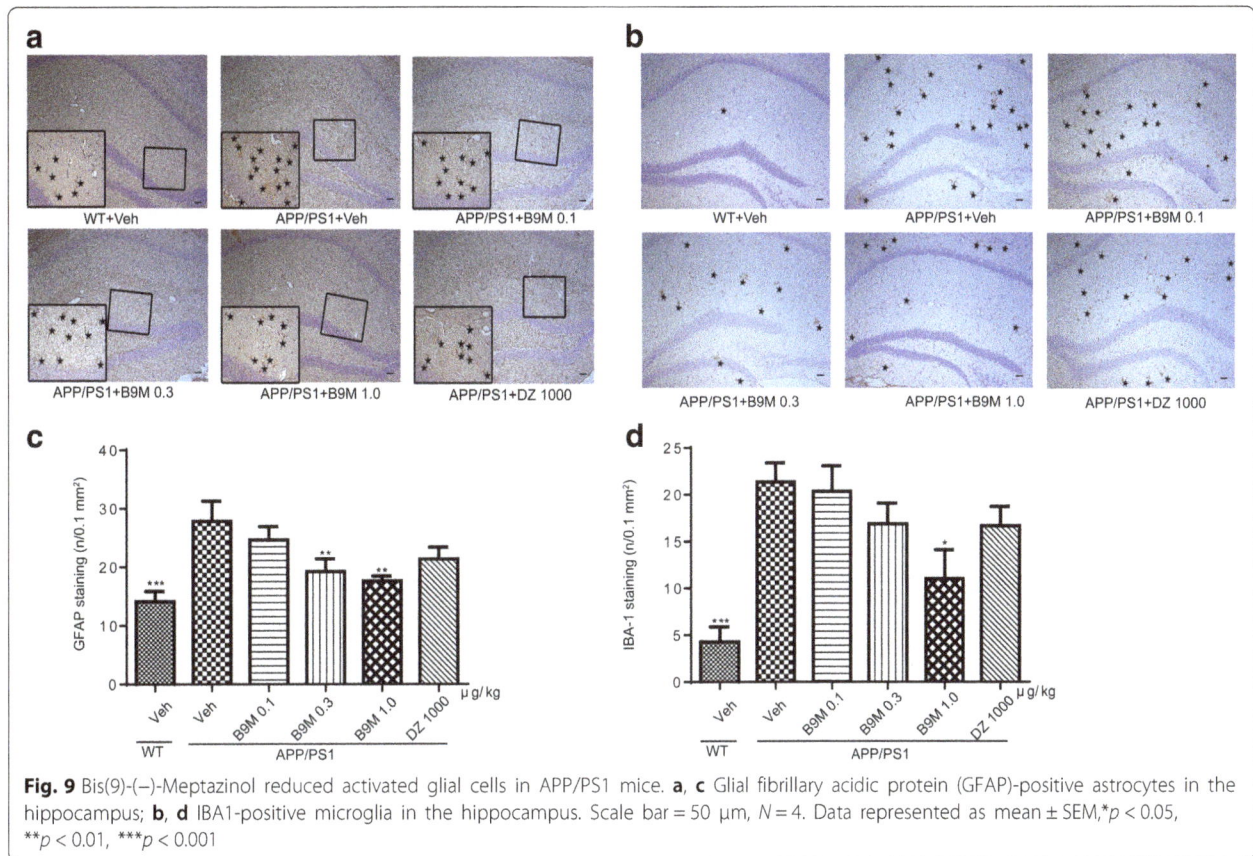

Fig. 9 Bis(9)-(−)-Meptazinol reduced activated glial cells in APP/PS1 mice. **a, c** Glial fibrillary acidic protein (GFAP)-positive astrocytes in the hippocampus; **b, d** IBA1-positive microglia in the hippocampus. Scale bar = 50 μm, N = 4. Data represented as mean ± SEM,*p < 0.05, **p < 0.01, ***p < 0.001

such as Aβ deposition during the course of the disease. Over the last two decades, the immunotherapies against Aβ were developed to treat AD. However, phase III trials of several anti-Aβ monoclonal antibodies failed to improve cognitive function in patients. Wang et al. demonstrated that the agent was not effective in removing Aβ plaques due to the saturation of antibody with soluble Aβ [29]. Our results showed that dual-binding AChEI B9M could inhibit AChE and reduce Aβ deposits, and might be better for late stage AD owning to the sustained symptomatic improvement and Aβ plaques reduction.

In addition, it has been found that the proliferation of microglia and astrocytes exists around Aβ deposition in the brain of AD model mice [24, 30] and in AD human brains [31]. Therefore, in order to clarify the effect of B9M on Aβ deposition-induced glial activation in APP/PS1 mice, we performed immunohistochemical staining of brain tissue with microglia and astrocyte-specific antibodies. Our results indicated that microglia and astrocyte activation reduced following B9M treatment at the dose of 1 μg/kg.

Conclusion

In summary, this paper offers essential preclinical evidences that dual-binding site AChE inhibitor B9M can effectively improve cognition ability and significantly reduce Aβ plaques in APP/PS1 mice. And the optimal concentration of B9M is one in a thousand of that of Donepezil acted as the control treatment. The present data, together with our previous findings, suggest that B9M is a potential novel therapeutic strategy for AD by improving symptoms and slowing disease progression.

Acknowledgements
We would like to thank all individuals participating in the study.

Funding
This work was supported by grants from the National Natural Science Foundation of China (No. 81503174, 81573415, 81573401, 81503044, 81373395) for financial support. All founding were used for the design, collection, analysis and interpretation of data and in writing in the manuscript.

Authors' contributions
SYH and HWY wrote the manuscript. WH and ZYF searched and selected the studies. SYH, WY, XJR, HLN and ZR participated in the acquisition of data and statistical analysis. QZB and XQ participated in the interpretation of data. All authors read and approved the final manuscript.

Competing interests
The authors declare that they have no competing interest.

Author details
¹Department of Pharmacology and Chemical Biology, Institute of Medical Sciences, Shanghai JiaoTong University School of Medicine, Shanghai 200025, People's Republic of China. ²Department of Medicinal Chemistry, School of Pharmacy, Fudan University, Shanghai, People's Republic of China.

References

1. Kocahan S, Dogan Z. Mechanisms of Alzheimer's disease pathogenesis and prevention: the brain, neural pathology, N-methyl-D-aspartate receptors, tau protein and other risk factors. Clin Psychopharmacol Neurosci. 2017;15(1):1–8.
2. Hunter S, Brayne C. Do anti-amyloid beta protein antibody cross reactivities confound Alzheimer disease research? J Negat Results Biomed. 2017;16(1):1.
3. Xie C, Miyasaka T. The role of the carboxyl-terminal sequence of tau and MAP2 in the pathogenesis of dementia. Front Mol Neurosci. 2016;9:158.
4. Kempuraj D, et al. Neuroinflammation Induces Neurodegeneration. J Neurol Neurosurg Spine. 2016;1(1):1003.
5. Wang CH, Wang LS, Zhu N. Cholinesterase inhibitors and non-steroidal anti-inflammatory drugs as Alzheimer's disease therapies: an updated umbrella review of systematic reviews and meta-analyses. Eur Rev Med Pharmacol Sci. 2016;20(22):4801–17.
6. Magistri M, et al. The BET-Bromodomain inhibitor JQ1 reduces inflammation and tau phosphorylation at Ser396 in the brain of the 3xTg model of Alzheimer's disease. Curr Alzheimer Res. 2016;13(9):985–95.
7. Yang RY, et al. DL0410 can reverse cognitive impairment, synaptic loss and reduce plaque load in APP/PS1 transgenic mice. Pharmacol Biochem Behav. 2015;139:15–26.
8. Nikolic K, et al. Drug design for CNS diseases: Polypharmacological profiling of compounds using Cheminformatic, 3D-QSAR and virtual screening methodologies. Front Neurosci. 2016;10:265.
9. Wang Y, Wang H, Chen HZ. AChE inhibition-based multi-target-directed ligands, a novel pharmacological approach for the symptomatic and disease-modifying therapy of Alzheimer's disease. Curr Neuropharmacol. 2016;14(4):364–75.
10. Korabecny J, et al. 7-Methoxytacrine-p-Anisidine hybrids as novel dual binding site acetylcholinesterase inhibitors for Alzheimer's disease treatment. Molecules. 2015;20(12):22084–101.
11. Hebda M, et al. Synthesis, molecular modelling and biological evaluation of novel heterodimeric, multiple ligands targeting Cholinesterases and amyloid Beta. Molecules. 2016;21(4):410.
12. Unzeta M, et al. Multi-target directed donepezil-like ligands for Alzheimer's disease. Front Neurosci. 2016;10:205.
13. Guzior N, et al. Recent development of multifunctional agents as potential drug candidates for the treatment of Alzheimer's disease. Curr Med Chem. 2015;22(3):373–404.
14. Xie Q, et al. Bis-(–)-nor-meptazinols as novel nanomolar cholinesterase inhibitors with high inhibitory potency on amyloid-beta aggregation. J Med Chem. 2008;51(7):2027–36.
15. Zhou L, et al. Dynamic alteration of neprilysin and endothelin-converting enzyme in age-dependent APPswe/PS1dE9 mouse model of Alzheimer's disease. Am J Transl Res. 2017;9(1):184–96.
16. Deacon RM. Assessing nest building in mice. Nat Protoc. 2006;1(3):1117–9.
17. Filali M, Lalonde R, Rivest S. Subchronic memantine administration on spatial learning, exploratory activity, and nest-building in an APP/PS1 mouse model of Alzheimer's disease. Neuropharmacology. 2011;60(6):930–6.
18. Gu XH, et al. The flavonoid baicalein rescues synaptic plasticity and memory deficits in a mouse model of Alzheimer's disease. Behav Brain Res. 2016;311:309–21.
19. Deng QS, et al. Disrupted-in-Schizophrenia-1 attenuates amyloid-beta generation and cognitive deficits in APP/PS1 transgenic mice by reduction of beta-site APP-cleaving enzyme 1 levels. Neuropsychopharmacology. 2016;41(2):440–53.
20. Volianskis A, et al. Episodic memory deficits are not related to altered glutamatergic synaptic transmission and plasticity in the CA1 hippocampus of the APPswe/PS1deltaE9-deleted transgenic mice model of ss-amyloidosis. Neurobiol Aging. 2010;31(7):1173–87.
21. Deacon RM, Bannerman DM, Rawlins JN. Anxiolytic effects of cytotoxic hippocampal lesions in rats. Behav Neurosci. 2002;116(3):494–7.
22. Taglialatela G, et al. Intermediate- and long-term recognition memory deficits in Tg2576 mice are reversed with acute calcineurin inhibition. Behav Brain Res. 2009;200(1):95–9.
23. Narahashi T, et al. Symposium overview: mechanism of action of nicotine on neuronal acetylcholine receptors, from molecule to behavior. Toxicol Sci. 2000;57(2):193–202.
24. Furman JL, et al. Targeting astrocytes ameliorates neurologic changes in a mouse model of Alzheimer's disease. J Neurosci. 2012;32(46):16129–40.
25. Thangavel R, et al. Expression of glia maturation factor in neuropathological lesions of Alzheimer's disease. Neuropathol Appl Neurobiol. 2012;38(6):572–81.
26. Meraz-Rios MA, et al. Inflammatory process in Alzheimer's disease. Front Integr Neurosci. 2013;7:59.
27. Liu T, et al. Bis(9)-(–)-nor-meptazinol as a novel dual-binding AChEI potently ameliorates scopolamine-induced cognitive deficits in mice. Pharmacol Biochem Behav. 2013;104:138–43.
28. Wesson DW, Wilson DA. Age and gene overexpression interact to abolish nesting behavior in Tg2576 amyloid precursor protein (APP) mice. Behav Brain Res. 2011;216(1):408–13.
29. Wang YJ, disease A. Lessons from immunotherapy for Alzheimer disease. Nat Rev Neurol. 2014;10(4):188–9.
30. Oddo S, et al. Amyloid deposition precedes tangle formation in a triple transgenic model of Alzheimer's disease. Neurobiol Aging. 2003;24(8):1063–70.
31. Venneti S, Wiley CA, Kofler J. Imaging microglial activation during neuroinflammation and Alzheimer's disease. J NeuroImmune Pharmacol. 2009;4(2):227–43.

19

Clinical features of Parkinson's disease with and without rapid eye movement sleep behavior disorder

Ye Liu[1†], Xiao-Ying Zhu[1†], Xiao-Jin Zhang[1], Sheng-Han Kuo[2], William G. Ondo[3] and Yun-Cheng Wu[1*]

Abstract

Background: Rapid eye movement sleep behavior disorder (RBD) and Parkinson's disease (PD) are two distinct clinical diseases but they share some common pathological and anatomical characteristics. This study aims to confirm the clinical features of RBD in Chinese PD patients.

Methods: One hundred fifty PD patients were enrolled from the Parkinson's disease and Movement Disorders Center in Department of Neurology, Shanghai General Hospital from January 2013 to August 2014. This study examined PD patients with or without RBD as determined by the REM Sleep Behavior Disorder Screening Questionnaire (RBDSQ), assessed motor subtype by Unified PD Rating Scale (UPDRS) III at "on" state, and compared the sub-scale scores representing tremor, rigidity, appendicular and axial. Investigators also assessed the Hamilton Anxiety Scale (HAMA), Hamilton Depression Scale (HAMD), Mini-Mental State Examination (MMSE), Clinical Dementia Rating (CDR), and Parkinson's disease Sleep Scale (PDSS).

Results: One hundred fourty one PD patients entered the final study. 30 (21.28%) PD patients had probable RBD (pRBD) diagnosed with a RBDSQ score of 6 or above. There were no significant differences for age, including age of PD onset and PD duration, gender, smoking status, alcohol or coffee use, presence of anosmia or freezing, UPDRS III, and H-Y stages between the pRBD+ and pRBD− groups. pRBD+ group had lower MMSE scores, higher PDSS scores, and pRBD+ PD patients had more prominent proportion in anxiety, depression, constipation, hallucination and a greater prevalence of orthostatic hypotension.

Conclusion: pRBD+ PD patients exhibited greater changes in non-motor symptoms. However, there was no increase in motor deficits.

Keywords: Rapid eye movement sleep behavior disorder, Parkinson's disease, Depression, Cognitive decline, Orthostatic hypotension, Motor deficits

Background

Rapid eye movement sleep (REM) is characterized by decreased or absent muscle tone (atonia), desynchronization of the electroencephalogram, with the presence of saw tooth waves, and autonomic instability. Rapid eye movement sleep behavior disorder (RBD) is a form of parasomnia during which patients develop limb or body movements, which correlate with dream enactment behavior. The abnormal physiology of RBD is loss of muscle atonia (paralysis) during otherwise intact REM sleep [1].

The standard RBD diagnostic criteria are based on the 2nd edition of the International Classification of Sleep Disorders (ICSD) [2], and polysomnology (PSG) is necessary for a definitive diagnosis. Nomura et al., determined that RBD rapid screening questionnaire (RBDSQ), which is completed by the patient, had a sensitivity of 84.2% and specificity of 96.2% to diagnose RBD when compared with standard RBD diagnostic criteria using PSG in PD at a cut off of 6 points (total score of RBDSQ is 13, and a score of 5 is the cut-off point for healthy individuals) [3]. Chahine

* Correspondence: yunchw@medmail.com.cn
Ye Liu and Xiao-Ying Zhu are co-first authors
†Equal contributors
[1]Department of Neurology, Shanghai General Hospital, Shanghai Jiao Tong University School of Medicine, No.100, Haining Road, Shanghai 200080, People's Republic of China
Full list of author information is available at the end of the article

et al. investigated the use of the RBDSQ plus Mayo Sleep questionnaire 1 (MSQ1) compared with PSG in PD patients. They found sensitivity was highest when the questionnaires were used in combination while specificity was highest for the RBDSQ used alone at a cut-off point of 7 [4]. Shen SS used the RBDSQ to diagnose RBD in Chinese patients, compared with PSG, and found a cutoff points at 6 had the best specificity and sensitivity [5].

RBD has a close relationship with neurodegenerative diseases, especially those with α-synucleinopathy pathology such as PD, dementia with Lewy bodies (DLB) and multiple system atrophy (MSA) [1, 6]. Recently, studies have indicated that PD patients with RBD might have some specific clinical features more commonly than those without RBD. Although data is mixed, PD patients with RBD have been reported to have worse decision-making [7], cognitive impairment [6], freezing, falls and rigidity [8, 9]. They also have a higher prevalence of orthostatic hypotension (OH) [8] and visual hallucinations (VH) [10]. However, there are no detailed data in PD patients with RBD in China. In this paper, we investigated the clinical features of PD patients with RBD in a tertiary referral center in China. The present study focused on the characteristics of motor and non-motor symptoms of PD with RBD compared to PD without RBD.

Methods
Patient selection
One hundred fifty PD patients were enrolled from the Parkinson's disease and Movement Disorder Center in the Department of Neurology, Shanghai General Hospital, Shanghai Jiao Tong University, Shanghai, China from January 2013 to August 2014. The diagnosis of PD was made by two movement disorder specialists according to the UK Parkinson's Disease Society (UKPDS) Brain Bank Criteria. Patients with severe dementia (CDR ≥ 2), or other central nervous system disorders were excluded from this study. The study was approved by the Institution's Ethics Committee and all recruited patients consented to participate in the study.

Patient evaluation
Of 150 patients, 5 patients were excluded because of probable DLB, 3 patients had probable MSA, and 1 patient had vascular Parkinsonism. A total of 141 patients were enrolled in the study. Patient evaluation was performed by movement disorder specialists. Parkinsonism staging was evaluated according to the Hoehn & Yahr staging scale. Part III of the Unified PD Rating Scale (UPDRS III) was performed during the "on" state. Motor subtype was analyzed by predominance of tremor or rigidity (UPDRS sub-scores) and predominance of limb or axial features (UPDRS sub-scores) [9], Hamilton Anxiety Scale (HAMA; cut-off point ≥8), Hamilton depression Scale (HAMD; cut-off point ≥8) and Mini-Mental State Examination (MMSE)

were used to evaluate the patient's mood and cognitive state. The patients whose MMSE score was lower than 17 (illiteracy) or lower than 20 (primary school level) or 24 (higher than middle school cultural level) [11] were considered to have dementia and were evaluated using the Clinical Dementia Rating (CDR). Patients whose CDR was higher than 2 were excluded from the study. Investigators used the REM Sleep Behavior Disorder Screening Questionnaire(RBDSQ)to detect clinical probable RBD (pRBD). We set the RBDSQ cut-off point at a score of 6 according to the highest sensitivity and specificity determined by a previous study [5]. The Parkinson's disease Sleep Scale (PDSS) was used to evaluate patient's sleep quality. Orthostatic hypotension (OH) was screened using a simple question:"Do you feel dizziness or weakness when you stand up?" If the answer was "yes", a blood pressure test from the supine to standing position was checked, a fall in systolic blood pressure of ≥20 mmHg, or in diastolic blood pressure of ≥10 mmHg, was diagnosed as OH. Other items including smoking, alcohol and coffee consumption, hyposmia or anosmia, constipation were also documented by question. Patients continued with their prescribed treatment regimen, they used anti-Parkinson drugs, anti-hypnotics or anti-depressants as necessary.

Statistical analysis
The data were analyzed using the Statistical Package for Social Sciences (SPSS) 19(IBM Co., USA). The data is presented as mean, counts and percentages, and the adjusted difference in means. Analysis of descriptive variables was performed using two-tailed t tests. Mann-Whitney U tests and X^2 tests were used where appropriate. A P-P plot was used to test normal distribution. A p value <0.05 was considered to be significant.

Results
Demographics
Among 141 patients, 74 were male (52.48%): 18 male (60%) in pRBD$^+$ group, and 56 male (50.45%) in pRBD$^-$ group (p = 0.655). Thirty patients (21.28%) were diagnosed with probable RBD (pRBD) based on a RBD screening questionnaire score ≥6. If the cut-off score was set at 7 or 5, the incidence of RBD was 17.02% and 26.24% respectively, with little difference in the clinical features (Table 3). The mean age in the pRBD$^+$ group was 68.33 ± 8.76 versus 69.32 ± 9.75 years in the pRBD$^-$ group (p = 0.618). Mean PD duration years is 4.13 ± 4.216 in pRBD$^+$ and 4.65 ± 3.570 in pRBD$^-$ group (p = 0.5). Smoking, alcohol and coffee consumption were infrequent in both groups (NS). There was no difference between the numbers of patients who took levodopa or dopamine agonists, and the levodopa equivalent dosage was similar in both

Table 1 Epidemiological characteristic of PD patients

	pRBD+	pRBD-	p
Patients number (n)	30	111	
Age (yr)	68.33 ± 8.76	69.32 ± 9.75	0.618
PD duration (yr)	4.13 ± 4.22	4.65 ± 3.57	0.500
Gender, male, n (%)	18 (60.00)	56 (50.45)	0.655
Smoking, n (%)	4 (13.3)	11 (9.91)	0.525
Alcohol, n (%)	0	9 (8.11)	0.204
Coffee, n (%)	1 (3.33)	5 (4.50)	1.0
Levodopa dose equivalent (mg/day)	353.53 ± 236.10	339.10 ± 272.08	0.531
Levodopa dose (mg/day)	325.00 ± 205.84	285.15 ± 250.09	0.221
Levodopa years	2.59 ± 3.08	3.03 ± 3.31	0.577
Dopa agonist dose (mg/day)	38.23 ± 51.01	33.19 ± 45.12	0.931
Dopa agonist years	0.91 ± 1.52	4.41 ± 29.21	0.479
TCA(Deanxit), n (%)	1 (0.033)	1 (0.009)	>0.90
Trihexyphenidyl, n (%)	4 (0.133)	18 (0.162)	>0.90
SSRI, n (%)	2 (0.067)	3 (0.027)	>0.75
BNZ, n (%)	6 (0.2)	3 (0.027)	<0.005

SSRI Selective Serotonin Reuptake Inhibitor
BNZ Benzodiazepines, n: number
The age, mean PD duration years, smoking, alcohol and coffee consumption rates, levodopa had no difference between two groups. However, the pRBD+ group had greater antidepressant and antihypnotic use

groups. However, the pRBD$^+$ group had greater antidepressant and anti-hypnotic use (Table 1).

Non-motor symptoms

pRBD$^+$ PD patients had significantly higher rates of anxiety (60% vs 22.52%, <0.001) and depression (63.33% vs 24.32%, $p < 0.001$) (Table 2), and a higher mean PDSS score (17.50 ± 9.60 vs 11.70 ± 8.55, p < 0.001) (Table 2). The pRBD$^+$ group had lower mean MMSE score (25.30 ± 3.91 vs. 26.75 ± 3.97, $p = 0.017$) (Table 3). When educational status was taken into account, a diagnosis of dementia was not significantly difference between two groups (16.67% vs 11.71%, $p = 0.538$) (Table 2). Constipation and OH were more prominent in the pRBD$^+$ group (Table 2).

There was no difference in the incidence of anosmia in pRBD$^+$ vs pRBD$^-$ group (46.67% vs 35.16%, $p = 0.247$) (Table 2). From PDSS item 7, we found that there were 13 patients who had visual hallucinations, 20% (6) in pRBD$^+$ group and 6.3% (7) in pRBD$^-$ group ($p = 0.032$) (Table 2).

Motor symptoms

The UPDRS III score was similar in the pRBD$^+$ and pRBD$^-$ groups (26.93 ± 14.62 vs 23.68 ± 15.93, $p = 0.174$). Mean H-Y stage was also similar between the two groups (2.40 ± 0.90 vs 2.26 ± 0.90, $p = 0.299$). When limb scores in UPDRS III was compared with axial scores, the ratio showed no difference between pRBD$^+$ and pRBD$^-$ groups (5.67 ± 4.22 vs 6.17 ± 4.61, $p = 0.734$). When rigidity scores in UPDRS III

Table 2 Clinical characteristics of PD patients

	pRBD+	pRBD-	p
Hoehn & Yahr stage	2.40 ± 0.90	2.26 ± 0.90	0.299
UPDRS III(total)	26.93 ± 14.62	23.68 ± 15.93	0.174
Bradykinesia (23–26)	8.87 ± 7.05	7.40 ± 6.11	0.292
Freezing, n (%)	8 (26.7)	25 (22.52)	0.750
LcompareA	5.67 ± 4.22	6.17 ± 4.61	0.734
RcompareT	3.01 ± 4.06	1.79 ± 2.08	0.320
PDSS	17.50 ± 9.60	11.70 ± 8.55	<0.001
MMSE	25.30 ± 3.91	26.75 ± 3.97	0.017
HAMA	7.53 ± 5.51	4.53 ± 6.38	0.002
HAMD	10.83 ± 8.60	5.39 ± 7.12	<0.001
Hallucination, n (%)	6 (20.00)	7 (6.30)	0.032
Dementia, n (%)	5(16.67)	13(11.71)	0.538
Anxiety, n (%)	18 (60.00)	25 (22.52)	<0.001
Depression, n (%)	19 (63.33)	27 (24.32)	<0.001
Hyposmia, %	46.67	35.16	0.247
Constipation, %	80.00	57.66	0.033
Orthostatic hypotension, n (%)	7 (23.33)	7 (6.30)	0.012

LcompareA (UPDRS III): UPDRS score in limb compare with axial; RcompareT (UPDRS III): UPDRS score in rigidity compare with tremor; n Number
The pRBD$^+$ PD patients had significantly higher rates of anxiety, depression and visual hallucinations rates. And they had a higher mean PDSS score. Dementia was not significantly difference between two groups. Constipation and OH were more prominent in the pRBD$^+$ group

Table 3 The clinical difference of RBD$^+$ vs RBD$^-$ patients while RBDSQ cutoff at 7, 6 and 5 in present study

	7 score	6 score	5 score
RBD incidence, n (%)	24 (17.02)	30 (21.28)	37 (26.24)
Age	–	–	–
PD duration	–	–	–
Gender	–	–	–
Dopamine use	–	–	–
Hypnosmia	–	–	–
Freezing	–	–	–
Hallucination	+	+	–
Constipation	+	+	+
HAMA	+	+	+
HAMD	+	+	+
PDSS	+	+	+
MMSE	+	+	+
Orthostatic hypotension	+	+	+
UPDRS III (total)	–	–	–
Bradykinesia (23–26)	–	–	–
LcompareA	–	–	–
RcompareT	–	–	–

If the cut off score was set at 7, 6, or 5, the clinical features had little difference. If the cut off score was set at 5 score, the hallucination rates would have no difference in two groups instead. The other features were same in the three condition

were compared with resting tremor score, the ratio was also not significantly different (3.01 ± 4.06 vs 1.79 ± 2.08, $p = 0.32$). Overall there was no difference between pRBD$^+$ group and pRBD$^-$ group for motor severity and motor subtype (Table 2). Freezing was also not different between the two groups (26.7% vs 22.52%, $p = 0.75$).

Discussion

Probable RBD is common in early PD and predicts future cognitive decline, particularly in attention and memory domains [12]. The pedunculopontine nucleus (PPN) and locus cerulean (LC)/ dorsal subcoeruleus (subCD) are compromised in both PD and RBD [13–15]. Autopsy studies show that the loss of cholinergic neurons of the PPN in PD has a significant negative correlation with the modified Hoehn and Yahr stage [16], and contribute to freezing and falls [16, 17]. Dysfunction of the PPN relates to visual hallucination (VH) [15]. A resting-state functional connectivity MRI (rs-fcMRI) study in RBD patient showed reduced connection between lateral geniculate nuclei LGN and visual association cortex [18]. PD patients with probable RBD showed smaller volumes than patients without RBD and than healthy controls in the pontomesencephalic tegmentum where cholinergic, GABAergic and glutamatergic neurons are located. It is additionally associated with

Table 4 Clinical features of PD with RBD patients

	Present study	Sixel-Doring 2014	Yoritaka 2009	Vibha 2011	Romenets 2012	Sommerauer 2014	Rolinski 2014
Patients(n)	141	158	150	134	98	59	475
RCP	6	no	b	b	no	no	5
RBD (%)	21.28	51.27	–	19.4	–	–	47.2
Male pro	–	–	+	–	+	–	+
older	–	–	+	–	+	–	–
MMSE	+	–	–	–	no	no	+
PDSS	+	no	no	+	no	no	a
Depression/anxiety	+	no	no	–	+	no	+
Dementia	–	no	–	no	ex	no	+
Hallucination	+	no	–	+	–	no	+
N-Tremor prominent	–	–	–	–	+	–	–
Axial/limb ratio	–	–	no	no	–	no	+
Constipation	+	no	+	no	–	no	+
Hyposmia	–	–	no	no	–	no	–
OH	+	no	–	no	+	no	+
PSG	N	Y	N	N	Y	Y	N

-: no difference, +: significant difference
Ex: dementia patient was excluded
Male pro Male prominent
No: no data
[a]Rolinski use Epworth Sleeping Scale instead of PDSS, difference is significant
[b]Yoritaka and Vibha use minimum clinical criteria of ICSD for RBD diagnosis instead
N No
N-tremor prominent Non-tremor prominent
OH Orthostatic hypotension
Y Yes
RCP RBDSQ cutoff points
Overall motor symptoms and signs were similar but we found significant difference between the two groups in many aspects of non-motor symptoms, including MMSE performance, visual hallucinations, depression, anxiety, orthostatic hypotension and constipation. Except for constipation, these results are consistent with most previous studies

more widespread atrophy in other subcortical and cortical regions [19]. The basal ganglia activity is changed across the sleep-wake cycle in RBD [20]. The appearance of RBD in PD may be related to regional gray matter changes in the left posterior cingulate and hippocampus but not localized to the brain stem [21].

Our study had compared motor and non-motor symptoms in PD patients with and without RBD. The results were similar if we used a RBDSQ cut off point at 6 or 7 (Table 3). Overall motor symptoms and signs were similar but we found significant difference between the two groups in many aspects of non-motor symptoms, including MMSE performance, visual hallucinations, depression, anxiety, orthostatic hypotension and constipation. Except for constipation, these results are consistent with most previous studies (detailed in Table 4) [7, 22–24]. Our findings are consistent with some studies that there are no difference between the motor symptoms [13, 23], however, some previous studies indicated that pRBD+ patients showed much more worse in the gait, balance or increased dyskinesia (Table 4) [8, 9, 22, 25].

In summary, this study systematically investigated the clinical features of PD patients with RBD. There are several potential weaknesses. We used the RBDSQ to detect RBD in PD patients which is easier and more readily available than PSG. The sample size is relatively small and it might have given false negatives and false positives for diagnosing RBD without PSG. We diagnosed the patient with anosmia and constipation only based on self-report and not using objective examination. Neurological image and electrophysiology will be valuable for further study.

Conclusions

The present study demonstrated that there were no significant differences in motor deficits in pRBD$^+$ PD patients, while the non-motor symptoms are prominent, such as mood, sleep, constipation, cognition and orthostatic hypotension. However, further studies and laboratory tests are needed to improve the understanding of RBD in PD.

Abbreviations

CDR: Clinical Dementia Rating; DLB: Dementia with Lewy bodies; HAMA: Hamilton Anxiety Scale; HAMD: Hamilton Depression Scale; ICSD: International Classification of Sleep Disorders; LC: Locus cerulean; MMSE: Mini-Mental State Examination; MSA: Multiple system atrophy; MSQ1: Mayo Sleep questionnaire 1; OH: Orthostatic hypotension; PD: Parkinson's disease; PDSS: Parkinson's disease Sleep Scale; PPN: Pedunculopontine nucleus; pRBD: Probable RBD; PSG: Polysomnology; RBD: Rapid eye movement sleep behavior disorder; RBDSQ: REM Sleep Behavior Disorder Screening Questionnaire; subCD: Dorsal subcoeruleus; VH: Visual hallucinations

Acknowledgments

This work was supported by the National Natural Science Foundation of China (NSFC) (81171205, 81371410) and the Biomedical Multidisciplinary Program of Shanghai Jiao Tong University (YG2014MS31, YG2015QN21, YG2016QN25).

Funding

National Natural Science Foundation of China, Biomedical Multidisciplinary Program of Shanghai Jiao Tong University.

Authors' contributions

YL, X-YZ and Y-CW mainly designed and drafted the manuscript. WGO and Y-CW were involved in critically revising the manuscript and provided intellectual thoughts. X-JZ attended the survey. S-HK modified the manuscript. All authors read and approved the final manuscript to be published.

Competing interests

The authors declare that they have no competing interests.

Author details

[1]Department of Neurology, Shanghai General Hospital, Shanghai Jiao Tong University School of Medicine, No.100, Haining Road, Shanghai 200080, People's Republic of China. [2]Department of Neurology, College of Physicians and Surgeons, Columbia University, New York, USA. [3]Methodist Neurological Institute, Houston, TX, USA.

References

1. Frenette E. REM sleep behavior disorder. Med Clin North Am. 2010;94:593–614.
2. Sateia MJ. International classification of sleep disorders-third edition: highlights and modifications. Chest. 2014;146:1387–94.
3. Nomura T, Inoue Y, Kagimura T, Uemura Y, Nakashima K. Utility of the REM sleep behavior disorder screening questionnaire (RBDSQ) in Parkinson's disease patients. Sleep Med. 2011;12:711–3.
4. Chahine LM, Daley J, Horn S, Colcher A, Hurtig H, Cantor C, Dahodwala N. Questionnaire-based diagnosis of REM sleep behavior disorder in Parkinson's disease. Mov Disord. 2013;28:1146–9.
5. Shen SS, Liu CF. [validation study of related questionnaires of REM sleep behavior disorder]. Graduation dissertation. China: Soochow Universtiy; 2012.
6. Vendette M, Gagnon JF, Decary A, Massicotte-Marquez J, Postuma RB, Doyon J, Panisset M, Montplaisir J. REM sleep behavior disorder predicts cognitive impairment in Parkinson disease without dementia. Neurology. 2007;69:1843–9.
7. Delazer M, Hogl B, Zamarian L, Wenter J, Ehrmann L, Gschliesser V, Brandauer E, Poewe W, Frauscher B. Decision making and executive functions in REM sleep behavior disorder. Sleep. 2012;35:667–73.
8. Romenets SR, Gagnon JF, Latreille V, Panniset M, Chouinard S, Montplaisir J, Postuma RB. Rapid eye movement sleep behavior disorder and subtypes of Parkinson's disease. Mov Disord. 2012;27:996–1003.
9. Postuma RB, Gagnon JF, Vendette M, Charland K, Montplaisir J. REM behaviour disorder in Parkinson's disease is associated with specific motor features. J Neurol Neurosurg Psychiatry. 2008;79:1117–21.
10. Wang G, Wan Y, Wang Y, Xiao Q, Liu J, Ma JF, Wang XJ, Zhou HY, Tan YY, Cheng Q, Chen SD. Visual hallucinations and associated factors in Chinese patients with Parkinson's disease: roles of RBD and visual pathway deficit. Parkinsonism Relat Disord. 2010;16:695–6.
11. Wang ZY, Zhang MY, Qiu GY, et al. Clinical application of Chinese edition of mini-mental state examination. Shanghai Arch Psychiatry. 1989;7(3):108–13.
12. Chahine LM, Xie SX, Simuni T, Tran B, Postuma R, Amara A, Oertel WH, Iranzo A, Scordia C, Fullard M, et al. Longitudinal changes in cognition in early Parkinson's disease patients with REM sleep behavior disorder. Parkinsonism Relat Disord. 2016;27:102–6.

13. Benninger DH, Michel J, Waldvogel D, Candia V, Poryazova R, van Hedel HJ, Bassetti CL. REM sleep behavior disorder is not linked to postural instability and gait dysfunction in Parkinson. Mov Disord. 2010;25:1597–604.

14. Heister DS, Hayar A, Garcia-Rill E. Cholinergic modulation of GABAergic and glutamatergic transmission in the dorsal subcoeruleus: mechanisms for REM sleep control. Sleep. 2009;32:1135–47.

15. Hepp DH, Ruiter AM, Galis Y, Voorn P, Rozemuller AJ, Berendse HW, Foncke EM, van de Berg WD. Pedunculopontine cholinergic cell loss in hallucinating Parkinson disease patients but not in dementia with Lewy bodies patients. J Neuropathol Exp Neurol. 2013;72:1162–70.

16. Rinne JO, Ma SY, Lee MS, Collan Y, Roytta M. Loss of cholinergic neurons in the pedunculopontine nucleus in Parkinson's disease is related to disability of the patients. Parkinsonism Relat Disord. 2008;14:553–7.

17. Fling BW, Cohen RG, Mancini M, Nutt JG, Fair DA, Horak FB. Asymmetric pedunculopontine network connectivity in parkinsonian patients with freezing of gait. Brain. 2013;136:2405–18.

18. Geddes MR, Tie Y, Gabrieli JD, McGinnis SM, Golby AJ, Whitfield-Gabrieli S. Altered functional connectivity in Lesional Peduncular Hallucinosis with REM sleep behavior disorder. Cortex. 2016;74:96–106.

19. Boucetta S, Salimi A, Dadar M, Jones BE, Collins DL, Dang-Vu TT. Structural brain alterations associated with rapid eye movement sleep behavior disorder in Parkinson's disease. Sci Rep. 2016;6:26782.

20. Tekriwal A, Kern DS, Tsai J, Ince NF, Wu J, Thompson JA. Abosch a.REM sleep behaviour disorder: prodromal and mechanistic insights for Parkinson's disease. J Neurol Neurosurg Psychiatry. 2017;88(5):445–51.

21. Lim JS, Shin SA, Lee JY, Nam H, Lee JY, Kim YK. Neural substrates of rapid eye movement sleep behavior disorder in Parkinson's disease. Parkinsonism Relat Disord. 2016;23:31–6.

22. Rolinski M, Szewczyk-Krolikowski K, Tomlinson PR, Nithi K, Talbot K, Ben-Shlomo Y, Hu MT. REM sleep behaviour disorder is associated with worse quality of life and other non-motor features in early Parkinson's disease. J Neurol Neurosurg Psychiatry. 2014;85:560–6.

23. Vibha D, Shukla G, Goyal V, Singh S, Srivastava AK, Behari M. RBD in Parkinson's disease: a clinical case control study from North India. Clin Neurol Neurosurg. 2011;113:472–6.

24. Lee JE, Kim KS, Shin HW, Sohn YH. Factors related to clinically probable REM sleep behavior disorder in Parkinson disease. Parkinsonism Relat Disord. 2010;16:105–8.

25. Ozekmekci S, Apaydin H, Kilic E. Clinical features of 35 patients with Parkinson's disease displaying REM behavior disorder. Clin Neurol Neurosurg. 2005;107:306–9.

20

AGE-induced neuronal cell death is enhanced in G2019S LRRK2 mutation with increased RAGE expression

Hyun Jin Cho[1], Chengsong Xie[2] and Huaibin Cai[2]* (iD)

Abstract

Background: Leucine-rich repeat kinase 2 (LRRK2) mutations represent the most common genetic cause of sporadic and familial Parkinson's disease (PD). Especially, LRRK2 G2019S missense mutation has been identified as the most prevalent genetic cause in the late-onset PD. Advanced glycation end products (AGEs) are produced in high amounts in diabetes and diverse aging-related disorders, such as cardiovascular disease, renal disease, and neurological disease. AGEs trigger intracellular signaling pathway associated with oxidative stress and inflammation as well as cell death. RAGE, receptor of AGEs, is activated by interaction with AGEs and mediates AGE-induced cytotoxicity. Whether AGE and RAGE are involved in the pathogenesis of mutant LRRK2 is unknown.

Methods: Using cell lines transfected with mutant LRRK2 as well as primary neuronal cultures derived from LRRK2 wild-type (WT) and G2019S transgenic mice, we compared the impact of AGE treatment on the survival of control and mutant cells by immunostaining. We also examined the levels of RAGE proteins in the brains of transgenic mice and PD patients by western blots.

Results: We show that LRRK2 G2019S mutant-expressing neurons were more sensitive to AGE-induced cell death compared to controls. Furthermore, we found that the levels of RAGE proteins were upregulated in LRRK2 G2019S mutant cells.

Conclusions: These data suggest that enhanced AGE-RAGE interaction contributes to LRRK2 G2019S mutation-mediated progressive neuronal loss in PD.

Keywords: Parkinson's disease, LRRK2, G2019S, AGE, RAGE, Neuronal death

Background

Parkinson's disease (PD) is the second most common neurodegenerative disease with progressive loss of pigmented dopaminergic (DA) neurons in the substantia nigra pars compacta (SNpc) [1]. Although the majority of PD cases are sporadic, genetic studies of familial PD patients have identified mutations in more than 15 genes as causal factors for PD [2, 3]. Among PD-related causal genes, leucine-rich repeat kinase 2 (LRRK2) is the most common genetic cause of sporadic and familial PD, as well as the late-onset PD [4]. Up to now, more than 100 mutations of LRRK2 have been reported to be related to

PD. Especially, the G2019S mutation has been identified as the most prevalent genetic cause of familial and sporadic PD [5]. Despite the relatively high prevalence, the penetrance of LRRK2 G2019S mutation is incomplete and age-dependent [5]. Therefore, it has been speculated that aging-related factors could also contribute to G2019S LRRK2-linked PD pathogenesis.

Advanced glycation end products (AGEs), raised from the reaction of sugars with certain amino acids or fats, are formed in high amounts in diabetes and also in the physiological organism during aging [6–9]. They have been implicated in numerous diabetes- and aging-related disorders such as cardiovascular disease, renal disease, and neurological disease by inducing oxidative stress, inflammation, and cell death [10–13]. Receptor of AGEs (RAGE), which belongs to the trans-membranous

* Correspondence: caih@mail.nih.gov
[2]Transgenics Section, Laboratory of Neurogenetics, National Institute on Aging, National Institutes of Health, Building 35, Room 1A112, MSC 3707, 35 Convent Drive, Bethesda, MD 20892–3707, USA
Full list of author information is available at the end of the article

receptor of the immunoglobulin superfamily, is activated by several ligands including amyloid beta oligomers, calcium-binding proteins (S100 Calgranulins), and high-mobility group box-1 protein (HMGB1) as well as AGEs [14, 15]. Moreover, RAGE reveals high expression levels in neurons in neurodegenerative disorders, such as PD and Alzheimer's disease (AD) [16]. In pathological environments, like PD and AD, RAGE expression is often up-regulated with increased amounts of its ligands as well. Engagement of RAGE by AGE has shown to generate reactive oxygen species (ROS) via RAGE-mediated intra-cellular signaling and to accelerate pro-inflammatory events in cells.

Based on these earlier studies, we hypothesized that AGE-RAGE interaction might contribute to progressive neuronal cell death in G2019S LRRK2 mutation-expressing cells. In this study, we used LRRK2 G2019S overexpressing mouse model for in vitro neuronal culture experiments and demonstrated that LRRK2 G2019S mutant-expressing neurons were more sensitive to AGE-induced toxicity compared to the controls. In addition, RAGE levels were upregulated in LRRK G2019S mutant cells, suggesting enhanced AGE-RAGE activation is involved in LRRK2 G2019S mutation-related progressive neuronal loss.

Methods

Cell line and mouse primary neuron culture

HEK293 cells were culture in Dulbecco's modified Eagle's medium (DMEM, Gibco) containing a high glucose concentration supplemented with 10% fetal bovine serum (FBS) and penicillin/streptomycin. For the transfection, Fugene HD (Roche) was used. Primary neurons from cortex and striatum were prepared from newborn pups (postnatal day 0) [17]. Briefly, cells were dissociated by papain (Worthington Biochemical Corp) solution and then placed in poly-D-lysine (BD Bioscience) plate in Basal Eagle Medium (Sigma-Aldrich) supplemented with 1 mM L-glutamine, B27, N2, and penicillin/streptomycin (Invitrogen). To prevent glial cell growth, arabinosylcytosine (Sigma-Aldrich) was used. The medium was changed every 2 days.

AGE preparation

To prepare AGE, BSA (50 mg/mL) was incubated with 0.5 M glucose in 0.2 M sodium phosphate buffer pH 7.4 for 10 weeks at 37 °C. The control sample of albumin was also incubated under same conditions but without glucose. All incubations were performed under sterile environments.

Cell death assays

To determine the number of viable HEK293 cells, trypan blue dye exclusion assay was performed. It is based on the principle that live cells possess intact cell membrane that excludes dye whereas dead cells do not. A 1:1 dilution of HEK293 cell suspension was mixed with 0.4% Trypan Blue solution (Bio-Rad) at room temperature for 1-2 min. Viable cells showed clear cytoplasm, whereas nonviable cells were blue. Cell mixtures were injected into the hemocytometer chamber, and counted under the microscope. To assess the survival of primary cultured neurons, we seeded the same number of neurons in each culture and randomly captured the images for about 100 MAP2-stained neurons in vehicle and AGR-treated groups. We counted the number of survived neurons based on the appearance of normal dendritic morphology, mainly the continuous and elaborated dendritic trees.

Generation of LRRK2 inducible transgenic mice

The cDNA fragments encoding full-length human G2019S LRRK2 mutant was inserted into a tetracycline operator-regulated gene expression vector, pPrP-tetP. To facilitate protein identification, C-termini of human G2019S LRRK2 protein were tagged by hemagglutinin (HA) epitope. The F1 transgenic mice were crossed with CaMKII-tTA mice to achieve high expression of LRRK2 G2019S in the forebrain [18]. The mice were fed regular diet ad libitum and housed in a 12 h light/dark cycle. All mouse work followed the guidelines approved by the Institutional Animal Care and Use Committees of the National Institute of Child Health and Human Development.

Immunofluorescence staining

For immunocytochemistry, cultured neurons were fixed with 4% paraformaldehyde (PFA) and permeabilized with 0.1% Triton X-100 in PBS. After blocking nonspecific staining using 10% goat serum (Sigma-Aldrich) for 1 h, cells were incubated with primary antibodies overnight. For immunohistochemistry, mice were perfused via cardiac infusion with 4% PFA in cold PBS. To prepare frozen sections, brain was removed and submerged in 30% sucrose for 24 h and then sectioned at 40 μm thickness using cryostat (Leica CM1950). Primary antibodies used included MAP2 (SantaCruz), GFAP (Sigma-Aldrich), and NeuN (Millipore). To detect RAGE protein, primary antibodies from SantaCruz and R&D were used. Anti-LRRK2 polyclonal antibodies (4EC9E and 4C84E) were kindly provided from Dr. Jean-Marc Taymans. Alexa 488 or 568-conjugated secondary antibody was incubated to visualize the staining. Fluorescent images were captured by a Zeiss confocal microscope (LSM 510 META).

Preparation of protein extracts and western blot

Mouse brain tissue was homogenized with 10 volumes of sucrose buffer (0.32 M sucrose, 1 mM $MgCl_2$, 1 mM $NaHCO_3$, and 0.5 mM $CaCl_2$) containing protease and phosphatase inhibitor cocktail (Roche). To obtain crude membrane fraction, homogenized brain samples were centrifuged at 1000 × g for 10 min to remove nuclear fraction and then supernatants were centrifuged at 20,000 × g for 20 min. The pellet fraction was dissolved in RIPA buffer by sonication and concentrations were measured by BCA assay. Proteins were analyzed by 4-12% NuPage BisTris-polyacrylamide gel electrophoresis (Invitrogen) in MOPS running buffer (Invitrogene) and transferred to polyvinylidene difluoride (PVDF) membranes. The signals were visualized by enhanced chemiluminescence development (Pierce) and quantified using Scion Image System (Frederick, MD).

Human brain tissues

Striatal tissues were obtained from the brain bank of Johns Hopkins University School of Medicine. Subjects or their legal representatives signed informed consents approved by the Johns Hopkins Institutional Review Boards. The diagnosis of PD was made based on the clinicopathological criteria including characteristic clinical features and on the presence of Lewy bodies within the pigmented neurons lost in the substantia nigra. The average age at death for the PD subjects included in this study was $80 + 6.9$ years old, while for the NPC subjects it was $85 + 6.6$ years old.

Statistical analysis

Statistical analysis was performed with GraphPad Prism 5 (GraphPad Software). Statistical significances were obtained by comparing means of different case using t test or ANOVA followed by Tukey's honestly significant difference test. Error bars indicate SD. $^{*}P < 0.05$; $^{**}P < 0.01$; $^{***}P < 0.001$.

Results

Characterization of AGE in cultured primary neurons

To test the toxic effects of AGEs generated for the cell viability assay, we first treated HEK293 cells with increasing dose of AGEs (Fig 1a). After treated with AGEs for 24 h, more HEK293 cells were lost at higher AGE dosages, whereas cells incubated with BSA showed no obvious cell death (Fig. 1a). Since LRRK2 is more abundant in the striatum [19], we cultured neurons from striatum of postnatal day 0 (P0) pups for AGE treatment. After 15 days in vitro culture (15 DIV), the cultured striatal neurons were incubated with AGEs at the concentrations of 0.0125, 0.025, 0.05, 0.1, and 0.2 µg/µl for 24 h and the cells were immuno-stained with anti-MAP2 and anti-GFAP antibodies to count the surviving neurons and astrocytes, respectively (Fig 1b). Cultured striatal neurons showed a number of neurites and healthy morphologies at the 0.0125 to 0.05 µg/µl AGE treatment. At the 0.1 µg/µl AGE-treated cases, we observed

fragmented neurites but not neuronal loss. By contrast, almost all MAP2-positive neurons were dead after incubated with 0.2 and 0.4 µg/µl AGE for 24 h. On the other hand, GFAP-positive astrocytes were less sensitive to AGEs on the same condition. Based on these findings, in the later experiments, we treated cultured striatal neurons with AGE at the concentrations of 0.1~0.15 µg/µl for 24 h.

LRRK2 G2019S-expressing neurons are more sensitive against AGE

Next, we cultured the striatal neurons (DIV 15) from the striatum of P0 G2019S LRRK2 transgenic (Tg) and wild-type (WT) LRRK2 Tg pups to investigate whether these neurons exhibit different vulnerability to AGEs at 0.1 and 0.15 µg/µl after 24 h treatment (Fig. 2a). We found more than 60% loss of G2019S LRRK2-expressing neurons compared to the WT LRRK2 cultures after treated with 0.1 µg/µl AGEs for 24 h (Fig. 2a, b). The surviving G2019S LRRK2-expressing neurons exhibited severe neurite fragmentation and condensed cell body, while control neurons showed only slight neurite fragmentation (Fig. 2a). After treated with AGEs at 0.15 µg/µl for 24 h, more severe loss of G2019S LRRK2-expressing neurons as well as WT neurons was observed (Fig. 2a, b). These data indicate that G2019S LRRK2-expressing neurons are much more sensitive to AGE –induced toxicity compared to neurons expressing WT LRRK2.

AGE-induced neuronal cell death is mediated by RAGE

We then investigated whether AGE-induced neuronal cell death in LRRK2 G2019S neurons is mediated by any specific intracellular signaling pathways. Receptor of AGE (RAGE) is reported to be expressed in aged brains. Therefore, we hypothesized that neuronal cell death triggered by AGE is mediated by RAGE. To test the role of RAGE, we neutralized RAGE function using anti-RAGE antiserum in LRRK2 G2019S neurons (Fig. 3a). As a result, severe cell death induced by 0.1 µg/µl AGE treatment was remarkably mitigated by pre-incubation of anti-RAGE antiserum (Fig. 3a, b). This event indicates that RAGE-related pathway participates AGE-induced neuronal cell death in LRRK2 G2019S mutation.

Upregulation of RAGE protein levels in G2019S LRRK2 samples

To test whether RAGE protein levels are regulated by G2019S LRRK2 expression, HEK293 cells were transfected with doxycycline (DOX)-activated G2019S LRRK2 expression constructs (Fig. 4a). We found enhanced RAGE protein levels in cells treated by DOX (Fig. 4a, b). Also, we observed increased levels of RAGE proteins in the G2019S LRRK2 expressing striatal neuron cultures compared to control neurons (Fig. 4c, d). Next, the

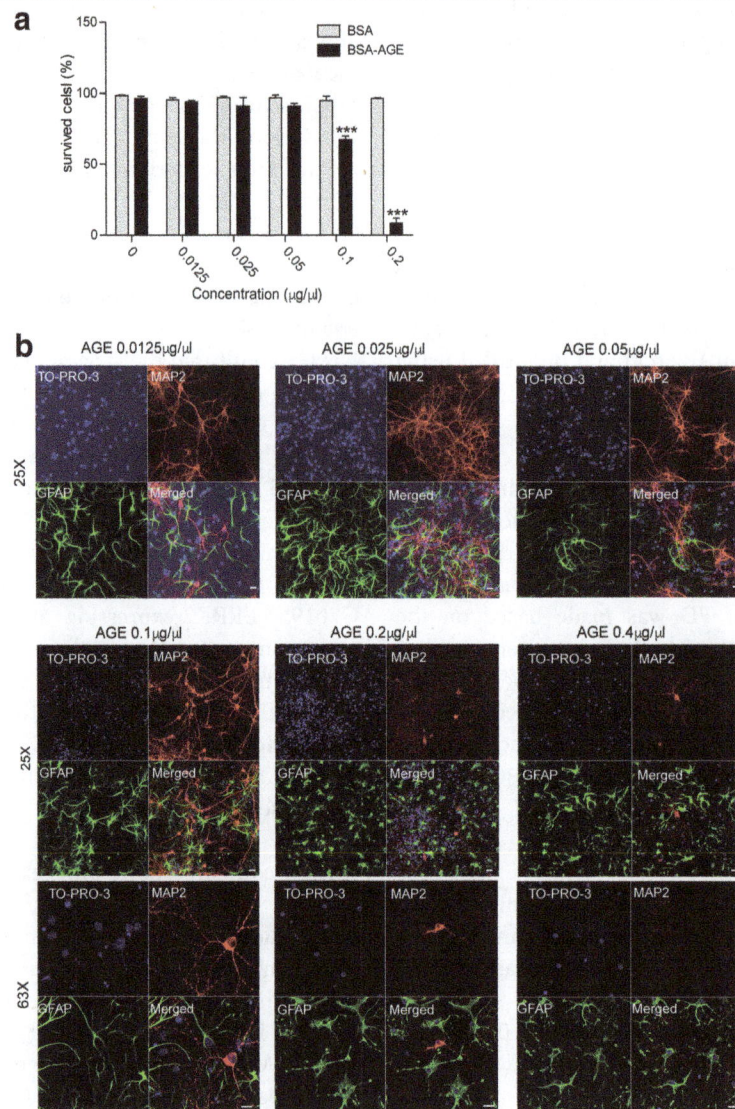

Fig. 1 Characterization of prepared AGEs. **a**. HEK293 cells were incubated with BSA or BSA-AGE in a dose-dependent manner (0, 0.125, 0.25, 0.5, 1, 2 µg/µl). After 24 h, cells were detached from the plates using trypsin. Harvested cells were counted by trypan blue staining. Survived cells were presented in the bar graph. Data are presented as mean ± SD for three independent experiments. ***P < 0.001. **b**. Representative images show AGE-treated neurons. Neurons were incubated with AGE in a dose-dependent manner (0, 0.125, 0.25, 0.5, 1, 2 µg/µl). After 24 h, primary striatal neurons (15 DIV) were immunostained with MAP2 (red) and GFAP (green) antibodies. Scale bar, 20 µm

striatal tissues from 3-month-old G2019S LRRK2 transgenic and littermate non-transgenic (nTG) mice were dissected and total proteins were extracted for analyses of RAGE expression. Since RAGE is a type I transmembrane protein, crude membrane proteins were also prepared to examine the RAGE protein levels. Significantly increased RAGE levels were presented in both total lysates and crude membrane extracts of the brains from G2019S LRRK2 mutant mice (Fig. 4e-g). Furthermore, immuno-staining with anti-RAGE antibody also confirmed the increase of RAGE levels in the cultured striatal neurons from G2019S LRRK2 P0 pups compared to the WT LRRK2 (Fig. 4h, i). These results provide strong evidence of upregulated RAGE protein expression in the G2019S LRRK2-expressing mouse brains.

Increased level of RAGE protein in the brains of PD patients

Finally, we examined the levels of RAGE proteins in the human brain samples from sporadic PD patients and age-matched control subjects. We tested total protein lysates extracted from striatal tissues. As expected, significantly increased RAGE expression in the striatum from sporadic PD patients was detected by the western blotting (Fig. 5). This upregulation of RAGE protein

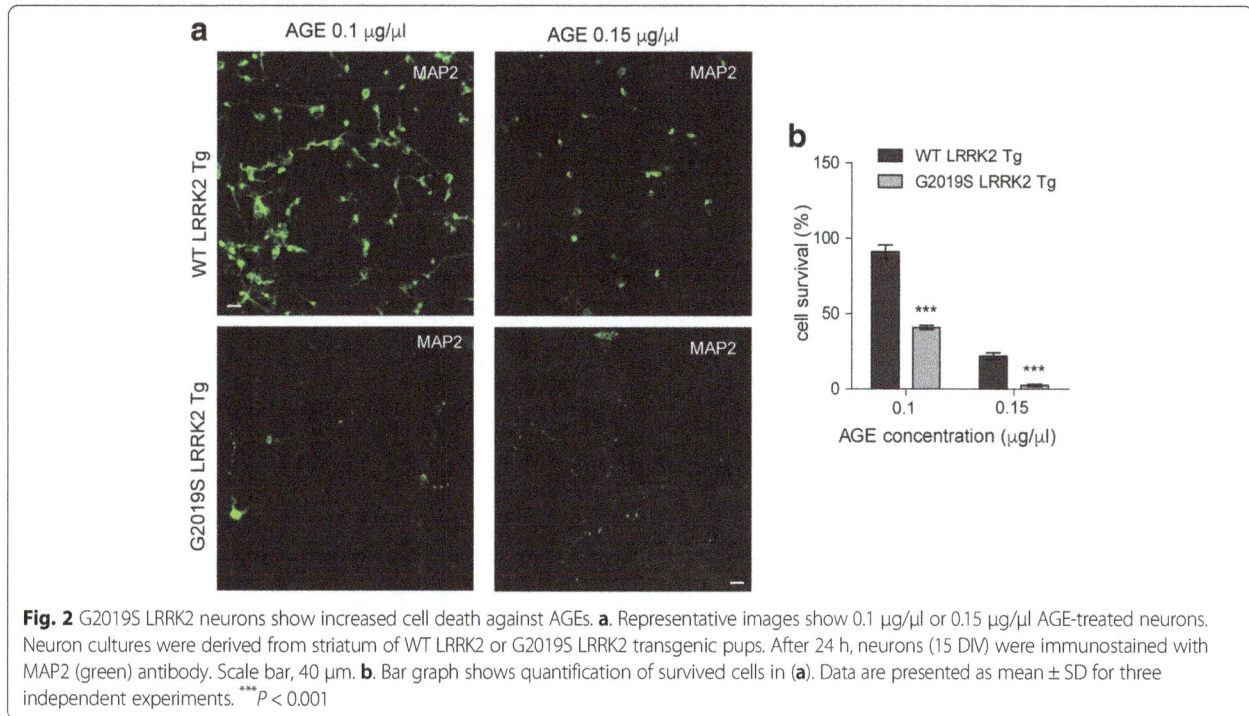

Fig. 2 G2019S LRRK2 neurons show increased cell death against AGEs. **a.** Representative images show 0.1 µg/µl or 0.15 µg/µl AGE-treated neurons. Neuron cultures were derived from striatum of WT LRRK2 or G2019S LRRK2 transgenic pups. After 24 h, neurons (15 DIV) were immunostained with MAP2 (green) antibody. Scale bar, 40 µm. **b.** Bar graph shows quantification of survived cells in (**a**). Data are presented as mean ± SD for three independent experiments. ***P < 0.001

levels in the striatum of PD patients supports the involvement of AGE-RAGE pathway in PD pathogenesis.

Discussion

Diverse mutations in LRRK2 underlie the most common genetic cause of familial and sporadic PD. Since the identification of PD-associated mutations in LRRK2, many studies have attempted to illustrate the potential pathogenic mechanisms of the neuronal cell death caused by mutant LRRK2, especially the G2019S mutation. Here, we demonstrated that AGE-induced toxicity in the striatal neurons was enhanced in the presence of

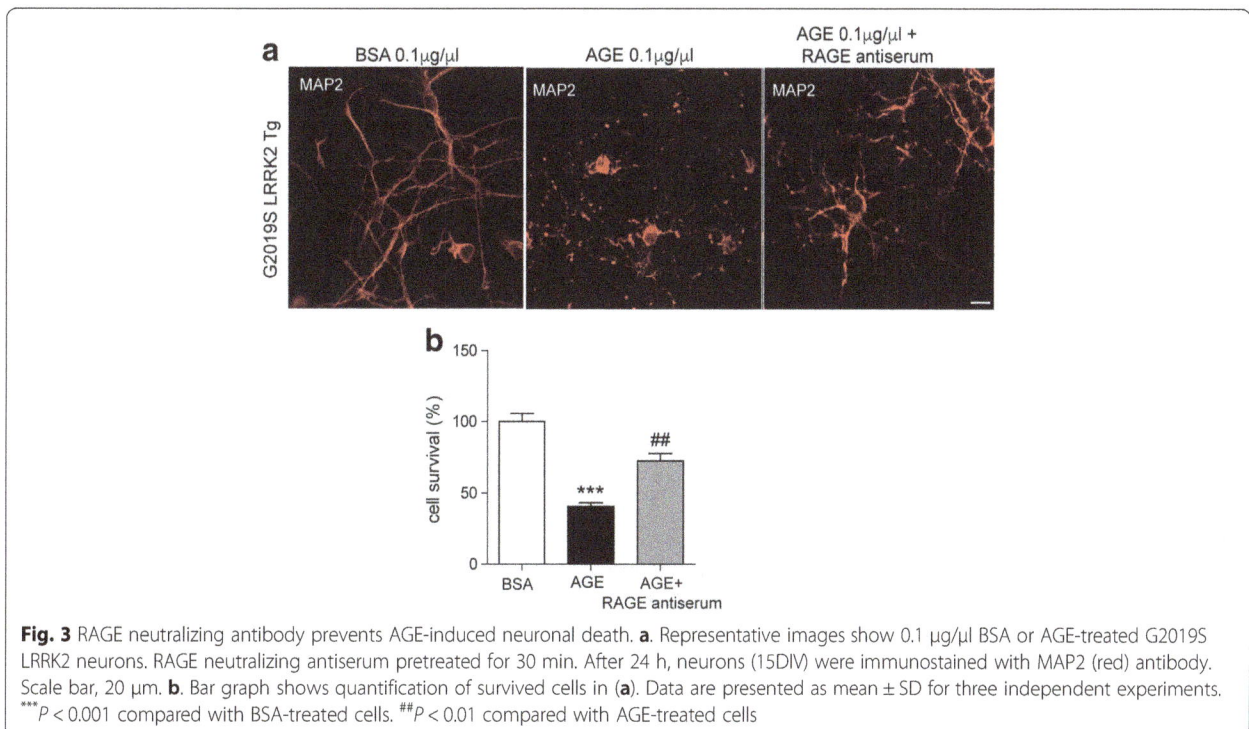

Fig. 3 RAGE neutralizing antibody prevents AGE-induced neuronal death. **a.** Representative images show 0.1 µg/µl BSA or AGE-treated G2019S LRRK2 neurons. RAGE neutralizing antiserum pretreated for 30 min. After 24 h, neurons (15DIV) were immunostained with MAP2 (red) antibody. Scale bar, 20 µm. **b.** Bar graph shows quantification of survived cells in (**a**). Data are presented as mean ± SD for three independent experiments. ***P < 0.001 compared with BSA-treated cells. ##P < 0.01 compared with AGE-treated cells

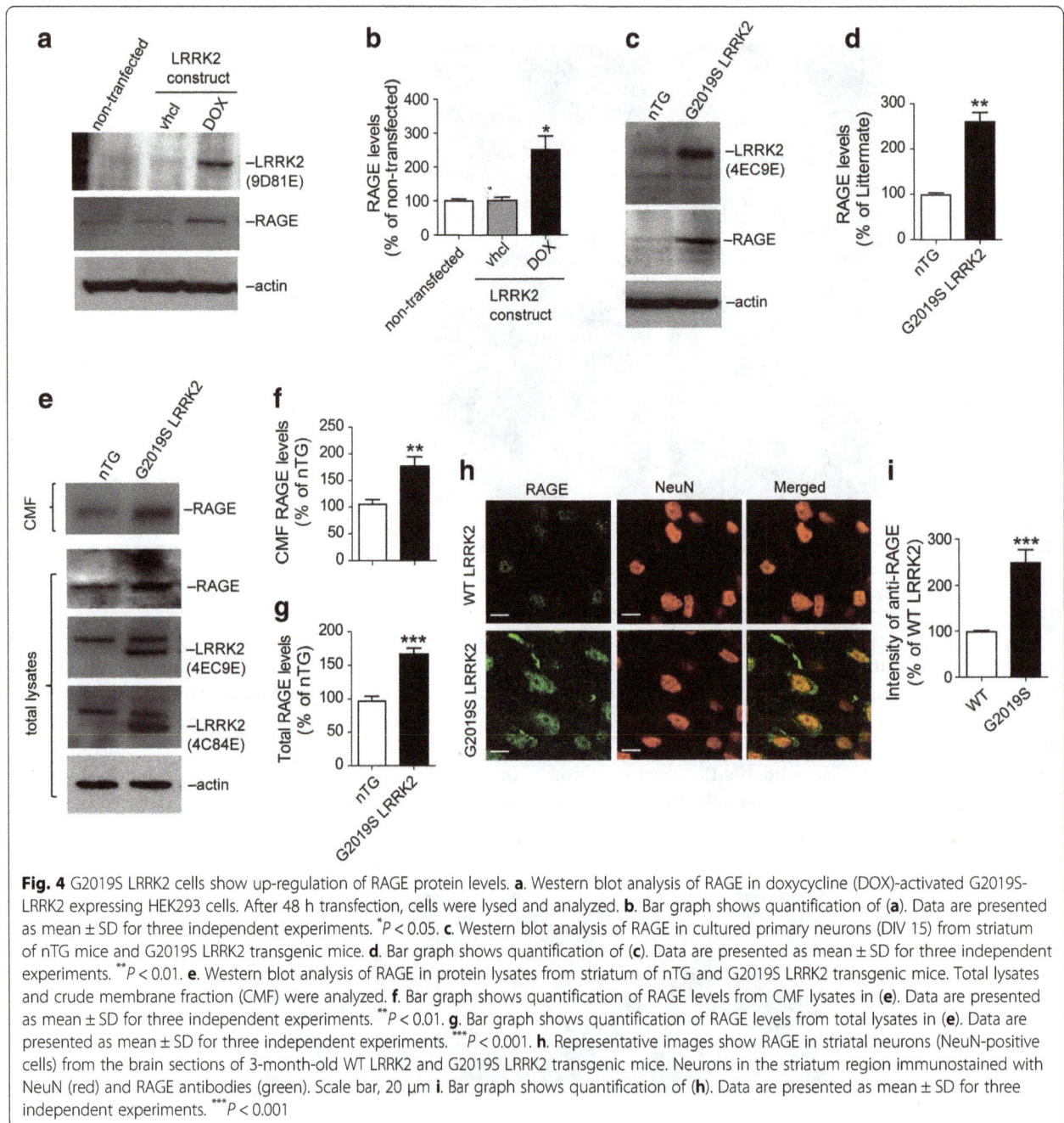

Fig. 4 G2019S LRRK2 cells show up-regulation of RAGE protein levels. **a.** Western blot analysis of RAGE in doxycycline (DOX)-activated G2019S-LRRK2 expressing HEK293 cells. After 48 h transfection, cells were lysed and analyzed. **b.** Bar graph shows quantification of (**a**). Data are presented as mean ± SD for three independent experiments. *$P < 0.05$. **c.** Western blot analysis of RAGE in cultured primary neurons (DIV 15) from striatum of nTG mice and G2019S LRRK2 transgenic mice. **d.** Bar graph shows quantification of (**c**). Data are presented as mean ± SD for three independent experiments. **$P < 0.01$. **e.** Western blot analysis of RAGE in protein lysates from striatum of nTG and G2019S LRRK2 transgenic mice. Total lysates and crude membrane fraction (CMF) were analyzed. **f.** Bar graph shows quantification of RAGE levels from CMF lysates in (**e**). Data are presented as mean ± SD for three independent experiments. **$P < 0.01$. **g.** Bar graph shows quantification of RAGE levels from total lysates in (**e**). Data are presented as mean ± SD for three independent experiments. ***$P < 0.001$. **h.** Representative images show RAGE in striatal neurons (NeuN-positive cells) from the brain sections of 3-month-old WT LRRK2 and G2019S LRRK2 transgenic mice. Neurons in the striatum region immunostained with NeuN (red) and RAGE antibodies (green). Scale bar, 20 μm **i.** Bar graph shows quantification of (**h**). Data are presented as mean ± SD for three independent experiments. ***$P < 0.001$

G2019S LRRK2. Furthermore, we found that the level of RAGE, the critical mediator of AGE-induced cell death, was upregulated in the G2019S LRRK2-expressing neurons. This finding was confirmed in diverse experimental systems, including G2019S LRRK2-expressing cell lines, primary neurons, and mouse brain extracts, as well as postmortem PD striatal tissues. These results reveal a previously unknown pathogenic mechanism of LRRK2 G2019S mutation in AGE/RAGE-mediated cytotoxicity.

We detected elevated protein levels of RAGE but not mRNA levels (data not shown) in G2019S LRRK2,

indicating the possibility that the upregulation of RAGE mRNA translation by G201S LRRK2, resulting from the pathologically enhanced kinase activity of G2019S mutation. Also, in support that increased RAGE protein levels are not the results from artificially over-expressed G2019S LRRK2, we checked the AGE-induced cell toxicity and RAGE levels in the wild-type LRRK2 over-expressing neurons. We found significant changes of RAGE levels between wild-type LRRK2 and G2019S LRRK2 overexpressing neurons, indicating that this event is not resulted from artificial transgene expression.

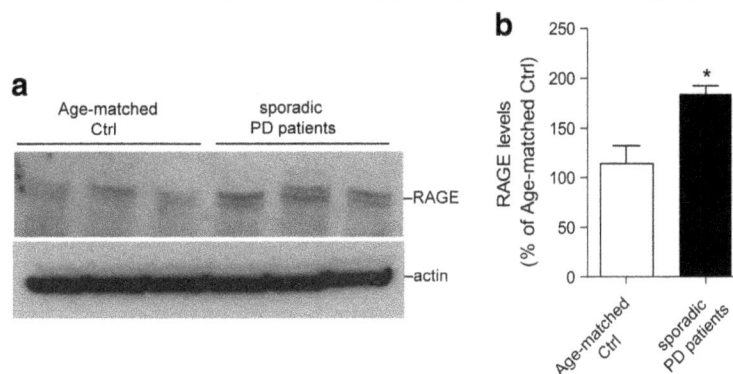

Fig. 5 Increased RAGE level in brains of sporadic PD patients. **a**. Western blot analysis of RAGE in total lysates from striatum of PD patients ($n = 3$) and age-matched control (Ctrl) subjects. ($n = 3$). **b**. Bar graph shows quantification of RAGE levels in (**a**). Data are presented as mean ± SD for three independent experiments. *$P < 0.05$

AGEs, the senescent protein derivatives are formed at accelerated rate under normal aging process, which elicit reactive oxygen species generation and inflammation, and subsequently alters diverse gene expressions, apoptotic neuronal cell death [20–22]. It has been reported that AGE-albumin, the most abundant AGE product, is synthesized and secreted from the cells and studied as a key inducer of host cell death in various neurodegenerative disorders by enhanced expression of RAGE [23]. Gomez et al. showed increased level of RAGE in the frontal cortex of sporadic PD brains [16]. In line with this early study, we found increased RAGE protein levels in the striatum of PD patients, as well as LRRK2 G2019S transgenic mice at 3 months of age.

Conclusions

In summary, we demonstrate that AGE-RAGE cascades are involved in G2019S LRRK2-mediated pathogenesis in PD. Our study suggests that targeted pharmacological interventions using inhibitors or antagonist, such as RAGE neutralizing antiserum, or inhibitors against AGE-RAGE intracellular signaling may serve as promising therapeutic strategies to slow down the progression of PD, especially, PD patients having G2019 LRRK2 mutation.

Acknowledgements
We want to thank members of Cai lab for their suggestions and technical assistance and Dr. Juan Troncoso from the Johns Hopkins University School of Medicine for providing the striatal tissues.

Funding
This work was supported by the intramural research programs of National Institute on Aging, National Institutes of Health (HC: AG000944).

Authors' contributions
HJC and HC wrote the manuscript. HJC performed immunostaining and western blot experiments. CX performed primary neuron cultures. HJC carried out data analyses. All authors read and approved the final manuscript.

Competing interests
The authors declare that they have no competing interests.

Author details
[1]Department of Biochemistry and Biomedical Sciences, Seoul National University, College of Medicine, 28 Yungun-dong, Jongro-gu, Seoul 110-799, South Korea. [2]Transgenics Section, Laboratory of Neurogenetics, National Institute on Aging, National Institutes of Health, Building 35, Room 1A112, MSC 3707, 35 Convent Drive, Bethesda, MD 20892–3707, USA.

References
1. Lee AJ, Hardy J, Revesz T. Parkinson's disease. Lancet. 2009;373(9680):2055–66.
2. Burbulla LF, Krüger R. Converging environmental and genetic pathways in the pathogenesis of parkinson's disease. J Neurol Sci. 2011;306(1-2):1–8.
3. Nalls MA, Pankratz N, Lill CM. Large-scale meta-analysis of genome-wide association data identifies six new risk loci for parkinson's disease. Nat Genet. 2014;46(9):989–93.
4. Simón-Sánchez J, Schulte C, Bras JM, et al. Genome- wide association study reveals genetic risk underlying parkinson's disease. Nat Genet. 2009;41(12):1308–12.
5. Healy DG, Falchi M, O'Sullivan SS, Bonifati V, et al. Phenotype, genotype, and worldwide genetic penetrance of LRRK2-associated Parkinson's disease: a case-control study. Lancet Neurol. 2008;7(7):583–90.
6. Ahmed N. Advanced glycation endproducts–role in pathology of diabetic complications. Diabetes Res Clin Pract. 2005;67(1):3–21.
7. Maillard LC. Action des acides amines sur les sucres: formation des melanoidines par voie methodique. C R Acad Sci (Paris). 1912;154:66–8.
8. Hodge JE. Dehydrated foods, chemistry of browning reactions in model systems. J Agric Food Chem. 1953;1(15):928–43.
9. Rahmadi A, Steiner N, Munch G. Advanced glycation endproducts as gerontotoxins and biomarkers for carbonyl-based degenerative processes in Alzheimer's disease. Clin Chem Lab Med. 2011;49(3):385–91.
10. Uribarri J, Cai W, Peppa M, et al. Circulating glycotoxins and dietary advanced glycation endproducts: two links to inflammatory response, oxidative stress, and aging. J Gerontol A Biol Sci Med Sci. 2007;62(4):427–33.
11. Van Puyvelde K, Mets T, Njemini R, et al. Effect of advanced glycation end product intake on inflammation and aging: a systematic review. Nutr Rev. 2014;72(10):638–50.
12. Munch G, Westcott B, Menini T, et al. Advanced glycation endproducts and their pathogenic roles in neurological disorders. Amino Acids. 2012;42(4):1221–36.
13. Clynes R, Moser B, Yan S, et al. Receptor for AGE (RAGE): weaving tangled webs within the inflammatory response. Curr Mol Med. 2007;7(8):743–51.

14. Herold K, Moser B, Chen Y, et al. Receptor for advanced glycation end products (RAGE) in a dash to the rescue: inflammatory signals gone awry in the primal response to stress. J Leukoc Biol. 2007;82(2):204–12.

15. Yan SS, Chen D, Yan S, et al. RAGE is a key cellular target for Abeta-induced perturbation in Alzheimer's disease. Front Biosci (Schol Ed). 2012;4:240–50.

16. Gomez A, Ferrer I. Involvement of the cerebral cortex in Parkinson disease linked with G2019S LRRK2 mutation without cognitive impairment. Acta Neuropathol. 2010;120(2):155–67.

17. Parisiadou L, Xie C, Cho HJ, et al. Phosphorylation of ezrin/radixin/moesin proteins by LRRK2 promotes the rearrangement of actin cytoskeleton in neuronal morphogenesis. J Neurosci. 2009;29(44):13971–80.

18. Lin X, Parisiadou L, Gu XL, et al. Leucine-rich repeat kinase 2 regulates the progression of neuropathology induced by Parkinson's-disease-related mutant alpha-synuclein. Neuron. 2009;64(6):807–27.

19. Cho HJ, Liu G, Jin SM, et al. MicroRNA-205 regulates the expression of Parkinson's disease-related leucine-rich repeat kinase 2 protein. Hum Mol Genet. 2013;22(3):608–20.

20. Ahmed N. Advanced glycation endproducts—role in pathology of diabetic complications. Diabetes Res Clin Pract. 2005;67(1):3–21.

21. Hodge JE. Dehydrated food, chemistry of browning reactions in model system. J Agric Food Chem. 1953;1(15):928–43.

22. Thorpe SR, Baynes JW. Maillard reaction products in tissue proteins: new products and new perspectives. Amino Acids. 2003;25(3-4):275–81.

23. Grillo MA, Colombatto S. Advanced glycation end-products (AGEs): involvement in aging and in neurodegenerative diseases. Amino Acids. 2008;35(1):29–36.

21

Ultra-High Field Diffusion MRI Reveals Early Axonal Pathology in Spinal Cord of ALS mice

Rodolfo G. Gatto[1]* ⓘ, Manish Y. Amin[2], Daniel Deyoung[2], Matthew Hey[3], Thomas H. Mareci[4] and Richard L. Magin[5]

Abstract

Background: Amyotrophic lateral sclerosis (ALS) is a disease characterized by a progressive degeneration of motor neurons leading to paralysis. Our previous MRI diffusion tensor imaging studies detected early white matter changes in the spinal cords of mice carrying the G93A-SOD1 mutation. Here, we extend those studies using ultra-high field MRI (17.6 T) and fluorescent microscopy to investigate the appearance of early structural and connectivity changes in the spinal cords of ALS mice.

Methods: The spinal cords from presymptomatic and symptomatic mice (80 to 120 days of age) were scanned (ex-vivo) using diffusion-weighted MRI. The fractional anisotropy (FA), axial (AD) and radial (RD) diffusivities were calculated for axial slices from the thoracic, cervical and lumbar regions of the spinal cords. The diffusion parameters were compared with fluorescence microscopy and membrane cellular markers from the same tissue regions.

Results: At early stages of the disease (day 80) in the lumbar region, we found, a 19% decrease in FA, a 9% decrease in AD and a 35% increase in RD. Similar changes were observed in cervical and thoracic spinal cord regions. Differences between control and ALS mice groups at the symptomatic stages (day 120) were larger. Quantitative fluorescence microscopy at 80 days, demonstrated a 22% reduction in axonal area and a 22% increase in axonal density. Tractography and quantitative connectome analyses measured by edge weights showed a 52% decrease in the lumbar regions of the spinal cords of this ALS mice group. A significant increase in ADC (23.3%) in the ALS mice group was related to an increase in aquaporin markers.

Conclusions: These findings suggest that the combination of ultra-high field diffusion MRI with fluorescent ALS mice reporters is a useful approach to detect and characterize presymptomatic white matter micro-ultrastructural changes and axonal connectivity anomalies in ALS.

Keywords: Amyotrophic Lateral Sclerosis, Spinal Cord, Ultra-high Field MRI, Diffusion Tensor Imaging, Yellow Fluorescent Protein, G93A-SOD1 mice, Axonal Degeneration, Tractography, Connectomics

Background

Amyotrophic lateral sclerosis (ALS) involves progressive deterioration of upper and lower motor neurons within the brainstem, corticospinal tracts, and anterior horn areas of the spinal cord (SC) [1]. It has been shown that genetic mutations in ALS patients lead to changes in molecular pathways and neuronal degeneration in selective groups of cells subsequently promoting abnormalities in genomic expressions [2] and axonal function [3]. Among the ALS transgenic animal models available, the G93A-SOD1 model is the most widely used to study the neurological deterioration associated with this disease [4].

Unfortunately, other than an increase in the number of available animal models [5–7], little progress has been made toward the early detection of ALS to improve the outcome of therapeutic interventions for these patients. However, a better way to understand the early changes occurring in cellular structures is to include transgenic mouse lines with constitutively expressed fluorescent protein. Thus, a specific neuronal population can be

* Correspondence: rgatto@uic.edu; rodogatto@gmail.com
[1]Department of Anatomy and Cell Biology, University of Illinois at Chicago, 808 S. Wood St. Rm 578 M/C 512, Chicago, IL 60612, USA
Full list of author information is available at the end of the article

visualized with quantitative fluorescence techniques to assess the morphological aspects of neuronal structures and to understand the role of axonal connectivity in neurological diseases [8–10]. One of the most commonly used fluorescent probes in research is the Thy1-YFP mouse model, expressing yellow fluorescent protein (YFP) in a subset of neurons across different brain structures and axon trajectories in specific layers of the cerebral cortex and spinal cord (SC) [11]. Although the study axonal degeneration with transgenic fluorescent ALS mice has been described in the past [12], such studies were mainly performed at the end stage of the disease with limited focus on changes in the SC white matter (WM) microstructure.

On the other hand, since the average life expectancy of ALS patients from the time of diagnosis ranges from two to five years, any meaningful improvement in the ALS survival rate would depend on the establishment of methods for the detection of early and critical pathogenic events. To this end, magnetic resonance imaging (MRI) provides the best non-invasive way to assess the appearance of neurodegenerative diseases at early presymptomatic stages [13, 14]. In addition, diffusion tensor imaging (DTI) provides substantial information on the organization of neural tissues [15]. As an example, the radial and axial diffusion parameters provide an index of axonal fiber tract integrity and fractional anisotropy gives a measure of brain tissue organization, which is important in the context of ALS. In the search for early ALS biomarkers, recent studies using tractography reconstructions related fiber track changes with a selective degeneration in WM axonal populations [16, 17]. Ultimately, improvements in the sensitivity and specificity of MRI diffusion methods have introduced new imaging biomarkers that could able to identify the changes occurring in the susceptible WM tissues caused by ALS [18].

Although several reports have shown that DTI methods can detect early alterations in WM, and extensive neuropathological evidence points towards early white matter structural alterations in ALS [19–23], the underlying link between the diffusion and the underlying axonal neuropathological process at early stages of the disease has not been fully elucidated. Thus, our study is designed to validate DTI markers obtained by ultra-high field MRI (UHF-MRI) and to characterize early changes in axonal ultrastructure and WM connectivity using an ex vivo tissue and a fluorescent ALS mouse.

Methods
Animals
All procedures used to obtain tissues followed an approved protocol from the animal care committee (ACC) at the University of Illinois in Chicago (UIC). C57BJ6 mice, overexpressing the SOD1 transgene with the G93A mutation, were obtained from the Jackson Laboratory

(JAX # 004435). The G93A-SOD1 mice have been extensively characterized as an animal model for ALS, developing motor symptoms at approximately 110 days of age and dying around 160 days [24, 25]. Based on these finding, we considered two groups of animals for this work: a presymptomatic group at postnatal day 80 (P80) and a symptomatic group at postnatal day 120 (P120). To evaluate morphologic axonal anomalies in the context of ALS, mice encoding a yellow fluorescent protein (YFP) transgene specifically associated with a neuronal Thy1 promoter was chosen (JAX#003709). Thus, we generated double transgenic mice (YFP, G93A-SOD1) and littermates carrying only the YFP transgene used as a control group. For this study, a total 18 animals (n=5 SCs per P80 and P120 YFP, G93A-SOD1 groups (10 SCs) and n=4 SCs per P80 and 120 YFP control groups (8 SCs), were used for scanning and further histological analysis. Mice had easy access to food and water and were checked daily to assess their level of well-being and health. In any situation of animal distress or pain, animals were euthanized in carbon dioxide using standard protocols.

Animal preparation for MRI imaging
Animals were rendered unconscious with CO_2 inhalation, then transcardiac perfused with a PBS and 4% paraformaldehyde (PFA) solution. A laminectomy was performed and the spinal cords were extracted intact then immersed in PFA (> 48 hours). Prior to imaging, the cords were soaked overnight in PBS to removed free fixative, then placed in individual 5 mm diameter NMR tubes (New Era #NEML5-7, 300-400 MHz) filled with fluorocarbon oil (Fluorinert®, 3M, Maplewood, MN). Each set of 9, 5-mm tubes (each containing a spinal cord) was positioned in a 20-mm diameter NMR tube (New Era # NE-L25-7) using a custom-made plastic tube holder. Images were acquired with a 17.6T vertical-bore Avance II scanner using a 20-mm RF coil, Micro-2.5 gradients, and Paravision 6.0 software (Bruker, Karlsruhe, Germany).

Diffusion weighted imaging and data processing
For each set of 9 spinal cords (2 imaging sessions) a total of 60 MRI slices were acquired in blocks of 20 slices, centered at the cervical, thoracic, and lumbar levels each, and oriented along the rostral-caudal axis of the spinal cord. Diffusion weighted images were acquired using a spin echo sequence with TR= 4000 ms and TE =28 ms, interleaved 0.15 mm thick slices, field of view = 20 x 20 x 3 mm^3 in each block of slices, in-plane acquisition matrix = 133 x 133, for an isotropic image resolution of 150 μm. For connectomics calculations ([26]), two images were acquired with b = 0 s/mm^2 and diffusion weighting was applied with b = 700 s/mm^2 in 12 directions, and b = 2500 s/mm^2 in 64 directions [27], with 3.5 ms gradient pulses and 17.5 ms separation. This

acquisition was averaged twice for a total acquisition time of 19 hrs. per set.

Diffusion data processing was performed using FSL [28] to calculate fractional anisotropy (FA), axial diffusivity (AD), and radial diffusivity (RD) [29]. The average apparent diffusion coefficient (ADC) over the 64 directions was calculated using b = 0 and b = 2500 s/mm². In addition, the calculation of the water displacement probability density function [30] was used to estimate white matter tracts. White matter regions-of-interest (ROIs), defined within slices at the top and bottom of each of spinal cord segments (cervical, thoracic, and lumbar), were manually outlined following the anterolateral distribution of the white matter on each slice (Fig. 1) using ImageJ software (NIH, Bethesda).

White matter connectivity

To determine white matter structural connectivity in the three regions of the spinal cords, deterministic tractography was performed using in-house software using 125 seeds per voxel, an angular threshold of 50°, and a step size of 75 μm. Fiber tracks were visualized with Trackvis (Version 0.6.1, Massachusetts General Hospital, Boston, MA). Using a network approach to define white matter integrity along the spinal cord, the top and bottom slices in each segment were used to define network nodes. White matter tracts were used to define network edges and the connectivity quantified using a dimensionless, scale-invariant edge weight (EW) [26].

Histology and immuno-fluorescence analysis

Although it is feasible to histologically examine all segments of the spinal cord (cervical and thoracic and lumbar), results from this and previous MRI diffusion ex-vivo studies [31] have shown predominant alterations in MRI diffusion at the lumbar segments of ALS mice. Thus, this study is focused in the histological analysis of white matter anomalies in the lumbar regions, specifically between the third and fifth lumbar segments (Fig. 2).

After MRI scanning, oil media was removed and spines were placed in progressive solutions of sucrose [5-30 %] for an additional 24 hrs for cryo-protection. After embedding in optical cutting temperature (OCT) polymer compound (Tissue Tek, Sakura, Finetek, cat #4583), 50 μm thick spinal cord sections were obtained using a microtome (Leica cryostat CM 1850 Cryostat, Buffalo Grove, IL). Based in our previous finding to detect early SC white matter (WM) changes [32], only coronal section of lumbar spinal cord were used for histological analysis. Spinal cord sections were mounted on slides (Fisher-brand Superforst, cat# 12-550-15) and dried for 15 minutes. Then, the OCT was removed by washing three times with Tris base buffer (TBS). Sections were permeabilized with Triton-X100 0.25 % for 10 minutes and blocked with 5 % goat serum for an hour in TBS. Spinal cord sections (50μm thickness) were mounted on slides. Slides were dried and mounted in Vecta-Shield mounting media (Vector Laboratories, Burlingame, CA). Images were acquired by confocal microscopy (Leica LMS-710 confocal microscope, Germany). Each coronal section in the lumbar spinal cord was

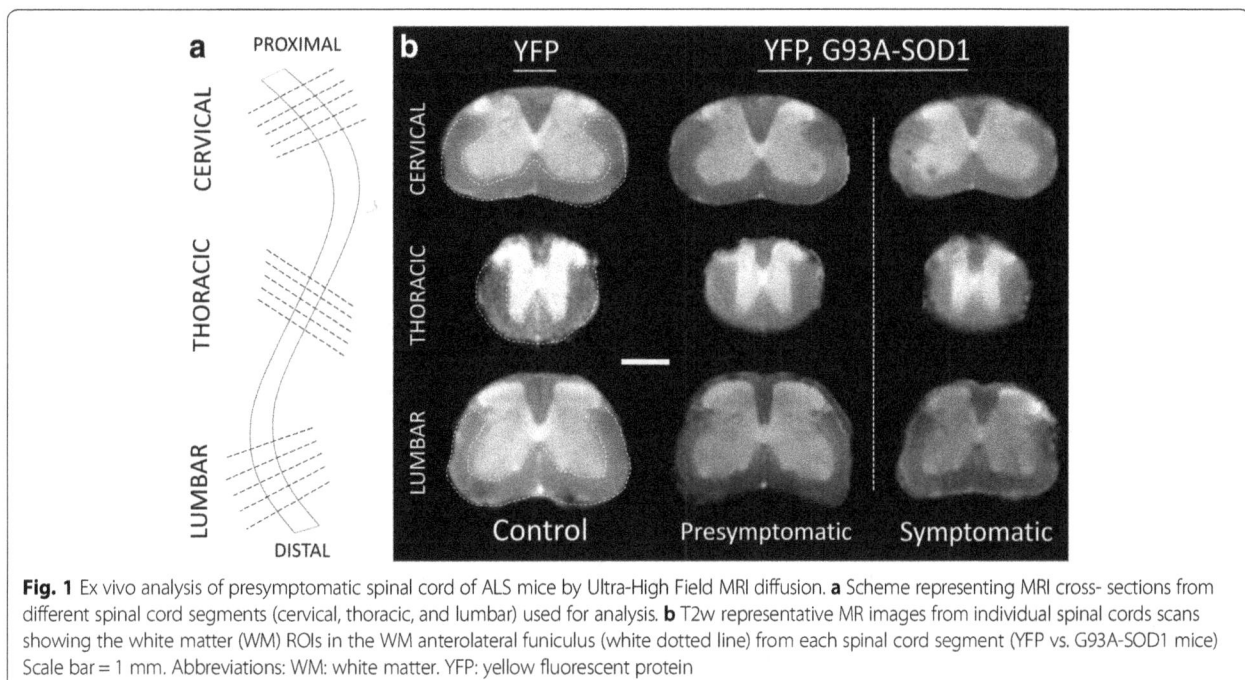

Fig. 1 Ex vivo analysis of presymptomatic spinal cord of ALS mice by Ultra-High Field MRI diffusion. **a** Scheme representing MRI cross- sections from different spinal cord segments (cervical, thoracic, and lumbar) used for analysis. **b** T2w representative MR images from individual spinal cords scans showing the white matter (WM) ROIs in the WM anterolateral funiculus (white dotted line) from each spinal cord segment (YFP vs. G93A-SOD1 mice) Scale bar = 1 mm. Abbreviations: WM: white matter. YFP: yellow fluorescent protein

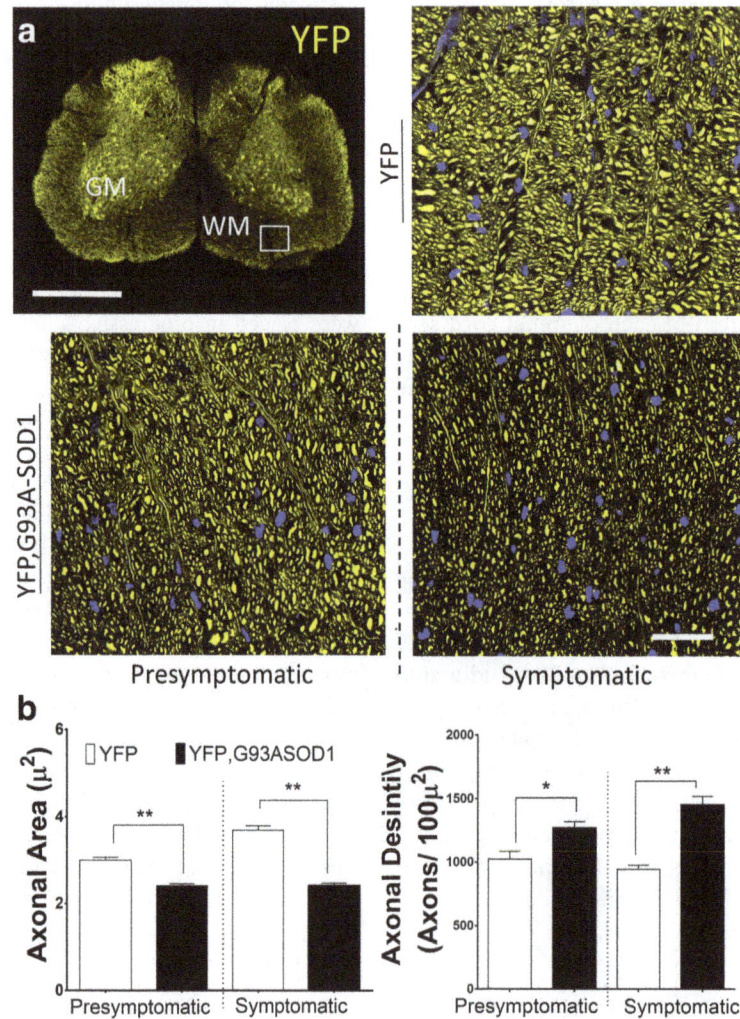

Fig. 2 Early axonal structural changes can be observed in spinal cord of ALS mice. **a** Spinal cord lumbar sections from an YFP, G93A-SOD1 mouse. Regions of Interest (ROI) were obtained from the anterior portion of the spinal cord (SC) white matter (WM) (white square area). Detailed changes in axonal diameter can be seen in the YFP, G93A-SOD1 mice. Note that each WM area in the histology pictures has an approximate voxel size (100×100 μm^2). Scale bar =1 mm. **b** Measurements from WM ROIs showed a significant (**$p < 0.01$) reduction in in axonal areas and an increase in the number of YFP-positive axons (axonal density contained within 100 μm^2) in the presymptomatic (P80) YFP, G93A-SOD1 mice. (* = $p < 0.05$); (** = $p < 0.01$) ($n = 4/5$ per group). Nuclear counterstaining with DAPI (blue). Scale bar =10 μm. Abbreviations: WM, white matter; GM, grey matter; YFP, yellow fluorescent protein

selected using similar anatomical reference following a spinal cords stereotaxic coordinates (The Spinal Cord: A Christopher and Dana Reeve Foundation Text and Atlas, 1st Ed, Watson & Paxinos, 2008). Confocal microscopy images and z stack images for three-dimensional reconstruction were obtained by background subtraction using negative controls samples without primary antibody and collected by two independent channels: 534 nm channel for the YFP yellow signal and 647 nm channel to detect fluorescent emission from antibodies from other markers. To evaluate the role of water permeability in ALS, we used anti aquaporin-4 staining (AQP4) (StressMarq Bioscence Inc., Victoria, BC) (Cat #SPC-505D, 1:400). Quantitative measures were obtained by counting the mean pixel value

per equal picture area using auto-threshold methods and the pixel aggregates of each figure compiled and tabulated for analysis. Briefly, the procedure divides the image into objects and background by taking an initial threshold. Averages of the number of pixels at, below, or above the threshold were computed and subsequent averages of these two values were used.

Statistical analysis

Quantitative data were tabulated and analyzed using GraphPad Prism 6 software (La Jolla, CA). Based on the results from pilot experiments, the group size of animals per experimental group were established using power analysis and sample size calculations. For quantitative analysis of YFP, and AQP4 fluorescence levels and MRI diffusion values (ADC, FA, AD and RD), one-way ANOVA and Tukey's post hoc tests were used to determine statistical differences among experimental animal groups (P80 and P120). A value of p < 0.05 was used to demonstrate statistical significance. Results were replicated by application of non-parametric statistical tools (Mann–Whitney test). Error bars in all the figures represent standard error of the mean (SEM).

Results

MRI diffusion demonstrate presymptomatic spinal cord changes of YFP, G93A-SOD1 mice

Previous clinical and animal diffusion imaging studies ALS SCs have shown that regional changes in parameters were more affected at the distal than proximal regions [14, 33]. Hence, we centered our MRI diffusion studies on the anterolateral white matter funiculi of three SC regions (cervical, thoracic and lumbar segments) (Fig. 1a). Manual segmentation of WM ROIs across diffusion maps from five SC slices were considered in this analysis, (Fig. 1b). Two time-points were considered; a presymptomatic stage (P80) and a symptomatic stage (P120). At presymptomatic stages (P80), we observed a significant reduction of FA in the cervical region ($p < 0.05$) in the YFP, G93A-SOD1 mice (YFP mice =0.60 +/- 0.01 versus YFP, G93A-SOD1 mice = 0.57 +/- 0.01) (- 6.6%) as well as in the thoracic regions ($p < 0.01$) (YFP mice = 0.66 +/- 0.01 versus YFP, G93A-SOD1 mice = 0.58 +/- 0.01) (- 12.6%) and lumbar region ($p < 0.001$) (YFP mice = 0.66 +/- 0.01 versus YFP, G93A-SOD1 mice = 0.53 +/- 0.03) (- 19.7%). A significant decrease in axial diffusion (AD) in the lumbar segment was seen at P80 (YFP mice = 6.7 +/- 0.1x10^{-4} mm^2/s versus YFP, G93A-SOD1 mice = 6.3 +/- 0.05x10^{-4} mm^2/s) ($p < 0.01$) (-8.7 %). These changes were decreased further on each spinal cord segment during the symptomatic stage. Presymptomatic results in radial diffusion (RD) demonstrate a significant ($p < 0.01$) increase not only in the lumbar levels (YFP mice = 2.0 +/- 0.1x10^{-4} mm^2/s versus YFP,G93A--SOD1 mice = 2.7 +/- 0.5x10^{-4} mm^2/s) ($p < 0001$) (+35 %) in the dorsal region (YFP mice = 2.5 +/- 0.1x10^{-4} mm^2/s versus YFP,G93A-SOD1 mice = 3.1 +/- 0.1x10^{-4} mm^2/s) ($p < 0001$) (+24.8%) and cervical levels (YFP mice = 2.2 +/- 0.2x10^{-4} mm^2 /s versus YFP, G93A-SOD1 mice = 2.52 +/- 0.9x10^{-4} mm^2/s) (p<001) (+16.1 %). Overall, these DTI findings demonstrated that lumbar changes in diffusion across axonal structures in this ALS mice can be detected before symptoms manifest (Fig. 4a).

Presymptomatic changes in white matter diffusion are linked to axonal structural anomalies

Alterations in axonal features from spinal cords (SC) in G93A-SOD1 mice associated to a fluorescent reporter has been previously reported [12]. However, the results from these studies only carried descriptive findings and no specific quantitative analysis has been done. To determine the structural changes underlying the WM alterations in diffusion observed in previous MRI scans, we focused our histological analysis on the anterolateral region at the lumbar SC section from YFP and YFP, G93A-SOD1 mice (Fig. 2a). To make results equivalent to the voxel size performed during the MRI sessions (voxel size = 100 x100 µm^2) we performed structural analysis using confocal fluorescence images with similar size. Specifically, for morphological evaluations we manually registered WM ROIs for each animal and group following similar topography and guided by stereotaxic coordinates [34]. Measurements from each groups showed a significant ($p < 0.01$) reduction (-22.1 %) in axonal areas in the YFP, G93A-SOD1 mice at P80 (YFP mice = 2.9 +/- 0.06 µm^2 versus. YFP, G93A-SOD1 mice= 2.3 +/-0.05 µm^2) and -41.9% P120 (YFP mice = 3.69 +/-0.09 µm^2 versus YFP, G93A-SOD1 mice = 2.4 +/-0.05 µm^2) (n > 2000 axons per group). Nonetheless, we also observed a significant ($p < 0.05$) increase in the number YFP-positive axons delimited within each ROI (Axonal Density) in the YFP, G93ASOD1 mice group (+21.6 %) at P80 (YFP mice 1024 +/- 61 axons/100µm^2 vs YFP, G93A-SOD1 mice 1272 +/- 48 axons/100µm^2) and more significant ($p < 0.01$) increase (+42.4 %) at P120 (Fig. 2b). All together, these results point towards a significant remodeling of the SC axonal structures at early stage of the disease.

Presymptomatic structural changes in axonal fibers are associated with alterations in axonal connectivity

Using tractography reconstructions and histological confocal reconstructions we have demonstrated a critical impact of ALS towards axonal connectivity. Specifically, tractography methods showed early anomalies in fiber organization in the YFP, G93A-SOD1 mice and histological reconstructions evaluated the specific structural anomalies across individual axons (Fig. 3a and b). Among new techniques has been developed for quantitative connectome analysis [35], edges weights (EW) analysis has been introducing the concept of the adjustment and quantitation of connection strengths [36] as calculated from our data set (Fig. 4b). Results from this analysis showed an early significant decrease of this parameters ($p < 0.01$) at P80, at the cervical levels (YFP mice = 0.024 +/- 0.002 versus YFP, G93A-SOD1 mice = 0.0136 +/- 0.004) ($p < 0.05$) (-43.5 %), as well as in the SC lumbar regions (YFP mice = 0.039 +/- 0.0001 versus YFP, G93A-SOD1 mice = 0.023 +/- 0.0004) (p<0.01) (-40.9 %), (Fig. 4c).

Early ADC anomalies in the spinal cord of the ALS mice are coupled with changes in water transport protein membranes

The role of ADC in SC ALS tissue has been described before but it changes in the early stages of the disease

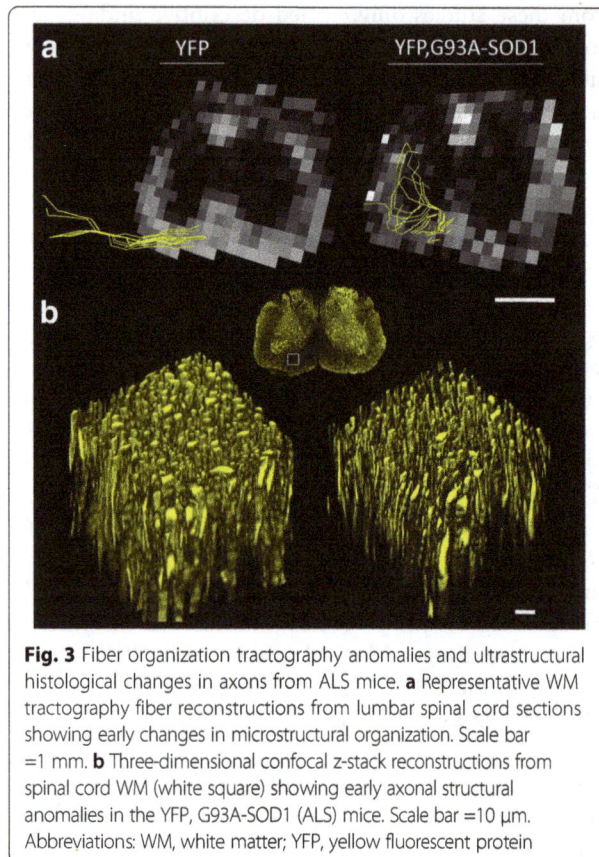

Fig. 3 Fiber organization tractography anomalies and ultrastructural histological changes in axons from ALS mice. **a** Representative WM tractography fiber reconstructions from lumbar spinal cord sections showing early changes in microstructural organization. Scale bar =1 mm. **b** Three-dimensional confocal z-stack reconstructions from spinal cord WM (white square) showing early axonal structural anomalies in the YFP, G93A-SOD1 (ALS) mice. Scale bar =10 μm. Abbreviations: WM, white matter; YFP, yellow fluorescent protein

remain unknown [16, 37]. Measurements from our experimental model have shown early changes of this parameter particularly at the thoracic (YFP mice = 3.2 +/- 0.1×10^{-4} mm^2 /s versus YFP, G93A-SOD1 mice = 3.8 +/- 0.1×10^{-4} mm^2/s) (p<001), (+16.4 %) and lumbar level (YFP mice = 3.2 +/- 0.1×10^{-4} mm^2 /s versus YFP, G93A-SOD1 mice = 3.53 +/- 0.9×10^{-4} mm^2/s) (p<001) (+23.3 %) (Fig. 5a). The complex nature of diffusional water exchange in diverse neuropathological conditions is associated to changes in membrane permeability [38, 39]. One of the factors regulating this water diffusion process is determined by the transmembrane proteins (aquaporin channels) [40]. Aquaporin 4 (AQP4) has shown a high prevalence in the central nervous system (CNS). Quantitative IHC analysis revealed a significant (*p* < 0.001) increase of AQP4 in the ALS mice SC at the presymptomatic stage (P80) (YFP mice = 541.6 +/- 131.5 a.u. vs YFP, G93A-SOD1 mice = 5403 +/-176 a.u.) (1-2 fold increase) predominantly in the extra-axonal compartment (Fig. 5b and c).

Discussion

ALS is characterized by a selective loss of motor neurons in the brain and spinal cord [41]. Although the underlying mechanism of the disease is unknown, pathological observations and experimental data establish that alterations in

synaptic and neuronal function occur well before neuronal death [41], supporting the principal role of axonal degeneration in the neuropathological process [3]. The earlier compromise of motor axons, and alterations in water diffusion in the spinal cords from an animal model of ALS have been increasingly gaining attention [42–44]. An unproven hypothesis of early axonal structural changes has been proposed to explain the preponderance of early phenotype and symptoms in ALS and other neurodegenerative diseases [10, 45]. Furthermore, our previous MRI studies demonstrated that early axonal injury in the G93A-SOD1 mice model occurred at the lower level of the spinal cord and that such microstructural changes could be monitored using DTI [31]. Moreover, *in vivo* UHF-MRI diffusion studies have a critical advantage for longitudinal studies acquired with high spatial resolution [46]. From the medical perspective, using DTI to gain an understanding of the ultrastructural changes occurring during the early stage of ALS may improve the detection and treatment of this disease at earlier stages [10, 47].

Previous work G93ASOD1 mice were not able to demonstrate presymptomatic changes in DTI diffusion parameters using 7T and 9.4T MRI instruments in combination with conventional histology [18, 48–52] (Table 1). To the best of our knowledge, this study is the first to use UHF-MRI at 17.6T to interrogate the WM microstructure of the spinal cord from an ALS mouse model. The combination of higher signal to noise ratios (SNR) available at higher magnetic fields [53, 54], and the histological detail provided by an ALS transgenic mice expressing a neuronal specific endogenous fluorescent protein (YFP), enhanced the detection of early changes in DTI parameters and WM microstructure (Figs. 1b and 4a). Thus, we have identified presymptomatic changes in MRI diffusion are based on alterations in of morphological axonal features, such as a reduction in axonal areas and increase in axonal density (Fig. 2).

Besides the increased number of mechanisms responsible for the alteration of axonal function in ALS [3, 55, 56], the microstructural alterations causing the changes the diffusion signal in ALS are still not well-known. Changes in axonal are widely used in diverse scientific and clinical scenarios [57–59]. Nonetheless, such tractography features are an under representation of the real neuropathological changes occurring inside a single voxel (Fig. 3). Thus, such non-quantitative parameters have to be perfected and validated before can be used to make further decisions in clinical scenarios [60–63].

Although the micro-anatomical anomalies displayed in this work could explain the early changes in diffusion in ALS, the analysis of axonal connectivity could unveil a further insight in the real axonal disconnection problem observed in many neurodegenerative diseases [57, 59].

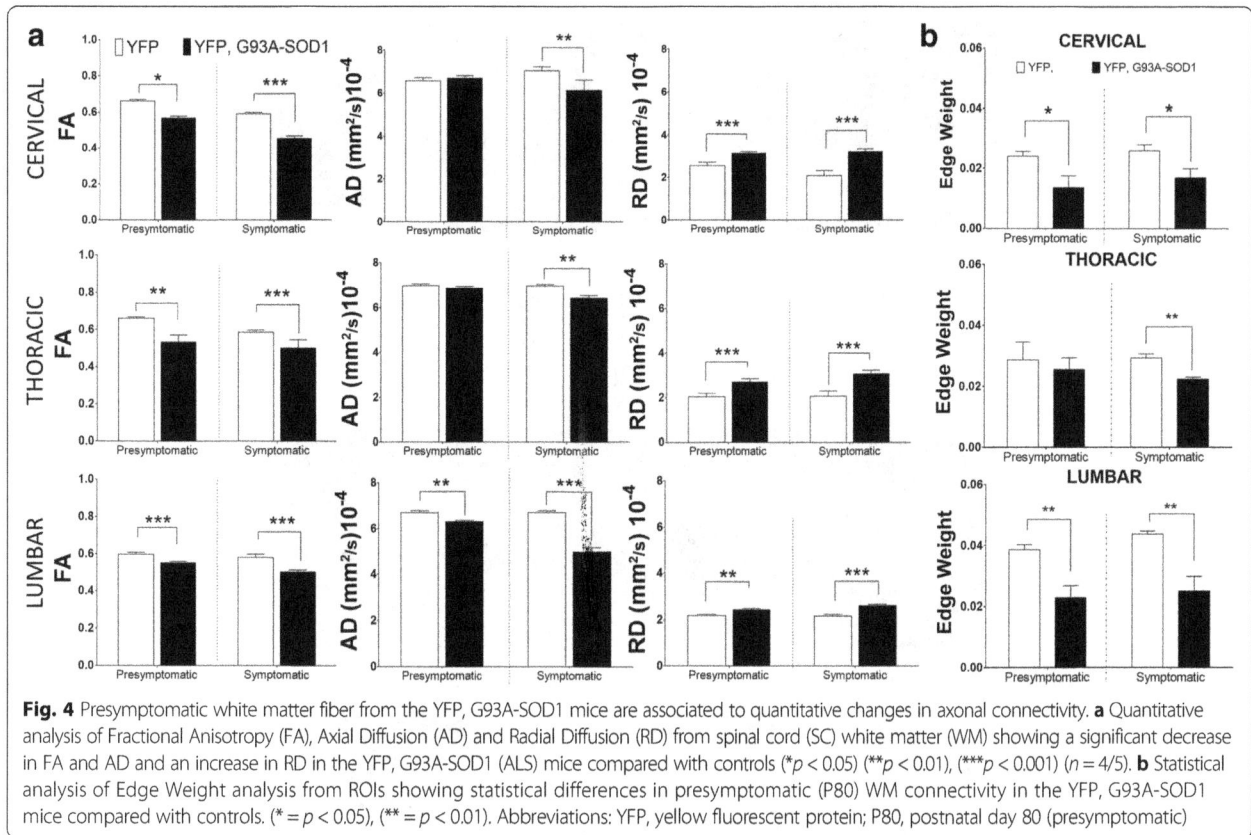

Fig. 4 Presymptomatic white matter fiber from the YFP, G93A-SOD1 mice are associated to quantitative changes in axonal connectivity. **a** Quantitative analysis of Fractional Anisotropy (FA), Axial Diffusion (AD) and Radial Diffusion (RD) from spinal cord (SC) white matter (WM) showing a significant decrease in FA and AD and an increase in RD in the YFP, G93A-SOD1 (ALS) mice compared with controls (*$p < 0.05$) (**$p < 0.01$), (***$p < 0.001$) ($n = 4/5$). **b** Statistical analysis of Edge Weight analysis from ROIs showing statistical differences in presymptomatic (P80) WM connectivity in the YFP, G93A-SOD1 mice compared with controls. (* = $p < 0.05$), (** = $p < 0.01$). Abbreviations: YFP, yellow fluorescent protein; P80, postnatal day 80 (presymptomatic)

Obtained by diffusion path probabilities, such techniques can estimate the connection strengths across different WM regions (nodes) enabling the reconstruction of connectomes, consistent with CNS networks properties, mapped by previous imaging modalities and post-mortem brain studies [64]. Using quantitative techniques measuring the diffusion properties along edge voxels, such as edge weight (EW) analysis [26, 36], we evaluated the early axonal disconnection in this animal model (Fig. 4b). Specifically, we addressed how structural information across spinal cord axons was linked and early impacted by ALS. These results have pointed to an early disconnection predominantly in cervical and lumbar regions, as observed in two thirds of ALS patients with upper and lower limbs symptoms (spinal form) [65].

In addition to the microstructural changes observed during early stages, another point of attention are the events related to alteration in cellular and membrane water exchange and their relationship with changes in MRI diffusion signals [66–68]. One of the mechanisms to maintain the osmotic balance across cellular membranes in the central nervous system is regulated by an intricate mechanism of water permeably controlled by membrane channels called Aquaporin (AQP) [69–73]. Although many structural alterations can be the cause of changes in water

diffusion across cellular membranes, recent work has shown a significant link between AQPs and the MRI apparent diffusion coefficient (ADC) [67]. Although such parameter has been found highly impaired in ALS models [74], changes in ADC has not be fully characterized in early stages of ALS. In that regard, our studies have demonstrated that changes in AQP4 and ADC are present at earlier stages of the disease (Fig. 5a and b). Moreover, based in our histological finding such increase in AQP4 channel expression could reveal additional anomalies across different cellular types located in the non- axonal compartment (Fig. 5c). Nevertheless, the specific role of AQP channels and their contribution to the water exchange and MRI diffusion in the early stages of ALS remains to be determined [75, 76].

Overall, this work proposes new insights to understand the biological nature of changes in MRI diffusion parameters during early stages of ALS (Fig. 6). Although previous MRI work has demonstrated a decrease in SC volume in ALS patients at symptomatic stages [77, 78], one of the limitations by our current MRI and histological techniques of axonal quantification is the exclusive assessment of ROIs without accounting for the volume reduction of the entire CNS structure (SC) interrogated. Moreover, recent findings using alternative diffusion techniques have demonstrated a similar increase

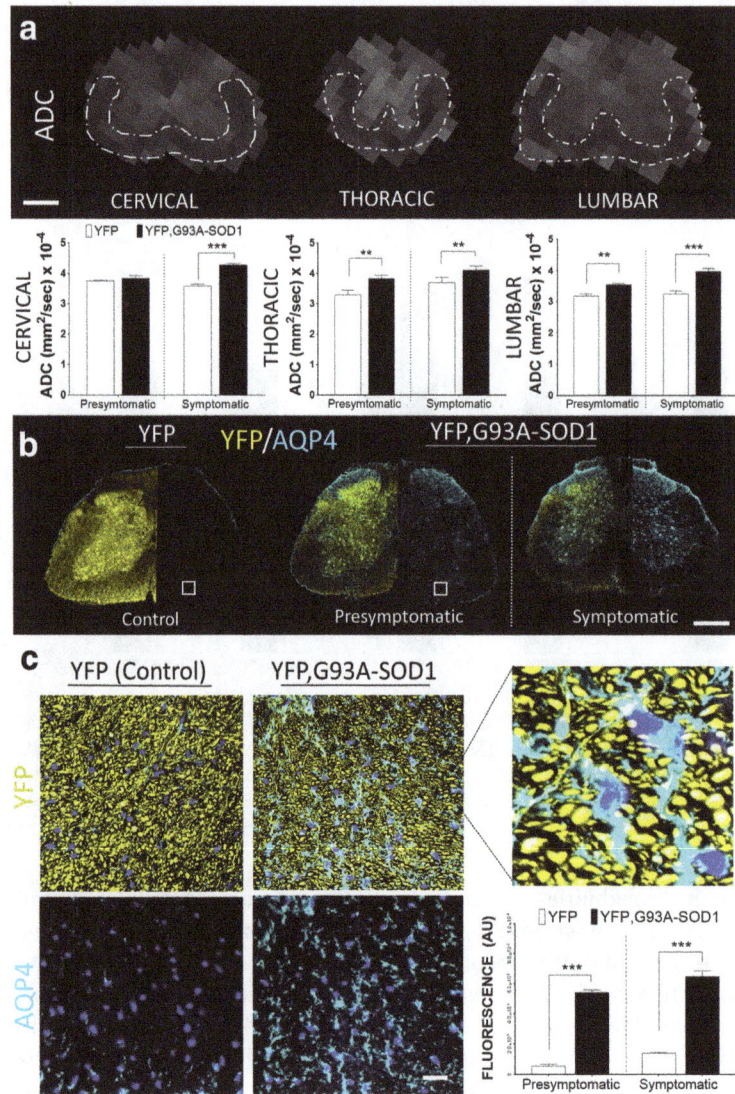

Fig. 5 Changes MRI diffusion are coupled with aquaporin expression anomalies in ALS white matter. **a** Quantitative measurements from apparent diffusion coefficient (ADC) spinal cord maps showing an increase in lower SC segments (dorsal and lumbar levels) in the ALS mice. **b** Progressive changes in aquaporin 4 (AQP4) expression can be seen in the presymptomatic and symptomatic YFP, G93A-SOD1 mice. Scale bar = 1 mm. **c** Further analysis of SC white matter (WM) shows a significant increase in AQP4 expression in the presymptomatic ALS mice compared to control, mostly located in the extra- axonal compartment. (*** = $p < 0.001$). Nuclear counterstaining with DAPI (blue). Scale bar = 10 µm. Abbreviations: YFP, yellow fluorescent protein; P80, postnatal day 80 (Presymptomatic); P120, postnatal day 120 (Symptomatic)

in axonal densities during early stages of neurodegenerative diseases [79] pointing to an increase in the total number of axons per volume unit of WM tissues at early stage among different neurodegenerative diseases. Among the different mechanisms to explain the early structural changes, one is related to the specific susceptibility of subsets of neurons by the mutated G93A-SOD1 protein, producing an axonal dying-back mechanism [3, 41, 80]. Another theory is the relative impairment in the glial cell population [81], and both are considered the subject of future DTI in vivo studies.

Another limitation in the co-registration of UHF-MRI and histological techniques is the mismatch between the resolution of the MRI signal (100 µm) and the maximum optical resolution given by the laser confocal systems and fluorescent probe used in our biological preparations (1/2 the wavelength of the excitation light, where YFP = 0.534 microns). Hence, results from a single reconstructed tract from DTI data (Fig. 3a) represents an area of approx. 100-200 axons/voxel (Fig. 3b). Moreover, considering the overall WM axonal sizes (1-20 microns) and the mosaic expression of the YFP tag in this particular

Table 1 Previous Spinal Cord Studies in ALS Using Diffusion Tensor Imaging (DTI)

Research group		Experimental Setup		MRI instrument	ROI	SC Level	Diffusion Coefficients			
Author	Year	Animal Models & Subjects	Cohort				FA	AD	RD	MD
Gatto et al. [28]	2018	B6JL G93A-SOD1 P40 (PS)	G93A-SOD1 WT (n = 5) (Ex-Vivo)	9.4 T Bruker Agilent	WM(ALF) GM	C,D,L	Decrease(WM) Increase(GM)	Decrease(WM) Increase (GM)	Increase(WM) Decrease(GM)	Increased(WM) Decrease(GM)
Fukuri et al. [81]	2017	Clinical	ALS patients (n = 38) Patient controls (n = 8)	3 T Siemens MAGNETROM	WM	C5	Decrease	Not Evaluated	Not Evaluated	Unchanged
Mancuzzo et al. [15]	2017	B6JL G93A-SOD1 P50,P56,P70(PS) & P84,P105,P128 (S)	G93A-SOD1 (n = 7) WT (n = 7) (In-Vivo)	7 T Bruker BioSpec	D,DR,DLV, VR,VL	L	Decrease	Unchanged (PS) Decrease (S)	Unchanged	Decrease
Rasoanandrianina et al. [82]	2017	Clinical	ALS patients (n = 10), Patient controls (n = 20)	3 T Siemens MAGNETROM	WM (CST, PST) GM	C2-C5	Decrease WM	Decrease(WM) Increase (GM)	Increase(WM) Increase(GM)	Not Evaluated
Budrewicz et al. [83]	2016	Clinical	ALS patients (n = 15), Patient controls (n = 10)	1.5 T GE Medical systems	ACST,PCST, LCST, GM	C1-C5	Decrease	Not Evaluated	Not Evaluated	Not Evaluated
Figini et al. [17]	2016	B6JL - G93A-SOD1 P70 (PS) & P119 (S)]	G93A-SOD1 (n = 7) vs WT-SOD1 (n = 7) (In-Vivo)	7 T Bruker BioSpec	VMT, dT, VLT, DLT, GM	L	Decrease	Unchanged (PS) Decrease (S)	Increase	Increase
Caron et al. [46]	2015	129Sv G93A-SOD1 P105,P133,P154 (S) & C57 SOD1-G93A P44 (PS); P105,P133,P154 (S)	C57 G93A-SOD1 (n = 6) 129Sv G93A-SOD1(n = 5) WT (n = 6,5) (In-Vivo) & C57 G93A-SOD1 (n = 16) 129Sv G93A-SOD1(n = 16) WT(n = 16) (Ex-Vivo)	7 T Bruker BioSpec	VMT,VLT,DLT, dT	L	Decrease	Unchanged (PS) Decrease (S)	Increase	Not Evaluated
Iglesias et al. [84]	2015	Clinical	ALS patients (n = 20) Patient controls (n = 19)	3 T Siemens	PMT, CST	C5- D1	Decrease	Unchanged	Increase	Increase
Wang et al. [10]	2014	Clinical	ALS patients (n = 24), Patient controls (n = 16)	1.5 T GE healthcare	ST, LCST	C1-C2	Decrease	Not Evaluated	Not Evaluated	Not Evaluated
Romano et al. [85]	2014	Clinical	ALS patients (n = 14) Patient controls (n = 14)	1.5 T Siemens	CST	C,D,L	Decrease	Unchanged	Increase	Increase
El Mendill et al. [86]	2014	Clinical	ALS patients (n = 14) Patient controls (n = 15)	3 T Siemens Trio	CST	C2 to T6	Decrease	Unchanged	Increase	Increase
Cohen- Adad et al. [87]	2013	Clinical	ALS patients (n = 29) Patient controls (n = 21)	3 T Siemens Trio	PSCT, LSCT	C2 to T2	Decrease	Decrease/ Unchanged	Increase	Not Evaluated
Kim et al. [18]	2011	B6JL G93A-SOD1 P84 (S)	G93A-SOD1 WT (n = 5) (In-Vivo)	4.7 T Oxford Instruments	VLT, dT	C & L	Decrease	Decrease	Increase	Not Evaluated
Underwood et al. [12]	2011	C57 G93A-SOD1 P145 (S)	G93A-SOD1 (n = 6) G93A-SOD1 (n = 6) (In-Vivo)	16.4 T Bruker	DF,VF,VLF, DLF	D12-L1	Decrease	Decrease	Increase	Not Evaluated
Nair et al. [11]	2010	Clinical	ALS patients (n = 14) Patient controls (n = 15)	3 T Siemens Trio	CST	C1-C6	Decrease	Unchanged	Increase	Increase

Table 1 Previous Spinal Cord Studies in ALS Using Diffusion Tensor Imaging (DTI) *(Continued)*

Research group		Experimental Setup					Diffusion Coefficients			
Author	Year	Animal Models & Subjects	Cohort	MRI instrument	ROI	SC Level	FA	AD	RD	MD
Agosta et al. [30]	2009	Clinical	ALS patients (n = 17) Patient controls (n = 20)	1.5 T Siemens Avanto	CST	C2-C3	Decrease	Not Evaluated	Not Evaluated	Increase
Valsalina et al. [88]	2007	Clinical	ALS patients (n = 28) Patient controls (n = 20)	1.5 T Siemens Avanto	CST	C2-C3	Decrease	Not Evaluated	Not Evaluated	Decrease
Rossi et al. [89]	2007	Clinical	ALS patients (n = 1) Patient controls (n = 8)	1.5 T and 3 T Scanner	CST	C	Decrease	Not Evaluated	Not Evaluated	Decrease

Summary of previous studies using DTI to investigate microstructural changes in ALS spinal cord
Abbreviations: *FA* Fractional Anisotropy *SC* Spinal Cord, *C* Cervical segment, *D* Dorsal segment, *L* Lumbar segment, *RD* Radial Diffusion, *AD* Axial Diffusion, *MD* Mean Diffusion, *ROI* Region of interest, *CST* Corticospinal Tracts, *LCST* Lateral Corticospinal Tracts, *PCST* Posterior Corticospinal Tract, *ACST* Anterior Corticospinal Tract, *CMG* Central Grey matter, *ST* Spinothalamic Tract, *PMT* Posterior Medial Tract, *CMG* Central Grey Matter, *ST* Spinothalamic Tracts, *PMT* Posterior Medial Tract, *VMT* Ventromedial Tract, *PS* Presymptomatic, *S* Symptomatic, *dT* Dorsal Tract, *VLT* Ventrolateral Tract, *DLT* Dorsolateral Tract, *DF* Dorsal Funiculi, *VF* Ventral Funiculi, *VLF* Ventrolateral Funiculi, *DLF* Dorsolateral Funiculi.[Source: PubMed. Key words: ALS / DTI /Spinal Cord /Diffusion Tensor imaging]

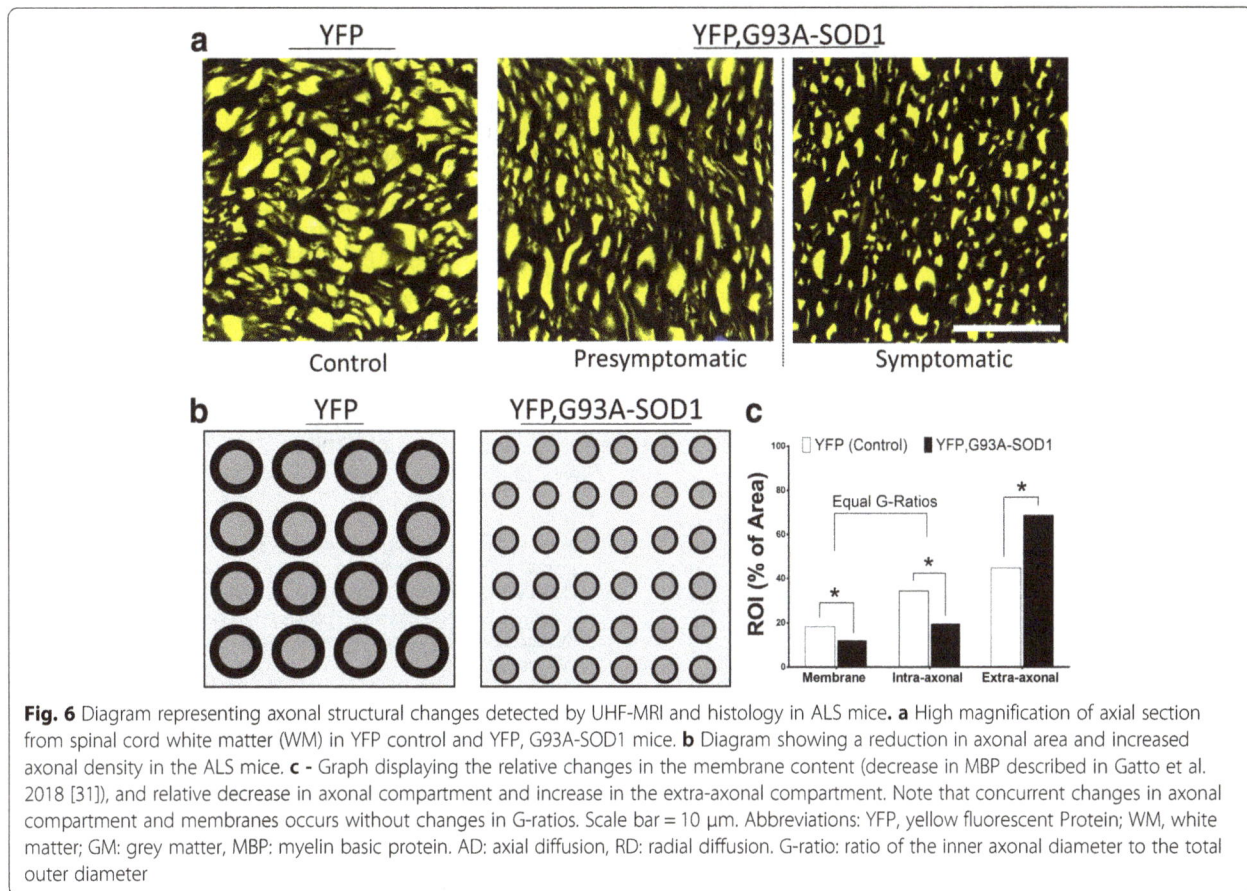

Fig. 6 Diagram representing axonal structural changes detected by UHF-MRI and histology in ALS mice. **a** High magnification of axial section from spinal cord white matter (WM) in YFP control and YFP, G93A-SOD1 mice. **b** Diagram showing a reduction in axonal area and increased axonal density in the ALS mice. **c** - Graph displaying the relative changes in the membrane content (decrease in MBP described in Gatto et al. 2018 [31]), and relative decrease in axonal compartment and increase in the extra-axonal compartment. Note that concurrent changes in axonal compartment and membranes occurs without changes in G-ratios. Scale bar = 10 μm. Abbreviations: YFP, yellow fluorescent Protein; WM, white matter; GM: grey matter, MBP: myelin basic protein. AD: axial diffusion, RD: radial diffusion. G-ratio: ratio of the inner axonal diameter to the total outer diameter

fluorescent animal (only 10-30% of the neuronal population) the current model clearly underrepresent the real number of axonal elements per voxel area (approx. 400-1000 axons/voxel).

Our studies have shown that UHF-MRI and DTI techniques are useful tools to detect early changes in the microstructural features of ALS (Table 2). Yet, our current techniques have some limitations due to the small range of b-values studied. In addition, the involvement of different cell populations as described in this work points towards the existence of an anomalous water diffusion process in a porous biological material marking the need for higher b-values and the use of more complex diffusion models [82–84] to evaluate the complex WM neuroanatomical changes occurring during the development of ALS [23]. Finally, more extensive neurobiological work should be done in order to validate each bioimaging marker during the early stages of this disease.

Conclusions

This work demonstrates that the combination of UHF-MRI and fluorescent mouse reporters is a useful approach to detect and characterize microstructural changes and axonal connectivity anomalies in ALS. Using a transgenic mouse fluorescent reporter, our studies were able to identify changes in axonal size, density and connectivity in the spinal cord of ALS mice before the disease was fully manifest. We found that anomalies in diffusion markers captured by DTI are possibly connected with alterations in cellular and molecular markers observed in our fluorescent ALS mice. We described early WM changes using connectomics as an additional method to evaluate early axonal connectivity anomalies in ALS.

Table 2 Presymptomatic UHF-MRI Diffusion Bioimaging Markers at 17.6T and Histological Findings in ALS Mice Spinal Cord

MRI markers	White Matter Microstructure	Histology/Molecular Markers
FA ↓	Axonal Organization	YFP labeled axons
RD ↑	Myelin Content	MBP ↓*
AD ↓	Axonal Degeneration	YFP labeled axons
EW ↓	Axonal Connectivity	YFP labeled axons
ADC ↑	Transmembrane Water Diffusion	AQP4 ↑↑

Presymptomatic white matter changes in UHF-MRI diffusion can be associated to biological and molecular markers of axonal ultrastructure & connectivity and other cellular compartments

Abbreviations: *ALS* Amyotrophic lateral Sclerosis, *WM* White matter, *ADC* Apparent diffusion coefficient, *RD* Radial Diffusivity, *AD* Axial diffusivity, *FA* Fractional Anisotropy, *EW* Edge Weight, *AQP4* Aquaporin 4, *MBP* Myelin Basic Protein, *YFP* Yellow fluorescent Protein. (* Presymptomatic changes in MBP seen in Gatto et al. 2018 [28])

We believe this investigation is a step in the characterization of early bioimaging markers to detect and eventually monitor future treatments in patients with ALS.

Abbreviations

AD: Axial diffusion; ALS: Amyotrophic lateral Sclerosis; AQP4: Aquaporin 4; DTI: Diffusion Tensor Imaging; FA: Fractional anisotropy; G93A-SOD1: transgenic mice with the overexpression of human mutant gene copper zinc superoxide dismutase identified in familiar forms of ALS patients; GM: Grey matter; G-ratio: ratio of the inner axonal diameter to the total outer diameter; RD: Radial diffusion; SC: Spinal Cord; UHF-MRI: Ultra-High Field MRI; WE: Weight edge connectomics; WM: White matter

Acknowledgements

We would like to especially acknowledge Dr. Gerardo Morfini for providing chemicals and materials used in our experiments and Ehsan Tavassoli for proofreading the manuscript.

Funding

This study was supported in part by a Chicago Biomedical Consortium (CBC) postdoctoral fellowship grant (Award #085740) to RG at the University of Illinois in Chicago. Data collection was supported by the Magnetic Laboratory Visiting Scientist Program (Award VSP #278) of the National High Magnetic Field Laboratory (NHMFL) and Advanced Magnetic Resonance Imaging and Spectroscopy (AMRIS) to RG. A portion of this work was performed in the McKnight Brain Institute at the National High.

Authors' contributions

RG conceived and designed the experiments. RG performed all the animal tissue collection, histology experiments and data analysis. RG and MA performed all the MRI imaging experiments. RG and RM wrote the manuscript. Algorithms of axonal connectivity described in the manuscript has been implemented by MA and developed by TM at of the University of Florida. DD and MH processed and compiled all the connectomics data. All authors read and approved the final manuscript.

Competing interests

The authors declare that they have no competing interests.

Author details

[1]Department of Anatomy and Cell Biology, University of Illinois at Chicago, 808 S. Wood St. Rm 578 M/C 512, Chicago, IL 60612, USA. [2]Department of Physics, University of Florida, Gainesville, FL, USA. [3]Department of Applied Physiology and Kinesiology, University of Florida, Gainesville, FL, USA. [4]Department of Biochemistry and Molecular Biology, University of Florida, Gainesville, FL, USA. [5]Department of Bioengineering, University of Illinois at Chicago, Chicago, IL, USA.

References

1. Mehta P, Antao V, Kaye W, Sanchez M, Williamson D, Bryan L, Muravov O, Horton K, Division of T, Human Health Sciences AfTS, et al. Prevalence of amyotrophic lateral sclerosis - United States, 2010-2011. MMWR Suppl. 2014;63:1–14.
2. de Oliveira GP, Alves CJ, Chadi G. Early gene expression changes in spinal cord from SOD1(G93A) Amyotrophic Lateral Sclerosis animal model. Front Cell Neurosci. 2013;7:216.
3. Morfini GA, Bosco DA, Brown H, Gatto R, Kaminska A, Song Y, Molla L, Baker L, Marangoni MN, Berth S, et al. Inhibition of fast axonal transport by pathogenic SOD1 involves activation of p38 MAP kinase. PLoS One. 2013;8:e65235.
4. Gurney ME, Pu H, Chiu AY, Dal Canto MC, Polchow CY, Alexander DD, Caliendo J, Hentati A, Kwon YW, Deng HX, et al. Motor neuron degeneration in mice that express a human Cu,Zn superoxide dismutase mutation. Science. 1994;264:1772–5.
5. Fogarty MJ, Klenowski PM, Lee JD, Drieberg-Thompson JR, Bartlett SE, Ngo ST, Hilliard MA, Bellingham MC, Noakes PG. Cortical synaptic and dendritic spine abnormalities in a presymptomatic TDP-43 model of amyotrophic lateral sclerosis. Sci Rep. 2016;6:37968.
6. Liu Y, Pattamatta A, Zu T, Reid T, Bardhi O, Borchelt DR, Yachnis AT, Ranum LP. C9orf72 BAC Mouse Model with Motor Deficits and Neurodegenerative Features of ALS/FTD. Neuron. 2016;90:521–34.
7. Nolan M, Talbot K, Ansorge O. Pathogenesis of FUS-associated ALS and FTD: insights from rodent models. Acta Neuropathol Commun. 2016;4:99.
8. Oglesby E, Quigley HA, Zack DJ, Cone FE, Steinhart MR, Tian J, Pease ME, Kalesnykas G. Semi-automated, quantitative analysis of retinal ganglion cell morphology in mice selectively expressing yellow fluorescent protein. Exp Eye Res. 2012;96:107–15.
9. Bannerman PG, Hahn A. Enhanced visualization of axonopathy in EAE using thy1-YFP transgenic mice. J Neurol Sci. 2007;260:23–32.
10. Gatto RG, Chu Y, Ye AQ, Price SD, Tavassoli E, Buenaventura A, Brady ST, Magin RL, Kordower JH, Morfini GA. Analysis of YFP(J16)-R6/2 reporter mice and postmortem brains reveals early pathology and increased vulnerability of callosal axons in Huntington's disease. Hum Mol Genet. 2015;24:5285–98.
11. Porrero C, Rubio-Garrido P, Avendano C, Clasca F. Mapping of fluorescent protein-expressing neurons and axon pathways in adult and developing Thy1-eYFP-H transgenic mice. Brain Res. 2010;1345:59–72.
12. King AE, Blizzard CA, Southam KA, Vickers JC, Dickson TC. Degeneration of axons in spinal white matter in G93A mSOD1 mouse characterized by NFL and alpha-internexin immunoreactivity. Brain Res. 2012;1465:90–100.
13. Wang Y, Liu L, Ma L, Huang X, Lou X, Wang Y, Wu N, Liu T, Guo X. Preliminary study on cervical spinal cord in patients with amyotrophic lateral sclerosis using MR diffusion tensor imaging. Acad Radiol. 2014;21:590–6.
14. Nair G, Carew JD, Usher S, Lu D, Hu XP, Benatar M. Diffusion tensor imaging reveals regional differences in the cervical spinal cord in amyotrophic lateral sclerosis. Neuroimage. 2010;53:576–83.
15. Underwood CK, Kurniawan ND, Butler TJ, Cowin GJ, Wallace RH. Non-invasive diffusion tensor imaging detects white matter degeneration in the spinal cord of a mouse model of amyotrophic lateral sclerosis. Neuroimage. 2011;55:455–61.
16. Evans MC, Serres S, Khrapitchev AA, Stolp HB, Anthony DC, Talbot K, Turner MR, Sibson NR. T(2)-weighted MRI detects presymptomatic pathology in the SOD1 mouse model of ALS. J Cereb Blood Flow Metab. 2014;34:785–93.
17. Ong HH, Wehrli FW. Quantifying axon diameter and intra-cellular volume fraction in excised mouse spinal cord with q-space imaging. Neuroimage. 2010;51:1360–6.
18. Marcuzzo S, Bonanno S, Figini M, Scotti A, Zucca I, Minati L, Riva N, Domi T, Fossaghi A, Quattrini A, et al. A longitudinal DTI and histological study of the spinal cord reveals early pathological alterations in G93A-SOD1 mouse model of amyotrophic lateral sclerosis. Exp Neurol. 2017;293:43–52.
19. Boillee S, Vande Velde C, Cleveland DW. ALS: a disease of motor neurons and their nonneuronal neighbors. Neuron. 2006;52:39–59.
20. Figini M, Scotti A, Marcuzzo S, Bonanno S, Padelli F, Moreno-Manzano V, Garcia-Verdugo JM, Bernasconi P, Mantegazza R, Bruzzone MG, Zucca I. Comparison of Diffusion MRI Acquisition Protocols for the In Vivo Characterization of the Mouse Spinal Cord: Variability Analysis and Application to an Amyotrophic Lateral Sclerosis Model. PLoS One. 2016;11:e0161646.

21. Kim JH, Wu TH, Budde MD, Lee JM, Song SK. Noninvasive detection of brainstem and spinal cord axonal degeneration in an amyotrophic lateral sclerosis mouse model. NMR Biomed. 2011;24:163–9.

22. Ozdinler PH, Benn S, Yamamoto TH, Guzel M, Brown RH Jr, Macklis JD. Corticospinal motor neurons and related subcerebral projection neurons undergo early and specific neurodegeneration in hSOD1G(9)(3)A transgenic ALS mice. J Neurosci. 2011;31:4166–77.

23. Saberi S, Stauffer JE, Schulte DJ, Ravits J. Neuropathology of Amyotrophic Lateral Sclerosis and Its Variants. Neurol Clin. 2015;33:855–76.

24. Heiman-Patterson TD, Deitch JS, Blankenhorn EP, Erwin KL, Perreault MJ, Alexander BK, Byers N, Toman I, Alexander GM. Background and gender effects on survival in the TgN(SOD1-G93A)1Gur mouse model of ALS. J Neurol Sci. 2005;236:1–7.

25. Durand J, Amendola J, Bories C, Lamotte d'Incamps B. Early abnormalities in transgenic mouse models of amyotrophic lateral sclerosis. J Physiol Paris. 2006;99:211–20.

26. Colon-Perez LM, Spindler C, Goicochea S, Triplett W, Parekh M, Montie E, Carney PR, Price C, Mareci TH. Dimensionless, Scale Invariant, Edge Weight Metric for the Study of Complex Structural Networks. PLoS One. 2015;10:e0131493.

27. Jones DK. The effect of gradient sampling schemes on measures derived from diffusion tensor MRI: a Monte Carlo study. Magn Reson Med. 2004;51:807–15.

28. Jenkinson M, Beckmann CF, Behrens TE, Woolrich MW, Smith SM. Fsl. Neuroimage. 2012;62:782–90.

29. Basser PJ, Mattiello J, LeBihan D. MR diffusion tensor spectroscopy and imaging. Biophys J. 1994;66:259–67.

30. Callaghan P, Eccles CD, Xia Y. NMR microscopy of dynamic displacements: k-space and q-space imaging. Journal of Physics E: Scientific Instruments. 1988;21:820–2.

31. Gatto RG, Li W, Magin RL. Diffusion tensor imaging identifies presymptomatic axonal degeneration in the spinal cord of ALS mice. Brain Res. 2018;1679:7.

32. Tallon C, Russell KA, Sakhalkar S, Andrapallayal N, Farah MH. Length-dependent axo-terminal degeneration at the neuromuscular synapses of type II muscle in SOD1 mice. Neuroscience. 2015;312:179–89.

33. Agosta F, Rocca MA, Valsasina P, Sala S, Caputo D, Perini M, Salvi F, Prelle A, Filippi M. A longitudinal diffusion tensor MRI study of the cervical cord and brain in amyotrophic lateral sclerosis patients. J Neurol Neurosurg Psychiatry. 2009;80:53–5.

34. Watson CP, G.; Kayalioglu, G.: The Spinal Cord : A Christopher and Dana Reeve Foundation Text and Atlas. 1st Edition edn. London: Academic Press 2008; 2008.

35. Preti MG, Bolton TA, Van De Ville D. The dynamic functional connectome: State-of-the-art and perspectives. Neuroimage. 2016;160:41–54.

36. Colon-Perez LM, Couret M, Triplett W, Price CC, Mareci TH. Small Worldness in Dense and Weighted Connectomes. Front Phys. 2016;4

37. Niessen HG, Angenstein F, Sander K, Kunz WS, Teuchert M, Ludolph AC, Heinze HJ, Scheich H, Vielhaber S. In vivo quantification of spinal and bulbar motor neuron degeneration in the G93A-SOD1 transgenic mouse model of ALS by T2 relaxation time and apparent diffusion coefficient. Exp Neurol. 2006;201:293–300.

38. Ye AQ, Hubbard Cristinacce PL, Zhou FL, Yin Z, Parker GJ, Magin RL. Diffusion tensor MRI phantom exhibits anomalous diffusion. Conf Proc IEEE Eng Med Biol Soc. 2014;2014:746–9.

39. Nilsson M, Latt J, van Westen D, Brockstedt S, Lasic S, Stahlberg F, Topgaard D. Noninvasive mapping of water diffusional exchange in the human brain using filter-exchange imaging. Magn Reson Med. 2013;69:1573–81.

40. Agre P. The aquaporin water channels. Proc Am Thorac Soc. 2006;3:5–13.

41. Fischer LR, Culver DG, Tennant P, Davis AA, Wang M, Castellano-Sanchez A, Khan J, Polak MA, Glass JD. Amyotrophic lateral sclerosis is a distal axonopathy: evidence in mice and man. Exp Neurol. 2004;185:232–40.

42. Kawamura Y, Dyck PJ, Shimono M, Okazaki H, Tateishi J, Doi H. Morphometric comparison of the vulnerability of peripheral motor and sensory neurons in amyotrophic lateral sclerosis. J Neuropathol Exp Neurol. 1981;40:667–75.

43. Bradley WG, Good P, Rasool CG, Adelman LS. Morphometric and biochemical studies of peripheral nerves in amyotrophic lateral sclerosis. Ann Neurol. 1983;14:267–77.

44. Hammad M, Silva A, Glass J, Sladky JT, Benatar M. Clinical, electrophysiologic, and pathologic evidence for sensory abnormalities in ALS. Neurology. 2007;69:2236–42.

45. Murmu RP, Li W, Holtmaat A, Li JY. Dendritic spine instability leads to progressive neocortical spine loss in a mouse model of Huntington's disease. J Neurosci. 2013;33:12997–3009.

46. Brennan FH, Cowin GJ, Kurniawan ND, Ruitenberg MJ. Longitudinal assessment of white matter pathology in the injured mouse spinal cord through ultra-high field (16.4 T) in vivo diffusion tensor imaging. Neuroimage. 2013;82:574–85.

47. Kamagata K, Kerever A, Yokosawa S, Otake Y, Ochi H, Hori M, Kamiya K, Tsuruta K, Tagawa K, Okazawa H, et al. Quantitative Histological Validation of Diffusion Tensor MRI with Two-Photon Microscopy of Cleared Mouse Brain. Magn Reson Med Sci. 2016;15:416–21.

48. Caron I, Micotti E, Paladini A, Merlino G, Plebani L, Forloni G, Modo M, Bendotti C. Comparative Magnetic Resonance Imaging and Histopathological Correlates in Two SOD1 Transgenic Mouse Models of Amyotrophic Lateral Sclerosis. PLoS One. 2015;10:e0132159.

49. El Mendili MM, Cohen-Adad J, Pelegrini-Issac M, Rossignol S, Morizot-Koutlidis R, Marchand-Pauvert V, Iglesias C, Sangari S, Katz R, Lehericy S, et al. Multi-parametric spinal cord MRI as potential progression marker in amyotrophic lateral sclerosis. PLoS One. 2014;9:e95516.

50. Cohen-Adad J, El Mendili MM, Morizot-Koutlidis R, Lehericy S, Meininger V, Blancho S, Rossignol S, Benali H, Pradat PF. Involvement of spinal sensory pathway in ALS and specificity of cord atrophy to lower motor neuron degeneration. Amyotroph Lateral Scler Frontotemporal Degener. 2013;14:30–8.

51. Valsasina P, Agosta F, Benedetti B, Caputo D, Perini M, Salvi F, Prelle A, Filippi M. Diffusion anisotropy of the cervical cord is strictly associated with disability in amyotrophic lateral sclerosis. J Neurol Neurosurg Psychiatry. 2007;78:480–4.

52. Rossi C, Boss A, Lindig TM, Martirosian P, Steidle G, Maetzler W, Claussen CD, Klose U, Schick F. Diffusion tensor imaging of the spinal cord at 1.5 and 3.0 Tesla. Rofo. 2007;179:219–24.

53. Behr VC, Weber T, Neuberger T, Vroemen M, Weidner N, Bogdahn U, Haase A, Jakob PM, Faber C. High-resolution MR imaging of the rat spinal cord in vivo in a wide-bore magnet at 17.6 Tesla. MAGMA. 2004;17:353–8.

54. Pallebage-Gamarallage M, Foxley S, Menke RAL, Huszar IN, Jenkinson M, Tendler BC, Wang C, Jbabdi S, Turner MR, Miller KL, Ansorge O. Dissecting the pathobiology of altered MRI signal in amyotrophic lateral sclerosis: A post mortem whole brain sampling strategy for the integration of ultra-high-field MRI and quantitative neuropathology. BMC Neurosci. 2018;19:11.

55. Shang Y, Huang EJ. Mechanisms of FUS mutations in familial amyotrophic lateral sclerosis. Brain Res. 2016;1647:65–78.

56. Sharma A, Lyashchenko AK, Lu L, Nasrabady SE, Elmaleh M, Mendelsohn M, Nemes A, Tapia JC, Mentis GZ, Shneider NA. ALS-associated mutant FUS induces selective motor neuron degeneration through toxic gain of function. Nat Commun. 2016;7:10465.

57. Agosta F, Pagani E, Petrolini M, Caputo D, Perini M, Prelle A, Salvi F, Filippi M. Assessment of white matter tract damage in patients with amyotrophic lateral sclerosis: a diffusion tensor MR imaging tractography study. AJNR Am J Neuroradiol. 2010;31:1457–61.

58. Iwata NK, Aoki S, Okabe S, Arai N, Terao Y, Kwak S, Abe O, Kanazawa I, Tsuji S, Ugawa Y. Evaluation of corticospinal tracts in ALS with diffusion tensor MRI and brainstem stimulation. Neurology. 2008;70:528–32.

59. Steinbach R, Loewe K, Kaufmann J, Machts J, Kollewe K, Petri S, Dengler R, Heinze HJ, Vielhaber S, Schoenfeld MA, Stoppel CM. Structural hallmarks of amyotrophic lateral sclerosis progression revealed by probabilistic fiber tractography. J Neurol. 2015;262:2257–70.

60. Campbell JS, Pike GB. Potential and limitations of diffusion MRI tractography for the study of language. Brain Lang. 2014;131:65–73.

61. Thomas C, Ye FQ, Irfanoglu MO, Modi P, Saleem KS, Leopold DA, Pierpaoli C. Anatomical accuracy of brain connections derived from diffusion MRI tractography is inherently limited. Proc Natl Acad Sci U S A. 2014;111:16574–9.

62. Daducci A, Dal Palu A, Descoteaux M, Thiran JP. Microstructure Informed Tractography: Pitfalls and Open Challenges. Front Neurosci. 2016;10:247.

63. Mukherjee P, Chung SW, Berman JI, Hess CP, Henry RG. Diffusion tensor MR imaging and fiber tractography: technical considerations. AJNR Am J Neuroradiol. 2008;29:843–52.

64. Sotiropoulos SN, Zalesky A. Building connectomes using diffusion MRI: why, how and but. NMR Biomed. 2017;

65. Wijesekera LC, Leigh PN. Amyotrophic lateral sclerosis. Orphanet J Rare Dis. 2009;4:3.

66. Obata T, Kershaw J, Kuroiwa, D.; Shibata, S.; , Yoichiro, A.; , Yasui, M.; Aoki I: Effect of Cell Membrane Water Permeability on Diffusion-Weighted MR Signal: A Study Using Expression-Controlled Aquaporin4 Cells. In

International Society for Magnetic Resonance in Medicine 20th Annual Meeting Melbourne, Australia. Proc. Intl. Soc. Mag. Reson. Med; 2012: 1830.

67. Mukherjee A, Wu D, Davis HC, Shapiro MG. Non-invasive imaging using reporter genes altering cellular water permeability. Nat Commun. 2016;7:13891.

68. Beaulieu C. The basis of anisotropic water diffusion in the nervous system - a technical review. NMR Biomed. 2002;15:435–55.

69. Amiry-Moghaddam M, Ottersen OP. The molecular basis of water transport in the brain. Nat Rev Neurosci. 2003;4:991–1001.

70. Foglio E, Rodella LF. Aquaporins and neurodegenerative diseases. Curr Neuropharmacol. 2010;8:112–21.

71. Oklinski MK, Skowronski MT, Skowronska A, Rutzler M, Norgaard K, Nieland JD, Kwon TH, Nielsen S. Aquaporins in the Spinal Cord. Int J Mol Sci. 2016;17:2050.

72. Vitellaro-Zuccarello L, Mazzetti S, Bosisio P, Monti C, De Biasi S. Distribution of Aquaporin 4 in rodent spinal cord: relationship with astrocyte markers and chondroitin sulfate proteoglycans. Glia. 2005;51:148–59.

73. Oshio K, Binder DK, Yang B, Schecter S, Verkman AS, Manley GT. Expression of aquaporin water channels in mouse spinal cord. Neuroscience. 2004;127:685–93.

74. Nicaise C, Soyfoo MS, Authelet M, De Decker R, Bataveljic D, Delporte C, Pochet R. Aquaporin-4 overexpression in rat ALS model. Anat Rec (Hoboken). 2009;292:207–13.

75. Dai J, Lin W, Zheng M, Liu Q, He B, Luo C, Lu X, Pei Z, Su H, Yao X. Alterations in AQP4 expression and polarization in the course of motor neuron degeneration in SOD1G93A mice. Mol Med Rep. 2017;16:1739–46.

76. Bataveljic D, Nikolic L, Milosevic M, Todorovic N, Andjus PR. Changes in the astrocytic aquaporin-4 and inwardly rectifying potassium channel expression in the brain of the amyotrophic lateral sclerosis SOD1(G93A) rat model. Glia. 2012;60:1991–2003.

77. de Albuquerque M, Branco LM, Rezende TJ, de Andrade HM, Nucci A, Franca MC Jr. Longitudinal evaluation of cerebral and spinal cord damage in Amyotrophic Lateral Sclerosis. Neuroimage Clin. 2017;14:269–76.

78. Grolez G, Kyheng M, Lopes R, Moreau C, Timmerman K, Auger F, Kuchcinski G, Duhamel A, Jissendi-Tchofo P, Besson P, et al. MRI of the cervical spinal cord predicts respiratory dysfunction in ALS. Sci Rep. 2018;8:1828.

79. Benitez A, Jensen JH, Helpern JA. Axonal Density and Myelin Integrity in Cognitice Decline: A diffusional Kurtosis Imaging Study. In: Alzheimer's Association International Conference; July 17, vol. 2017. London: Alzheimer & Dementia; 2018. p. P774–5.

80. Dadon-Nachum M, Melamed E, Offen D. The "dying-back" phenomenon of motor neurons in ALS. J Mol Neurosci. 2011;43:470–7.

81. Lasiene J, Yamanaka K. Glial cells in amyotrophic lateral sclerosis. Neurol Res Int. 2011;2011:718987.

82. Liang Y, Ye AQ, Chen W, Gatto RG, Colon-Perez L, Mareci TH, Magin RL. A fractal derivative model for the characterization of anomalous diffusion in magnetic resonance imaging. Commun Nonlinear Sci Numer Simul. 2016;39:529–37.

83. Magin RL, Akpa BS, Neuberger T, Webb AG. Fractional Order Analysis of Sephadex Gel Structures: NMR Measurements Reflecting Anomalous Diffusion. Commun Nonlinear Sci Numer Simul. 2011;16:4581–7.

84. Magin RL, Ingo C, Colon-Perez L, Triplett W, Mareci TH. Characterization of Anomalous Diffusion in Porous Biological Tissues Using Fractional Order Derivatives and Entropy. Microporous Mesoporous Mater. 2013;178:39–43.

85. Fukui Y, Hishikawa N, Sato K, Nakano Y, Morihara R, Shang J, Takemoto M, Ohta Y, Yamashita T, Abe K. Detecting spinal pyramidal tract of amyotrophic lateral sclerosis patients with diffusion tensor tractography. Neurosci Res. 2017;

86. Rasoanandrianina H, Grapperon AM, Taso M, Girard OM, Duhamel G, Guye M, Ranjeva JP, Attarian S, Verschueren A, Callot V. Region-specific impairment of the cervical spinal cord (SC) in amyotrophic lateral sclerosis: A preliminary study using SC templates and quantitative MRI (diffusion tensor imaging/inhomogeneous magnetization transfer). NMR Biomed. 2017;30

87. Budrewicz S, Szewczyk P, Bladowska J, Podemski R, Koziorowska-Gawron E, Ejma M, Slotwinski K, Koszewicz M. The possible meaning of fractional anisotropy measurement of the cervical spinal cord in correct diagnosis of amyotrophic lateral sclerosis. Neurol Sci. 2016;37:417–21.

88. Iglesias C, Sangari S, El Mendili MM, Benali H, Marchand-Pauvert V, Pradat PF. Electrophysiological and spinal imaging evidences for sensory dysfunction in amyotrophic lateral sclerosis. BMJ Open. 2015;5:e007659.

89. Romano A, Guo J, Prokscha T, Meyer T, Hirsch S, Braun J, Sack I, Scheel M. In vivo waveguide elastography: effects of neurodegeneration in patients with amyotrophic lateral sclerosis. Magn Reson Med. 2014;72:1755–61.

22

Nicorandil potentiates sodium butyrate induced preconditioning of neurons and enhances their survival upon subsequent treatment with H_2O_2

Parisa Tabeshmehr[1,2], Haider Kh Husnain[3], Mahin Salmannejad[4], Mahsa Sani[4], Seyed Mojtaba Hosseini[1,2,4*] and Mohammad Hossein Khorraminejad Shirazi[1,2]

Abstract

Background: Extensive loss of donor neural stem cell (NSCs) due to ischemic stress and low rate of differentiation at the site of cell graft are two of the major issues that hamper optimal outcome in NSCs transplantation studies. Given that histone deacetylases (HDACs) modulate various cellular processes by deacetylating histones and non-histone proteins, we hypothesized that combined treatment with small molecules, sodium butyrate (NaB; a known HDAC inhibitor) and nicorandil, will enhance the rate neuronal differentiation of NSCs besides their preconditioning to resist oxidative stress.

Methods: NSCs derived from 14-day old Sprague Dawley rat ganglion eminence were characterized for tri-lineage differentiation. Treatment with 1 mM NaB significantly changed their culture characteristics while continuous treatment for 10 days enhanced their neural differentiation. NaB treatment also preconditioned the cells for their resistance to oxidative stress.

Results: The highest rate of neural differentiation and preconditioning effect was achieved when the NSCs were treated concomitantly with NaB and nicorandil. Cell proliferation assay showed that concomitant treatment with NaB and nicorandil retarded their rate of proliferation.

Conclusion: These data conclude that preconditioning of NSCs with NaB and nicorandil effectively enhances their differentiation capacity besides preconditioning the cells to support their survival under ischemic conditions.

Keywords: Apoptosis, Neural stem cells, Oxidative stress, Preconditioning

Background

Neural stem cells (NSCs) isolated from the adult and fetal nervous tissue, have been extensively studied for tri-lineage differentiation potential including neurons, oligodendrocytes and astrocytes in vitro as well as post-engraftment in experimental animal models [1]. One of the major problems during the experimental animal studies is the extensive apoptosis of donor NSCs post-engraftment due to the ischemic stress. It might also be the consequence of nutrient deprivation and oxidative load caused by the free radicals [2]. Regardless of the underlying cause, the altered oxidative load remains a significant determinant of the cell fate and function. The biochemical cues and inflammatory response emanating from the ischemic tissue activate redox-sensitive signaling pathways in the cells thus lowering the oxidative load to favor cell proliferation [3]. These molecular changes activate PI3K/Akt signaling via oxidative inactivation of PTEN thus promoting cell proliferation. On the contrary, as the concentration of reactive oxygen species (ROS) increases in the cells, the intracellular environment becomes more conducive for differentiation instead of supporting cell proliferation. This molecular

* Correspondence: hoseini2010m@gmail.com
[1]Student Research Committee, Shiraz University of Medical Sciences, Shiraz, Iran
[2]Cell & Molecular Medicine Student Research Group, Medical Faculty, Shiraz University of Medical Sciences, Shiraz, Iran
Full list of author information is available at the end of the article

mechanism holds true for both neural progenitor cells and glial precursor cells [4].

Histone deacetylases (HDACs) are modulators of gene expression profile and thus influence the various intracellular processes encompassing from survival to differentiation by deacetylating both histone and non-histone proteins [5]. Hence, treatment of NSCs with small molecule HDAC inhibitors (HDACi) exerts neuroprotective effects and stimulates neurogenesis [6, 7]. A series of small molecules including valproic acid (VPA), sub-eroylanilidec hydroxamic acids (SAHA), benzamide (MS-275), M344 and the short-chain fatty acid sodium butyrate (NaB) have been studied to modulate neural differentiation of stem cells [5, 8]. HDACi treatment of NSCs under pro-proliferation culture conditions leads to long-term changes in the cell fate in vitro by different mechanisms including inhibition of DNA synthesis [9] and by G1-phase arrest of the cell cycle [5]. HDACi also promote transcriptional changes in NSCs by increasing Cdk inhibitor genes p21 and p27 transcription and elevated H3K9 acetylation at proximal promoter regions of p21 and p27 [5].

Apurinic pyrimidinic endonuclease-1/Redox effector factor-1 (APE-1/Ref-1) is crucial for cellular response to oxidative stress [10]. This is achieved by N-terminus lysine reaction with the nucleic acids and nucleophosmin besides base excision repair through C-terminus initiating enzymatic activity. The anti-apoptotic function of APE1 under oxidative stress has been confirmed via activation of nuclear factor-kappa B (NF-kB) signaling [11, 12]. Nicorandil is a stimulator of the APE1 pathway in the neurons subjected to oxidative stress [13, 14]. The present study was designed to determine the combined protective effect of NaB and nicorandil on NSCs under oxidative stress. We hypothesized that serial treatment of NSCs with NaB (HDACi) followed by nicorandil (as the APE1 stimulator) would promote neuronal differentiation of NSCs that would be preconditioned to resist oxidative stress.

Methods

The present study conformed to the Guideline for the Care and Use of Laboratory Animals and all the experimental animal procedures were performed strictly in accordance with protocol approved by Ethical Committee of Shiraz University of Medical Sciences, Iran. All surgical manipulations were carried out under general anesthesia. The results shown in the manuscript are replicate of five experiments."

NSCs isolation and culture

NSCs were obtained from 14-day old Sprague Dawley rat ganglion eminence as described earlier (Additional file 1).

One week after isolation, sphere-like colonies of neurospheres were observed that were trypsinized as single cells and passaged into new culture flasks at 50000 cells/ml concentration (Additional file 1).

Characterization of NSCs

NSCs were characterized for tri-lineage differentiation into neurons, astrocytes and oligodendrocytes as described earlier (Additional file 1).

Preconditioning with histone deacetylase inhibitor

For the differentiation NSCs using HDACi alone, the cells were treated with freshly prepared 1 mM NaB in distilled water (Cat# B5887, Sigma Aldrich, St. Louis, USA). NaB treatment was performed at 2 h after NSCs passage as single cell culture. Neural differentiation of NSCs was assessed by flow cytometry and immunocytochemistry on day-7 after NaB treatment.

For flow cytometry, the cells were fixed with 4% paraformaldehyde for 20 min at 4 °C. Subsequently, the cells were incubated with MAP-2 specific primary antibody (1:1000, cat # ab5392, Abcam, Cambridge, UK) at room temperature. After one hour, the cells were washed with phosphate buffer saline (PBS) and the primary antigen-antibody reaction was detected by incubating the cells for 1 h at room temperature with fluorescently conjugated secondary antibody diluted in 5% goat serum. The MAP-2 positive cells were analyzed by flow cytometry (BD Bioscience, San Jose, USA). For microscopic analysis of MAP-2 positive cells, the cells were stained with 4′,6-diamidino-2-phenylindole (DAPI; 1:1000; Millipore S7113, Billerica, USA) and observed using fluorescence microscope (Olympus BX53; Tokyo, Japan). The MAP-2 positive neurons were counted in various microscopic fields and compared with the untreated control group.

Cell cluster and neurosphere count

The NSCs derived cell clusters and neurospheres were counted as described earlier [5]. One week after HDACi treatment, 10 randomly selected microscopic fields were counted using an inverted microscope (Olympus; Tokyo, Japan). The inclusion criteria was set as small cell cluster an aggregation of cell count > 4 cells but cell aggregation diameter of < 50 μm. For neurospheres, the diameter was set as more than 50 μm. The number of small cell clusters and neurospheres were compared with the control group [5].

Cell proliferation assay

5-Bromo-2′-deoxyuridine (BrdU) immunocytochemistry was performed to assess NSCs proliferation after NaB treatment. In brief, after NaB treatment, 1×10^5 cells in 96-well plates were incubated with 25 μM BrdU (Cat #B5002; Sigma-Aldrich; St.Louis, USA). After 16 h, the cells were washed and fixed with 4% paraformaldehyde for 20 min at 4 °C and later treated with 1 N HCl for 15 min at 37 °C. Subsequently, the cells were incubated with anti-BrdU specific primary antibody (Cat# B8434; 1:1000; Sigma-Aldrich; St. Louis, USA) in 0.1% triton and 2.5% BSA in PBS. The cells were kept at room temperature for 2 h followed by washing ×3 with PBS. The primary antigen-antibody reaction was detected with the Alexa flour-488 conjugated secondary antibody. The cells were incubated with the secondary antibody at 37 °C for 1 h, washed and observed using fluorescence microscope (Olympus BX53; Tokyo, Japan). Cell proliferation was measured by BrdU+/total number of cells in NaB treated group.

The data was analyzed by unpaired t-test using Prism 8.00 software.

Treatment with nicorandil

To determine the activation of the APE1 pathway, 12.5 µM nicorandil was added to the cells as described earlier [14].

Induction of apoptosis using H_2O_2

For induction of apoptosis, 500 µM H_2O_2 was added to the culture media for one hour at one hour after nicorandil treatment [15].

MTT assay

The viability of the preconditioned and control cells were assessed by MTT assay at 24 h after their exposure to H_2O_2. Briefly, NSCs culture media in different treatment groups was supplemented with 10 µl of 5 mg/ml 3-(4,5-Dimethyl-2-thiazolyl)-2,5-diphenyl-2H-tetrazolium bromide (MTT) (Cat# M2128; Sigma-Aldrich; St. Louis, USA). The cells were then incubated at 37 °C for 4 h. At the end of the incubation period, the medium was removed, treated with acidic isopropanol (0.1 N HCl in isopropanol) and the samples were read using spectrophotometer at wavelength 570 nm [16]. The survival of the cells in control group (which was exposed to H_2O_2 without small molecule treatment) was considered as 100% and the other treatment groups were compared with the control. In accordance with the calculations, group survival of

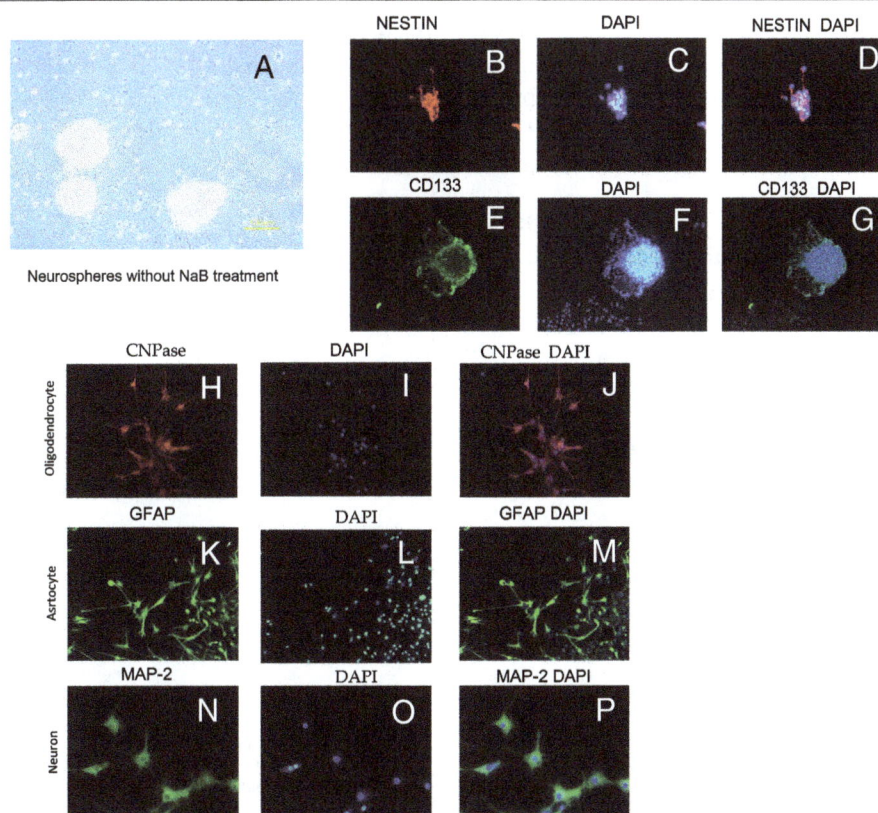

Fig. 1 Neural stem cell culture and characterization. **a** Phase contrast image of neural stem cells (NSCs) derived aggregates of neurospheres after 5–7 days of in vitro culture in NuroCult NS-A medium. The cells were maintained at 37 °C and 5%CO$_2$ culture conditions. Immunocytochemistry of NSCs for CD133 (**b-d**) and Nestin expression (**e-g**) using specific antibodies for the respective antigen. Differentiation of NSCs to oligodendrocyte and astrocyte was assessed by immunostaining for CNPase (Oligodendrocytes specific marker; **h-j**) and GFAP (astrocytes specific marker; **k-m**) expression using specific antibodies for the respective antigen. The cells were subjected to tri-lineage differentiation assay in vitro. (**n-p**) The neural differentiation of NSCs was confirmed by MAP-2 antibody staining

more than 100% represents the treatment as protective against H_2O_2 stress.

Annexin-V staining and flow cytometry

The resistance of the HDACi induced neurons to H_2O_2 treatment was assessed by flow cytometry using Annexin-V Apoptosis detection kit in combination with propidium iodide (PI) according to manufacturer's instructions (Cat# 14085; Abcam; Cambridge, UK). Briefly, 5×10^5 cells with or without HDACi treatment were incubated with Annexin V-FITC/PI for 1 h at room temperature. After washing ×3 with PBS, the cells were harvested using Trypsin-EDTA. After washing ×2 with PBS, the cells were analyzed by flow cytometry (BD Bioscience, San Jose, USA) in FITC channel (488). The cells were stained with PI to discriminate the necrotic cells from the apoptotic cells and measured by flow cytometry. The apoptotic cells were defined as the ones staining positive for Annexin-V.

Colorimetric analysis and immunocytochemistry for caspase-3

The activity of caspase-3 was measured using caspase-3 Assay kit (Cat# ab39401; Abcam, Cambridge, USA) according to the manufacturer's instructions. Immunocytochemistry for caspase 3 was performed with anti-caspase-3 antibody (Cat# MAB10753; Sigma Aldrich; St. Louis, USA).

Statistical analysis

Data were presented as mean ± STD. For quantitative analysis, data was analyzed with unpaired t-test and one-way ANOVA with post-hoc analysis using SPSS 16.00. A value of p 0.05 was considered as statistically significant.

Results

NSCs culture and characterization

The isolated NSCs were cultured in NeuroCult NS-A media (Cat# 05750; Stem Cell Technology, Vancouver; Canada) and maintained at 37 °C and 5% CO_2. After 5 days in the culture, NSCs started to form spherical cell aggregates or the neurospheres (Fig. 1a). The spherical cell aggregates were clearly distinguishable from the extraneous particulate material in the culture based on their morphology at higher magnification. Fluorescence immunocytochemistry with specific primary antibodies revealed their positivity for both Nestin (Fig. 1b-d) and CD133 expression (Fig. 1e-g). The neurospheres were dissociated into single cells and cultured in differentiating media for tri-lineage differentiation assay. Fluorescence immunocytochemistry showed their successful differentiation into neurons; oligodendrocytes and astrocytes as was evident from positivity for CNPase (for oligodendrocytes) and GFAP (for astrocytes) (Fig. 1h-j and k-m).

NSCs sphere formation and proliferation

Treatment with NaB clearly changed the culture characteristics of NSCs in comparison with the untreated control NSCs that were maintained under similar culture conditions. The most obvious difference between the two groups of cells was that NaB treatment markedly reduced their ability to form neurospheres despite significantly enhanced rate of cluster formation ($p < 0.05$ vs control) (Fig. 2a-b). A continuous treatment for 10 days promoted neuronal differentiation of the clusters which had elongated morphology with distinct cell body, dendrite and axon (Fig. 2c). Neural differentiation was confirmed by MAP-2 expression using fluorescence immunocytochemistry (Fig. 3a-c) and flow cytometry (Fig. 3d-e). As compared to the control non-treated cells, 78.1% cells differentiated into neurons after 10 days treatment with NaB (Fig. 3d-e). The flow cytometry data showed that NaB treatment for HDAC inhibition significantly enhanced the neural differentiation.

Cell viability

An interesting feature of our study was that NaB treatment preconditioned the cells towards subsequent exposure to H_2O_2. The viability of NaB treated cells was significantly higher as compared to the non-preconditioned cells upon

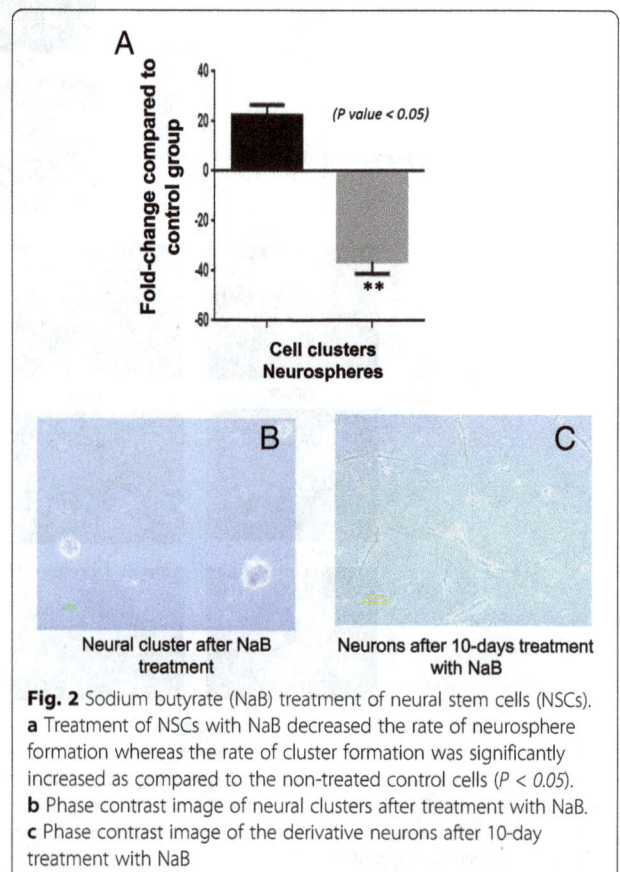

Fig. 2 Sodium butyrate (NaB) treatment of neural stem cells (NSCs). **a** Treatment of NSCs with NaB decreased the rate of neurosphere formation whereas the rate of cluster formation was significantly increased as compared to the non-treated control cells ($P < 0.05$). **b** Phase contrast image of neural clusters after treatment with NaB. **c** Phase contrast image of the derivative neurons after 10-day treatment with NaB

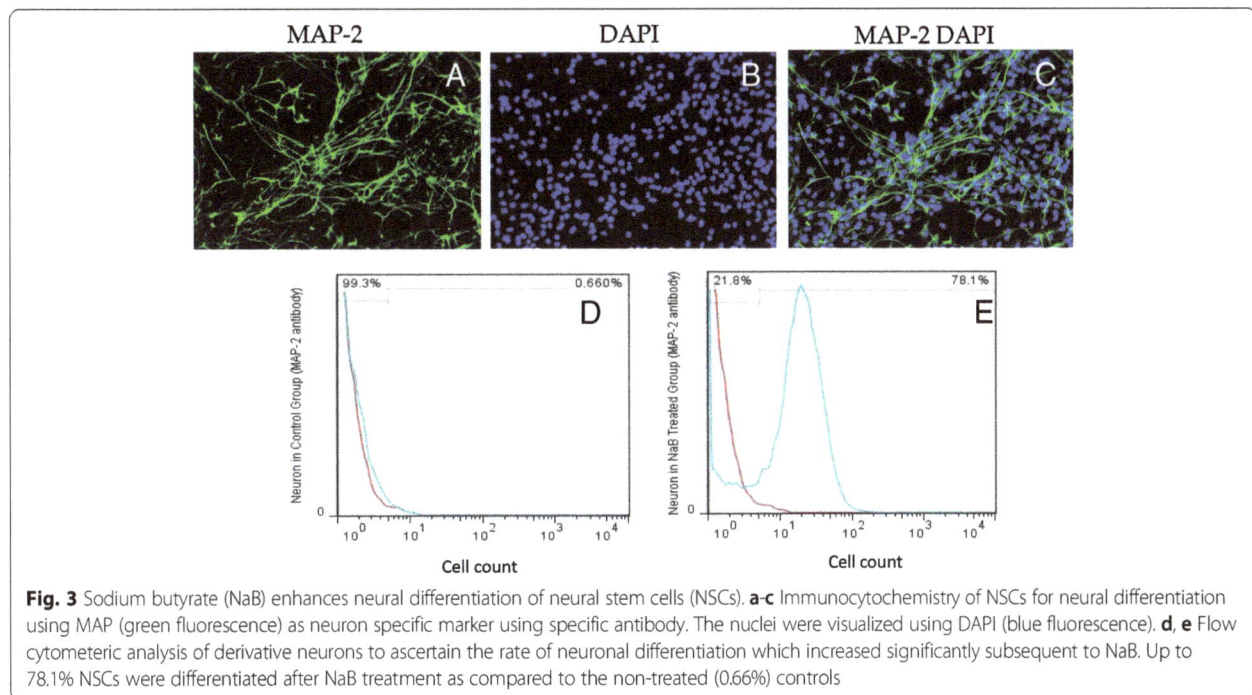

Fig. 3 Sodium butyrate (NaB) enhances neural differentiation of neural stem cells (NSCs). **a-c** Immunocytochemistry of NSCs for neural differentiation using MAP (green fluorescence) as neuron specific marker using specific antibody. The nuclei were visualized using DAPI (blue fluorescence). **d, e** Flow cytometeric analysis of derivative neurons to ascertain the rate of neuronal differentiation which increased significantly subsequent to NaB. Up to 78.1% NSCs were differentiated after NaB treatment as compared to the non-treated (0.66%) controls

subsequent exposure to H_2O_2. However, preconditioning with NaB in the presence of nicorandil significantly enhanced the cell viability further as compared to the control as well as NaB alone treated cells as assessed by MTT assay ($p < 0.05$; Fig. 4).

Caspase-3 activity and annexin-V assays

Caspase-3 plays an important role in cell apoptosis and initiates the execution-phase of the apoptosis [17]. Hence, caspase-3 activity was measured to identify the apoptotic cells in different treatment cell groups upon exposure to H_2O_2 (Fig. 5a). The caspase-3 activity was significantly higher in the non-treated cell group upon exposure to H_2O_2 as compared to the NaB and combined (NaB + nicorandil) treatment groups whereas least activity of caspase-3 was observed in the combined (NaB + nicorandil) treatment group. Untreated cells without exposure to H_2O_2 were used as baseline control (Fig. 5a). These results were well supported by Annexin-V flow cytometry assay which showed that the percentage of Annexin-V positive cells was 19.3% in the untreated control cells upon exposure to oxidative stress as compared to 16.3% in NaB preconditioned cells and 10.6% in the combined (NaB and nicorandil) treatment group ($p < 0.005$ vs control; Fig. 5b-g). PI staining combined with flow cytometry showed that the more than 99% cell death was due to apoptosis (Fig. 5f-g).

Cell proliferation assay by BrdU labeling

To assess the proliferation of NSCs after NaB treatment, the cells were labeled with BrdU. The number of the

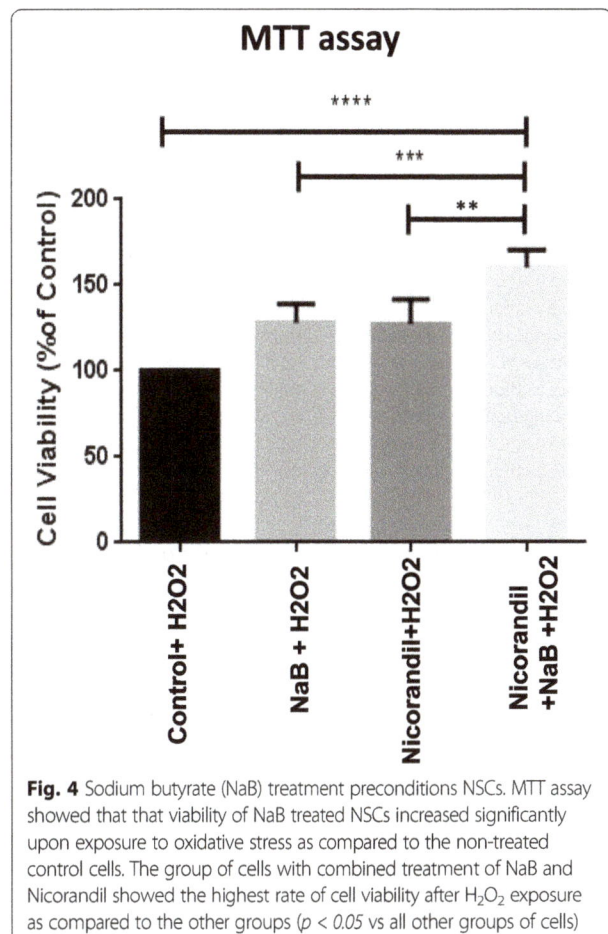

Fig. 4 Sodium butyrate (NaB) treatment preconditions NSCs. MTT assay showed that that viability of NaB treated NSCs increased significantly upon exposure to oxidative stress as compared to the non-treated control cells. The group of cells with combined treatment of NaB and Nicorandil showed the highest rate of cell viability after H_2O_2 exposure as compared to the other groups ($p < 0.05$ vs all other groups of cells)

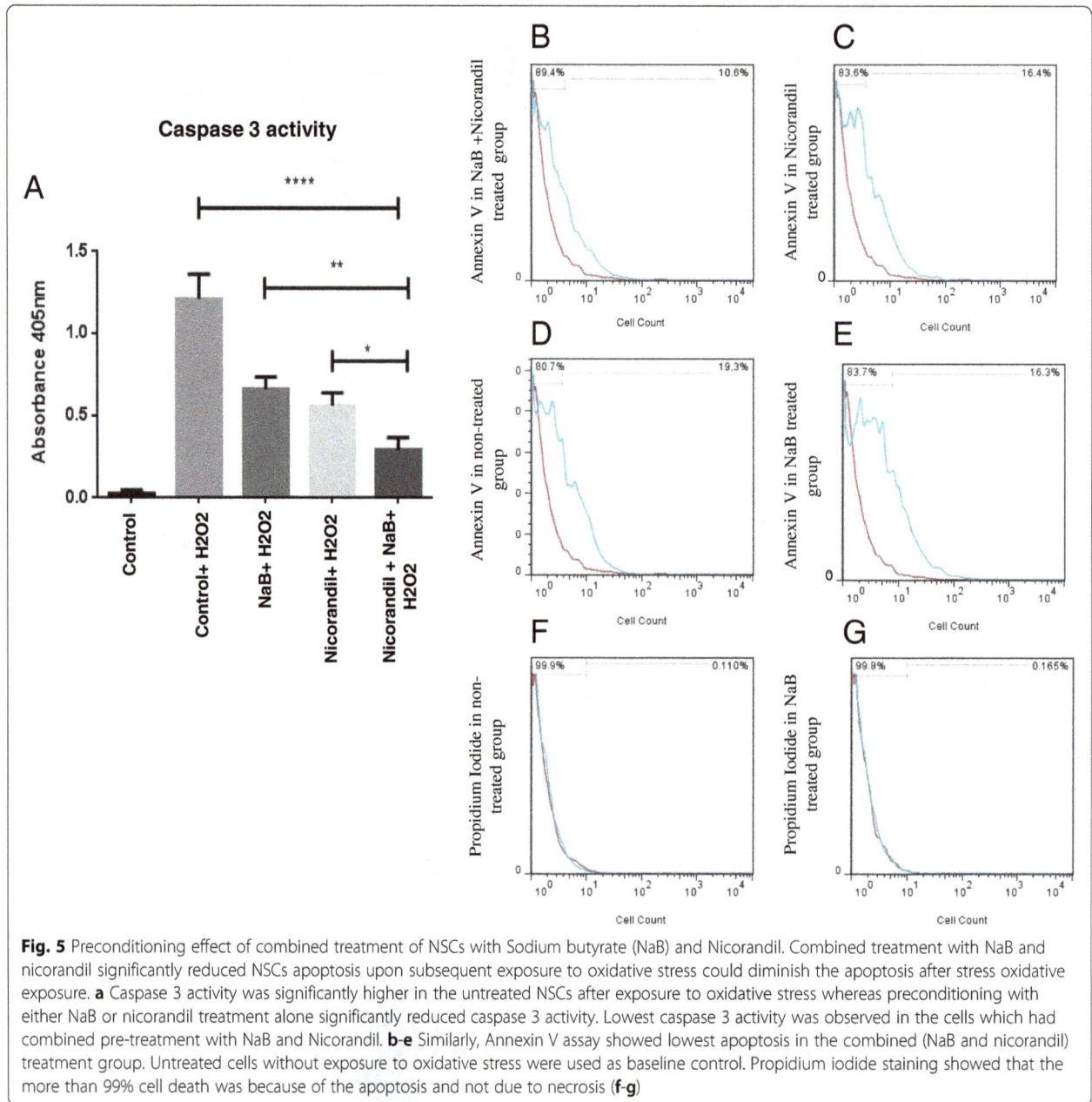

Fig. 5 Preconditioning effect of combined treatment of NSCs with Sodium butyrate (NaB) and Nicorandil. Combined treatment with NaB and nicorandil significantly reduced NSCs apoptosis upon subsequent exposure to oxidative stress could diminish the apoptosis after stress oxidative exposure. **a** Caspase 3 activity was significantly higher in the untreated NSCs after exposure to oxidative stress whereas preconditioning with either NaB or nicorandil treatment alone significantly reduced caspase 3 activity. Lowest caspase 3 activity was observed in the cells which had combined pre-treatment with NaB and Nicorandil. **b–e** Similarly, Annexin V assay showed lowest apoptosis in the combined (NaB and nicorandil) treatment group. Untreated cells without exposure to oxidative stress were used as baseline control. Propidium iodide staining showed that the more than 99% cell death was because of the apoptosis and not due to necrosis (**f-g**)

NaB treated cells positive for (Brdu⁺/total cells) was (1.06 ± 0.04) as compared to the untreated control group (1.18 ± 0.10; $p < 0.05$) (Fig. 6).

Discussion

The main finding of our study is that NSCs treated with NaB successfully produce preconditioned neurons while subsequent treatment with nicorandil accentuates the preconditioning effect of NaB and enhances their survival upon subsequent exposure to H_2O_2.

The rate of neuronal differentiation of NSCs without teratogenicity and the ability of the differentiated cells to survive in the ischemic environment post-engraftment are two of the major challenges in stem cell-based therapy [18, 19]. Spontaneous malignant transformation of NSCs after long-term culture has been attributed to their extensive proliferation potential [20]. Molecular studies have shown constitutively higher NFkB activity, enhanced VEGF expression and adoption of tumorgenic phenotype in NSCs under growth factor-free culture conditions (in the absence of EGF and bFGF) [21]. Neutralization of VEGF significantly reduces the proliferation potential of NSCs in the growth factor-free culture and promotes their differentiation [22]. Various strategies have been adopted to promote their rate of neuronal differentiation. For example, alleviation of

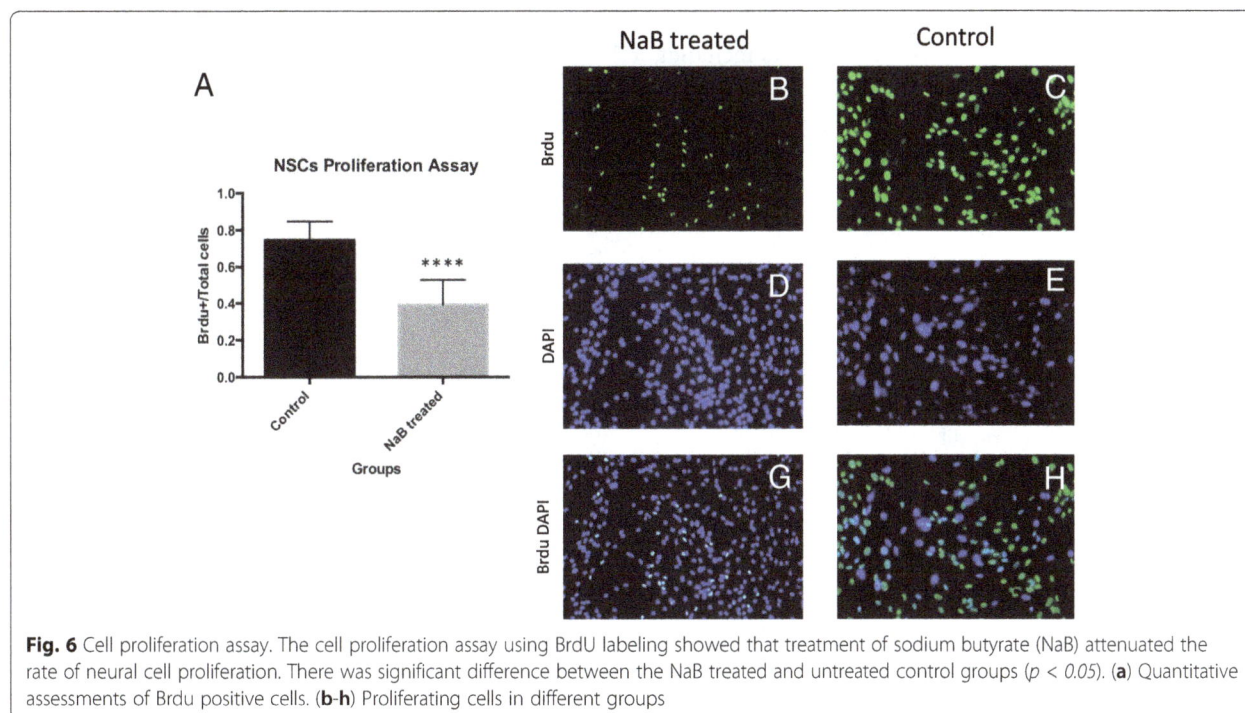

Fig. 6 Cell proliferation assay. The cell proliferation assay using BrdU labeling showed that treatment of sodium butyrate (NaB) attenuated the rate of neural cell proliferation. There was significant difference between the NaB treated and untreated control groups ($p < 0.05$). (**a**) Quantitative assessments of Brdu positive cells. (**b-h**) Proliferating cells in different groups

hypoxia in the developing cortex through angiogenesis promotes neurogenic differentiation of NSCs [23]. Similarly, exploiting the critical role of cell cycle regulators to prepare the cells for differentiation via cell cycle exit, double knock-down of cyclin dependent kinase (cdk)2 and cdk4 significantly enhances neuronal differentiation of neuronal precursors both in vivo and in culture conditions [24]. Supported by the loss-of-function studies, both cell proliferation and survival are significantly affected by the class-I HDACs [25, 26]. HDACi treatment stops the proliferation and sphere-forming potential of NSCs and supports their neural differentiation [27–29]. These data vividly support our findings that treatment with NaB enhances neural differentiation of NSCs. We observed that NaB effectively suppressed the rate of NSCs proliferation as was evident from increased cell cluster formation and their reduced sphere-forming ability. At molecular levels, previous studies have shown that NaB inhibits deacetylation of the lysine and arginine residues on the N-terminus of histones with concomitant increase in p21 which is responsible for antiproliferative effects of the HDACi [30–33]. Their exit from cell cycle is accompanied by change of fate as a result of which NSCs become committed to tri-neural lineage fate, with neural differentiation as the dominant prospect [8, 34]. A recent study has shown that proneural genes *Ngn2* and *NeuroD1* are elevated during HDACi treatment with a consequent increase in neural differentiation [35]. Our results are in agreement with the published reports and show that NaB induce

significantly higher neural differentiation of NSCs in comparison with the non-treated control NSCs as determined by MAP-2 antigen expression.

Besides exit from cell cycle and neural differentiation, cytoprotection afforded by NaB was the cardinal feature of our study. The NaB treated cells were more resistant to H_2O_2 induced apoptosis than the untreated control cells ($p < 0.05$ vs untreated control cells) as determined by MTT and caspase-3 assays. Neuroprotective effects of NaB have also been reported in the retinal glial cells cultured under serum-free conditions at par with erythropoietin [36]. Mechanistic studies have shown that cytoprotection with NaB was mediated via activation of PI3K/Akt signaling [37]. Treatment with NaB significantly reduced the number of apoptotic neurons during cerebral ischemia-reperfusion injury in experimental mouse model. The authors have reported significantly elevated Bcl2 and phosphorylated Akt, and reduced caspase-3 and Bax expression as compared to the non-treated experimental animals. Enhanced resistance to oxidative stress has also been reported in rat hippocampus via elevated levels of thiorexidine binding protein-2 (TBP-2) after NaB treatment which was attributed to antioxidant effects of TBP-2 [38]. We observed that combined treatment of NSCs with NaB and nicorandil was more cytoprotective as compared to treatment of the cells with either of the two molecules alone. Nicorandil is a small molecule capable of stimulating APE1/Ref1 activity in the cells which is responsible for cell reaction to DNA damage and oxidative stress [39].

The cytoprotective effects of APE1/Ref1 have been attributed to modulation of transcription factors including activator protein-1 (AP-1), NF-κB, p53, cAMP response element binding protein (CREB), and hypoxia-inducible factor-1α (HIF-1α) [14, 40, 41]. Based on these data, we propose that nicorandil treatment activated APE1 in the neurons after treatment with HDACi. Further studies are warranted to fully understand the underlying molecular mechanism and efficacy of the combined cytoprotective effects of NaB and nicorandil.

Notwithstanding the interesting data, the study has some limitations. Firstly, we focused only on the apoptosis markers for evaluation of the preconditioning effects of NaB and nicorandil. Although H_2O_2 has been widely accepted as an inducer of apoptosis in various cell-based studies, it may induce cell death by multiple mechanisms [42–44]. Study of the oxidative stress markers would have enhanced the significance of the data. Secondly, future studies will be required to understand the mechanism of cytoprotection afforded by the combined treatment with NaB and nicorandil using HDAC-mutant cells, loss-of-function and gain-of-function studies to understand the role of p21 in proliferation of the preconditioned cells besides their cell cycle marker expression profile.

Conclusion

In conclusion, combined treatment with NaB and nicorandil is effective to enhance neural commitment of NSCs and cytoprotection of the derivative neural cells.

Abbreviations

APE-1: Apurinic pyrimidinic endonuclease-1; bFGF: Basic fibroblast growth factor; cGMP: cyclic guanosine-3',-5'-monophasphate; EGF: Epidermal growth factor; HDACi: Histone deacetylases inhibitors; HDACs: Histone deacetylases; iPSCs: Induced pluripotent stem cells; MCAO: Middle cerebral artery occlusion; MS-275: Benzamide; NaB: Sodium butyrate; NSCs: NSCs; PBS: Phosphate buffered saline; Ref-1: Redox effector factor-1; SAHA: Assuberoylanilidec hydroxamic acid; TUNEL: dUTP nick end labeling; VEGF: Vascular endothelial growth factor; VPA: Valproic acid

Acknowledgments

The authors wish to thank Cell& Molecular Medicine lab members for discussing about the data and also Stem Cell lab members in anatomy department.

Funding

The authors thank Shiraz University of Medical Sciences research deputy of the Cell & Molecular Medicine lab for financial support.

Authors' contributions

PT, MS and M.Salmannejad has contributed in performing the experiment, KhHH has the central role in paper writing and SMH designed the experiment, revised the paper and contributed in performing the experiment. All authors read and approved the final manuscript.

Competing interests

The authors declare that they have no competing interests.

Author details

[1]Student Research Committee, Shiraz University of Medical Sciences, Shiraz, Iran. [2]Cell & Molecular Medicine Student Research Group, Medical Faculty, Shiraz University of Medical Sciences, Shiraz, Iran. [3]Department of Basic Sciences, SRU, Riyadh, Saudi Arabia. [4]Stem Cell Laboratory, Department of Anatomy, Shiraz University of Medical Sciences, Shiraz, Iran.

References

1. Zhao Y, Zuo Y, Jiang J, Yan H, Wang X, Huo H, et al. Neural stem cell transplantation combined with erythropoietin for the treatment of spinal cord injury in rats. Exp Thera Med. 2016;12(4):2688–94.
2. Lee IH, Huang SS, Chuang CY, Liao KH, Chang LH, Chuang CC, Su YS, Lin HJ, Hsieh JY, Su SH, Lee OK. Delayed epidural transplantation of human induced pluripotent stem cell-derived neural progenitors enhances functional recovery after stroke. Sci Rep. 2017;7(1):1943.
3. Bjugstad KB, Rael LT, Levy S, Carrick M, Mains CW, Slone DS, et al. Oxidation-reduction potential as a biomarker for severity and acute outcome in traumatic brain injury. Oxid Med Cell Longev. 2016;2016:9.
4. Lu J, Xie L, Liu C, Zhang Q, Sun S. PTEN/PI3k/AKT regulates macrophage polarization in emphysematous mice. Scand J Immunol. 2017;85(6):395-405. doi:10.1111/sji.12545.
5. Zhou Q, Dalgard CL, Wynder C, Doughty ML. Histone deacetylase inhibitors SAHA and sodium butyrate block G1-to-S cell cycle progression in neurosphere formation by adult sub-ventricular cells. BMC Neurosci. 2011;12(1):1.
6. Hsing CH, Hung SK, Chen YC, Wei TS, Sun DP, Wang JJ, et al. Histone deacetylase inhibitor trichostatin a ameliorated endotoxin-induced neuro-inflammation and cognitive dysfunction. Mediat Inflamm. 2015;27:2015.
7. Ziemka-Nalecz M, Jaworska J, Sypecka J, Polowy R, Filipkowski RK, Zalewska T. Sodium butyrate, a Histone Deacetylase inhibitor, exhibits Neuroprotective/Neurogenic effects in a rat model of neonatal hypoxia-ischemia. Mol Neurobiol. 2017;54(7):5300-18.
8. Siebzehnrubl FA, Buslei R, Eyupoglu IY, Seufert S, Hahnen E, Blumcke I. Histone deacetylase inhibitors increase neuronal differentiation in adult forebrain precursor cells. Exp Brain Res. 2007;176(4):672–8.
9. Alvarez AA, Field M, Bushnev S, Longo MS, Sugaya K. The effects of histone deacetylase inhibitors on glioblastoma-derived stem cells. J Mol Neurosci. 2015;55(1):7–20.
10. Fung H, Demple B. A vital role for Ape1/Ref1 protein in repairing spontaneous DNA damage in human cells. Mol Cell. 2005;17:463–70.
11. Domenis R, Bergamin N, Gianfranceschi G, Vascotto C, Romanello M, Rigo S, et al. The redox function of APE1 is involved in the differentiation process of stem cells toward a neuronal cell fate. PLoS One. 2014;9(2):e89232.
12. Poletto M, Vascotto C, Scognamiglio PL, Lirussi L, Marasco D. Role of the unstructured N-terminal domain of the hAPE1 (human apurinic/apyrimidinic endonuclease-1) in the modulation of its interaction with nucleic acids and NPM1 (nucleophosmin). Biochem J. 2013;452:545–57.
13. Jason M, Kaski JC. Vasodilator therapy: nitrates and Nicorandil. Cardiovasc Drugs Ther. 2016; 10.1007/s10557-016-6668-z.
14. Georgiadis MM, Chen Q, Meng J, Guo C, Wireman R, Reed A, et al. Small molecule activation of apurinic/apyrimidinic endonuclease 1 reduces DNA damage induced by cisplatin in cultured sensory neurons. DNA Repair (Amst). 2016;41:32–41.

15. Zhou Y, Wang Q, Evers BM, Chung DH. Signal transduction pathways involved in oxidative stress-induced intestinal epithelial cell apoptosis. Pediatric Res. 2005;58(6):1192–7.

16. So EC, Chen YC, Wang SC, Wu CC, Huang MC, Lai MS, et al. Midazolam regulated caspase pathway, endoplasmic reticulum stress, autophagy, and cell cycle to induce apoptosis in MA-10 mouse Leydig tumor cells. Onco Targets Ther. 2016;9:2519.

17. Boland K, Flanagan L, Prehn JH. Paracrine control of tissue regeneration and cell proliferation by Caspase-3. Cell Death Dis. 2013;4(7):e725.

18. Amariglio N, Hirshberg A, Scheithauer BW, et al. Donor-derived brain tumor following neural stem cell transplantation in an ataxia telangiectasia patient. PLoS Med. 2009;6:e1000029.

19. Radtke C, Redeker J, Jokuszies A, et al. In vivo transformation of neural stem cells following transplantation in the injured nervous system. J Reconstr Microsurg. 2010;26:211–2.

20. Wu W, He Q, Li X, Zhang X, Lu A, Ge R, et al. Long-term cultured human neural stem cells undergo spontaneous transformation to tumor-initiating cells. Int J Biol Sci. 2011;7:892–901.

21. Kaus A, Widera D, Kassmer S, Peter J, Zaenker K, Kaltschmidt C, et al. Neural stem cells adopt tumorigenic properties by constitutively activated NF-kappaB and subsequent VEGF up-regulation. Stem Cells Dev. 2010;19(7):999–1015.

22. Zhao LN, Wang P, Liu YH, Cai H, Ma J, Liu LB, Xi Z, Li ZQ, Liu XB, Xue YX. Mir-383 inhibits proliferation, migration and angiogenesis of glioma-exposed endothelial cells in vitro via vegf-mediated fak and src signaling pathways. Cellular signalling. 2017;30:142-53.

23. Lange C, Garcia MT, Decimo I, Bifari F, Eelen G, Quaegebeur A, et al. Relief of hypoxia by angiogenesis promotes neural stem cell differentiation by targeting glycolysis. EMBO J. 2016;35(9):924–41.

24. Lim S, Kaldis P. Loss of Cdk2 and Cdk4 induces a switch from proliferation to differentiation in neural stem cells. Stem Cells. 2012;30:1509–20.

25. Dokmanovic M, Clarke C, Marks PA. Histone Deacetylase inhibitors: overview and perspectives. Mol Cancer Res. 2007;5(10):981–9.

26. Lagger G. O'Carro II D, Rembold M et al. essential function of histone deacetylase 1 in proliferation control and CDK inhibitor repression. EMBO J. 2002;21:2672–81.

27. Marks PA, Jiang X. Histone deacetylase inhibitors in programmed cell death and cancer therapy. Cell Cycle. 2005;4(4):549–51.

28. Marks PA, Xu WS. Histone deacetylase inhibitors: potential in cancer therapy. J Cell Biochem. 2009;107(4):600–8.

29. Elmi M, Matsumoto Y, Zeng ZJ, Lakshminarasimhan P, Yang W, Uemura A, et al. TLX activates MASH1 forinduction of neuronal lineage commitment of adult hippocampal neuroprogenitors. Mol Cell Neurosci. 2010;45(2):121–31.

30. Roth SY, Denu JM, Allis CD. Histone acetyltransferases. Annu Rev Biochem. 2001;70:81–120.

31. Gregory PD, Wagner K, Horz W. Histone acetylation and chromatin remodeling. Exp Cell Res. 2001;265:195–202.

32. Thiagalingam S, Cheng KH, Lee HJ, Mineva N, Thiagalingam A, Ponte JF. Histone deacetylases: unique players in shaping the epigenetic histone code. Ann N Y Acad Sci. 2003;983:84–100.

33. Richon VM, Sandhoff TW, Rifkind RA, Marks PA. Histone deacetylase inhibitor selectively induces p21WAF1 expression and gene-associated histone acetylation. Proc Natl Acad Sci U S A. 2000;97:10014–9.

34. Hsieh J, Nakashima K, Kuwabara T, Mejia E, Gage FH. Histone deacetylase inhibition-mediated neuronal differentiation of multipotent adult neural progenitor cells. Proc Natl Acad Sci U S A. 2004;101(47):16659–64.

35. Chu W, Yuan J, Huang L, Xiang X, Zhu H, Chen F, et al. Valproic acid arrests proliferation but promotes neuronal differentiation of adult spinal NSPCs from SCI rats. Neurochem Res. 2015;40(7):1472–86.

36. Biermann J, Boyle J, Pielen A, Lagrè WA. Histone deacetylase inhibitors sodium butyrate and valproic acid delay spontaneous cell death in purified rat retinal ganglion cells. Mol Vis. 2011;17:395–403.

37. Sun J, Wang F, Li H, Zhang H, Jin J, Chen W, et al. Neuroprotective effect of sodium butyrate against cerebral ischemia/reperfusion injury in mice. Biomed Res Int. 2015 May;7:2015.

38. Valvassori SS, Dal-Pont GC, Steckert AV, Varela RB, Lopes-Borges J, Mariot E, et al. Sodium butyrate has an antimanic effect and protects the brain against oxidative stress in an animal model of mania induced by ouabain. Psychiatry Res. 2016;235:154–9.

39. Georgiadis MM, Luo M, Gaur RK, Delaplane S, Li X, Kelley MR. Evolution of the redox function in mammalian apurinic/apyrimidinic endonuclease. Mutat Res. 2008;643:54–63.

40. Luo M, Zhang J, He H, Su D, Chen Q, Gross ML, et al. Characterization of the redox activity and disulfide bond formation in apurinic/apyrimidinic endonuclease. Biochemist. 2012;51:695–705.

41. Park MS, Kim CS, Joo HK, Lee YR, Kang G, Kim SJ, et al. Cytoplasmic localization and redox cysteine residue of APE1/Ref-1 are associated with its anti-inflammatory activity in cultured endothelial cells. Mol Cells. 2013;36:439–45.

42. Idris NM1, Ashraf M, Ahmed RP, Shujia J, Haider KH. Activation of IL-11/STAT3 pathway in preconditioned human skeletal myoblasts blocks apoptotic cascade under oxidant stress. Regen Med. 2012;7(1):47–57.

43. Niagara MI, Haider HK, Jiang S, Ashraf M. Pharmacologically preconditioned skeletal myoblasts are resistant to oxidative stress and promote angiomyogenesis via release of paracrine factors in the infarcted heart. Circ Res. 2007;100(4):545–55.

44. Xiang J, Wan C, Guo R, Guo D. Is hydrogen peroxide a suitable apoptosis inducer for all cell types? Biomed Res Int. Volume 2016, Article ID 7343965, 6-pages. http://dx.doi.org/10.1155/2016/7343965.

23

Neurodegeneration-associated FUS is a novel regulator of circadian gene expression

Xin Jiang[1,2], Tao Zhang[1,2], Haifang Wang[1], Tao Wang[1], Meiling Qin[1], Puhua Bao[1], Ruiqi Wang[1], Yuwei Liu[1], Hung-Chun Chang[1], Jun Yan[1] and Jin Xu[1*]

Abstract

Background: Circadian rhythms are oscillating physiological and behavioral changes governed by an internal molecular clock, and dysfunctions in circadian rhythms have been associated with ageing and various neurodegenerative diseases. However, the evidence directly connecting the neurodegeneration-associated proteins to circadian control at the molecular level remains sparse.

Methods: Using meta-analysis, synchronized animals and cell lines, cells and tissues from FUS R521C knock-in rats, we examined the role of FUS in circadian gene expression regulation.

Results: We found that FUS, an oscillating expressed nuclear protein implicated in the pathogenesis of amyotrophic lateral sclerosis (ALS) and frontotemporal dementia (FTD), exerted a novel feedback route to regulate circadian gene expression. *Nr1d1*-encoded core circadian protein REV-ERBα bound the *Fus* promoter and regulated the expression of *Fus*. Meanwhile, FUS was in the same complex as PER/CRY, and repressed the expression of E box-containing core circadian genes, such as *Per2*, by mediating the promoter occupancy of PSF-HDAC1. Remarkably, a common pathogenic mutant FUS (R521C) showed increased binding to PSF, and caused decreased expression of *Per2*.

Conclusions: Therefore, we have demonstrated FUS as a modulator of circadian gene expression, and provided novel mechanistic insights into the mutual influence between circadian control and neurodegeneration-associated proteins.

Keywords: FUS, ALS, FTD, Circadian rhythm, Gene regulation

Background

Circadian rhythms are oscillating physiological and behavioral changes governed by an internal molecular clock, and rely on two transcriptional feedback loops to regulate the expression of various core circadian genes [1–3]. BMAL1 and CLOCK transcriptionally activate E-box-containing genes, including *Per*, *Cry* and *Nr1d1/2*. When the protein products of *Per*, *Cry* and *Nr1d1/2* build up, *Nr1d1/2*-encoded REV-ERBα/β can repress the transcription of *Bmal1* by binding to retinoic acid–related orphan receptor response (ROR) elements in the *Bmal1* promoter [4, 5], and PER and CRY proteins can join a mega-transcriptional repressor complex with BMAL1 and CLOCK to shut down the expression of E-box-containing genes [6–11]. The strength of these two major transcriptional feedback loops can be further fine-tuned by additional transcriptional co-regulators [12–14]. For example, RNA/DNA-binding protein PSF (also known as splicing factor proline and glutamine rich) could act as a transcriptional co-repressor by recruiting SIN3A-HDAC1 to rhythmically deacetylate *Per1* promoter and repress the transcription of *Per1*[12].

There is a plethora of evidence connecting circadian rhythm dysfunction to neurodegeneration [15, 16]. However, except for Ataxin-2 in *Drosophila* circadian loco-motor behavior regulation [17, 18], there is little evidence mechanistically links neurodegenerative disease-associated proteins to the regulation of circadian clock. FUS is a nuclear protein implicated in the pathogenesis of ALS and FTD [19–21]. Mutations in FUS cause early onset of ALS,

---

* Correspondence: jin.xu@ion.ac.cn
[1]Institute of Neuroscience, State Key Laboratory of Neuroscience, CAS Key laboratory of Primate Neurobiology, Shanghai Institutes for Biological Sciences, Chinese Academy of Sciences, New Life Science Bldg, 320 Yue Yang Road, Shanghai 200031, China
Full list of author information is available at the end of the article

and the accumulation of FUS is a common feature in FTD neuropathology [21]. Furthermore, sleep disorders are known to affect some ALS and FTD patients [22–24]. *Fus* is suggested as a potential circadian regulated gene with oscillating mRNA expression in mouse liver, prefrontal cortex, skeletal muscle and other tissues [25, 26]; however, its regulation by circadian clock has never been characterized and its role in circadian regulation is unknown. In this study, we found that FUS is not only transcriptionally regulated by REV-ERBα, but also modulates the expression of *Per* and *Cry*. Therefore, our study provides novel insights into mutual regulation between circadian control and neurodegeneration-related proteins.

Methods

Animals

All animal works were performed in accordance with the regulations by the Animal Care and Use Committee of the Institute of Neuroscience, Shanghai Institutes for Biological Sciences.

The detailed procedures for the establishment of the FUS-R521C knock-in rats via CRISPR/Cas9, and the characterization of the animals were described elsewhere (T.Z. et al, *Neurobiology of Aging*, in press; Additional file 1). Briefly, Cas9 mRNA, single guide RNA (sgRNA) targeting the C-terminus of rat *Fus* gene, and donor DNA were injected into the cytoplasm of zygotes of the Sprague Dawley rats (Additional file 1: Figure S1). The sequence for sgRNA and donor DNA are: TGAGCACAGACAGGATCGCA (sgRNA), TTAATCTAACAAATAATTTTTTCTTTCAGG GGTGAGCACAG ACAGGATTGCAGGGAGAGGCCATATTAGCCTGACTCCTGAAG TTCTGGAACAGCTCTTC (donor DNA). The presence of inserted mutation was determined by PCR followed by sequencing. The potential off-target effects in F0 (founder) rats were estimated using Cas-OFFinder [27] and assessed by PCR-sequencing. Multiple rounds of breeding were carried out to eliminate off potential off target effects. The *Nr1d1* knock-out mice were described previously [5].

Cell culture, transfection and synchronization

Rat embryonic fibroblasts (REFs) were collected from E13.5-15.5 embryos using pregnant rats from heterozygous R521C FUS knock-in rats mating pairs. Mouse embryonic fibroblasts (MEFs) were collected from E13.5-E15.5 embryos using pregnant mice from heterozygous *Nr1d1* knock-out mice mating pairs. REFs, MEFs, HEK293T cells (ATCC) and Neuro-2a (ATCC) cells were cultured at 37 °C in 5% CO_2 in DMEM (for REFs and HEK293T cells, Gibco c11965) or DMEM/F-12 (for Neuro-2a cells, Gibco c11330) medium, supplemented with 10% fetal bovine serum (Gibco, 10099) and antibiotics (Penicillin and streptomycin, HyClone, SV30010).

Cells were transfected using Lipofectamine 2000 reagent (Invitrogen, 11668) for over-expression or Lipofectamine

RNAiMAX (Invitrogen, 13778) for gene silencing. Control plasmids (GFP) or scrambled siRNA (Ctrl) were used to make sure equal amount of the constructs were transfected in each condition. Typically, cells were harvested 48 hrs for over-expression and 72 hrs for RNAi silencing after transfection.

Neuro-2a cell were synchronized as described previously [13]. Briefly, 48 hrs after siRNA silencing or 24 hrs after over-expression, the cultural medium for transfected cells were changed to 50% horse serum (Gibco, 16050)-50% DMEM/F12 for 2 hrs followed by culturing in 1%-FBS-containing DMEM for 22 hrs before harvesting. For REFs synchronization, 48 hrs after transfection, cells were cultured in DMEM (with 1% FBS and antibiotics) containing 10μM forskolin (Sigma, F3917) for 2 hrs, followed by culturing in the low serum condition until the end of the experiment (DMEM with 1% FBS) as described [28]. The synchronization of MEFs was as described [29, 30]. MEFs were treated with 100nM Dexamethasone for 1 hr when cells reach confluence, then the cells were cultured in the low serum condition (DMEM with 1% FBS) for 36 hr followed by harvesting.

Circadian tissue collection

For Fig. 1a-c, 7-week-old male wild-type C57BL/6 mice (SLAC Laboratory Animal, Shanghai) were maintained in a light-tight, ventilated, temperature (22 °C) and humidity (60%)-controlled animal facility with free access to food and water. The lighting schedule was 12 hr light:12 hr dark (lights on at 7 a.m.). To measure the endogenous circadian gene oscillation, entrained mice were then released to a constant low irradiance light condition (~30 Lux, measured at the bottom of cage) for one week. Starting at CT-8 (circadian time), five mice were sacrificed every 4 hrs, for 24 hrs. Tissues were quickly dissected and frozen immediately in solid carbon dioxide for further analysis.

For Fig. 1d, the detailed method for sleep deprivation (SD) was as described [31]. Briefly, SD was initiated at ZT-0 hr (Zeitgeber time), ZT-6 hr, ZT-12 hr and ZT-18 hr by gentle-handing method for 5.5 hrs, mice were then sacrificed within the next 30 min.

For Fig. 2d, 3.5-month-old *Nr1d1*-knockout mice and littermate wild-type control mice were entrained in the 12 hr:12 hr light:dark condition for more than a week then released to constant dark condition for five days. Three pairs of littermate mice were sacrificed at CT-0 hr and two pairs of mice were sacrificed at CT-12 hr under the dim red light. Tissues were quickly dissected and frozen immediately in solid carbon dioxide for further analysis.

Dual-luciferase assay

Firefly luciferase reporter constructs directed by the intact mouse *Fus* promoter (~1.5kb upstream) or the

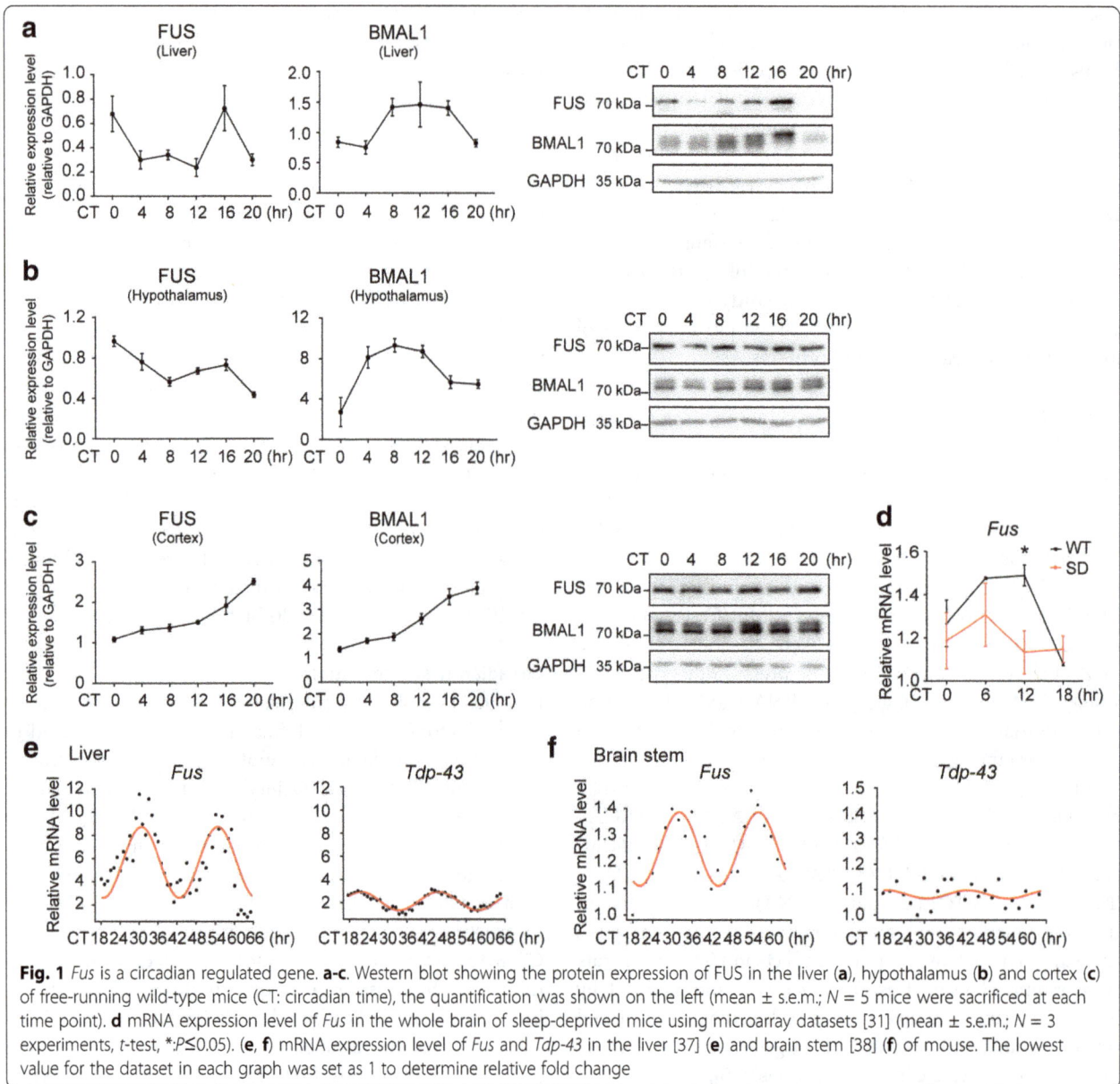

Fig. 1 *Fus* is a circadian regulated gene. **a-c.** Western blot showing the protein expression of FUS in the liver (**a**), hypothalamus (**b**) and cortex (**c**) of free-running wild-type mice (CT: circadian time), the quantification was shown on the left (mean ± s.e.m.; $N = 5$ mice were sacrificed at each time point). **d** mRNA expression level of *Fus* in the whole brain of sleep-deprived mice using microarray datasets [31] (mean ± s.e.m.; $N = 3$ experiments, *t*-test, *:$P \leq 0.05$). (**e**, **f**) mRNA expression level of *Fus* and *Tdp-43* in the liver [37] (**e**) and brain stem [38] (**f**) of mouse. The lowest value for the dataset in each graph was set as 1 to determine relative fold change

promoter with predicted REV-ERBα-binding site (350 bp [32]) deleted were PCR amplified from mouse genomic DNA and cloned into firefly luciferase reporter vector (pGL3-Basic Vector, Promega, E1751). Firefly luciferase reporter constructs directed by mouse *Per2* promoter (1.7 kb) [33] was a gift from Dr. Hung-Chun Chang's lab. Cells were transfected with firefly luciferase reporter with renilla luciferase reporter (pRL-SV40 Vector, Promega, E2231) as internal control. According to the technical manual of Dual-Luciiferase Reporter Assay System (Promega, E1910), 48 hrs after transfection, cells were eventually lysed with Passive Lysis Buffer. Then, transferred 20μL of cell lysate into 100μL of LARII reagent

and the luminescence of firefly luciferase reporter was read by the tube luminometer (Titertek Berthold). Next, added 100μL of Stop & Glo reagent and put the tube back to the luminometer again and read the luminescence for internal renilla luciferase control. For each experiment, samples were analyzed in duplicates. Sequences of siRNAs were listed in Additional file 2: Table S1.

Plasmids, siRNA, and Antibodies
FLAG-mouse REV-ERBα and FLAG-PSF, FUS, R521C and 1-360 FUS were generated by PCR cloning. The primary antibodies used are: rabbit anti-PSF (Sigma,

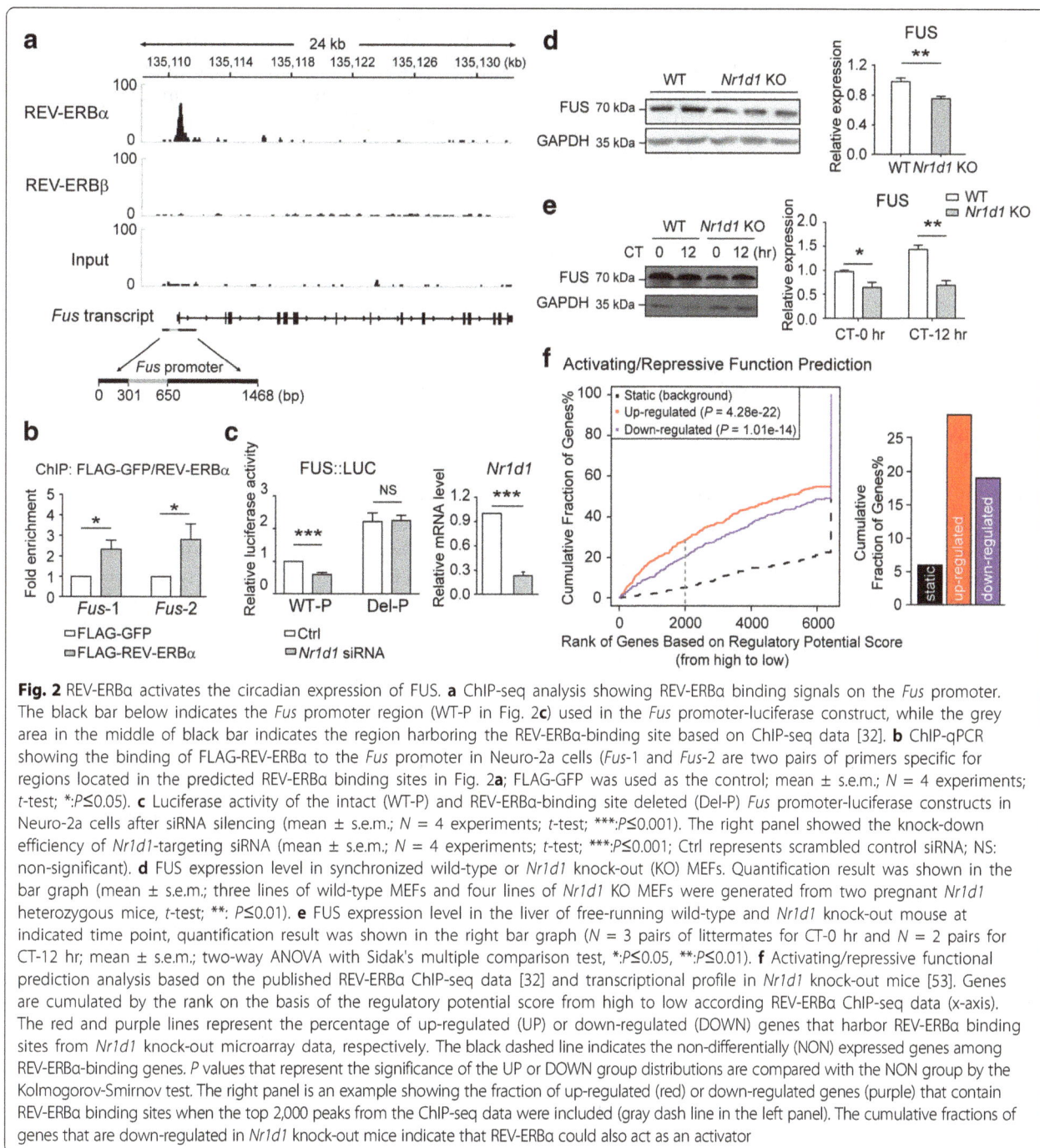

Fig. 2 REV-ERBα activates the circadian expression of FUS. **a** ChIP-seq analysis showing REV-ERBα binding signals on the *Fus* promoter. The black bar below indicates the *Fus* promoter region (WT-P in Fig. 2**c**) used in the *Fus* promoter-luciferase construct, while the grey area in the middle of black bar indicates the region harboring the REV-ERBα-binding site based on ChIP-seq data [32]. **b** ChIP-qPCR showing the binding of FLAG-REV-ERBα to the *Fus* promoter in Neuro-2a cells (*Fus*-1 and *Fus*-2 are two pairs of primers specific for regions located in the predicted REV-ERBα binding sites in Fig. 2**a**; FLAG-GFP was used as the control; mean ± s.e.m.; $N = 4$ experiments; t-test; *:$P \leq 0.05$). **c** Luciferase activity of the intact (WT-P) and REV-ERBα-binding site deleted (Del-P) *Fus* promoter-luciferase constructs in Neuro-2a cells after siRNA silencing (mean ± s.e.m.; $N = 4$ experiments; t-test; ***:$P \leq 0.001$). The right panel showed the knock-down efficiency of *Nr1d1*-targeting siRNA (mean ± s.e.m.; $N = 4$ experiments; t-test; ***:$P \leq 0.001$; Ctrl represents scrambled control siRNA; NS: non-significant). **d** FUS expression level in synchronized wild-type or *Nr1d1* knock-out (KO) MEFs. Quantification result was shown in the bar graph (mean ± s.e.m.; three lines of wild-type MEFs and four lines of *Nr1d1* KO MEFs were generated from two pregnant *Nr1d1* heterozygous mice, t-test; **: $P \leq 0.01$). **e** FUS expression level in the liver of free-running wild-type and *Nr1d1* knock-out mouse at indicated time point, quantification result was shown in the right bar graph ($N = 3$ pairs of littermates for CT-0 hr and $N = 2$ pairs for CT-12 hr; mean ± s.e.m.; two-way ANOVA with Sidak's multiple comparison test, *:$P \leq 0.05$, **:$P \leq 0.01$). **f** Activating/repressive functional prediction analysis based on the published REV-ERBα ChIP-seq data [32] and transcriptional profile in *Nr1d1* knock-out mice [53]. Genes are cumulated by the rank on the basis of the regulatory potential score from high to low according REV-ERBα ChIP-seq data (x-axis). The red and purple lines represent the percentage of up-regulated (UP) or down-regulated (DOWN) genes that harbor REV-ERBα binding sites from *Nr1d1* knock-out microarray data, respectively. The black dashed line indicates the non-differentially (NON) expressed genes among REV-ERBα-binding genes. P values that represent the significance of the UP or DOWN group distributions are compared with the NON group by the Kolmogorov-Smirnov test. The right panel is an example showing the fraction of up-regulated (red) or down-regulated genes (purple) that contain REV-ERBα binding sites when the top 2,000 peaks from the ChIP-seq data were included (gray dash line in the left panel). The cumulative fractions of genes that are down-regulated in *Nr1d1* knock-out mice indicate that REV-ERBα could also act as an activator

PLA0181; WB: 1:2,000, IP: 1:100; ChIP: 1:100), mouse anti-FUS (Santa Cruz, sc-4H11; WB: 1:1,000), mouse anti-DYKDDDDK-Tag (FLAG) (Abmart, M2008; WB:1:5,000), mouse anti-DYKDDDDK-Tag conjugated protein A/G beads (Abmart, M200018; IP and ChIP: 35uL beads per each assay), mouse anti-PSF antibody (Sigma, P2860; WB: 1:1,000), rabbit anti-CLOCK (Cell Signaling Technology, D45B10; WB:1:3,000), rabbit anti-BMAL1 (CST, D2L7G; WB: 1:3,000), rabbit anti-PER2 (Abcam, ab179813; WB: 1:1,000), mouse anti-ACTIN (Abmart, M20010; WB: 1:5,000), rabbit anti HDAC1 (Abcam, ab7028; ChIP: 1:150; WB: 1:2,000), mouse anti-TUBULIN (Abmart, T40103; WB: 1:5,000), mouse-anti GAPDH (Proteintech, 60004-1-Ig; WB: 1:10,000). Primer sequences are included in Additional file 2: Table S1.

Immunoblotting, immunoprecipitation and chromatin-immunoprecipitation

The procedure for western blotting was as described previously [34]. Briefly, animal tissue samples or cultured cells were lysed in RIPA buffer (150 mM NaCl, 50 mM Tris buffer (pH=8.0), 1% NP-40, 1% deoxycholate and 0.1% SDS) with protease inhibitors (Roche, 5892970001). After centrifugation at 12,000 rpm for 15 min at 4 °C, the concentration of soluble fraction was measured by BCA Protein Assay Kit (Tiangen) and the soluble fraction was boiling in 5× loading buffer at 100 °C for 15 min. Around 40 μg of protein was loaded per lane for western blotting.

The procedure for immunoprecipitation was described previously with minor modification [35]. Briefly, transfected HEK293T cells (10 cm-plate, 48 hrs after transfection) or the whole brain of rats were lysed in NP-40 buffer (150mM NaCl, 1% NP-40, 50 mM Tris buffer (pH=8.0) and 0.25% deoxycholate) with protease inhibitors. After centrifugation at 12,000 rpm for 15 min at 4 °C, 1 mg of protein lysates were pre-cleaned with IgG for one hour, followed by incubation with the mouse anti-DYKDDDDK-Tag conjugated protein A/G beads (Abmart, M200018) overnight. Pre-cleaned brain lysates were incubated with primary antibodies or control IgG overnight, followed by incubation with protein A/G sepharose beads (Santa Cruz, sc2003) for one hour. The beads were then washed and immunoprecipitated proteins were eluted by boiling in loading buffer.

ChIP assays were performed with serum-shocked synchronized Neuro-2a cells as previously described [36]. Briefly, Neuro-2a cells cultured in 15-cm plates were washed twice by PBS and cross-linked with 1% formaldehyde for 15 min. Cross-linked cells were washed by ice-cold PBS and collected. The nuclear fractions were extracted by high-salt buffer followed by sonication three times for 10s at the maximum setting (SCIENTZ, Scientz-II D). The fragmentation of sonicated chromatin was evaluated by agarose gel electrophoresis and the sonication condition was optimized to achieve ideal fragment size of 200 – 1,000 bp. After centrifugation for 10 min at 12,000 rpm, the supernatants were immunocleared with 2μg sheared salmon sperm DNA (Sigma, D1626), IgG and protein A/G sepharose beads for 2 hrs at 4 °C, and immunoprecipitated with indicated antibodies overnight followed by incubation with salmon sperm DNA and protein A/G sepharose beads. Precipitates were de-crosslinked at 65 °C for 8 hrs and DNA was purified with Universal DNA Purification Kit (Tiangen, DP214) and used in quantitative PCR. For qPCR, 1.5 μL from 60 μL DNA extraction were used with specific primer pairs (Additional file 2: Table S1) and SYBR Green (BIO-RAD, 170888).

Bioinformatics analysis

For Fig. 1d, *Fus* expression pattern in sleep deprived mouse brain was obtained from GSE9442 [31]. For Fig.1e and f, mouse liver and brain stem circadian microarray data were from GSE119237 [37] and GSE54650 [38] respectively. The circadian oscillation of gene expression was determined by fitting the circadian time-series data to cosine functions with 24 hours' period and shifting phases as described previously [26]. For Fig. 2a, REV-ERBα and REV-ERBβ ChIP-seq data in mouse liver were mapped to mouse genome (mm9) by bowtie2 program [39] (default parameters). MACS program [40] was applied to identify the binding sites (MACS 1.4.2, default parameter) from ChIP-seq data. For Fig. 2f, BETA program [41] were applied to evaluate the activating/repressive function of REV-ERBα in mouse liver from the genome-wide data (with parameters:--df=0.05 -d 30000 -k BSF --da 500).

Statistical analysis

Data are presented as mean ± s.e.m. and were analyzed by Prism 7 software (GraphPad). Two-tailed unpaired *t*-test was used to compare the means of two groups. One-way ANOVA followed by Newman-Keuls multiple comparisons test was used for multiple comparisons. Two-way ANOVA followed by Sidak multiple comparison test was used for analysis gene expression in various time points.

Results

FUS is a circadian clock-regulated gene

We first examined the protein expression of FUS in various mouse tissues, including the peripheral circadian clock center liver [42, 43], hypothalamus which harbors central circadian pacemaker suprachiasmatic nucleus[44], and cortex (Fig. 1a-c). FUS expression showed clear circadian oscillation although the patterns varied in different tissues. Since sleep deprivation (SD) affects the expressions of many core circadian genes [31, 45, 46], we compared the expression of *Fus* in the normal and SD conditions by a meta-analysis of published microarray datasets [31] (Fig. 1d). The basal level of *Fus* mRNA was decreased and oscillation amplitude was diminished in sleep-deprived mice (Fig. 1d). These results suggested that the expression of *Fus* was regulated by circadian clock. Furthermore, the oscillation of *Fus* expression was much stronger than *Tdp-43*, another ALS and FTD-associated nuclear protein [47–50] in mice, suggesting that FUS may exert a more active role in circadian rhythm (Fig. 1e, f).

To investigate the underlying mechanism of circadian regulation of *Fus*, we performed a bioinformatics analysis of published ChIP-seq datasets of core circadian proteins and found that only REV-ERBα, not even REV-ERBβ, bound within a 350 bp region in the *Fus* promoter [32], although the *Fus* promoter lacked a consensus REV-ERBα-binding site, the retinoic acid–related orphan receptor response (ROR) element (Fig. 2a, Additional file 3: Table S2). We confirmed the binding of REV-ERBα to the *Fus* promoter using chromatin immunoprecipitation (Fig. 2b). Silencing the gene encoding REV-ERBα, *Nr1d1*, reduced the expression from the *Fus* promoter, and deletion of the REV-ERBα-binding region relieved the effect of *Nr1d1* silencing (Fig. 2c). Intriguingly, removing the 350 bp region containing the REV-ERBα-binding site led to a REV-ERBα-independent increase of *Fus* promoter-luciferase activity, indicating that this region harbored a repressor-responsive element. Furthermore, the protein expression of FUS was reduced in *Nr1d1* knock-out MEF cells (Fig. 2d) as well as in the liver of *Nr1d1* knock-out mice (Fig. 2e), although the number of *Nr1d1* knock-out mice in our experiment was restricted by limited availability due to reduced fertility of these mice [5, 51]. Although REV-ERBα was usually reported as a transcriptional repressor [32], it regulated FUS as an activator in a way very similar to a *Drosophila Nr1d1* homolog, E75 [52], suggesting its versatile action depending on the presence of other transcriptional co-factors. To evaluate the global transcriptional regulation by REV-ERBα, we conducted an activating/repressive functional prediction analysis [41] based on the published REV-ERBα ChIP-seq data [32] and transcriptional profile from the *Nr1d1* knock-out mice [53], and found that REV-ERBα could activate a large number of genes it binds (Fig. 2f). These results indicate that *Fus* is a REV-ERBα-regulated circadian gene.

FUS regulates the expression of core circadian genes

The diurnal expression of core circadian genes, such as *Per* and *Cry*, are regulated by complicated negative feedback loops involving transcriptional and post-translational regulation [1–3]. Since FUS is nuclear protein known to regulate gene expression [54], we assessed whether FUS may affect the expression patterns of some key genes in circadian control. We knocked-down the expression of endogenous *Fus* in synchronized Neuro-2a cells and found the mRNA levels of *Per2* and *Cry1* were generally increased with silenced expression of FUS at various time points during a diurnal cycle (Fig. 3a-c). Conversely, restoring the expression of FUS blunted the activation of *Per2* and *Cry1* by FUS depletion (Fig. 3d, e). These results suggest that FUS is a potential circadian regulator.

FUS facilitates the recruitment of co-repressor complex to the promoters of *Per* genes

We have previously shown that FUS interacts with PSF [35]. Interestingly, PSF is in the PER/CRY, BMAL1, CLOCK protein complex and negatively regulates the expression of *Per1* by recruiting the Sin3A-HDAC1 complex

[12]. Using co-immunoprecipitation assay, we found that FUS could similarly bind PER2, BMAL1, and CLOCK (Fig. 4a). To evaluate the possibility that FUS and PSF may cooperatively repress *Per2* promoter-luciferase activity, we transfected PSF, in the presence or absence of FUS RNAi construct, and found that over-expression of PSF could reduce the *Per2* activation by FUS RNAi (Fig. 4b). Next, we found that while the knock-down of either FUS or PSF led to increased *Per2* promoter-luciferase activity, double knock-down did not produce an additive effect, suggesting that PSF and FUS operate through a common repressor complex (Fig. 4c). After analyzing the promoter loading of PSF at different circadian time in synchronized Neuro-2a cells, we found that during the observation window between 22 to 40 hrs after synchronization, the 28-hr time point showed the peak PSF binding (Fig. 4d). We then assessed the effect of FUS on the loading of PSF and HDAC1 onto the promoters of *Per1*, and *Per2* at this time point. FUS depletion led to reduced promoter occupancy of PSF and HDAC1 (Fig. 4e, f). Collectively, our results indicate that FUS may facilitate the recruitment of co-repressor complex PSF-HDAC1 to the promoters of *Per* genes.

Mutation in *Fus* leads to abnormal circadian gene expression

Mutations in *Fus* cause early onset of ALS and FTD [19–21, 55–57]. To evaluate whether pathogenic mutations may affect circadian regulation by FUS, we examined the expression of *Per2* and *Bmal1* in REFs derived from FUS R521C knock-in rats available in the lab. R521C is one of the most common FUS point mutations [58–61]. Both the *Per2* promoter activity and mRNA expression were decreased (Fig. 5a, b). We then assessed the interaction between PSF and FUS-R521C. We found that FUS-R521C showed a much stronger binding to PSF than the wild-type FUS and the binding between FUS and PSF required the C-terminus of FUS (Fig. 5c). Furthermore, we confirmed the increased binding between FUS R521C and PSF in the brain tissue from FUS-R521C knock-in rats (Fig. 5d). We have also detected the binding between PSF and other two C-terminus-located FUS pathogenic mutations, R518K and P525L (Fig. 5e). Surprisingly, unlike R521C, FUS P525L showed significantly weaker binding with PSF than wild-type FUS (more in Discussion). Taken together, our results suggest that mutations in *Fus* could lead to abnormal circadian gene expression.

Discussion

In summary, we have identified ALS/FTD-associated FUS as a novel modulator for the circadian gene expression. The FUS expression is positively regulated by REV-ERBα. Meanwhile, FUS is a component of the

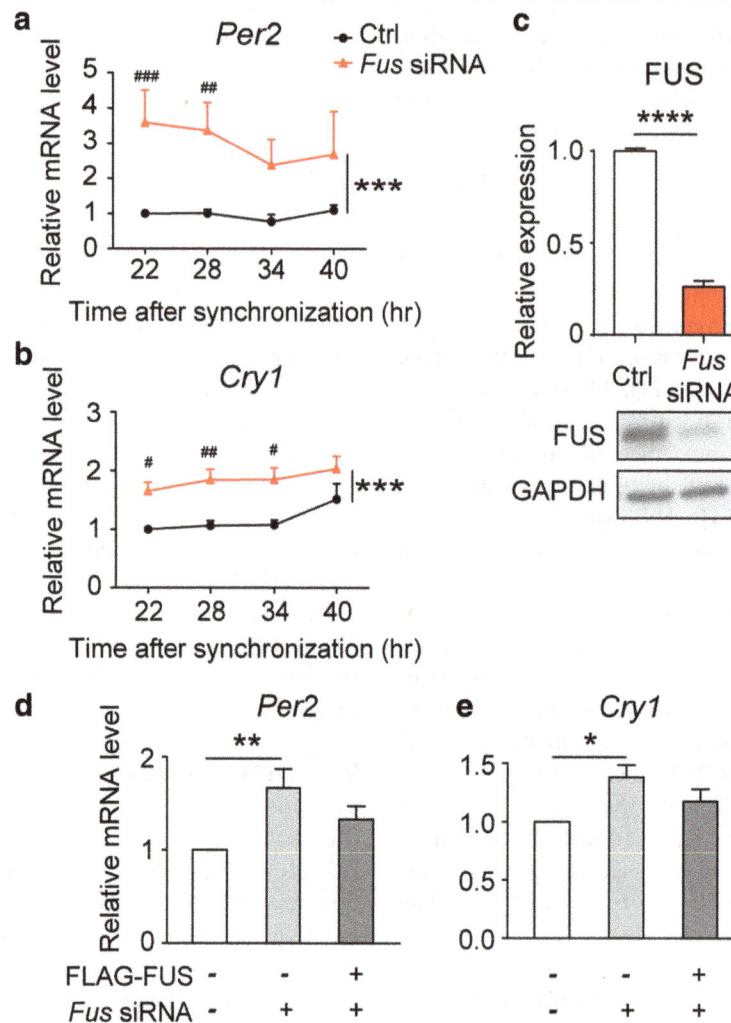

Fig. 3 FUS regulates the expression of core circadian genes. **a, b** mRNA expression levels of *Per2* (**a**) and *Cry1* (**b**) in synchronized Neuro-2a cells after siRNA silencing (mean ± s.e.m.; N = 4-6 experiments; two-way ANOVA with Sidak's multiple comparison test, * represents the significant P-value of overall two-way ANOVA analysis, ***:$P \leq 0.001$, # represents the significant P-value of Sidak's multiple comparison test, #:$P \leq 0.05$, ##:$P \leq 0.01$, ###:$P \leq 0.001$). **c** Western blot showing the knock-down efficiency of *Fus*-targeting siRNA (mean ± s.e.m.; N = 3-4 experiments; t-test; ****: $P \leq 0.0001$). **d, e** RT-qPCR showing the mRNA expression of *Per2* and *Cry1* in cells with indicated transfection conditions in serum shock-synchronized Neuro-2a cells (mean ± s.e.m.; N = 8-9 experiments; One-way ANOVA with Newman-Keuls multiple comparisons test; *:$P \leq 0.05$; **:$P \leq 0.01$)

PER-CRY-BMAL1-CLOCK mega-complex, and it represses the expression of *Per* by recruiting PSF-HDAC1. Therefore, besides transcriptionally repressing *Bmal1*, REV-ERBα could negatively regulate the expression of *Per* genes via the action of FUS.

The regulation of FUS by REV-ERBα suggests that dysregulated circadian clock could lead to the abnormal expression of FUS, as demonstrated by the reduction of FUS expression in sleep-deprived mice (Fig. 1d). Since the change in *Fus* expression is detrimental to neuronal health and contributes to the pathogenesis of ALS and FTD [58, 62, 63], our results have provided new mechanistic insights into the role of circadian dysfunction as a risk factor for neurodegeneration. Because of the

importance of FUS, dramatic fluctuation of FUS would not be desirable for the organism. It is not surprising to observe the moderate but reproducible regulation of FUS by REV-ERBα. In addition, it is possible that other circadian regulators may also participate in the regulation of FUS expression.

Although we have described a mechanism related to the transcriptional regulation by FUS, other functions of FUS could also contribute to circadian gene regulation. For example, FUS is a key regulator in RNA splicing [64, 65]. However, published RNA splicing targets by FUS do not contain core circadian genes [64]. Whether the RNA-binding property of FUS is involved in circadian gene regulation remains to be elucidated.

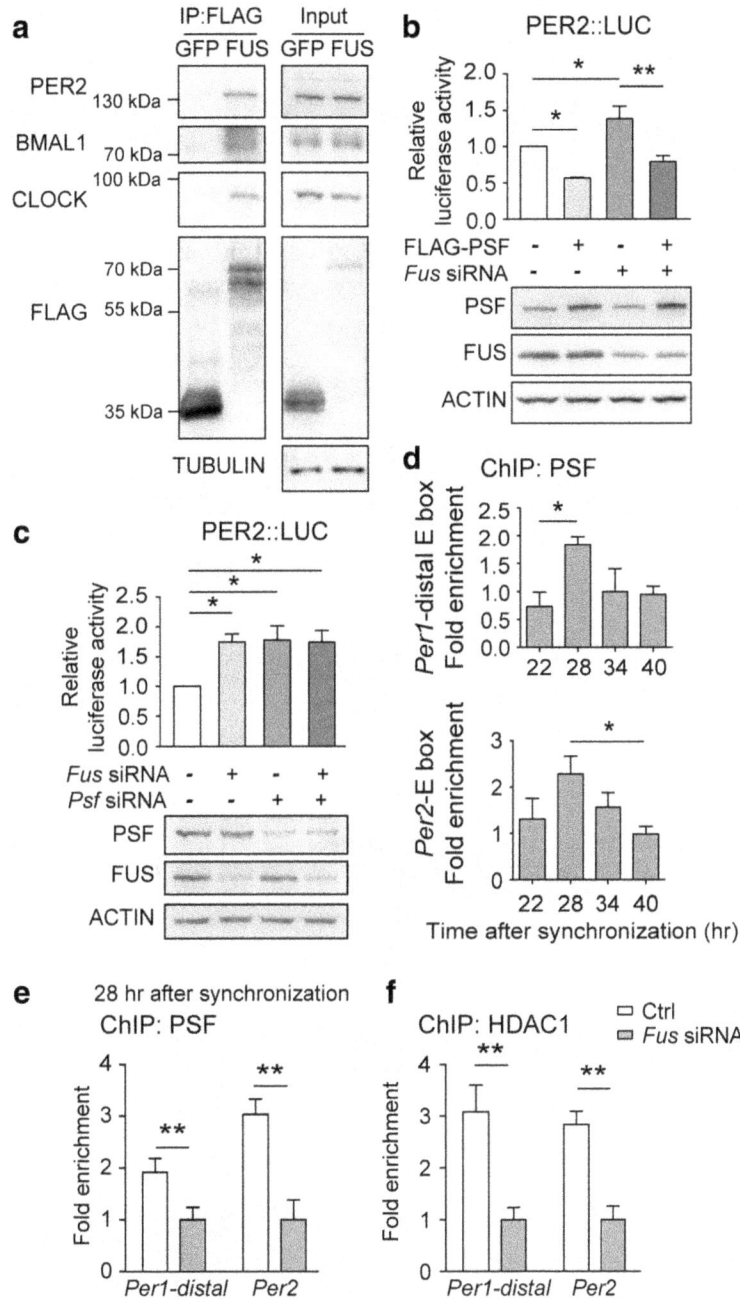

Fig. 4 FUS is in the repressor complex and mediates the recruitment of PSF-HDAC1 to the promoters of E box-containing genes. **a** Co-immunoprecipitation of FLAG-FUS with PER2, BMAL1 and CLOCK in HEK293T cells. **b, c** *Per2* promoter-luciferase reporter activity in synchronized Neuro-2a cells after transfection and siRNA silencing with indicated conditions. Cells were first transfected with indicated RNAi constructs at 0 hr, followed by expression plasmid transfection at 24 hr if needed. Cells were synchronized at the 48 hr point for 2 hrs, and harvested for analysis at the 72 hr time point (mean ± s.e.m.; $N = 3$ experiments in duplicates; One-way ANOVA followed by Newman-Keuls multiple comparisons test; *:$P \leq 0.05$, **:$P \leq 0.01$). **d** ChIP-qPCR showing the promoter loading of PSF relative to IgG control. Neuro-2a cells were harvested at indicated time points after serum shock synchronization (mean ± s.e.m.; $N = 3$-5 experiments; One-way ANOVA followed by Dunnett's multiple comparison test; *:$P \leq 0.05$). **e, f** ChIP-qPCR showing the effect of FUS silencing on the binding of endogenous PSF (**e**) or HDAC1 (**f**) onto the E box-containing promoters of circadian genes. Neuro-2a cells were harvested at 28 hrs after serum shock synchronization (IgG as the ChIP control, mean ± s.e.m.; $N = 3$-5 experiments; t-test; **:$P \leq 0.01$)

Our data suggest that the FUS C-terminus, a mutation hot spot [66], may mediate the binding between FUS and the PSF-containing protein complex. Consistent with a recent report [67], pathogenic mutations such as R518K and P525L (Fig. 5e) could affect the binding between FUS and PSF. Therefore, some pathogenic

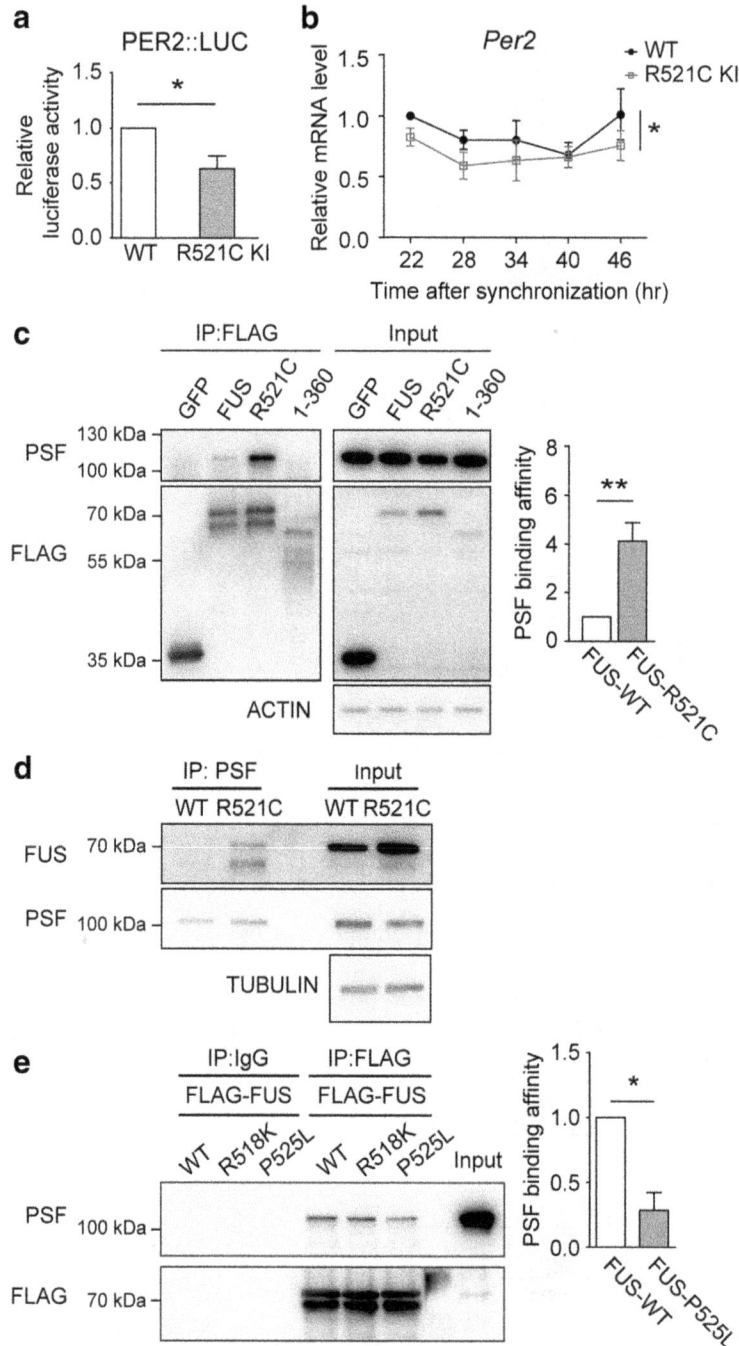

Fig. 5 The pathogenic R521C mutation of FUS leads to abnormal expression of core circadian genes. **a** Luciferase activity of transfected PER2-promoter-luciferase in the wild-type (WT) and FUS R521C knock-in (KI) REFs (mean ± s.e.m.; N = 3 experiments; t-test; *:P≤0.05). **b** mRNA expression levels of *Per2* in synchronized REFs (mean ± s.e.m.; N = 6 experiments; two-way ANOVA, *:P≤0.05). **c** Co-immunoprecipitation of FLAG-GFP, wild-type or R521C-FUS and a FUS C-terminus deletion construct (1-360 residues) with endogenous PSF in HEK293T cells (mean ± s.e.m.; N = 5 experiments; t-test; **:P≤0.01). **d** Co-immunoprecipitation of endogenous PSF with FUS in the whole brain tissue of the wild-type and FUS R521C knocked-in rats. **e** Co-immunoprecipitation of FLAG-tagged wild-typed and R518K and P525L FUS with endogenous PSF in HEK293T cells (mean ± s.e.m.; N = 3 experiments, t-test, *:P≤0.05)

mutations in *Fus* will conceivably lead to altered recruitment of the repressor complex and affect the transcription of core circadian genes. It will be of great interest in the future to determine whether FUS mutation-induced circadian gene dysregulation may contribute to or further exacerbate the neurodegeneration process.

Conclusions

We have identified ALS/FTD-associated FUS as a modulator of circadian gene expression, and provided new mechanistic evidence supporting the mutual influence between circadian disturbance and neurodegeneration.

Abbreviations

Per: Period; *Cry*: Cryptochrome; *Nr1d1*: Nuclear receptor subfamily 1 group D member 1; PSF: PTB-associated splicing factor; HDAC1: Histone deacetylase 1; SIN3A: SIN3 transcription regulator family member A; GAPDH: Glyceraldehyde 3-phosphate dehydrogenase; NS: Non-significant; KO: Knock-out; KI: Knock-in; SD: sleep deprivation; CT: circadian time; RT-qPCR: Reverse transcription-quantitative polymerase chain reaction

Acknowledgements

We thank Dr. Ying Xu (Soochow University) for providing the *Nr1d1* knock-out mice.

Funding

This work was supported by Hundreds of Talents Program to J.X. and H.C.C, Chinese Academy of Sciences; Shanghai Pujiang Talent Program (12PJ1410000) and National Natural Science Foundation of China grant (81771425) to J.X.; Chinese Academy of Sciences Strategic Priority Research Program Grant (XDB02060006) and National Natural Science Foundation of China Grant (31571209) to J.Y.; Natural Science Foundation of Shanghai Grant (16ZR1448800) to H.F.W.

Authors' contributions

XJ and JX designed research, XJ, TZ, HFW, TW, MLQ, PBH, RQW, YWL performed research, XJ, TZ and JX analyzed data, and HFW and JY performed bioinformatics analysis. HCC contributed crucial reagents and provided key discussion. JX and XJ wrote the paper with input from co-authors. All authors read and approved the final manuscript.

Competing interests

The authors declare that they have no competing interests.

Author details

¹Institute of Neuroscience, State Key Laboratory of Neuroscience, CAS Key laboratory of Primate Neurobiology, Shanghai Institutes for Biological Sciences, Chinese Academy of Sciences, New Life Science Bldg, 320 Yue Yang Road, Shanghai 200031, China. ²University of Chinese Academy of Sciences, Shanghai 200031, China.

References

1. Takahashi JS. Transcriptional architecture of the mammalian circadian clock. Nat Rev Genet. 2016;18:164–79.
2. Dibner C, Schibler U, Albrecht U. The Mammalian Circadian Timing System: Organization and Coordination of Central and Peripheral Clocks. Ann Rev Physiol. 2010;72:517–49.
3. Novak B, Tyson JJ. Design principles of biochemical oscillators. Nat Rev Mol Cell Biol. 2008;9:981–91.
4. Zhang Y, Fang B, Emmett MJ, Damle M, Sun Z, Feng D, Armour SM, Remsberg JR, Jager J, Soccio RE, et al. GENE REGULATION. Discrete functions of nuclear receptor Rev-erbalpha couple metabolism to the clock. Science. 2015;348:1488–92.
5. Preitner N, Damiola F, Lopez-Molina L, Zakany J, Duboule D, Albrecht U, Schibler U. The orphan nuclear receptor REV-ERBalpha controls circadian transcription within the positive limb of the mammalian circadian oscillator. Cell. 2002;110:251–60.
6. Gekakis N, Staknis D, Nguyen HB, Davis FC, Wilsbacher LD, King DP, Takahashi JS, Weitz CJ. Role of the CLOCK protein in the mammalian circadian mechanism. Science. 1998;280:1564–9.
7. Kume K, Zylka MJ, Sriram S, Shearman LP, Weaver DR, Jin X, Maywood ES, Hastings MH, Reppert SM. mCRY1 and mCRY2 are essential components of the negative limb of the circadian clock feedback loop. Cell. 1999;98:193–205.
8. Shearman LP, Sriram S, Weaver DR, Maywood ES, Chaves I, Zheng B, Kume K, Lee CC, van der Horst GT, Hastings MH, Reppert SM. Interacting molecular loops in the mammalian circadian clock. Science. 2000;288:1013–9.
9. Lee C, Etchegaray JP, Cagampang FR, Loudon AS, Reppert SM. Posttranslational mechanisms regulate the mammalian circadian clock. Cell. 2001;107:855–67.
10. Kim J, Kwak P, Weitz CJ. Specificity in Circadian Clock Feedback from Targeted Reconstitution of the NuRD Corepressor. Molecular Cell. 2014;56:738–48.
11. Padmanabhan K, Robles MS, Westerling T, Weitz CJ. Feedback regulation of transcriptional termination by the mammalian circadian clock PERIOD complex. Science. 2012;337:599–602.
12. Duong HA, Robles MS, Knutti D, Weitz CJ. A molecular mechanism for circadian clock negative feedback. Science. 2011;332:1436–9.
13. Chang HC, Guarente L. SIRT1 mediates central circadian control in the SCN by a mechanism that decays with aging. Cell. 2013;153:1448–60.
14. Asher G, Gatfield D, Stratmann M, Reinke H, Dibner C, Kreppel F, Mostoslavsky R, Alt FW, Schibler U. SIRT1 regulates circadian clock gene expression through PER2 deacetylation. Cell. 2008;134:317–28.
15. Musiek ES, Xiong DD, Holtzman DM. Sleep, circadian rhythms, and the pathogenesis of Alzheimer disease. Exp Mol Med. 2015;47:e148.
16. Videnovic A, Lazar AS, Barker RA, Overeem S. The clocks that time us'--circadian rhythms in neurodegenerative disorders. Nat Rev Neurol. 2014;10:683–93.
17. Lim C, Allada R. ATAXIN-2 activates PERIOD translation to sustain circadian rhythms in Drosophila. Science. 340:875–9.
18. Zhang Y, Ling J, Yuan C, Dubruille R, Emery P. A role for Drosophila ATX2 in activation of PER translation and circadian behavior. Science. 2013;340:879–82.
19. Kwiatkowski TJ Jr, Bosco DA, Leclerc AL, Tamrazian E, Vanderburg CR, Russ C, Davis A, Gilchrist J, Kasarskis EJ, Munsat T, et al. Mutations in the FUS/TLS gene on chromosome 16 cause familial amyotrophic lateral sclerosis. Science. 2009;323:1205–8.
20. Vance C, Rogelj B, Hortobagyi T, De Vos KJ, Nishimura AL, Sreedharan J, Hu X, Smith B, Ruddy D, Wright P, et al. Mutations in FUS, an RNA processing protein, cause familial amyotrophic lateral sclerosis type 6. Science. 2009;323:1208–11.
21. Deng H, Gao K, Jankovic J. The role of FUS gene variants in neurodegenerative diseases. Nat Rev Neurol. 2014;10:337–48.
22. Ahmed RM, Newcombe RE, Piper AJ, Lewis SJ, Yee BJ, Kiernan MC, Grunstein RR. Sleep disorders and respiratory function in amyotrophic lateral sclerosis. Sleep Med Rev. 26:33–42.
23. Bonakis A, Economou NT, Paparrigopoulos T, Bonanni E, Maestri M, Carnicelli L, Di Coscio E, Ktonas P, Vagiakis E, Theodoropoulos P, Papageorgiou SG. Sleep in frontotemporal dementia is equally or possibly more disrupted, and at an earlier stage, when compared to sleep in Alzheimer's disease. J Alzheimers Dis. 38:85–91.

24. Liguori C, Placidi F, Albanese M, Nuccetelli M, Izzi F, Marciani MG, Mercuri NB, Bernardini S, Romigi A. CSF beta-amyloid levels are altered in narcolepsy: a link with the inflammatory hypothesis? J Sleep Res. 23:420–4.

25. Kornmann B, Schaad O, Bujard H, Takahashi JS, Schibler U. System-driven and oscillator-dependent circadian transcription in mice with a conditionally active liver clock. PLoS Biol. 2007;5:e34.

26. Yan J, Wang H, Liu Y, Shao C. Analysis of Gene Regulatory Networks in the Mammalian Circadian Rhythm. PLoS Comput Biol. 2008;4:e1000193.

27. Bae S, Park J, Kim JS. Cas-OFFinder: a fast and versatile algorithm that searches for potential off-target sites of Cas9 RNA-guided endonucleases. Bioinformatics. 2014;30:1473–5.

28. Yagita K, Okamura H. Forskolin induces circadian gene expression of rPer1, rPer2 and dbp in mammalian rat-1 fibroblasts. FEBS Lett. 2000;465:79–82.

29. Balsalobre A, Damiola F, Schibler U. A serum shock induces circadian gene expression in mammalian tissue culture cells. Cell. 1998;93:929–37.

30. Balsalobre A, Brown SA, Marcacci L, Tronche F, Kellendonk C, Reichardt HM, Schutz G, Schibler U. Resetting of circadian time in peripheral tissues by glucocorticoid signaling. Science. 2000;289:2344–7.

31. Maret S, Dorsaz S, Gurcel L, Pradervand S, Petit B, Pfister C, Hagenbuchle O, O'Hara BF, Franken P, Tafti M. Homer1a is a core brain molecular correlate of sleep loss. Proc Natl Acad Sci USA. 2007;104:20090–5.

32. Cho H, Zhao X, Hatori M, Yu RT, Barish GD, Lam MT, Chong LW, DiTacchio L, Atkins AR, Glass CK, et al. Regulation of circadian behaviour and metabolism by REV-ERB-alpha and REV-ERB-beta. Nature. 2012;485:123–7.

33. Travnickova-Bendova Z, Cermakian N, Reppert SM, Sassone-Corsi P. Bimodal regulation of mPeriod promoters by CREB-dependent signaling and CLOCK/BMAL1 activity. Proc Natl Acad Sci USA. 2002;99:7728–33.

34. Xu J, Kao SY, Lee FJ, Song W, Jin LW, Yankner BA. Dopamine-dependent neurotoxicity of alpha-synuclein: a mechanism for selective neurodegeneration in Parkinson disease. Nat Med. 2002;8:600–6.

35. Wang T, Jiang X, Chen G, Xu J. Interaction of amyotrophic lateral sclerosis/frontotemporal lobar degeneration-associated fused-in-sarcoma with proteins involved in metabolic and protein degradation pathways. Neurobiol Aging. 2015;36:527–35.

36. Shang Y, Hu X, DiRenzo J, Lazar MA, Brown M. Cofactor dynamics and sufficiency in estrogen receptor-regulated transcription. Cell. 2000;103:843–52.

37. Zhang R, Lahens NF, Ballance HI, Hughes ME, Hogenesch JB. A circadian gene expression atlas in mammals: implications for biology and medicine. Proc Natl Acad Sci USA. 2014;111:16219–24.

38. Hughes ME, DiTacchio L, Hayes KR, Vollmers C, Pulivarthy S, Baggs JE, Panda S, Hogenesch JB. Harmonics of circadian gene transcription in mammals. PLoS genetics. 2009;5:e1000442.

39. Langmead B, Salzberg SL. Fast gapped-read alignment with Bowtie 2. Nature methods. 2012;9:357–9.

40. Zhang Y, Liu T, Meyer CA, Eeckhoute J, Johnson DS, Bernstein BE, Nussbaum C, Myers RM, Brown M, Li W, Liu XS. Model-based Analysis of ChIP-Seq (MACS). Genome Biol. 2008;9:R137.

41. Wang S, Sun HF, Ma J, Zang CZ, Wang CF, Wang J, Tang QZ, Meyer CA, Zhang Y, Liu XS. Target analysis by integration of transcriptome and ChIP-seq data with BETA. Nat Protoc. 2013;8:2502–15.

42. Damiola F, Le Minh N, Preitner N, Kornmann B, Fleury-Olela F, Schibler U: Restricted feeding uncouples circadian oscillators in peripheral tissues from the central pacemaker in the suprachiasmatic nucleus. Genes Dev 2000, 14:2950-2961.

43. Mohawk JA, Green CB, Takahashi JS. Central and peripheral circadian clocks in mammals. Annu Rev Neurosci. 2012;35:445–62.

44. Eastman CI, Mistlberger RE, Rechtschaffen A. Suprachiasmatic nuclei lesions eliminate circadian temperature and sleep rhythms in the rat. Physiol Behav. 1984;32:357–68.

45. Franken P, Thomason R, Heller HC, O'Hara BF. A non-circadian role for clock-genes in sleep homeostasis: a strain comparison. BMC Neurosci. 2007;8:87.

46. Wisor JP, O'Hara BF, Terao A, Selby CP, Kilduff TS, Sancar A, Edgar DM, Franken P. A role for cryptochromes in sleep regulation. BMC Neurosci. 2002;3:20.

47. Arai T, Hasegawa M, Akiyama H, Ikeda K, Nonaka T, Mori H, Mann D, Tsuchiya K, Yoshida M, Hashizume Y, Oda T. TDP-43 is a component of ubiquitin-positive tau-negative inclusions in frontotemporal lobar degeneration and amyotrophic lateral sclerosis. Biochem Biophys Res Commun. 2006;351:602–11.

48. Neumann M, Sampathu DM, Kwong LK, Truax AC, Micsenyi MC, Chou TT, Bruce J, Schuck T, Grossman M, Clark CM, et al. Ubiquitinated TDP-43 in frontotemporal lobar degeneration and amyotrophic lateral sclerosis. Science. 2006;314:130–3.

49. Cairns NJ, Neumann M, Bigio EH, Holm IE, Troost D, Hatanpaa KJ, Foong C, White CL 3rd, Schneider JA, Kretzschmar HA, et al. TDP-43 in familial and sporadic frontotemporal lobar degeneration with ubiquitin inclusions. Am J Pathol. 2007;171:227–40.

50. Mackenzie IR, Bigio EH, Ince PG, Geser F, Neumann M, Cairns NJ, Kwong LK, Forman MS, Ravits J, Stewart H, et al. Pathological TDP-43 distinguishes sporadic amyotrophic lateral sclerosis from amyotrophic lateral sclerosis with SOD1 mutations. Ann Neurol. 2007;61:427–34.

51. Chomez P, Neveu I, Mansen A, Kiesler E, Larsson L, Vennstrom B, Arenas E. Increased cell death and delayed development in the cerebellum of mice lacking the rev-erbA(alpha) orphan receptor. Development. 2000;127:1489–98.

52. Jaumouille E, Machado Almeida P, Stahli P, Koch R, Nagoshi E. Transcriptional regulation via nuclear receptor crosstalk required for the Drosophila circadian clock. Curr Biol. 2015;25:1502–8.

53. Fang B, Everett LJ, Jager J, Briggs E, Armour SM, Feng D, Roy A, Gerhart-Hines Z, Sun Z, Lazar MA. Circadian Enhancers Coordinate Multiple Phases of Rhythmic Gene Transcription In Vivo. Cell. 2014;159:1140–52.

54. Tan AY, Riley TR, Coady T, Bussemaker HJ, Manley JL. TLS/FUS (translocated in liposarcoma/fused in sarcoma) regulates target gene transcription via single-stranded DNA response elements. Proc Natl Acad Sci U S A. 2012;109:6030–5.

55. Neumann M, Rademakers R, Roeber S, Baker M, Kretzschmar HA, Mackenzie IR. A new subtype of frontotemporal lobar degeneration with FUS pathology. Brain. 2009;132:2922–31.

56. Seelaar H, Klijnsma KY, de Koning I, van der Lugt A, Chiu WZ, Azmani A, Rozemuller AJ, van Swieten JC. Frequency of ubiquitin and FUS-positive, TDP-43-negative frontotemporal lobar degeneration. J Neurol. 2010;257:747–53.

57. Urwin H, Josephs KA, Rohrer JD, Mackenzie IR, Neumann M, Authier A, Seelaar H, Van Swieten JC, Brown JM, Johannsen P, et al. FUS pathology defines the majority of tau- and TDP-43-negative frontotemporal lobar degeneration. Acta Neuropathol. 2010;120:33–41.

58. Huang C, Zhou H, Tong J, Chen H, Liu Y-J, Wang D, Wei X, Xia X-G. FUS Transgenic Rats Develop the Phenotypes of Amyotrophic Lateral Sclerosis and Frontotemporal Lobar Degeneration. PLoS Genetics. 2011;7:e1002011.

59. Sharma A, Lyashchenko AK, Lu L, Nasrabady SE, Elmaleh M, Mendelsohn M, Nemes A, Tapia JC, Mentis GZ, Shneider NA. ALS-associated mutant FUS induces selective motor neuron degeneration through toxic gain of function. Nat Commun. 2016;7:10465.

60. Qiu H, Lee S, Shang Y, Wang WY, Au KF, Kamiya S, Barmada SJ, Finkbeiner S, Lui H, Carlton CE, et al. ALS-associated mutation FUS-R521C causes DNA damage and RNA splicing defects. J Clin Invest. 2014;124:981–99.

61. Huang C, Tong J, Bi F, Wu Q, Huang B, Zhou H, Xia XG. Entorhinal cortical neurons are the primary targets of FUS mislocalization and ubiquitin aggregation in FUS transgenic rats. Hum Mol Genet. 2012;21:4602–14.

62. Mitchell JC, McGoldrick P, Vance C, Hortobagyi T, Sreedharan J, Rogelj B, Tudor EL, Smith BN, Klasen C, Miller CC, et al. Overexpression of human wild-type FUS causes progressive motor neuron degeneration in an age- and dose-dependent fashion. Acta Neuropathol. 2013;125:273–88.

63. Sabatelli M, Moncada A, Conte A, Lattante S, Marangi G, Luigetti M, Lucchini M, Mirabella M, Romano A, Del Grande A, et al. Mutations in the 3' untranslated region of FUS causing FUS overexpression are associated with amyotrophic lateral sclerosis. Hum Mol Genet. 2013;22:4748–55.

64. Lagier-Tourenne C, Polymenidou M, Hutt KR, Vu AQ, Baughn M, Huelga SC, Clutario KM, Ling SC, Liang TY, Mazur C, et al. Divergent roles of ALS-linked proteins FUS/TLS and TDP-43 intersect in processing long pre-mRNAs. Nat Neurosci. 2012;15:1488–97.

65. Rogelj B, Easton LE, Bogu GK, Stanton LW, Rot G, Curk T, Zupan B, Sugimoto Y, Modic M, Haberman N, et al. Widespread binding of FUS along nascent RNA regulates alternative splicing in the brain. Sci Rep. 2012;2:603.

66. Lattante S, Rouleau GA, Kabashi E. TARDBP and FUS mutations associated with amyotrophic lateral sclerosis: summary and update. Hum Mutat. 2013;34:812–26.

67. Ishigaki S, Fujioka Y, Okada Y, Riku Y, Udagawa T, Honda D, Yokoi S, Endo K, Ikenaka K, Takagi S, et al. Altered Tau Isoform Ratio Caused by Loss of FUS and SFPQ Function Leads to FTLD-like Phenotypes. Cell Rep. 2017;18:1118–31.

24

Cognitive characteristics in Chinese non-demented PD patients based on gender difference

Ke Yang[1†], Bo Shen[1†], Da-ke Li[1], Ying Wang[1], Jue Zhao[1], Jian Zhao[1], Wen-Bo Yu[1], Zhen-yang Liu[1], Yi-lin Tang[1], Feng-tao Liu[1], Huan Yu[1], Jian Wang[1], Qi-hao Guo[1*] and Jian-jun Wu[1,2*]

Abstract

Background: Cognitive impairment is one of the non-motor symptoms in Parkinson's disease (PD). In the present study, we aim to examine the cognitive function of non-demented Parkinson's disease patients and compare the results between male and female patients as well as control groups in search of any gender effect.

Methods: Sixty PD Patients (30 males and 30 females) from the Movement Disorders Clinic at Huashan Hospital Affiliated to Fudan University were recruited to participate in the study. One hundred age and gender matched control subjects without neurological or psychiatric disorders were voluntarily recruited. The participants were administered measures of cognition in five domains including memory, language, spatial processing abilities, attention and executive function.

Results: PD patients attained significantly lower scores in the visual spatial function, language and attention/executive function compared with the control group. Anti-parkinsonian treated patients performed worse in Rey-copy score, Clock Drawing Test (CDT) and Verbal Fluency-City than untreated ones. In regard to gender differences, though no general cognitive differences were found in Mini-mental State Examination (MMSE), men surpassed women on Boston naming test (BNT) while women were superior on Auditory Verbal Learning Test-long (AVLT) delayed cued recall test.

Conclusions: Cognitive impairments were common in PD patients even in the absence of dementia. PD patients with anti-parkinsonian medication had worse cognitive impairment than untreated patients. Genders may have different manifestations of cognitive impairment in PD patients.

Keywords: Parkinson's disease, Cognition, Gender effect, Cognitive deficits

Background

Parkinson's disease (PD) has been considered a debilitating motor disorder, and the non-motor symptoms are gaining more and more attention. Cognitive impairment is a major non-motor symptoms, which greatly influence the quality of life [1]. It is estimated that 25% untreated 'de novo' patients have cognitive impairment of varying degrees. Some changes in cognition are subtle thus inconspicuous to the patients and their caregivers [2, 3]. Various studies have been conducted to measure specific cognitive functions in PD patients, such as executive abilities, working memory, visuospatial processing, language and attentional processes [4–6]. However, no agreement has been reached as to a definite neuropsychological profile of non-demented PD patients. Besides, it is reported that more men than women are diagnosed with PD, suggesting a gender difference in PD [7, 8]. Although a few studies addressed the gender differences in PD as well as the influence of estrogen on dopaminergic neurons and related pathways in the brain, most of them adopted general cognitive screening tools such as Mini-mental State Examination (MMSE) or Montreal Cognitive Assessment (MocA), little is known as to the specific cognitive domains influenced by gender [9–12]. Therefore, knowledge about differences in cognition between men and

* Correspondence: dr.guoqihao@126.com; jungliw@gmail.com
†Ke Yang and Bo Shen contributed equally to this work.
[1]Department of Neurology and Institute of Neurology, Huashan Hospital, Fudan University, 12 Wulumuqi Zhong Road, Shanghai 200040, China
Full list of author information is available at the end of the article

women with PD and about the pathophysiology under-lying those differences may enhance the accuracy and ef-fectiveness of clinical assessment and treatment of the disease.

The current study examined the five domains of cogni-tive function in non-demented PD patients who were not treated with anticholinergic medications and normal con-trols, with special emphasis on the comparison between male and female patients. Meanwhile, we performed sub-group analysis regarding medical treatment of PD patients, aiming to eliminate the possible confounding effects of medication and making the groups more com-parable. As the effect of anti-parkinsonism medication on cognitive function was complicated and controversial [13–15].

Methods
Subjects
Patients were recruited from the Movement Disorders Clinic at Huashan Hospital Affiliated to Fudan University. All patients fulfilled the UK PD Society Brain Bank (PDSBB) diagnostic criteria for PD [16]. A total of 60 PD patients were recruited to participate in the study, including 30 males and 30 females. Every participant underwent a comprehensive neuro-psychological assessment as part of a longitudinal study of cognition in PD patients. None of the patients complained of cognitive decline or visual hallucination. Dementia and depression were ruled out according to Diagnostic and Statistical Manual of

Mental Disorders IV criteria [17]. Patients with the his-tory of drug or alcohol abuse, cardiovascular disease, insulin - dependent diabetes, head trauma as well as those who underwent surgical relief of PD symptoms were excluded. One hundred age- and gender- matched control subjects with no neurological or psychiatric disorders were voluntar-ily recruited. The study was approved by the ethics commit-tee of Huashan Hospital and written informed consent was obtained from each subject included in the study after the procedure was fully explained. Demographic and clinical data of all the PD patients are summarized in Table 1.

Procedure
All the evaluations were conducted or supervised by a licensed clinical neurologist. Stage of illness was de-termined using the Hoehn and Yahr scale [18]. PD duration was defined as the time between disease on-set (self-reported onset of the first cardinal motor manifestation of Parkinsonism, i.e., rest tremor, rigid-ity, or bradykinesia) and the time of neuropsycho-logical evaluation. The severity of the motor symptoms was assessed using part III of the Unified PD Rating Scale (UPDRS) (examined in the medica-tion "off" phase) [19].

Participants were asked to provide information on their use of medication. Thirty-one of the patients were on anti-parkinsonian treatment at the time of investiga-tion and 29 were untreated. Treatment included MAO-B inhibitors ($n = 4$), L-dopa monotherapy ($n = 9$), dopamine agonist monotherapy ($n = 7$), a combination of

Table 1 Clinical and Demographic Description of PD patients

	PD ($n = 60$)	Male PD ($n = 30$)	Female PD ($n = 30$)
Age(yr)	59.05 ± 9.55	58.67 ± 10.23	59.43 ± 8.98
Age of onset(yr)	54.97 ± 10.42	54.4 ± 11.38	55.53 ± 9.53
Handedness(L/R)(n)	0/60	0/30	0/30
Educational level(yr)	12.86 ± 2.97	13.1 ± 2.94	12.61 ± 3.03
Duration of illness(yr)	4.22 ± 5.33	4.37 ± 4.85	4.07 ± 5.85
Hoehn and Yahr stage	1.73 ± 0.8	1.92 ± 0.81	1.54 ± 0.76
UPDRS—Part III ("off" medication)	24.81 ± 12.04	24.42 ± 13.32	25.19 ± 10.92
Medication(n)	31/60	15/30	16/30
MAOI-B	4	1	3
Dopamine agonist	7	2	5
Levodopa	9	5	4
Levodopa and dopamine agonist	12	7	5
Levodopa and MAOI-B	2	1	1
Dopamine agonist and MAOI-B	1	1	0
Medication(equivalent)	472.74 ± 293.16	483.73 ± 293.69	460.28 ± 302.34
BDI	12.44 ± 9.06	12.48 ± 10.88	12.39 ± 7.08
MMSE	28.98 ± 1.07	28.97 ± 0.81	29 ± 1.29

Note. *UPDRS* Unified parkinson's disease rating scale, *MAOI-B* Monoamine oxidase inhibitor type B, *BDI* Beck depression inventory, *MMSE* Mini-mental state examination

L-dopa and dopamine agonist ($n = 12$), a combination of L-dopa and MAO-B inhibitors ($n = 2$), or a combination of dopamine agonist and MAO-B inhibitors ($n = 1$). No patients were asked to change their medication for this study, nor were any receiving psychoactive or anticholinergic medication. Levodopa-equivalent daily dose (LEDD) was calculated according to standard conversion formula [20].

Neuropsychological tests were conducted in the morning under the "on" status, which was 30 to 60 min after taking the anti-parkinsonism medication. Subjects were allowed to take breaks when needed, in order to maximize performances. All tests were conducted according to standard procedure as outlined in test manuals. The test battery, which required approximately 2.0 h to complete, included a screening test of MMSE for global cognitive efficiency [21]. Five cognitive domains were evaluated: memory, language, spatial processing abilities, attention and executive function. All the tests were administered and scored according to published procedures which were shown in Table 2.

Data analysis

Statistical analysis was performed using the Statistical Package for Social Science (SPSS version 18 for windows, Baltimore). For comparisons, the Student's T test was applied as the variables met the normal distribution, whereas the Manne Whitney test was used for the variables that did not meet the norms for using parametric statistics. Multiple linear regression was used to evaluate the effects of gender on cognitive function. A value of $P < 0.05$ was considered statistically significant.

Results

Demographic and clinical characteristics of participants

Demographic and clinical data of all the PD patients are summarized in Table 1. There was no significant difference between male and female patients, with respect to age, education, years of illness duration, mean UPDRS-III score, proportion of treatment, levodopa equivalent dose or disease severity. In the comparison of treated and untreated PD patients, we found much longer disease duration in the treated PD group, without any other demographic difference. The controls did not differ on age, education background or the dementia screening.

Cognitive performance

The results of neuropsychological tests in PD patients and controls are reported in Table 3. PD patients and controls did not differ on age, education background or the dementia screening (MMSE, $p = 0.71$). It is worth mentioning that under medication-naïve condition, male patients scored significantly worse in the MMSE (male-MMSE 28.43 ± 0.65, female-MMSE 29.20 ± 1.15, $p = 0.014$). The comparison between these two groups on specific cognitive measures revealed some differences. Three out of five domains were involved: the visual spatial function, language and attention/executive function. Specifically, PD patients attained significantly lower scores in AVLT-sum 1 to 5 (verbal memory, $p = 0.000$), Clock Drawing Test (Visual spatial function, $p = 0.004$), Verbal Fluency-City (Language, $p = 0.000$), Verbal Fluency-Alternative (Language, $p = 0.003$), Symbol Digit Modality Test (Attention/ executive function, $p = 0.000$) and Trail Making Test-A (Attention/ executive function, p = 0.000). Comparing with untreated

Table 2 Cognitive Tests

Cognitive domains	Tests	Descriptions
Verbal memory	AVLT [45]	A list of 12 items is presented three times, each followed by free recall testing. After an interference test lasting 5 min, free recall of the list for the fourth time (short delayed free recall). After another 20 min, free and cued recall for the fifth time (long delayed free and cued recall), and choose the right items from a total of 24 (recognition). (Max score of recognition = 24, the rest = 12)
Spatial processing ability	Rey-copy [46]	Copy one complex line-drawing figure without reminding later recall. (Max score = 36)
	CDT [47]	Draw a clock and mark the time 1:50. (Max score = 30)
Non-verbal memory	Rey-delayed recall [46]	20–25 min after copying, recall the complex line-drawing figure. Identify the color of print in which a color name is written rather than the reading of the name itself. (Max score = 110)
Language	BNT [48]	Name 30 line drawings of common objects shown sequentially, each within 20s. (Max score = 30)
	VFT(animals, cities, alternatives) [48]	Name as many animals as possible within 1 min; same for cities and animal-city alternatives.
Attention/executive function	SDMT	Numbers ranging from 1 to 9, with each digit matched to a different geometrical symbol. Write down the digit according to the symbol as quickly as possible.
	TMT [49]	Scan and connect either all numbers (Trail A), or alternating numbers and letters (Trail B), distributed in a spatial array.
	Stroop [50]	Identify the color of print in which a color name is written rather than the reading of the name itself. (Max score = 110)

Note. *AVLT* Auditory verbal learning test, *Rey-copy* Copy of Rey-Osterrieth complex figure, *CDT* Clock drawing test, *Rey-delayed recall* Delayed recall of Rey-Osterrieth complex figure, *BNT* Boston naming test, *VFT* Verbal fluency tasks, *SDMT* Symbol digit modality test, *TMT* Trail making test, *Stroop* Stroop color word interference test

Table 3 Cognitive performance of patients and control (Mean ± SD)

	PD($n = 60$)	Control($n = 100$)	Significance
Age	59.05 ± 9.55	58.2 ± 7.57	$p = 0.412$
Education	12.86 ± 2.97	12.63 ± 3.24	$p = 0.665$
MMSE	28.98 ± 1.07	29.03 ± 0.69	$p = 0.71$
Verbal memory			
AVLT-short delayed free recall	4.91 ± 1.93	5.29 ± 2.5	$p = 0.234$
AVLT-long delayed free recall	4.47 ± 1.66	4.72 ± 2.72	$p = 0.20$
AVLT-long delayed cued recall	4.57 ± 2.06	4.69 ± 2.57	$p = 0.819$
AVLT-sum 1 to 5	15.53 ± 5.12	26.17 ± 8.15	$p = 0.000$
AVLT-recognition	20.02 ± 3.47	20.35 ± 2.89	$p = 0.53$
Non-verbal memory			
Rey-delayed recall	15.6 ± 7.58	15.16 ± 6.5	$p = 0.74$
Visuospatial function			
Rey-copy (time)	178.42 ± 61.11	165.57 ± 68.41	$p = 0.24$
Rey-copy (score)	32.98 ± 3.88	34.16 ± 1.74	$p = .944$
CDT	22.72 ± 6.05	25.81 ± 6.3	$p = 0.004*$
Language			
VFT (animals)	16.1 ± 3.6	19.43 ± 19.22	$p = 0.19$
VFT (cities)	13.76 ± 5.35	17.39 ± 5.82	$p = 0.00*$
VFT (alternative)	14.46 ± 5.2	17.11 ± 5.02	$p = 0.003*$
BNT	23.03 ± 3.66	23.63 ± 3.81	$p = 0.34$
Attention/executive function			
SDMT	31.88 ± 11.91	43.61 ± 11.6	$p = 0.00*$
Stroop (time)	77.95 ± 26.27	75.98 ± 24.22	$p = 0.63$
Stroop (score)	46.66 ± 4.61	46.58 ± 7.86	$p = 0.94$
TMT-A	71.37 ± 33.5	55.77 ± 24.8	$p = 0.00*$
TMT-B	164.61 ± 59.16	150.55 ± 74.35	$p = 0.23$

Note. *MMSE* Mini-mental state examination, *AVLT* Auditory verbal learning test, *Rey-delayed recall* Delayed recall of Rey-Osterrieth complex figure, *Rey-copy* Copy of Rey-Osterrieth complex figure, *CDT* Clock drawing test, *VFT* Verbal fluency tasks, *BNT* Boston naming test, *SDMT* Symbol digit modality test, *Stroop* Stroop color word interference test, *TMT* Trail making test
*$p < 0.05$

PD, those with anti-Parkinsonism medication exhibited worse performance in Rey-copy score, Clock Drawing Test and Verbal Fluency-City. In the treated PD group, decreased score in Rey-copy test was observed, while there was no significant difference in the untreated group comparing with the controls (Table 4). Except for that, both treated and untreated PD patients displayed the same distinction in cognition tests with total PD patients as described above.

Table 5 summarizes the results of analyses of each gender, respectively. When compared with control, both male and female patients showed worse performance in Auditory Verbal Learning Test-sum (AVLT) 1 to 5 (Verbal memory, $p = 0.000$ for both male and female patients) and Symbol Digit Modality Test (Attention/ executive function, p = 0.000 for both male and female patients). Specifically, male patients performed worse on Verbal Fluency Test-Animals (Language, p = 0.000), Verbal Fluency-Cities (Language, $p = 0.000$) and Verbal Fluency-Alternatives (Language, $p = 0.001$), while female patients attained worse scores on Clock Drawing Test (Visual spatial function, $p = 0.019$), Boston Naming Test (Language, $p = 0.02$) and Trail Making Test-A (Attention/ executive function, $p = 0.003$).

Between male and female participants, the comparison of cognitive performance is also reported in Table 5. In the control group, males performed better on Verbal Fluency-City (Language, $p = 0.01$) and Verbal Fluency-Alternative (Language, $p = 0.046$). In the PD patient group, although male and female patients did not differ on the dementia screening test, male patients performed worse on AVLT-long delayed cued recall test (Verbal memory, $p = 0.031$) and BNT test ($p = 0.003$).

We have conducted multiple linear regression using age, gender, educational level, UPDRS-III and BECK as

Table 4 Cognitive Performance of PD patients with and without treatment

	Treated PD (n = 31)	Untreated PD (n = 29)	Controls (n = 100)	P-value[a]	P-value[b]	P-value[c]
Age	57.03 ± 10.19	61.21 ± 8.46	58.2 ± 7.57	0.591	0.061	0.111
Gender(male)	15/31	15/29	38/100	0.402	0.204	1.000
Disease duration	6.16 ± 6.36	2.13 ± 2.79				0.000*
Education	12.70 ± 3.12	13.04 ± 2.85	12.63 ± 3.24	0.765	0.512	0.774
MMSE	29.13 ± 1.12	28.83 ± 1.00	29.03 ± 0.69	0.137	0.350	0.135
Verbal memory						
AVLT-short delayed free recall	5.04 ± 1.99	4.79 ± 1.90	5.29 ± 2.5	0.439	0.264	0.734
AVLT-long delayed free recall	4.55 ± 1.84	4.38 ± 1.47	4.72 ± 2.72	0.699	0.502	0.994
AVLT-sum 1 to 5	15.10 ± 5.83	15.96 ± 4.33	26.17 ± 8.15	0.000*	0.000*	0.378
AVLT-recognition	20.27 ± 3.95	19.78 ± 3.00	20.35 ± 2.89	0.585	0.355	0.788
Non-verbal memory						
Rey-delayed recall	13.86 ± 6.15	17.63 ± 8.67	15.16 ± 6.5	0.347	0.206	0.102
Visuospatial function						
Rey-copy (time)	175.21 ± 58.78	181.75 ± 64.34	165.57 ± 68.41	0.268	0.162	0.854
Rey-copy (score)	31.62 ± 4.82	34.44 ± 1.58	34.16 ± 1.74	0.006*	0.503	0.016*
CDT	20.41 ± 7.15	25.04 ± 3.52	25.81 ± 6.3	0.000*	0.252	0.004*
Language						
VFT (animals)	16.17 ± 3.23	16.03 ± 4.01	19.43 ± 19.22	0.358	0.193	0.632
VFT (cities)	15.10 ± 5.42	12.38 ± 5.00	17.39 ± 5.82	0.021*	0.000*	0.012*
VFT (alternative)	14.33 ± 4.01	14.59 ± 6.27	17.11 ± 5.02	0.009*	0.003*	0.715
BNT	23.10 ± 3.41	22.96 ± 3.98	23.63 ± 3.81	0.337	0.323	1.000
Attention/executive function						
SDMT	31.14 ± 13.92	32.62 ± 9.70	43.61 ± 11.6	0.000*	0.000*	0.602
Stroop (time)	76.17 ± 29.36	79.72 ± 23.15	75.98 ± 24.22	0.699	0.339	0.323
Stroop (score)	46.79 ± 4.56	46.52 ± 4.73	46.58 ± 7.86	0.027*	0.088	0.827
TMT-A	75.21 ± 44.69	67.66 ± 18.71	55.77 ± 24.8	0.004*	0.001*	0.873
TMT-B	163.96 ± 66.04	165.21 ± 53.15	150.55 ± 74.35	0.278	0.063	0.762

Note. *MMSE* Mini-mental state examination, *AVLT* Auditory verbal learning test, *Rey-delayed recall* Delayed recall of Rey-Osterrieth complex figure, *Rey-copy* Copy of Rey-Osterrieth complex figure, *CDT* Clock drawing test, *VFT* Verbal fluency tasks, *BNT* Boston naming test, *SDMT* Symbol digit modality test, *Stroop* Stroop color word interference test, *TMT* Trail making test
[a]Comparison between Treated PD and Control
[b]Comparison between Untreated PD and Control
[c]Comparison between Treated PD and Untreated PD
*$p < 0.05$

independent variables, eliminating the cofounders of age, educational level, UPDRS and BECK (Table 6). Considering the purpose of our article, we only demonstrated the β value and P value of gender. After adjustment of other cofounding factors, gender difference had significant effects on the AVLT-long delayed cued recall and BNT test, consistent with the results of student T test and Manne Whitney test.

More supporting data could be accessed through emails with the corresponding authors.

Discussion

PD patients frequently encounter neuropsychological problems. The present study has confirmed the previously reported cognitive impairment in cognitive domains including attention/executive function, visuospatial function, verbal memory and language. These aspects of cognition were all affected by the disease to varying degrees.

Dysexecutive syndrome is the most prominent prototype of early cognitive impairment in PD [22]. Deficits in this domain could be sensitively detected by measures of SDMT, which showed abnormality in this study. Our result was also in accordance with previous studies documenting visuospatial impairments by evidence of poor performance of PD patients in CDT [23]. Poor performance on free recall tasks but near normal performance on recognition and cued recall tasks in our study concur

Table 5 Comparison of cognitive performance between PD Patients and control by gender respectively (Mean ± SD)

	Male PD (n = 30)	Male Control (n = 38)	Female PD (n = 30)	Female Control (n = 62)	P-value[a]	P-value[b]	P-value[c]	P-value[d]
MMSE	28.97 ± 0.81	28.97 ± 0.79	29 ± 1.29	29.06 ± 0.62	$p = 0.97$	$p = 0.97$	$p = 0.705$	$p = 0.54$
Verbal memory								
AVLT-short delayed free recall	4.55 ± 1.68	4.74 ± 2.48	5.29 ± 2.12	5.63 ± 2.46	$p = 0.92$	$p = 0.53$	$p = 0.153$	$p = 0.083$
AVLT-long delayed free recall	4.14 ± 1.51	4.29 ± 2.56	4.79 ± 1.76	4.98 ± 2.8	$p = 0.99$	$p = 0.99$	$p = 0.133$	$p = 0.216$
AVLT-long delayed cued recall	3.96 ± 1.56	4.11 ± 2.33	5.13 ± 2.32	5.07 ± 2.66	$p = 0.99$	$p = 0.91$	$p = 0.031*$	$p = 0.075$
AVLT-sum 1 to 5	15.07 ± 4.32	24.37 ± 8.67	15.97 ± 5.84	27.27 ± 7.67	$p = 0.000*$	$p = 0.000*$	$p = 0.506$	$p = 0.083$
AVLT-recognition	20.52 ± 4.01	19.68 ± 2.04	19.5 ± 2.79	20.77 ± 3.26	$p = 0.287$	$p = 0.09$	$p = 0.29$	$p = 0.069$
Non-verbal memory								
Rey-delayed recall	17.16 ± 7.14	15.13 ± 7.08	14.15 ± 7.82	15.17 ± 6.18	$p = 0.27$	$p = 0.51$	$p = 0.154$	$p = 0.978$
Visuospatial function								
Rey-copy (time)	178.07 ± 67.9	159.35 ± 66.09	178.73 ± 55.47	169.4 ± 70.08	$p = 0.27$	$p = 0.53$	$p = 0.968$	$p = 0.485$
Rey-copy(score)	33.08 ± 4.13	34.11 ± 1.75	32.9 ± 3.72	34.19 ± 1.74	$p = 0.49$	$p = 0.49$	$p = 0.867$	$p = 0.807$
CDT	23 ± 4.29	25.82 ± 9.05	22.5 ± 7.22	25.8 ± 3.83	$p = 0.16$	$p = 0.019*$	$p = 0.766$	$p = 0.989$
Language								
VFT (animals)	16.45 ± 3.39	18.03 ± 5.42	15.77 ± 3.83	20.6 ± 25.66	$p = 0.48$	$p = 0.31$	$p = 0.472$	$p = 0.556$
VFT (cities)	13.9 ± 4.75	19.26 ± 5.77	13.63 ± 5.96	15.8 ± 5.43	$p = 0.000*$	$p = 0.12$	$p = 0.852$	$p = 0.01*$
VFT (alternatives)	14 ± 4.34	18.34 ± 5.41	14.9 ± 5.95	16.05 ± 4.46	$p = 0.001*$	$p = 0.36$	$p = 0.511$	$p = 0.046*$
BNT	24.45 ± 2.93	24 ± 4.65	21.62 ± 3.81	23.4 ± 3.21	$p = 0.65$	$p = 0.02*$	$p = 0.003*$	$p = 0.45$
Attention/executive function								
SDMT	31.97 ± 12.25	43.33 ± 12.24	31.79 ± 11.78	43.84 ± 11.17	$p = 0.000*$	$p = 0.000*$	$p = 0.957$	$p = 0.849$
Stroop (time)	83.43 ± 31.6	76.68 ± 18.87	72.83 ± 19.24	75.56 ± 27.05	$p = 0.29$	$p = 0.62$	$p = 0.126$	$p = 0.827$
Stroop (score)	46.04 ± 5.32	47.35 ± 12.15	47.23 ± 3.83	46.11 ± 3.42	$p = 0.60$	$p = 0.16$	$p = 0.327$	$p = 0.451$
TMT-A	64.1 ± 21.64	54.11 ± 22.81	78.89 ± 42.3	56.8 ± 26.09	$p = 0.074$	$p = 0.003*$	$p = 0.101$	$p = 0.601$
TMT-B	164.79 ± 69	152.84 ± 55.07	164.41 ± 47.71	149.11 ± 84.58	$p = 0.43$	$p = 0.38$	$p = 0.646$	$p = 0.81$

Note. *MMSE* Mini-mental state examination, *AVLT* Auditory verbal learning test, *Rey-delayed recall* Delayed recall of Rey-Osterrieth complex figure, *Rey-copy* Copy of Rey-Osterrieth complex figure, *CDT* Clock drawing test, *VFT* Verbal fluency tasks, *BNT* Boston naming test, *SDMT* Symbol digit modality test, *Stroop* Stroop color word interference test, *TMT* Trail making test

[a]Comparison between Male PD and Male Control
[b]Comparison between Female PD and Female Control
[c]Comparison between Male PD and Female PD
[d]Comparison between Male Control and Female Control
*$p < 0.05$

with the hypothesis that verbal memory impairment in PD has been manifested as retrieval difficulty more than encoding problems [22]. Although the majority of studies showed that language remain relatively intact in PD, we found it was impaired compared to the control group in the verbal fluency test. Verbal fluency combines the ability to retrieve the correct information and suppress the incorrect response. According to O'Brien's report, dysfunction of various domains does not occur in isolation, but presents in association with each other [24]. In fact, though impairment in substantia nigra is most pronounced in PD, areas affected by the disease are widespread, including ventral tegmental area, dorsal raphe nucleus, hypothalamus, thalamus, hippocampus, cerebral cortex, the temporal, frontal, anterior cingulate and insular cortices [25]. Thus, it is not surprising that the

cognitive deficits are due to cortical pathology and subcortical circuitry dysfunction as a whole and deficits in language may be the result of deterioration of the other cognitive functions as a whole. In addition to that, PD patients with anti-parkinsonism medication had extra deficits in Rey-copy score and stroop3 test score, which may due to the longer disease duration ($p = 0.000$) or medical effects. These results displayed a possible vulnerability of PD patients to the effects of disease duration and medication on Rey-copy score and stroop3 test.

In regard to gender differences in PD, epidemiological survey showed that the ratio of men and women who had the disease is approximately 2:1, suggesting a biological diversity [18]. However, not many studies considered gender when examining cognition in PD patients.

Table 6 Effects of gender on cognitive tests based on multiple linear regression

	Adjusted R^2	P	Standardized β(gender)	P (gender)
MMSE	−0.027	0.587	−0.033	0.830
Verbal memory				
AVLT-short delayed free recall	0.005	0.403	0.099	0.511
AVLT-long delayed free recall	0.118	0.070	0.129	0.361
AVLT-long delayed cued recall	0.127	0.065	0.331	0.025*
AVLT-sum 1 to 5	0.044	0.235	0.037	0.799
AVLT-recognition	0.007	0.399	−0.074	0.634
Non-verbal memory				
Rey-delayed recall	0.143	0.059	−0.215	0.148
Visuospatial function				
Rey-copy (time)	0.194	0.017	−0.123	0.365
Rey-copy(score)	−0.084	0.900	−0.091	0.567
CDT	0.175	0.058	0.155	0.341
Language				
VFT (animals)	−0.042	0.680	−0.133	0.386
VFT (cities)	0.040	0.250	−0.101	0.490
VFT (alternatives)	−0.108	0.992	0.029	0.856
BNT	0.175	0.025	−0.386	0.007*
Attention/executive function				
SDMT	0.053	0.212	−0.011	0.938
Stroop (time)	0.091	0.113	−0.203	0.159
Stroop (score)	0.079	0.136	0.070	0.625
TMT-A	0.337	0.001	0.173	0.163
TMT-B	0.192	0.019	0.057	0.675

There were some studies investigated the gender differences with a remarkable number of participants, but the lack of control groups did not permit to determine if these differences could be specific to PD patients [26, 27]. The present study highlights the role of gender differences associated with cognitive functions. The conclusion was strengthened by the study design of age and education matched control groups. Our study showed a disparity between male and female patients in two domains of cognition. Male patients surpassed female patients on BNT, a measure less commonly used to assess frontal lobe dysfunction [28], while female patients were superior on verbal retrieval test, reflecting the impairment of hippocampus [29]. Since no significant differences were observed in these two measures between male and female controls, it is reasonable to infer that gender-based differences existed in PD patients. In a cross-sectional study of the effect of gender on BNT which recruited 1111 healthy elderly subjects, there was also a tendentiously while non-significantly higher score of males ($p = 0.08$) [30]. Meanwhile, it reveals that age and educational level had more powerful effect on BNT. On the other hand, other studies found no effect of gender on the BNT. Therefore,

there was possibility that the gender difference in BNT was due to the natural difference between men and women, which was unrelated to PD.

One consideration centers on our results is the role estrogen plays in the pathogenesis of PD. Even though the menopausal condition at experiment might be heterogeneous of the female PD patients in our cohort, the lifetime cumulative level of estrogen also played an important part in the pathogenesis of Parkinson's disease [31, 32]. According to other's reports, it is still a mystery as to the mechanism of estrogen acting on the dopaminergic system [33, 34]. In addition, the changes in other neurotransmitter systems, such as cholinergic, noradrenergic, serotonergic, also contribute to the multiple neuropsychological impairments. The interactions of these neurotransmitter systems make the role of estrogen even more complex. Another frequently-used theory to explain the gender differences is "cognitive reserve", which posits that premorbid condition may generate distinctions in clinical presentation [35–37]. Although the subjects in our study have been adjusted for education, it may not be sufficient to rule out the impact of other socioeconomic factors such as occupation, income and social status. Thus better performance in verbal memory by female patients may indicate a larger cognitive reserve in this aspect. Likewise, advantages in naming by male patients may suggest a later onset of impairment and greater reserve of prefrontal function than female counterpart. The gender differences might also be associated with neural organization [38]. Some studies shown that greater bihemispheric representation were more prominent in women taking verbal memory task and men taking visuospatial task [39, 40]. Others found right hemispheric lateralization for males and bilateralization for females [41, 42]. Though no consensus has been reached, differences in neural lateralization render certain aspects of cognition more sensitive to neuropathological changes in a gender-specific manner, which lead to dissimilar manifestation in male and female patients.

When interpreting these data, several limitations should be acknowledged. First of all, the relatively small sample size may limit the generalization of these data. As several studies pointed out, normal elderly women performed better in tests involving verbal components [37, 43].Thus, whether female PD patients' better performance in RVLT-long delayed cued recall was due to the influence of the disease needs further study with larger sample size. Secondly, as Cronin-Golomb described, side of disease onset may also influence the cognition of the patients [44]. Should this be the case, more detailed division of participants by both gender and side of disease onset would provide stronger evidence. Finally, another limitation is the influence of medication. Though anticholinergic medications were ruled out and levodopa equivalent dose were well matched between groups, the underlying effect of dopaminergic medication may still change the natural pathological development of neurodegeneration.

In conclusion, our study indicates that cognitive impairment was common in PD patients even in the absence of dementia. PD patients who underwent anti-parkinsonian treatment had worse cognitive impairment than untreated ones. In light of the above mentioned observations, we hypothesized that genders may have a different presentation of cognitive impairment in PD patients. Sex influences on brain anatomy, chemistry and functions are poorly understood. Increased knowledge on possible gender effects in PD would provide an enhanced insight in underlying pathological mechanisms, and has potential implications for the diagnosis and treatment of PD.

Acknowledgements
This work was supported by grants 81571232 and 81371413 from the National Natural Science Foundation of China (to Jian Wang), grant 81301136 from the National Natural Science Foundation of China (to Huan Yu). Project 2016YFC1306500 from Ministry of Science and technology of China (to Jian Wang), project XBR20134042 from Shanghai Municipal Health Bureau (to Huan Yu), project 15ZR1435800 from the Science and Technology Commission of Shanghai Municipality (to Jian-jun Wu).

Fundings
This work was supported by grants 81571232 and 81371413 from the National Natural Science Foundation of China (to Jian Wang), grant 81301136 from the National Natural Science Foundation of China (to Huan Yu). Project 2016YFC1306500 from Ministry of Science and technology of China (to Jian Wang), project XBR20134042 from Shanghai Municipal Health Bureau (to Huan Yu), Grant form Jingan District JA2015-Z002 (to Jian-jun Wu).

Authors' contributions
KY and BS were involved in the manuscript preparation, writing of the first draft, and statistical analysis with design and execution. DL, YW, JZ, JZ, W-BY, ZL, YT were involved in the initiation of the project, data collection, and review of the manuscript. HY, FL and JW were involved in organization and execution of the project, review and revision of the manuscript. JW and QG were involved in the conception, planning and supervising the execution of the research project, and critical revision final review of the manuscript. All authors read and approved the final manuscript.

Competing interests
The authors declare that they have no competing interests.

Author details
[1] Department of Neurology and Institute of Neurology, Huashan Hospital, Fudan University, 12 Wulumuqi Zhong Road, Shanghai 200040, China.
[2] Department of Neurology, Jing'an District Center Hospital of Shanghai, 259 Xikang Road, Shanghai 20040, China.

References
1. Schrag A, Jahanshahi M, Quinn N. What contributes to quality of life in patients with Parkinson's disease? J Neurol Neurosurg Psychiatry. 2000;69(3): 308–12.
2. Muslimovic D, et al. Cognitive profile of patients with newly diagnosed Parkinson disease. Neurology. 2005;65(8):1239–45.
3. Aarsland D, Bronnick K, Fladby T. Mild cognitive impairment in Parkinson's disease. Curr Neurol Neurosci Rep. 2011;11(4):371–8.
4. Aarsland D, et al. Risk of dementia in Parkinson's disease: a community-based, prospective study. Neurology. 2001;56(6):730–6.
5. Allain H, et al. Procedural memory and Parkinson's disease. Dementia. 1995; 6(3):174–8.
6. Brown RG, Marsden CD. Cognitive function in Parkinson's disease: from description to theory. Trends Neurosci. 1990;13(1):21–9.
7. Dluzen DE, McDermott JL. Gender differences in neurotoxicity of the nigrostriatal dopaminergic system: implications for Parkinson's disease. J Gend Specif Med. 2000;3(6):36–42.
8. Van Den Eeden SK, et al. Incidence of Parkinson's disease: variation by age, gender, and race/ethnicity. Am J Epidemiol. 2003;157(11):1015–22.
9. Lyons KE, et al. Gender differences in Parkinson's disease. Clin Neuropharmacol. 1998;21(2):118–21.
10. Braak H, et al. Cognitive status correlates with neuropathologic stage in Parkinson disease. Neurology. 2005;64(8):1404–10.
11. Nazem S, et al. Montreal cognitive assessment performance in patients with Parkinson's disease with "normal" global cognition according to mini-mental state examination score. J Am Geriatr Soc. 2009;57(2):304–8.
12. Riedel O, et al. Cognitive impairment in 873 patients with idiopathic Parkinson's disease. Results from the German study on epidemiology of Parkinson's disease with dementia (GEPAD). J Neurol. 2008;255(2):255–64.
13. MacDonald AA, et al. Differential effects of Parkinson's disease and dopamine replacement on memory encoding and retrieval. PLoS One. 2013;8(9):e74044.

14. Edelstyn NM, et al. Effect of disease severity and dopaminergic medication on recollection and familiarity in patients with idiopathic nondementing Parkinson's. Neuropsychologia. 2010;48(5):1367–75.

15. Hanna-Pladdy B, Pahwa R, Lyons KE. Paradoxical effect of dopamine medication on cognition in Parkinson's disease: relationship to side of motor onset. J Int Neuropsychol Soc. 2015;21(4):259–70.

16. Daniel SE, Lees AJ. Parkinson's disease society brain Bank, London: overview and research. J Neural Transm Suppl. 1993;39:165–72.

17. Runeson BS, Rich CL. Diagnostic and statistical manual of mental disorders, 3rd ed. (DSM-III), adaptive functioning in young Swedish suicides. Ann Clin Psychiatry. 1994;6(3):181–3.

18. Hoehn MM, Yahr MD. Parkinsonism: onset, progression and mortality. Neurology. 1967;17(5):427–42.

19. Goetz CG, et al. Movement Disorder Society-sponsored revision of the unified Parkinson's disease rating scale (MDS-UPDRS): scale presentation and clinimetric testing results. Mov Disord. 2008;23(15):2129–70.

20. Tomlinson CL, et al. Systematic review of levodopa dose equivalency reporting in Parkinson's disease. Mov Disord. 2010;25(15):2649–53.

21. Folstein MF, Folstein SE, McHugh PR. "Mini-mental state". A practical method for grading the cognitive state of patients for the clinician. J Psychiatr Res. 1975;12(3):189–98.

22. Higginson CI, et al. The relationship between executive function and verbal memory in Parkinson's disease. Brain Cogn. 2003;52(3):343–52.

23. Cormack F, et al. Pentagon drawing and neuropsychological performance in dementia with Lewy bodies, Alzheimer's disease, Parkinson's disease and Parkinson's disease with dementia. Int J Geriatr Psychiatry. 2004;19(4):371–7.

24. O'Brien TJ, et al. The contribution of executive control on verbal-learning impairment in patients with Parkinson's disease with dementia and Alzheimer's disease. Arch Clin Neuropsychol. 2009;24(3):237–44.

25. Tomer R, Levin BE, Weiner WJ. Side of onset of motor symptoms influences cognition in Parkinson's disease. Ann Neurol. 1993;34(4):579–84.

26. Locascio JJ, Corkin S, Growdon JH. Relation between clinical characteristics of Parkinson's disease and cognitive decline. J Clin Exp Neuropsychol. 2003; 25(1):94–109.

27. Solla P, et al. Gender differences in motor and non-motor symptoms among Sardinian patients with Parkinson's disease. J Neurol Sci. 2012;323(1–2):33–9.

28. Green J, et al. Cognitive impairments in advanced PD without dementia. Neurology. 2002;59(9):1320–4.

29. Balthazar ML, et al. Learning, retrieval, and recognition are compromised in aMCI and mild AD: are distinct episodic memory processes mediated by the same anatomical structures? J Int Neuropsychol Soc. 2010;16(1):205–9.

30. Zec RF, et al. A cross-sectional study of the effects of age, education, and gender on the Boston naming test. Clin Neuropsychol. 2007;21(4):587–616.

31. Simon KC, et al. Reproductive factors, exogenous estrogen use, and risk of Parkinson's disease. Mov Disord. 2009;24(9):1359–65.

32. Gatto NM, et al. Lifetime exposure to estrogens and Parkinson's disease in California teachers. Parkinsonism Relat Disord. 2014;20(11):1149–56.

33. Liu B, Dluzen DE. Oestrogen and nigrostriatal dopaminergic neurodegeneration: animal models and clinical reports of Parkinson's disease. Clin Exp Pharmacol Physiol. 2007;34(7):555–65.

34. Janowsky JS. The role of androgens in cognition and brain aging in men. Neuroscience. 2006;138(3):1015–20.

35. Stern Y. What is cognitive reserve? Theory and research application of the reserve concept. J Int Neuropsychol Soc. 2002;8(3):448–60.

36. Barnes LL, et al. Gender, cognitive decline, and risk of AD in older persons. Neurology. 2003;60(11):1777–81.

37. Beinhoff U, et al. Gender-specificities in Alzheimer's disease and mild cognitive impairment. J Neurol. 2008;255(1):117–22.

38. Ripich DN, et al. Gender differences in language of AD patients: a longitudinal study. Neurology. 1995;45(2):299–302.

39. Volf NV, Razumnikova OM. Sex differences in EEG coherence during a verbal memory task in normal adults. Int J Psychophysiol. 1999;34(2):113–22.

40. Clements AM, et al. Sex differences in cerebral laterality of language and visuospatial processing. Brain Lang. 2006;98(2):150–8.

41. Antonova E, et al. The relationship between brain structure and neurocognition in schizophrenia: a selective review. Schizophr Res. 2004; 70(2–3):117–45.

42. Gur RC, et al. An fMRI study of sex differences in regional activation to a verbal and a spatial task. Brain Lang. 2000;74(2):157–70.

43. Proust-Lima C, et al. Gender and education impact on brain aging: a general cognitive factor approach. Psychol Aging. 2008;23(3):608–20.

44. Cronin-Golomb A. Parkinson's disease as a disconnection syndrome. Neuropsychol Rev. 2010;20(2):191–208.

45. Guo Q, et al. A comparison study of mild cognitive impairment with 3 memory tests among Chinese individuals. Alzheimer Dis Assoc Disord. 2009; 23(3):253–9.

46. Caffarra P, et al. Rey-Osterrieth complex figure: normative values in an Italian population sample. Neurol Sci. 2002;22(6):443–7.

47. Guo Q, Fu J, Yuan J, et al. A study of validity of a new scoring system of clock drawing test. Chin J Neurol. 2008;41(4):234–7.

48. Lucas JA, et al. Mayo's older African Americans normative studies: norms for Boston naming test, controlled oral word association, category fluency, animal naming, token test, WRAT-3 reading, trail making test, Stroop test, and judgment of line orientation. Clin Neuropsychol. 2005;19(2):243–69.

49. Zhao Q, et al. The Shape Trail test: application of a new variant of the trail making test. PLoS One. 2013;8(2):e57333.

50. Steinberg BA, et al. Mayo's older Americans normative studies: age- and IQ-adjusted norms for the trail-making test, the Stroop test, and MAE controlled oral word association test. Clin Neuropsychol. 2005;19(3–4):329–77.

25

Direct conversion of mouse astrocytes into neural progenitor cells and specific lineages of neurons

Kangmu Ma[1,3†], Xiaobei Deng[1†], Xiaohuan Xia[1†], Zhaohuan Fan[1], Xinrui Qi[1], Yongxiang Wang[1,3], Yuju Li[1,3], Yizhao Ma[1], Qiang Chen[1,3], Hui Peng[3], Jianqing Ding[4], Chunhong Li[1], Yunlong Huang[1,3*], Changhai Tian[1,3*] and Jialin C. Zheng[1,2,3,5*]

Abstract

Background: Cell replacement therapy has been envisioned as a promising treatment for neurodegenerative diseases. Due to the ethical concerns of ESCs-derived neural progenitor cells (NPCs) and tumorigenic potential of iPSCs, reprogramming of somatic cells directly into multipotent NPCs has emerged as a preferred approach for cell transplantation.

Methods: Mouse astrocytes were reprogrammed into NPCs by the overexpression of transcription factors (TFs) Foxg1, Sox2, and Brn2. The generation of subtypes of neurons was directed by the force expression of cell-type specific TFs Lhx8 or Foxa2/Lmx1a.

Results: Astrocyte-derived induced NPCs (AiNPCs) share high similarities, including the expression of NPC-specific genes, DNA methylation patterns, the ability to proliferate and differentiate, with the wild type NPCs. The AiNPCs are committed to the forebrain identity and predominantly differentiated into glutamatergic and GABAergic neuronal subtypes. Interestingly, additional overexpression of TFs Lhx8 and Foxa2/Lmx1a in AiNPCs promoted cholinergic and dopaminergic neuronal differentiation, respectively.

Conclusions: Our studies suggest that astrocytes can be converted into AiNPCs and lineage-committed AiNPCs can acquire differentiation potential of other lineages through forced expression of specific TFs. Understanding the impact of the TF sets on the reprogramming and differentiation into specific lineages of neurons will provide valuable strategies for astrocyte-based cell therapy in neurodegenerative diseases.

Keywords: Astrocytes, iNPCs, Reprogramming, Transcription factor, Neuronal lineage, Cholinergic neurons, Dopaminergic neurons, Lhx8, Foxa2, Lmx1a

Background

Neural progenitor cells (NPCs) exist throughout life and are able to proliferate and generate neurons, astrocytes, and oligodendrocytes in the central nervous systems (CNS) [1]. Recently, NPCs have also been shown to modulate immune response and protect neurons in the CNS [2, 3]. Due to their regenerative potentials, NPCs have been implicated in the treatment of neurodegenerative diseases [4, 5]. However, limited number and restricted anatomical locations have reduced the feasibility of using NPCs as a therapeutic approach. NPCs derived from human fetal tissues/embryonic stem cells may serve as an alternative cell source. However, this approach receives criticism over ethical concerns. The emerging field of cell reprogramming gives NPC-based therapy a boost because it avoids the aforementioned problems. Therefore, reprogrammed NPCs appear to be an attractive novel strategy for the treatment of neurodegenerative disorders [6–9].

* Correspondence: yhuan1@unmc.edu; ctian@unmc.edu; jialinzheng@tongji.edu.cn
†Kangmu Ma, Xiaobei Deng and Xiaohuan Xia contributed equally to this work.
[1]Center for Translational Neurodegeneration and Regenerative Therapy, Shanghai Tenth People's Hospital affiliated to Tongji University School of Medicine, Shanghai 200072, China
Full list of author information is available at the end of the article

Two common approaches are used to reprogram somatic cells into induced neural progenitor cells (iNPCs). The first one is to generate iNPCs through induced pluripotent stem cells (iPSCs), more primitive stem cells than NPCs [4, 10–17]. Because iPSCs derive from autologous tissues, the usage of iPSCs will prevent the deleterious immune reactions initiated by cell transplantation or replacement. However, iPSCs have also been noted to demonstrate variable potencies for neuronal differentiation as well as high risk of teratoma formation [4, 10], both of which pose challenges for clinical use. The second approach is the direct conversion of somatic cells into self-renewable and lineage-restricted NPCs by ectopic expression of defined transcription factors (TFs). Since 2011, we, along with other groups, have reported that defined TFs sets can reprogram somatic cells into iNPCs [13, 17–23]. Because the initial cell sources and the TFs sets used in these studies were not uniform, the resulting iNPCs showed variable NPC properties such as their distinct differentiation potentials for subtypes of neurons.

Because astrocytes are the most abundant type of cells within the CNS and reactive astrogliosis are present in all neurodegenerative disorders [24–26], astrocytes have become a key cell source for cell reprogramming [27]. Our previous data has suggested that astrocyte-derived iPSCs possess more tendencies for neuronal differentiation than fibroblast-derived iPSCs [17]. In the current studies, we used a set of TFs previously used for fibroblast-derived iNPC reprogramming [19]. We demonstrated that this set of TFs could successfully reprogram mouse astrocytes into tripotent iNPCs (AiNPCs). The AiNPCs expressed NPC-specific genes, acquired characteristic NPC functions, including self-renewal and proliferation. Interestingly, AiNPCs seemed to have a regional fate commitment with restricted forebrain differentiation competency. The subtype specification studies further suggested that the differentiation of AiNPCs is biased to favor the glutamatergic and GABAergic lineages over the dopaminergic lineage. Interestingly, the regional and lineage commitment of AiNPCs could be overwritten by additional overexpression of key TFs specific for neuronal subtype differentiation. For example, Lhx8 could induce cholinergic neuron differentiation and Foxa2/Lmx1a could induce midbrain dopaminergic neuronal differentiation. Together, our data provide further understanding on astrocyte-based cell reprogramming for the development of future therapies in neurodegenerative diseases.

Methods
Mice and astrocyte culture
E/Nestin:EGFP mice (kindly provided by Dr. Richard J. Miller from Northwestern University, Chicago, IL) are housed and bred in the Comparative Medicine animal facilities at the University of Nebraska Medical Center (UNMC).

All procedures were conducted according to protocols approved by the Institutional Animal Care and Use Committee of the UNMC. E/Nestin:EGFP positive transgenic pups were identified by direct fluoresce visualization under a IVIS optical imaging system and validated by genotyping. Astrocytes were isolated from cortices of E/Nestin:EGFP transgenic mice at postnatal day 7 as previously described [28]. Briefly, cortices were dissected out after removing cerebellum, olfactory bulb, meninges, and peripheral blood vessels. After washed twice with HBSS, cortices were digested at 37 °C for 20 min in 0.25% trypsin solution supplemented with 0.05% DNase I. Digestion was stopped by FBS (Invitrogen). The tissue sediment was centrifuged at 375 g for 5 min at room temperature (RT) and washed twice with HBSS. After trituration, cells were cultured in DMEM/F12 with 10% FBS, 50 U penicillin and 50 mg/mL streptomycin at 37 °C. The culture medium was replaced every 3 days. Cells were subjected to three passages for purification purpose. Astrocyte purity was tested by immunostaining with antibodies against GFAP (DAKO) and GLAST (Sigma).

Reagents
For adherent NPC cultures, tissue culture dishes or plates were coated with 100 µg/mL Poly-D-Lysine (Sigma) and 5 µg/mL Fibronectin (Sigma). Mouse AiNPCs and control NPCs were cultured in NPC favoring medium (NPCM), which contains NeuroCult® NSC Basal Medium (Stem Cell Technologies), NeuroCult® NSC Proliferation Supplements (Stem Cell Technologies), 20 ng/mL bFGF (BioWalkersville), 20 ng/mL EGF (BioWalkersville) and 2 µg/mL heparin (Sigma). AiNPCs and control NPCs were passaged with TrypLE™ select (Invitrogen). Plat-E packaging cells were cultured in DMEM with high glucose (Gibco) containing 10% heat inactivated FBS, 50 U penicillin and 50 mg/mL streptomycin, 1 µg/mL puromycin (Sigma) and 10 µg/mL blasticidin S (InvivoGen).

Control NPCs used in this study were generated from E15.5 mouse cortices. Briefly, the cortices were dissociated into single cells by triturating the tissue sediments with a 1 mL pipette. Cells were seeded into 100 mm non-coated Petri dishes (Fisher) at a density of 2×10^5 cells/mL in 10 mL of NPCM for primary neurosphere formation. Culture medium was replaced every other day. Neurospheres were passaged every 4–6 days when they reached 150 µm in diameter.

iPSC derived from mouse cortical astrocytes and fibroblasts were generated and characterized in our lab as previously described [17].

Retroviral vectors and retrovirus preparation
Plasmid encoding mouse Sox2 was purchased from Addgene (Plasmid #13367). Mouse Foxg1 (restriction enzymes: BamHI and XhoI), Brn2 (restriction enzymes:

BamHI and XhoI), Lhx8 (restriction enzymes: BamHI and SalI), Foxa2 (restriction enzymes: Xho1 and Sal1) and Lmx1a (restriction enzymes: BamH1 and SalI) were amplified from mouse control NPCs cDNA library. Each gene was individually cloned into pMXs-retroviral vectors (Cell Biolabs, RTV-010).

Retroviruses (pMXs) were generated with Plat-E packaging cells as previously described [11]. Constructed pMXs-based retroviral plasmids along with empty pMXs-vector control were introduced into Plat-E cells using Lipofectamine® LTX with Plus™ transfection reagent (Invitrogen) according to the protocol from the manufacturer. 24 h after transduction, medium was changed to astrocyte favoring medium for astrocyte transduction or NPCM for AiNPC transduction. 48 h after transfection, virus containing supernatants were filtered with 0.45 μm cellulose acetate filters (Fisher) and immediately used for astrocyte reprogramming.

Reprogramming of mouse astrocytes

NPC direct reprogramming was performed with an adopted and modified protocol as previously described [3]. Briefly, mouse astrocytes were incubated in the mixed virus-containing supernatants overnight. 10 μg/mL polybrene (Millipore) was added during the viral vector infection to increase the transduction efficiencies. A second round of infection was performed using the same mixed virus-containing supernatants. Infected astrocytes were changed to NPCM culture 1 day after the second infection. NPCM was replaced every 2 days. A drastic cell morphology change was observed from day 4 post infection. Patches of highly proliferating transduced cells formed dense networks and by day 28 bulging Nestin-EGFP⁺ colonies were found aggregated at the intersections of cell patches. On day 30 after retroviral transduction, bulged Nestin-EGFP⁺ colonies were manually picked, pooled, and suspended into single cells in Petri dishes. After culturing for 4–6 days, floating primary neurospheres were collected and re-plated into Poly-D-Lysine/Fibronectin coated 6 well plates. Upon 80% confluency, cells were collected and resuspended into single cells for a second round neurosphere formation in suspension culture. After 3 rounds of selection and enrichment, cells were passaged either in adherent culture or suspension culture according to the requirements of further experiments.

NPC Neurosphere formation assay

NPC neurosphere formation (self-renewal) assay was performed by suspending 1.0×10^4 cells with NPCM in a 60-mm non-coated Petri dish. Fresh medium was added into the suspension culture every other day. On day 5 neurospheres were collected and the number of neurospheres was counted under the bright field of a microscope.

Immunocytochemistry

Cells were fixed in 4% paraformaldehyde (Sigma) for 15 min at RT, rinsed 3 times with PBS (Fisher), and then incubated with permeabilizing/blocking buffer containing 5% goat serum (Vector Laboratories) and 0.2% Triton X-100 (Bio-Rad) in PBS for 60 min at RT. Primary antibodies were added overnight at 4 °C. The following day cells were washed 3 times with PBS and incubated with secondary antibodies (Molecular Probes) for 60 min at RT. Cells were counterstained with DAPI (Sigma-Aldrich). IgG control was used as negative controls for all immunocytochemical analysis. Images were captured using a Nikon Eclipse E800 microscope equipped with a digital imaging system and imported into Image-ProPlus, version 7.0 (Media Cybernetics, Sliver Spring, MD) for quantification. Images were imported into Image-Pro Plus, version 7.0 (Media Cybernetics, Silver Spring, MD), for quantification and 600–1,000 immunostained cells from 15 random fields per group were counted.

RNA isolation and qPCR analysis

Total RNA was isolated by RNA Purification Kit (Fermentas), and DNase I digestion was included (Qiagen) to remove genomic DNA. mRNA derived cDNA was generated through Oligo-dT priming with Transcriptor First Strand cDNA Synthesis Kit (Roche). RNase inhibitor was used to prevent RNA degradation during reverse transcription. Amplification was performed with SYBR Green PCR Master Mix (Applied Biosystems) and specific primer sets (Additional file 1: Table S2). All mRNA expression levels were normalized to GAPDH and calibrated on the control cells specified in each experiment.

Neuronal differentiation

Basic neuronal differentiation medium contained DMEM/F12 (without HEPEs), 1x N2 (Invitrogen), 1x B27 (Invitrogen), 1 μM cAMP (Sigma-Aldrich) and 0.2 mM Ascorbic Acid (Sigma-Aldrich). Spontaneous neuronal differentiation was carried out on Poly-D-Lysine/Fibronectin coated coverslip as previously described [29]. The single-cell spontaneous differentiation assay was performed by plating 10^4 cells/well on 24-well plates in basic neuronal differentiation medium, 10 ng/mL BDNF (R&D Systems), 10 ng/mL GDNF (PeproTech), 10 ng/mL IGF (PeproTech), 10 ng/mL CNTF (ProSpec) for 14 to 28 days. Medium was changed every 3 days. For ventral mesencephalic "inducing" differentiation, cells were treated with DMEM/F12 (without HEPEs), 1x N2, 1x B27, 100 ng/mL murine N-terminal fragment of SHH (R&D Systems) and murine 100 ng/mL FGF8 isoform b (R&D Systems) for 6 days followed by 14 days in DMEM/F12 (without HEPEs), 1 mM cAMP (Sigma) and 200 mM AA (Sigma). Medium was changed every 3 days.

Pyrosequencing and DNA methylation analysis

Genomic DNA was isolated using DNeasy Blood & Tissue Kit (Qiagen). Bisulfite treatment was carried out using 1000 ng of DNA and the EZ DNA Methylation-Direct kit (Zymo Research). This process deaminated unmethylated cytosine (C) residues to uracil (U) leaving methylated cytosine (^mC) residues unchanged. To perform PCR reactions, 32 ng of bisulfite-treated DNA was used as template. The PCR reactions were performed in a total volume of 25 µl for 35 cycles using 1.0 U FastStart Taq DNA Polymerase (Roche), 3.5 mM MgCl2 solution, 0.2 mM dNTPs, 0.24 µM sense primer, 0.18 µM antisense primer (Additional file 1: Table S3) under the following conditions: 95 °C for 30 s, 45 s at annealing temperature (Additional file 1: Table S3) and 72 °C for 1 min. Human lymphocyte genomic DNA (Roche) was used as a positive control (high methylation level) and was methylated using M. SssI (CpG) methylase kit (New England Biolabs) followed by sodium bisulfite treatment as described above. The negative control (low methylation level) was obtained by treating 1000 ng human lymphocyte genomic DNA with sodium bisulfite directly. All PCR products were electrophoresed and visualized under a Bio-Rad Laboratories Gel-Doc UV illuminator (Hercules). Methylation percentage of each CpG was determined using a Qiagen Pyromark Q24 pyrosequencer (Valencia) and sequencing primer (Additional file 1: Table S3), according to recommendations from manufacturer.

Statistical analyses

Data were evaluated statistically by the analysis of variance (ANOVA), followed by a Tukey's test for multiple comparisons (Graphpad Prism 5.0 software). Data were shown as mean ± SD, and significance was determined as $P < 0.05$. Means between two groups were compared with two-tailed, paired or unpaired Student's t tests.

Results

Conversion of mouse astrocytes into iNPCs

To facilitate the observation of the somatic reprogramming toward a neural progenitor fate, we used Nestin:EGFP transgenic mice, where Nestin positive cells expressed enhanced GFP fluorescence. Under the IVIS optical imaging system, Nestin:EGFP positive transgenic mice at postnatal day 7 showed strong EGFP signals in the brain (Fig. 1a). To reprogram EGFP negative astrocytes into EGFP positive iNPCs, we employed a set of TFs (Foxg1, Sox2, and Brn2) that were previously used in the reprogramming of fibroblast into iNPC (Fig. 1b) [19]. Control NPCs, which formed floating neurosphere, were derived from cortices of embryonic day 15.5 Nestin:EGFP transgenic mice. These NPCs served as positive controls for the fibroblast-derived iNPCs. Green fluorescence of Nestin:EGFP was readily detectable from those control

NPC neurospheres under fluorescent microscope, indicating the expression of Nestin, one of NPC-specific marker genes (Fig. 1c, d). For reprogramming, astrocytes were derived from cortices of Nestin:EGFP transgenic mice at postnatal day 7. Over 95% of cells in the primary culture were positive for glial fibrillary acidic protein (GFAP) and no Nestin, Sox2, Iba1 and Tuj1 staining was detected in the astrocyte cultures, suggesting the purity of astrocyte culture in the absence of NPCs, microglia and neurons (Fig. 1e, f; Additional file 1: Figure S1). This enriched astrocyte culture was negative for any EGFP signal and was used as the starting cells for somatic reprogramming (Fig. 1g, h). To reprogram astrocytes into NPCs, we transduced them with mixed retroviruses that individually expressed either Sox2, Brn2, or Foxg1 and subsequently changed the medium to NPCM. At 7 days after transduction, Nestin$^+$ cells emerged, which could be identified through EGFP expression. These EGFP$^+$ cells proliferated and formed neurospheres in the cultures. At 28 days after transduction, EGFP positive colonies were collected, dissociated into single cells, and sub-cultured in suspension as neurospheres (Fig. 1i, j). These neurospheres maintained strong EGFP fluorescence and could be continuously sub-cultured (Fig. 1k, l). Postnatal cultured astrocytes are known to form spherical clones in the presence of EGF and bFGF (Laywell et al., PNAS 2000). To rule out that the NPCs obtained from the transduced astrocyte cultures are not from Sox2, Brn2, and Foxg1 transduction but from spontaneously formed spherical clones, we used astrocytes transduced with the same titer of the retroviral vector and subsequently cultured with the same NPCM as the control cultures. No EGFP signal or neurospheres was observed in the control group (Fig. 1m, n) [30]. Therefore, we concluded that the NPCs obtained from the transduced astrocyte cultures were the result of Sox2, Brn2, and Foxg1 transduction. The transduction efficiency of Sox2, Brn2, and Foxg1 was validated by qPCR. Compared with those in the starting astrocytes, the overall gene expression levels of Sox2, Brn2, and Foxg1, which included both endogenous (from normal gene transcription) and exogenous (from retroviral vectors) in transduced astrocytes or reprogrammed NPCs, which we referred to as AiNPCs, were upregulated. Similarly, the NPC-specific gene nestin, neural lineage gene Mash1, and proliferation marker gene Ki67, were all upregulated. As expected, astrocyte-specific genes, including GFAP and S100b, were downregulated compared with those in the starting (Fig. 1o). To differentiate between endogenous and exogenous gene transcripts of Sox2, Brn2, and Foxg1, we designed primers specific for each transcript. Endogenous gene expression levels of Sox2, Brn2, and Foxg1 in transduced astrocytes or AiNPCs, were downregulated compared with those in the control group. In contrast, exogenous gene expression of Sox2, Brn2, and Foxg1 from

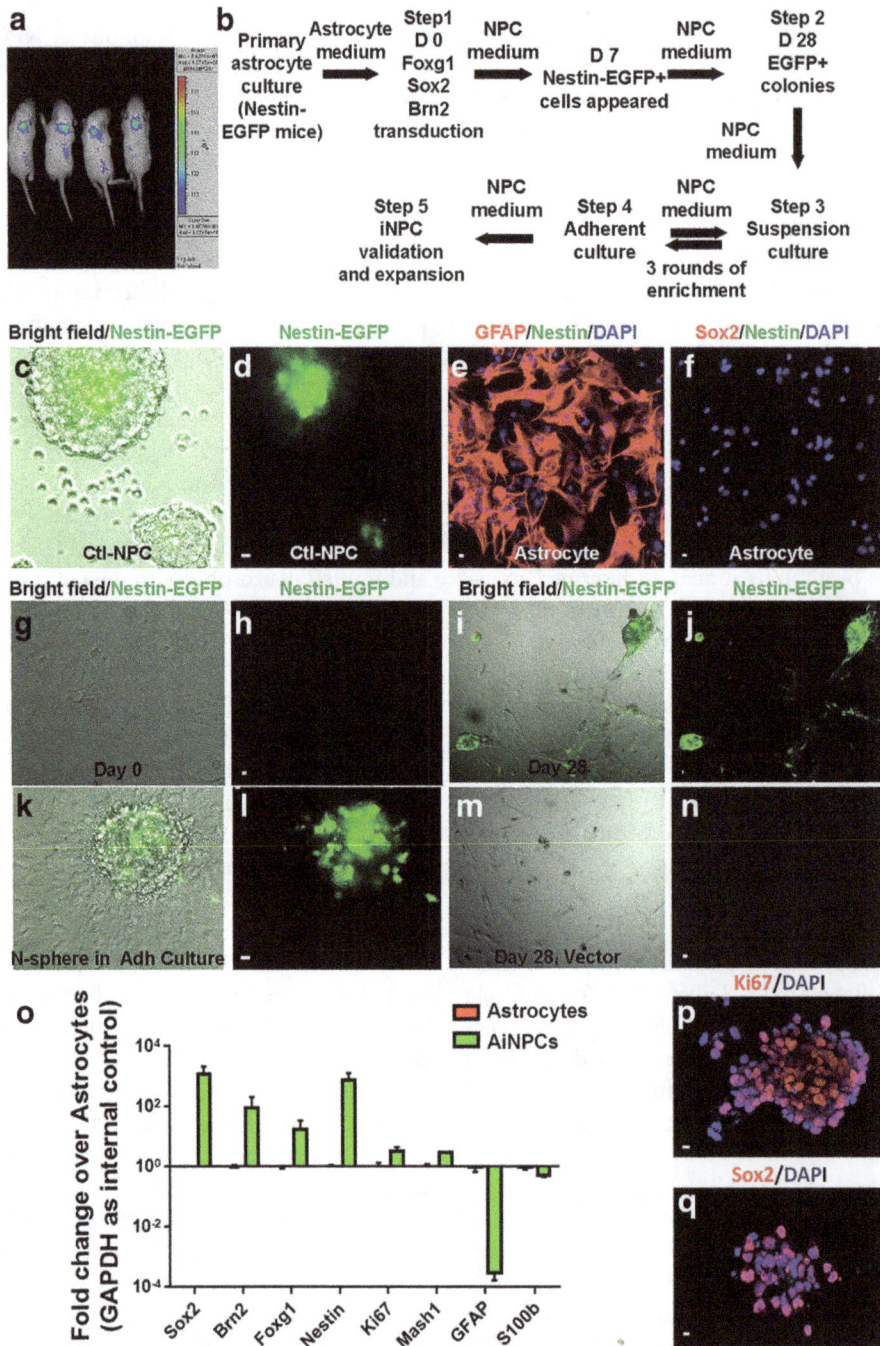

Fig. 1 Reprogramming of mouse astrocytes into AiNPCs. **a** Nestin:EGFP transgenic mice were imaged under IVIS optical imaging system. **b** Schematics for the reprogramming of astrocytes into AiNPCs. **c, d** Nestin-EGFP⁺ neurospheres were derived from E15.5 Nestin:EGFP transgenic mouse cortices in suspension culture. **e, f** Primary astrocyte cultures were positive for GFAP, but negative for Sox2 and Nestin. **g-n** Representative bright field and fluorescent pictures of cultures during generation of GFP⁺ NPC-like cells were shown. Step 1, day 0, astrocytes were in adherent culture before retrovirus-mediated Foxg1 + Sox2 + Brn2 transduction (**g, h**). Step 2, day 28, the cultures formed multiple bulged Nestin-EGFP⁺ colonies (**i, j**). Step 3 & 4, Nestin-EGFP⁺ primary neurospheres appeared and NPC-like cells migrated from neurospheres during adherent culture in poly-D-lysine- and fibronectin-coated dishes (**k, l**). Mock treated astrocytes showed minimum levels of Nestin-EGFP (**m, n**). **o** RNA of astrocytes and AiNPCs was collected and expression of NPC- and glial-specific genes was analyzed using qPCR. Data were normalized to GAPDH and presented as fold change compared with astrocytes. **p, q** AiNPCs were positive for Ki67 and Sox2. Scale bars represent 10 μm (**c-n, p, q**). Error bars denote s.d. from triplicate measurements (**o**)

the retroviral vectors in transduced astrocytes or AiNPCs were significantly upregulated compared with those in the control group, suggesting that the elevation of Sox2, Brn2, and Foxg1 transcript levels was mainly due to the exogenous expression of these genes (Additional file 1: Figure S2). Consistent with high mRNA levels of Sox2 and Ki67, AiNPCs showed strong immunoreactivities to Sox2 and Ki67, suggesting a very active proliferative status of AiNPCs (Fig. 1p, q).

Characterization of AiNPC

Next, we characterized the AiNPCs with multiple approaches. First, we examined whether the AiNPCs manifested any phenotypes of pluripotency. SSEA-1, a marker shared by embryonic stem cells (ESCs), induced pluripotent stem cells (iPSCs) and NPCs/iNPCs [13, 31], was expressed in AiNPCs at comparable levels to iPSCs (Fig. 2a, b, e, f). In contrast, Oct4, a pluripotency marker specific for iPSCs (Fig. 2c, d), was absent in AiNPCs (Fig. 2g, h). Consistent with the immunostaining data, AiNPC expressed comparable levels of SSEA-1 gene transcripts but expressed significantly lower levels of pluripotency mark genes Oct4 compared to iPSCs (Fig. 2i). Furthermore, other pluripotency markers Nanog and Zfp42 [3] were also expressed at

significantly lower levels in AiNPCs compared to iPSCs (Fig. 2i). Pyrosequencing on bisulfite-treated DNA showed the regulatory region on the promoter region of Oct4 [32], but not that of SSEA-1 was hypermethylated, confirming the transcriptional silencing of Oct4 (Fig. 2j, Additional file 1: Figure S3). Together, these data suggest that the AiNPCs likely do not go through the stage of the pluripotency.

Second, we tested whether AiNPCs shared key characteristics with control NPCs that generated from E15.5 mouse brains. Morphologically, AiNPCs highly resembled control NPCs isolated and cultured from E15.5 mice cortices in both suspension and adherent culture (Fig. 3a-d). Furthermore, AiNPCs were positive for NPC markers such as Nestin, Pax6, and Sox2, similar to control NPCs, suggesting that the AiNPCs possessed molecular characteristics of NPCs (Fig. 3e-h). In addition, the AiNPCs were similar in both nuclear-cytoplasmic ratio and efficiency in proliferative and self-renewal capacities with control NPCs (Fig. 3i-k). qPCR further revealed that AiNPCs expressed all endogenous NPC marker genes that we detected at levels close to the control NPCs, including Nestin, Sox1, Sox2, Sox3, Msi1, Ncan, Gpm6a, Bmi1, Blbp, Tox3, and Zbtb16 (Fig. 3l). In contrast, astrocytic marker gene expressions were suppressed after reprogramming (Fig. 3m). The DNA

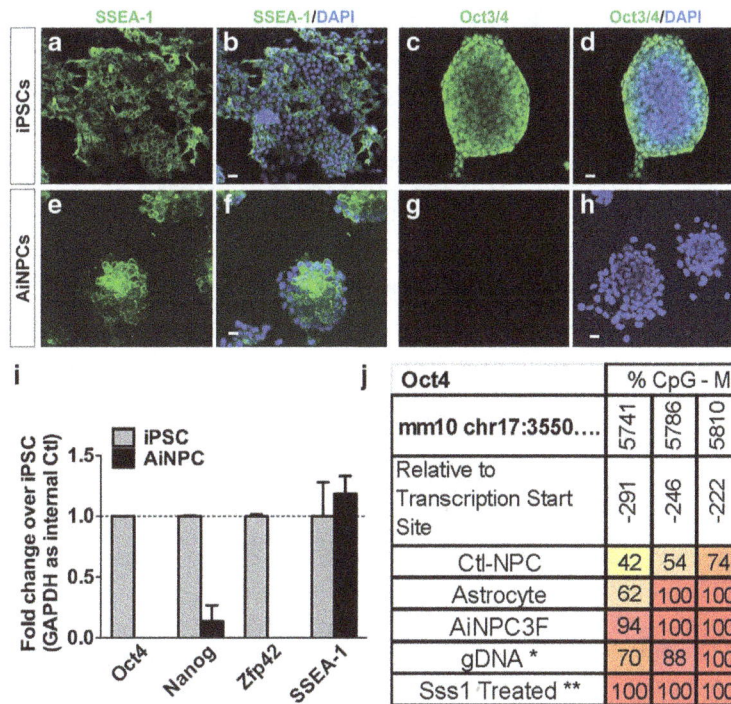

Fig. 2 Absence of pluripotency markers in AiNPCs. **a-h** iPSC and AiNPC cultures were fixed and immunostained for pluripotency markers SSEA-1 and Oct4. **i** RNA of cultured AiNPCs and control iPSCs was collected and expression of pluripotent-associated genes was analyzed using qPCR. Data were normalized to GAPDH and presented as fold change compared with control iPSCs. Error bars denote s.d. from triplicate measurements. **j** The Oct4 promoter regulatory region DNA methylation patterns of AiNPCs, control astrocytes, and control NPCs were analyzed using pyrosequencing method. *Human lymphocyte genomic DNA was used as a negative control for pyrosequencing. **Sss1 methyltranferase treated human lymphocyte genomic DNA was used for positive control. Scale bars represent 10 μm (**a-h**). Error bars denote s.d. from triplicate measurements (**i**)

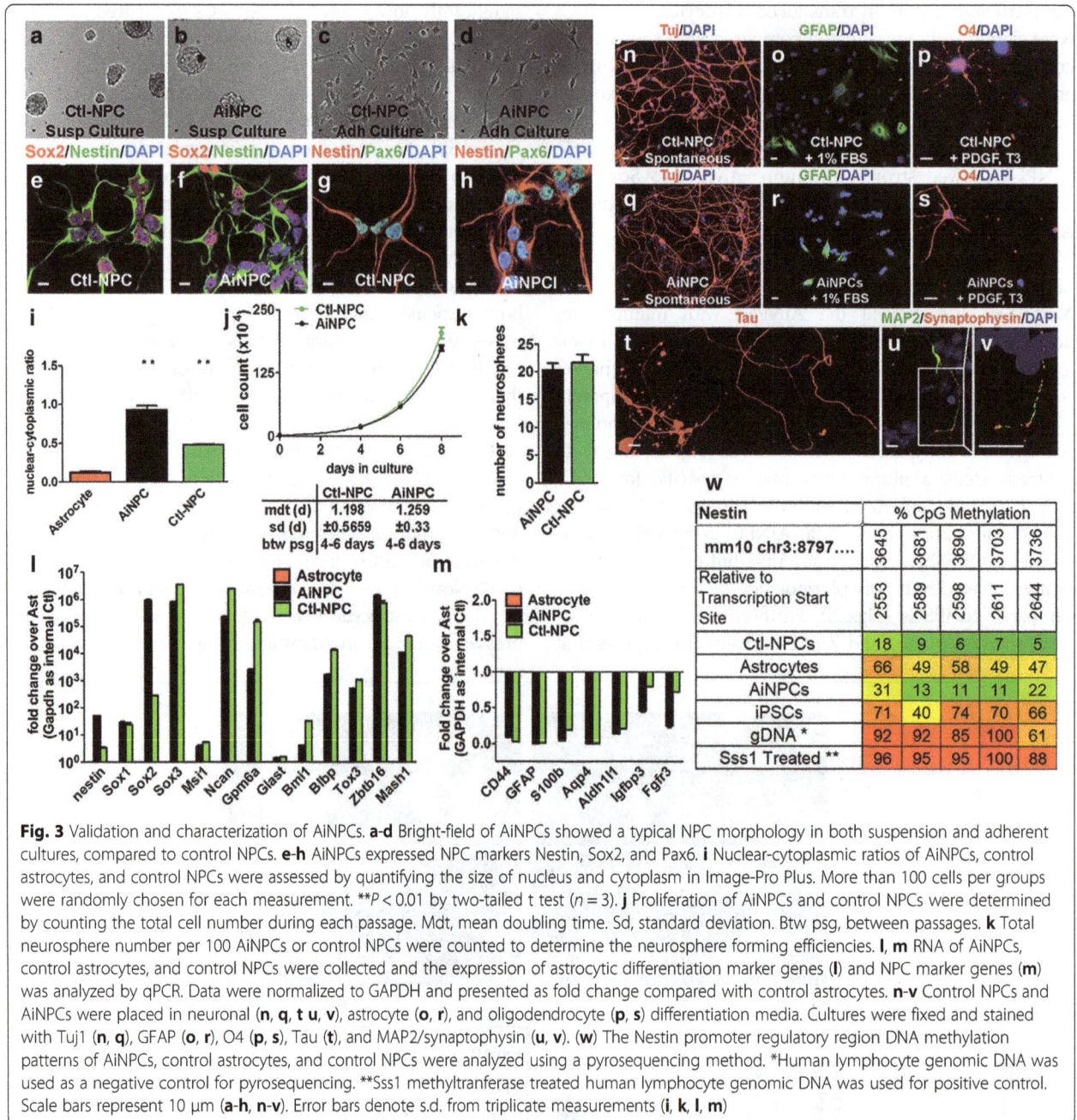

Fig. 3 Validation and characterization of AiNPCs. **a-d** Bright-field of AiNPCs showed a typical NPC morphology in both suspension and adherent cultures, compared to control NPCs. **e-h** AiNPCs expressed NPC markers Nestin, Sox2, and Pax6. **i** Nuclear-cytoplasmic ratios of AiNPCs, control astrocytes, and control NPCs were assessed by quantifying the size of nucleus and cytoplasm in Image-Pro Plus. More than 100 cells per groups were randomly chosen for each measurement. **P < 0.01 by two-tailed t test ($n = 3$). **j** Proliferation of AiNPCs and control NPCs were determined by counting the total cell number during each passage. Mdt, mean doubling time. Sd, standard deviation. Btw psg, between passages. **k** Total neurosphere number per 100 AiNPCs or control NPCs were counted to determine the neurosphere forming efficiencies. **l, m** RNA of AiNPCs, control astrocytes, and control NPCs were collected and the expression of astrocytic differentiation marker genes (**l**) and NPC marker genes (**m**) was analyzed by qPCR. Data were normalized to GAPDH and presented as fold change compared with control astrocytes. **n-v** Control NPCs and AiNPCs were placed in neuronal (**n, q, t u, v**), astrocyte (**o, r**), and oligodendrocyte (**p, s**) differentiation media. Cultures were fixed and stained with Tuj1 (**n, q**), GFAP (**o, r**), O4 (**p, s**), Tau (**t**), and MAP2/synaptophysin (**u, v**). (**w**) The Nestin promoter regulatory region DNA methylation patterns of AiNPCs, control astrocytes, and control NPCs were analyzed using a pyrosequencing method. *Human lymphocyte genomic DNA was used as a negative control for pyrosequencing. **Sss1 methyltransferase treated human lymphocyte genomic DNA was used for positive control. Scale bars represent 10 μm (**a-h, n-v**). Error bars denote s.d. from triplicate measurements (**i, k, l, m**)

methylation analysis of the promoter of Nestin revealed low methylation status in AiNPCs, confirming the activation of the endogenous Nestin gene (Fig. 3w). Finally, we looked at the multipotency of AiNPCs and found that similar to NPCs (Fig. 3n-v), AiNPCs spontaneously differentiated into Tuj1+ neurons, GFAP+ astrocytes, and O4+ oligodendrocytes after culturing in cell type-specific differentiation media for 14 days (Fig. 3n-s). In the prolonged differentiation cultures (3 weeks), positive labeling of MAP-2, Tau, and Synaptophysin was found, suggesting the presence of axons and neuronal presynaptic structures that are hallmarks of mature neurons (Fig. 3t-v). Together, these

extensive characterizations strongly support the NPC status of the AiNPCs.

The telencephalic-phenotype and neuronal subtype specification of AiNPCs

In the developing brain, gene expression pattern changes following a spatiotemporal order based on their embryonic anatomical locations [33, 34]. The gene expression pattern, collectively depicting the regional identity of NPCs, is known to closely associate with specific neuronal lineages [35], so we examined the region-specific gene expression patterns of the AiNPCs by qPCR. The expression levels of marker genes along the anterior-posterior axis confirmed the regional identities of the tissues isolated from the cortex, midbrain, or hindbrain (Fig. 4a). Based on the marker genes expression, control NPCs had a distinct cortical identity. Similarly, AiNPCs expressed markers of cortex but not that of midbrain or hindbrain. Telencephalic NPCs from midgestation mouse embryos (E10.5) were lineage-restricted and refractory to ventral mesencephalic cues for inducing dopaminergic neurons [29].

Next, we investigated the neuronal subtypes that could be derived from the AiNPCs. Interestingly, under spontaneous neuronal differentiation condition, AiNPCs were able to differentiate into VGLUT$^+$ glutamatergic neurons, GABA$^+$/Darpp32$^+$ inhibitory neurons, and ChAT$^+$ cholinergic neurons, but not TH$^+$ dopaminergic neurons (Fig. 4b-f). This specific pattern of neuronal subtype differentiation is supported by qPCR analysis of gene transcripts. The transcription levels of VGLUT1 (glutamatergic neuron), Gad65 and Darpp32 (GABAergic neuron), and Ache (cholinergic neuron) were at significantly higher levels in AiNPCs-differentiated cells collected at 14 days after differentiation, compared to AiNPCs-differentiated cells collected at 3 days after differentiation. In contrast, the transcription levels of TH (dopaminergic neuron marker) remained unchanged during differentiation (Fig. 4g). Quantification of Tuj1$^+$ cells expressing neuronal subtype-specific markers suggested that the differentiation of AiNPCs was predominantly toward the glutamatergic and GABAergic neurons, occasionally toward cholinergic neurons, but rarely toward dopaminergic neurons (Fig. 4h).

To test whether AiNPCs still lack dopaminergic differentiation capacity when put in a ventral mesencephalic "inducing" condition, we adapted a differentiation protocol that involved SHH and FGF8 [21, 29, 36] and found that in such condition the gene expression of AiNPCs still represented a distinct telencephalic pattern (Fig. 4i-m). The mouse astrocyte-derived iPSCs and iPSCs-derived NPCs were used as positive controls [37]. Unlike AiNPCs, the expression of regional markers associated with midbrain/rostral hindbrain and dopaminergic markers could be induced in NPCs derived from iPSCs in the same culture condition (Fig. 4n-p). This restricted neuronal subtype specification suggested that AiNPCs had committed to a telencephalic lineage that predominantly generated glutamatergic and GABAergic neurons.

The induction of cholinergic neuron differentiation by additional Lhx8 overexpression

Emerging evidence demonstrated that the loss of cholinergic neurons is directly linked with the pathogenesis of Alzheimer's disease (AD) [38, 39]. Inefficiency of cholinergic neuronal differentiation from iNPCs has become a critical roadblock for cell transplantation based therapeutic strategy of AD. Recent studies suggested that

Lhx8 is a key facilitator of cholinergic neurogenesis, therefore, we hypothesized that Lhx8 involves in the cell fate commitment of AiNPCs towards cholinergic lineage. To test the hypothesis, we first overexpressed Lhx8 in AiNPCs through the pMXs-retroviral vector. The overexpression of Lhx8 was confirmed in AiNPCs by qPCR at 4 days post transduction (Fig. 5a). After Lhx8 overexpression, no difference in proliferation as indicated by the CCK-8 analysis, was observed in AiNPCs except at the day 4, suggesting that Lhx8 has no effect on proliferation of AiNPCs (Fig. 5b). Importantly, through immunocytochemical analysis, we found that the percentage of ChAT$^+$ cholinergic neurons generated from AiNPCs was significantly increased following the overexpression of Lhx8 (Fig. 5c-i). In contrast, Lhx8 overexpression had no significant impact on the generation of other neuronal subtypes in our immunocytochemical analysis (Additional file 1: Figure S4). These immunocytochemical data were corroborated by qPCR that demonstrated significant increases of gene transcripts corresponding to the marker of cholinergic neurons (Ache) but not those of glutamatergic neurons (VGLUT1), GABAergic neurons (Gad65), and dopaminergic neurons (Th) (Fig. 5j). Together, these data suggested that Lhx8 specifically promotes the generation of cholinergic neurons from AiNPCs.

The induction of dopaminergic neuron differentiation by additional Foxa2 overexpression

Degeneration of midbrain dopaminergic neurons is a key pathological event of Parkinson's disease (PD). The cell-based therapy for PD requires high efficiency of dopaminergic neuron generation. To determine whether midbrain dopaminergic fate could be achieved from the forebrain-specific AiNPCs, we further included two more TFs, Foxa2 and Lmx1a, that are crucial in midbrain dopaminergic neuron differentiation [23, 40, 41]. We used pMX retroviral gene delivery system to transduce Foxa2 and Lmx1a into AiNPCs. The overexpression of Foxa2 and Lmx1a was evident in AiNPCs at 4 days post transduction (Fig. 6a, b). After cultured under ventral mesencephalic cue SHH and FGF8 for 1 week, AiNPCs acquired dopaminergic neurogenesis capability after the transduction of individual Foxa2, Lmx1a, or Foxa2/Lmx1a in combination (Fig. 6c-j). Interestingly, TH$^+$/Nurr1$^+$ dopaminergic neuron yields in Foxa2- and Foxa2/Lmx1a-transduced AiNPCs were significantly higher than Lmx1a-transduced AiNPCs (6 k, l), suggesting that Foxa2 is a stronger factor for dopaminergic neuronal induction compared with Lmx1a. qPCR analysis of the differentiated AiNPCs confirmed the predominant induction of dopaminergic genes (Th and Aadc) but not that of glutamatergic, GABAergic, and cholinergic genes (Fig. 6m).

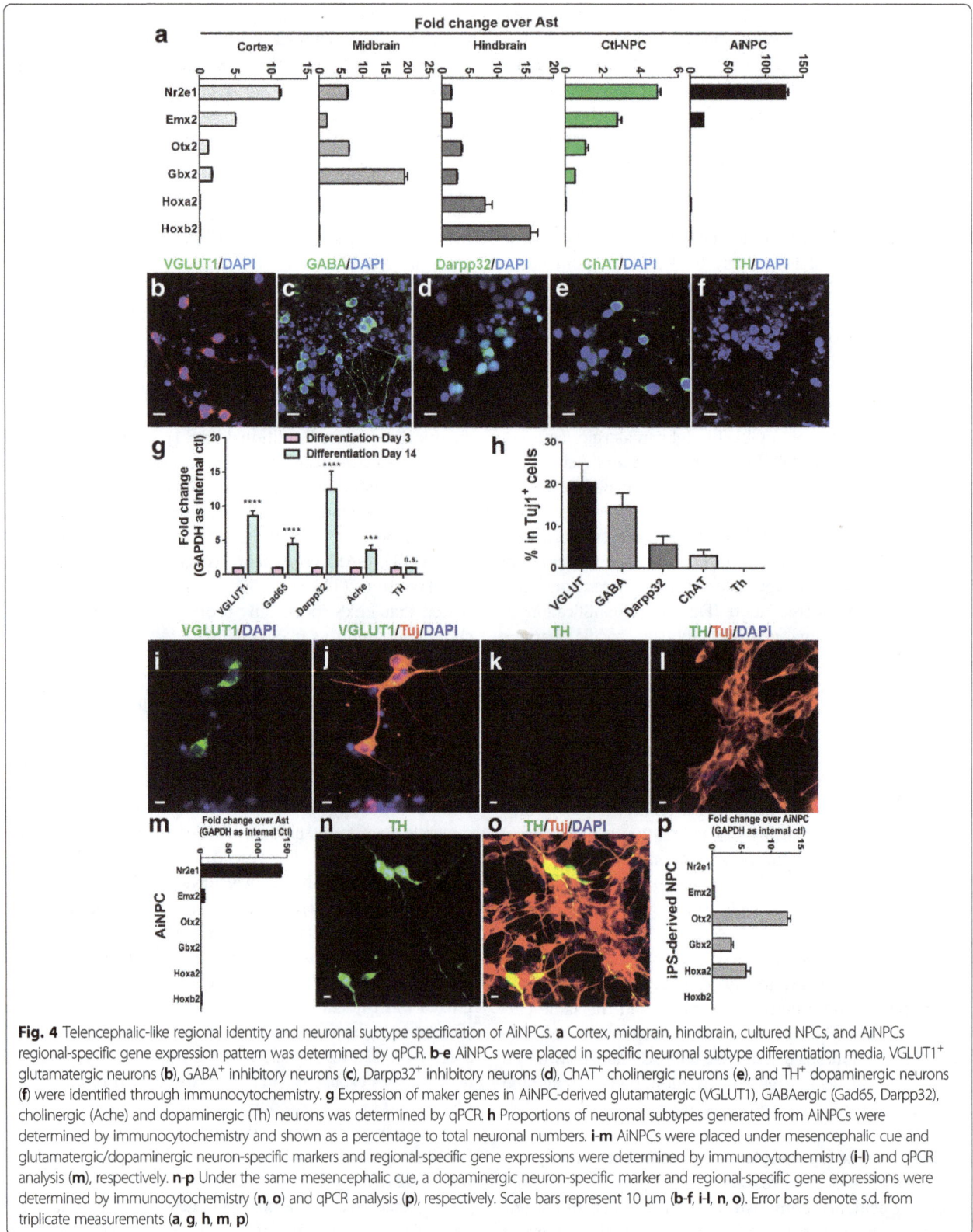

Fig. 4 Telencephalic-like regional identity and neuronal subtype specification of AiNPCs. **a** Cortex, midbrain, hindbrain, cultured NPCs, and AiNPCs regional-specific gene expression pattern was determined by qPCR. **b-e** AiNPCs were placed in specific neuronal subtype differentiation media, VGLUT1$^+$ glutamatergic neurons (**b**), GABA$^+$ inhibitory neurons (**c**), Darpp32$^+$ inhibitory neurons (**d**), ChAT$^+$ cholinergic neurons (**e**), and TH$^+$ dopaminergic neurons (**f**) were identified through immunocytochemistry. **g** Expression of maker genes in AiNPC-derived glutamatergic (VGLUT1), GABAergic (Gad65, Darpp32), cholinergic (Ache) and dopaminergic (Th) neurons was determined by qPCR. **h** Proportions of neuronal subtypes generated from AiNPCs were determined by immunocytochemistry and shown as a percentage to total neuronal numbers. **i-m** AiNPCs were placed under mesencephalic cue and glutamatergic/dopaminergic neuron-specific markers and regional-specific gene expressions were determined by immunocytochemistry (**i-l**) and qPCR analysis (**m**), respectively. **n-p** Under the same mesencephalic cue, a dopaminergic neuron-specific marker and regional-specific gene expressions were determined by immunocytochemistry (**n, o**) and qPCR analysis (**p**), respectively. Scale bars represent 10 μm (**b-f, i-l, n, o**). Error bars denote s.d. from triplicate measurements (**a, g, h, m, p**)

Discussion

Adult brain is known to have limited regeneration after injury. During neurodegenerative diseases, the limited regeneration is often not sufficient to compensate for the loss of neuronal functions [4, 42]. The reprogramming of somatic cells to replace the damaged neurons is

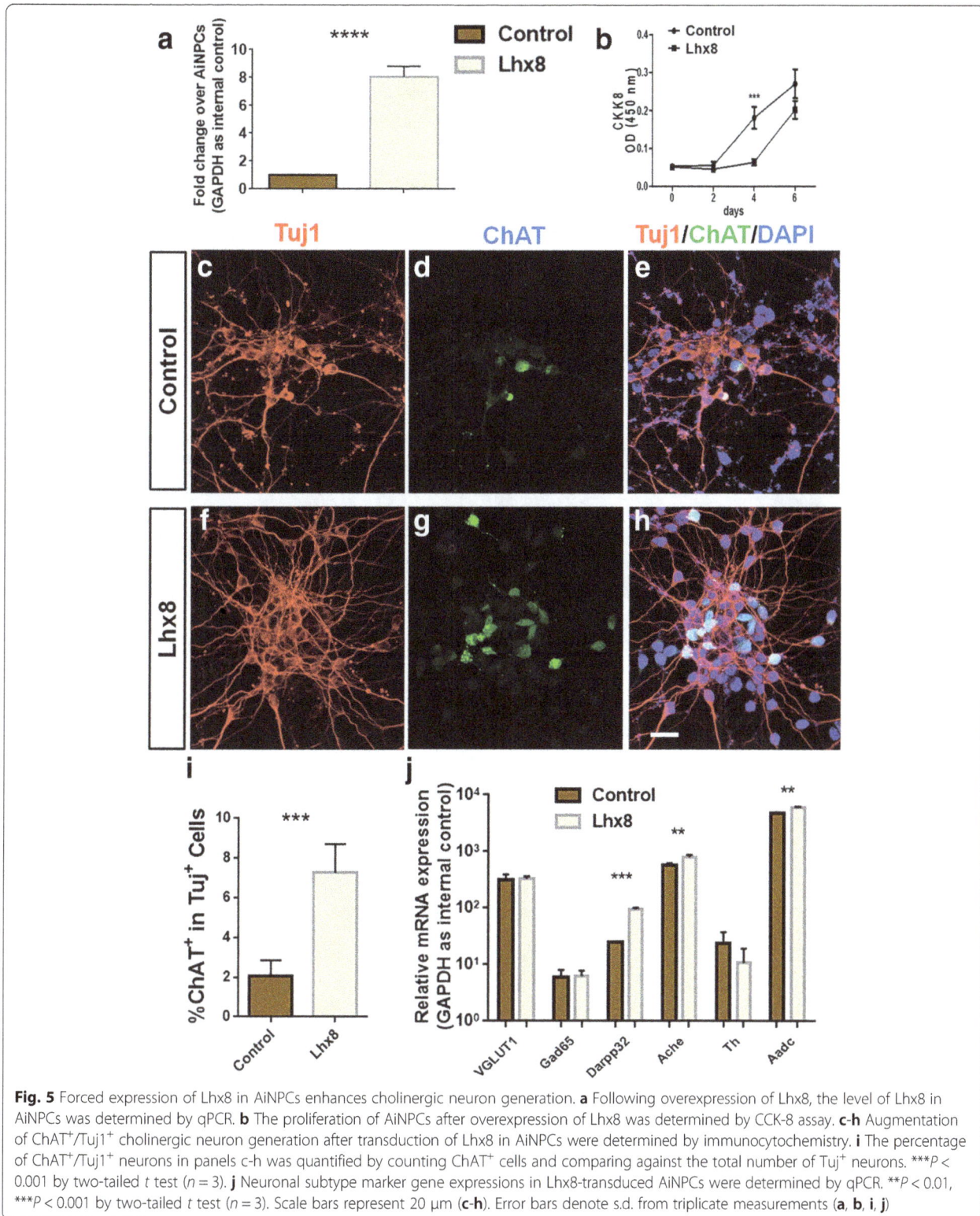

Fig. 5 Forced expression of Lhx8 in AiNPCs enhances cholinergic neuron generation. **a** Following overexpression of Lhx8, the level of Lhx8 in AiNPCs was determined by qPCR. **b** The proliferation of AiNPCs after overexpression of Lhx8 was determined by CCK-8 assay. **c-h** Augmentation of ChAT$^+$/Tuj1$^+$ cholinergic neuron generation after transduction of Lhx8 in AiNPCs were determined by immunocytochemistry. **i** The percentage of ChAT$^+$/Tuj1$^+$ neurons in panels c-h was quantified by counting ChAT$^+$ cells and comparing against the total number of Tuj$^+$ neurons. ***$P <$ 0.001 by two-tailed t test ($n = 3$). **j** Neuronal subtype marker gene expressions in Lhx8-transduced AiNPCs were determined by qPCR. **$P <$ 0.01, ***$P <$ 0.001 by two-tailed t test ($n = 3$). Scale bars represent 20 μm (**c-h**). Error bars denote s.d. from triplicate measurements (**a**, **b**, **i**, **j**)

a promising therapeutic strategy in treating neurodegenerative diseases [43, 44]. Recently, astrocyte-based reprogramming has received growing interest within the scientific community due to its abundance and regenerative capacity [21, 45–49]. Two main approaches are typically applied in these studies. One approach is to directly convert astrocytes into neuronal cells [45–47]. This approach may be more specific and less

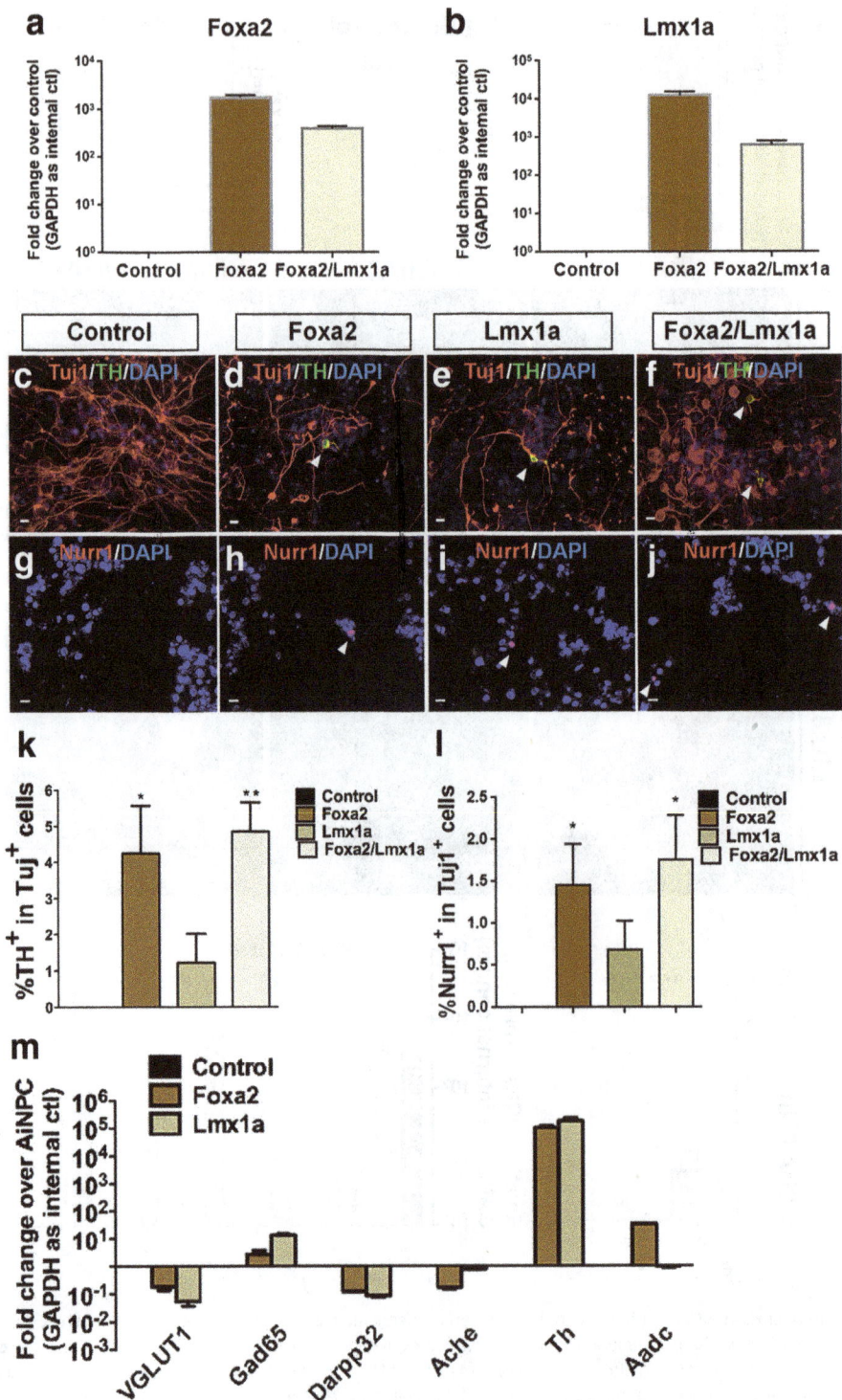

Fig. 6 Forced expression of Foxa2/Lmx1a in AiNPCs enhances dopaminergic neuron generation. **a**, **b** Following overexpression of Foxa2/Lmx1a, the levels of Foxa2 and Lmx1a in AiNPCs were determined by qPCR. **c-j** Augmentation of TH[+]/Nurr1[+] dopaminergic neuron generation after transduction of Foxa2 (**d**, **h**), Lmx1a (**e**, **i**), and Foxa2/Lmx1a (**f**, **j**) in AiNPCs were determined by immunocytochemistry. **k**, **l** The percentage of TH[+]/Nurr1[+] neurons in panels c-j was quantified by counting TH[+]/Nurr1[+] cells and comparing against the total number of Tuj[+] neurons. *$P < 0.05$, **$P < 0.01$ by two-tailed t test ($n = 3$). **m** Neuronal subtype marker gene expressions in Foxa2- and Lmx1a-transduced AiNPCs under mesencephalic cues were determined by qPCR. Scale bars represent 10 μm (**c-j**). Error bars denote s.d. from triplicate measurements (**a**, **b**, **k-m**)

tumorigenic. However, limitations in reprogramming efficiency and cell number curb broad functional recoveries in the brain. Another approach is to reprogram astrocytes into proliferative iNPCs [21, 49]. This approach could overcome the cell number limitation and is applied in the current study. Using retroviral vectors that overexpressed TFs Foxg1, Sox2, and Brn2, we successfully reprogramed mouse astrocytes into iNPCs without going through the stage of iPSCs. The AiNPCs exhibited typical NPCs' phenotype, including the self-renewal and the tripotency to differentiate into neurons, astrocytes, and oligodendrocytes under defined conditions. Interestingly, AiNPCs had robust expression of regional marker genes for forebrain but not for midbrain or hindbrain. Therefore, the AiNPCs were more readily differentiated into glutamatergic and GABAergic neurons, but not dopaminergic neurons. However, overexpression of Lhx8 and Foxa2/Lmx1a in AiNPCs promoted cholinergic and dopaminergic neuronal differentiation, respectively, suggesting that fate-committed AiNPCs can be shifted to other lineages through forced expression of specific TFs.

To date, various cell sources has been used to generate iNPCs, including fibroblasts, astrocytes, sertoli cells, and urine cells. The successful conversion of different types of somatic cells into iNPCs suggests a common iNPCs reprogramming path. Our current study suggests the same NPC transcriptional core network, used for mouse fibroblast reprogramming, can superimpose a NPC fate onto astrocytes [19]. Given the neural origin of astrocytes, it is possible that fewer TFs or even a single TF may be able to coerce astrocytes into the same NPC fate [49]. Cultured astrocytes are quite heterogeneous and may manifest a spectrum of phenotypes for NPC conversion. In specific culture conditions, developing or adult damaged brains might contain immature or reactive astrocytes, respectively, that exhibit neurosphere-forming ability [30, 50]. In our studies, the astrocytes are likely not in reactive status because we did not observe any EGFP+ neurospheres generated from the control astrocyte cultures even though growth factors were present. Furthermore, the protocols to generate reactive astrocytes usually need physical damage or chemical stimulation, which is not used in our culture conditions [51, 52]. We have previously activated the culture to generate a reactive phenotype, suggesting a lower activation status of our astrocyte culture [53]. It is possible that retroviral transduction diminished the efficiencies for NPC conversion. In addition, astrocyte cultures in our studies are derived from cortices of P7 mice, which are likely quite different from adult astrocytes. Caution needs to be taken to translate the findings to the adult brain and to the in vivo experiments.

Our study also confirm that Foxg1, Sox2, and Brn2 may be one of the master regulator sets for stabilizing the status of NPC, given that NPCs stand for a progenitor population with diverse fate restrictions in a region-specific manner [54, 55]. We cannot exclude the possibility that neuronal differentiation potential of AiNPCs could be altered by extended passages, where cell fate may be modulated by endogenous machinery. Nonetheless, throughout all AiNPCs passages, the AiNPCs manifested all cardinal properties of definitive NPCs: proliferating, self-renewal, tripotency and most importantly, a specific regional identity.

iNPCs theoretically could generate all known neuronal subtypes in the brain. Surprisingly, we found that AiNPCs are committed to a clear regional fate with the 3 factors-imposed transcriptional core network. The telencephalic fate commitment may be largely due to the inclusion of Foxg1, a critical denominator of ventral telencephalic fate during development. It starts to express when the anterior part of the neural plate is specified to telencephalon (E8.5), after the emergence of primitive NPCs at E7 [56–58]. NPCs interpret patterning cues of neuronal specification within a very short window (E8.5 to E10.5) at early stages of neural development [29] and Foxg1, whose expression is independent of SHH [59], acts autonomously to endow cells with intrinsic competency to obtain ventral telencephalic identity [57].

Our neuronal subtype specification studies suggested the spontaneous differentiation of AiNPCs is biased to favor glutamatergic/GABAergic neuronal differentiations. This trend follows a similar neural development program in vivo, that NPCs in the dorsal and ventral telencephalon majorly develop into glutamatergic and GABAergic neurons during brain development [60]. Similar patterns were also observed when differentiate telencephalic NPCs in vitro, confirming the differentiation preference of telencephalic NPCs bias to glutamatergic and GABAergic neurons [61]. Besides, a small proportion of cholinergic neurons could be differentiated from AiNPCs, whereas no dopaminergic neuron generation takes place, which further confirmed the telencephalic phenotype of AiNPCs. Our results suggested that the generation of other types of neurons from AiNPCs involves more regional-/subtype-specific TFs. Lhx8, a member of the LIM homeobox gene family, is selectively expressed in the medial ganglionic eminence [62]. Lhx8-null mice presented significantly less basal forebrain cholinergic neurons [63]. In our studies, significant increase in the generation of ChAT+ cholinergic neurons was found in Lhx8-overexpressed AiNPCs. These results confirm that Lhx8 positively regulates cholinergic differentiation. However, the efficiency of cholinergic neuron generation is still relatively low even with Lhx8 overexpression. For further enhancement of cholinergic neurons differentiation, approaches that modify the microenvironment of AiNPCs might be recruited, such as small molecule treatment, astrocyte co-culture and 3D scaffold culture, which are under investigation.

Foxa2 & Lmx1a are reported to determine the cell fate of dopaminergic neurons in midbrain cooperatively [64, 65]. We previously reported that a defined TFs set including Foxa2 could reprogram mouse fibroblasts into dopaminergic precursors efficiently [23]. Here, we demonstrated that Foxa2/Lmx1a could overwrite the telencephalic fate commitment of AiNPCs and direct the differentiation of AiNPCs into a mesodiencephalic dopaminergic fate. Interestingly, the influence of Foxa2 on the induction of DAs differentiation is significantly stronger than that of Lmx1a in our studies, suggesting Foxa2 plays its role more upstream and may regulate multiple downstream factors besides Lmx1a. Similar findings were reported that during the mouse midbrain development in vivo, Foxa family members (Foxa1 & Foxa2) function upstream of Lmx1a/b, together with other dopaminergic neuron determinant genes such as Nkx2.2 and TH to promote mesodiencephalic DA

differentiation [65]. Lmx1a can only specify mesodiencephalic dopaminergic fate within Foxa2$^+$ mesencephalic progenitors [66]. Thus, our and other independent groups' observations demonstrate the key gene network for the cell fate determination of DAs.

The reprogramming of somatic cells into proliferative iNPCs is a promising technique to prepare sufficient cells for cell replacement purpose. We previously reported the survival and maturation of reprogrammed dopaminergic precursors in MPTP-treated mouse brain. AiNPCs and their-derived cell-type specific precursors may broaden the precursor cell types suitable to be transplanted in neurodegenerative disease mouse models. These cells are not only able to achieve therapeutic effects through cell replacement, but also to modulate brain microenvironment for tissue repair and regeneration [67, 68]. Thus, the effects of AiNPCs transplantation and the underlying in vivo

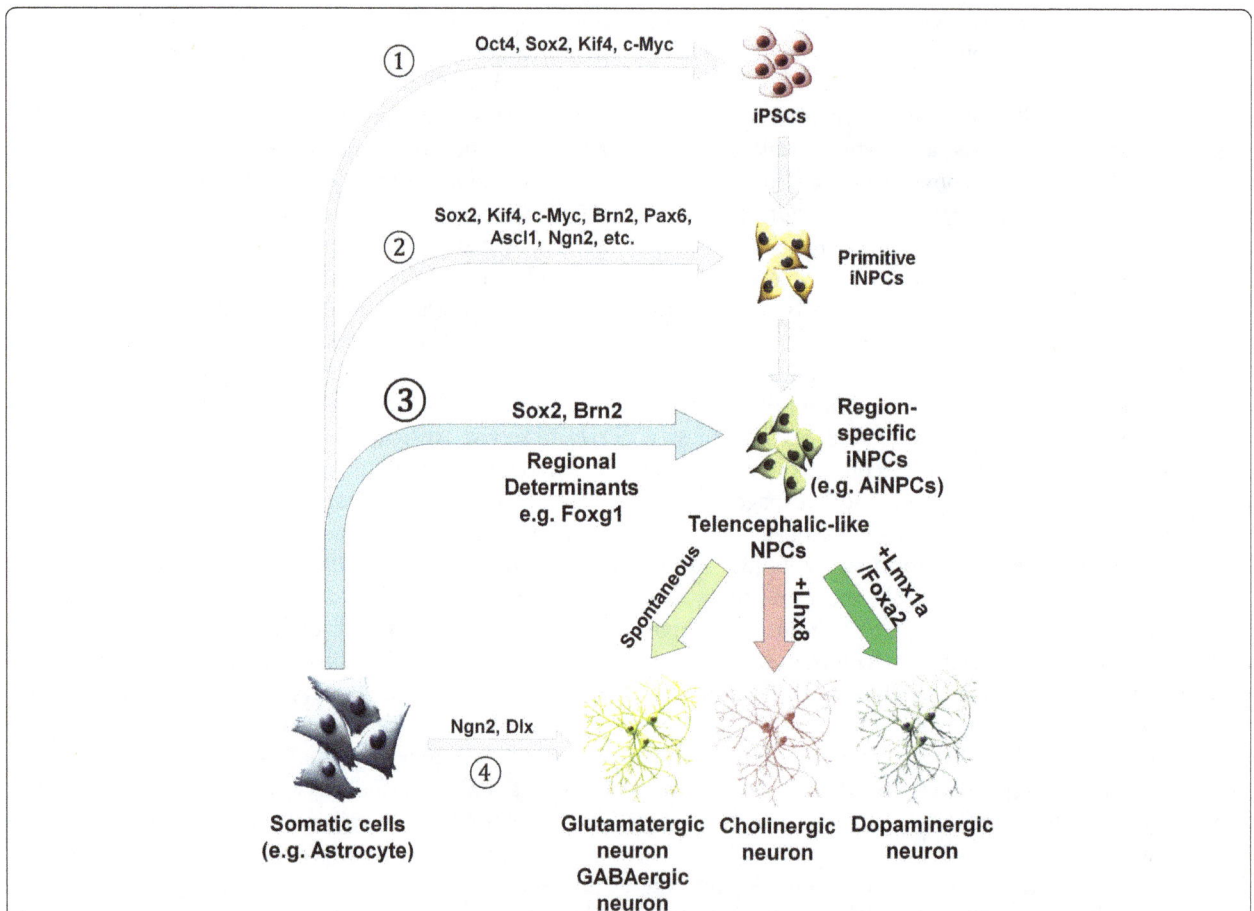

Fig. 7 Proposed model for reprogramming for iNPCs and differentiation for specific lineages of neurons. Combination of Yamanaka Factors (Oct4, Sox2, Klf4, c-Myc) and ESC media leads to iPSC dedifferentiation from somatic cells (Path 1). Direct conversion of somatic cells into iNPCs was achieved by transducing fibroblasts or astrocytes with NPC fate determinants (Path 2). Induced neurons are termed after terminally differentiated cells were directly converted into neurons (Path 4). We propose that somatic cells can be converted to regional-committed iNPCs with restricted neuronal subtype differentiation capacities (e.g. glutamatergic and GABAergic neurons for telencephalon). The transdifferentiation is achieved using NPC fate master regulators (e.g., Sox2 and Brn2) in addition to potent regional determinants (e.g. Foxg1 for telencephalon) (Path 3). The differentiation potential of AiNPC differentiation towards forebrain Gluamatergic and GABAergic neurons can be altered by the forced expression of TFs that promotes dedicated neuronal specifications (e.g., Lhx8 for cholinergic neurons and Foxa2/Lmx1a for midbrain dopaminergic neurons)

mechanisms remain open propositions, which is currently under investigation.

Conclusions

In summary, astrocyte is a promising candidate for iNPC direct conversion. Targeting astrocytes with specific viral-based transgene delivery to induce NPC fate is particularly attractive since it is able to target those pre-existing reactive astrocytes within the proximity of lesion areas and may have great therapeutic potentials in neurodegenerative diseases. Furthermore, Foxg1, Sox2, and Brn2 may be one of the master regulator sets for successfully superimposing NPC fate not only on fibroblasts but on astrocytes as well (Fig. 7). The AiNPCs demonstrate cardinal features of NPCs with ventral telencephalic identity and differentiation capacity. The limitations in differentiation potentials of AiNPCs could be overcome by factors promoting dedicated neuronal specifications. Because reactive astrogliosis is ubiquitous in neurodegenerative disorders, our results suggest astrocyte-iNPC reprogramming is a potentially promising strategy to boost brain regeneration. The identification of specific factors for neuronal subtype generation could offer valuable information for cell-based therapy for devastating neurodegenerative diseases.

Additional file

Additional file 1: Figure S1. The validation of primary astrocyte culture. A-C: Primary astrocyte cultures were positive for GFAP, but negative for Iba1 and Tuj1. Scale bars represent 20 μm. **Figure S2.** The validation of transcription factors transduction. A, B: The transduction was validated by examining the expression of endogenous (A) and exogenous (B) Sox2, Brn2, and Foxg1. Error bars denote s.d. from triplicate measurements. **Figure S3.** The methylation status of SSEA-1 promoter. The SSEA-1 promoter regulatory region DNA methylation patterns of AiNPCs, control astrocytes, control NPCs and astrocyte-derived iPSCs were analyzed using pyrosequencing method. *Human lymphocyte genomic DNA was used as a negative control for pyrosequencing. **Sss1 methyltranferase treated human lymphocyte genomic DNA was used for positive control. **Figure S4.** The effects of Lhx8 forced expression in the differentiation of neuronal subtypes from AiNPCs. A. The generation of VGLUT+ glutamatergic neurons, GABA+/Darpp32+ GABAergic neurons and TH+ dopaminergic neuron after transduction of Lhx8 in AiNPCs were determined by immunocytochemistry. B. The percentage of different subtypes of neurons was quantified by counting VGLUT+, GABA+, Darpp32+ and TH+ cells and comparing against the total number of cells. Scale bars represent 50 μm (A). Error bars denote s.d. from triplicate measurements (B). **Table S1.** Antibody List. **Table S2.** Primers for Marker Genes. **Table S3.** Pyrosequencing Primer Sequences. (DOCX 4248 kb)

Abbreviations

AD: Alzheimer's disease; AiNPCs: Astrocyte-derived induced neural progenitor cells; CNS: Central nervous system; iNPCs: Induced neuronal progenitor cells; iPSCs: Induced pluripotent stem cells; NPCs: Neural progenitor cells; PD: Parkinson's disease; TFs: Transcription factors

Acknowledgements

We kindly acknowledge Dr. Li Wu, Kristin Leland Wavrin, and Michael Price who provided valuable technical support, comments, and suggestions about the manuscript. We thank Dr. David Klinkebiel at the Epigenomics Core of UNMC to perform and assist in the analysis of DNA methylation data. We thank Julie Ditter, Robin Taylor, Myhanh Che, Na Ly, and Lenal Bottoms provided outstanding administrative support.

Funding

This work was supported in part by research grants from the National Basic Research Program of China (973 ProgramGrant No. 2014CB965001 to JZ), Innovative Research Groups of the National Natural Science Foundation of China (#81221001 to JZ), and Joint Research Fund for Overseas Chinese, Hong Kong and Macao Young Scientists of the National Natural Science Foundation of China (#81329002 to JZ), the National Institutes of Health: 2R56NS041858-15A1 (JZ), 1R01NS097195-01 (JZ), and R03 NS094071-01 (YH), the State of Nebraska, DHHS-LB606 Stem Cell 2009-10 to JZ.

Authors' contributions

Conceived and designed the experiments: JCZ CT KM XD. Performed the experiments: KM XD XX YX XQ YM HP YH YL QC HP KD. Analyzed the data: KM XD XX HP YH. Contributed reagents/materials/analysis tools: KM XD XX QC YX JD YL CT. Wrote the paper: KM XD XX YH CT JCZ. All authors read and approved the final manuscript.

Competing interests

The authors declare that they have no competing interests.

Author details

[1]Center for Translational Neurodegeneration and Regenerative Therapy, Shanghai Tenth People's Hospital affiliated to Tongji University School of Medicine, Shanghai 200072, China. [2]Collaborative Innovation Center for Brain Science, Tongji University, Shanghai 200092, China. [3]Departments of Pharmacology and Experimental Neuroscience, University of Nebraska Medical Center, Omaha, NE 68198-5930, USA. [4]Department of Neurology & Institute of Neurology, Ruijin Hospital affiliated to Shanghai Jiao Tong University School of Medicine, Shanghai 200025, China. [5]Department of Pathology and Microbiology, University of Nebraska Medical Center, Omaha, NE 68198-5930, USA.

References

1. Reynolds BA, Weiss S. Generation of neurons and astrocytes from isolated cells of the adult mammalian central nervous system. Science. 1992; 255(5052):1707–10.
2. Bonnamain V, Neveu I, Naveilhan P. In vitro analyses of the immunosuppressive properties of neural stem/progenitor cells using anti-CD3/CD28-activated T cells. Methods Mol Biol. 2011;677:233–43.
3. Mosher KI, et al. Neural progenitor cells regulate microglia functions and activity. Nat Neurosci. 2012;15(11):1485–7.
4. Amor S, et al. Inflammation in neurodegenerative diseases. Immunology. 2010;129(2):154–69.
5. Whitney NP, et al. Inflammation mediates varying effects in neurogenesis: relevance to the pathogenesis of brain injury and neurodegenerative disorders. J Neurochem. 2009;108(6):1343–59.
6. Rosenberg GA, et al. Tumor necrosis factor-a-induced gelatinase B causes delayed opening of the blood-brain barrier: an expanded therapeutic window. Brain Res. 1995;703:151–5.
7. Tapscott SJ, et al. MyoD1: a nuclear phosphoprotein requiring a Myc homology region to convert fibroblasts to myoblasts. Science. 1988; 242(4877):405–11.
8. Smith DK, et al. The therapeutic potential of cell identity reprogramming for the treatment of aging-related neurodegenerative disorders. Prog Neurobiol. 2017;157:212–29.
9. Lai S, et al. Direct reprogramming of induced neural progenitors: a new promising strategy for AD treatment. Transl Neurodegener. 2015;4:7.

10. Miura K, et al. Variation in the safety of induced pluripotent stem cell lines. Nat Biotechnol. 2009;27(8):743–5.

11. Takahashi K, Yamanaka S. Induction of pluripotent stem cells from mouse embryonic and adult fibroblast cultures by defined factors. Cell. 2006;126(4):663–76.

12. Karumbayaram S, et al. Directed differentiation of human-induced pluripotent stem cells generates active motor neurons. Stem Cells. 2009; 27(4):806–11.

13. Han DW, et al. Direct reprogramming of fibroblasts into neural stem cells by defined factors. Cell Stem Cell. 2012;10(4):465–72.

14. Koehler KR, et al. Extended passaging increases the efficiency of neural differentiation from induced pluripotent stem cells. BMC Neurosci. 2011; 12:82.

15. Kim JB, et al. Oct4-induced pluripotency in adult neural stem cells. Cell. 2009;136(3):411–9.

16. Wernig M, et al. Neurons derived from reprogrammed fibroblasts functionally integrate into the fetal brain and improve symptoms of rats with Parkinson's disease. Proc Natl Acad Sci U S A. 2008;105(15):5856–61.

17. Tian C, et al. Direct conversion of dermal fibroblasts into neural progenitor cells by a novel cocktail of defined factors. Curr Mol Med. 2012;12(2):126–37.

18. Thier M, et al. Direct conversion of fibroblasts into stably expandable neural stem cells. Cell Stem Cell. 2012;10(4):473–9.

19. Lujan E, et al. Direct conversion of mouse fibroblasts to self-renewing, tripotent neural precursor cells. Proc Natl Acad Sci U S A. 2012;109(7):2527–32.

20. Sheng C, et al. Direct reprogramming of Sertoli cells into multipotent neural stem cells by defined factors. Cell Res. 2012;22(1):208–18.

21. Corti S, et al. Direct reprogramming of human astrocytes into neural stem cells and neurons. Exp Cell Res. 2012;318(13):1528–41.

22. Kim J, et al. Direct reprogramming of mouse fibroblasts to neural progenitors. Proc Natl Acad Sci U S A. 2011;108(19):7838–43.

23. Tian C, et al. Selective generation of dopaminergic precursors from mouse fibroblasts by direct lineage conversion. Sci Rep. 2015;5:12622.

24. Barreto GE, et al. Astrocyte proliferation following stroke in the mouse depends on distance from the infarct. PLoS One. 2011;6(11):e27881.

25. Verkhratsky A, et al. Neurological diseases as primary gliopathies: a reassessment of neurocentrism. ASN Neuro. 2012;4(3):e00082.

26. Sirko S, et al. Reactive glia in the injured brain acquire stem cell properties in response to sonic hedgehog glia. Cell Stem Cell. 2013;12(4):426–39.

27. Torper O, et al. Generation of induced neurons via direct conversion in vivo. Proc Natl Acad Sci U S A. 2013;110(17):7038–43.

28. Walter L, et al. Astrocytes in culture produce anandamide and other acylethanolamides. J Biol Chem. 2002;277(23):20869–76.

29. Baizabal JM, et al. Telencephalic neural precursor cells show transient competence to interpret the dopaminergic niche of the embryonic midbrain. Dev Biol. 2011;349(2):192–203.

30. Laywell ED, et al. Identification of a multipotent astrocytic stem cell in the immature and adult mouse brain. Proc Natl Acad Sci U S A. 2000;97(25):13883–8.

31. Capela A, Temple S. LeX/ssea-1 is expressed by adult mouse CNS stem cells, identifying them as nonependymal. Neuron. 2002;35(5):865–75.

32. Western PS, et al. Male fetal germ cell differentiation involves complex repression of the regulatory network controlling pluripotency. FASEB J. 2010;24(8):3026–35.

33. Hebert JM, Fishell G. The genetics of early telencephalon patterning: some assembly required. Nat Rev Neurosci. 2008;9(9):678–85.

34. Rallu M, Corbin JG, Fishell G. Parsing the prosencephalon. Nat Rev Neurosci. 2002;3(12):943–51.

35. Rouaux C, Bhai S, Arlotta P. Programming and reprogramming neuronal subtypes in the central nervous system. Dev Neurobiol. 2012;72(7):1085–98.

36. Lee HK, et al. Regulation of distinct AMPA receptor phosphorylation sites during bidirectional synaptic plasticity. Nature. 2000;405(6789):955–9.

37. Tian C, et al. Reprogrammed mouse astrocytes retain a "memory" of tissue origin and possess more tendencies for neuronal differentiation than reprogrammed mouse embryonic fibroblasts. Protein Cell. 2011;2(2):128–40.

38. Blusztajn JK, Berse B. The cholinergic neuronal phenotype in Alzheimer's disease. Metab Brain Dis. 2000;15(1):45–64.

39. Mufson EJ, et al. Cholinergic system during the progression of Alzheimer's disease: therapeutic implications. Expert Rev Neurother. 2008;8(11):1703–18.

40. Panman L, et al. Transcription factor-induced lineage selection of stem-cell-derived neural progenitor cells. Cell Stem Cell. 2011;8(6):663–75.

41. Lee HS, et al. Foxa2 and Nurr1 synergistically yield A9 nigral dopamine neurons exhibiting improved differentiation, function, and cell survival. Stem Cells. 2010;28(3):501–12.

42. Peng H, et al. HIV-1-infected and/or immune-activated macrophage-secreted TNF-alpha affects human fetal cortical neural progenitor cell proliferation and differentiation. Glia. 2008;56(8):903–16.

43. Abeliovich A, Doege CA. Reprogramming therapeutics: iPS cell prospects for neurodegenerative disease. Neuron. 2009;61(3):337–9.

44. Chen Y, Pu J, Zhang B. Progress and challenges of cell replacement therapy for neurodegenerative diseases based on direct neural reprogramming. Hum Gene Ther. 2016;27(12):962–70.

45. Masserdotti G, et al. Transcriptional mechanisms of proneural factors and REST in regulating neuronal reprogramming of astrocytes. Cell Stem Cell. 2015;17(1):74–88.

46. Addis RC, et al. Efficient conversion of astrocytes to functional midbrain dopaminergic neurons using a single polycistronic vector. PLoS One. 2011; 6(12):e28719.

47. Berninger B, et al. Functional properties of neurons derived from in vitro reprogrammed postnatal astroglia. J Neurosci. 2007;27(32):8654–64.

48. Chouchane M, et al. Lineage reprogramming of Astroglial cells from different origins into distinct neuronal subtypes. Stem Cell Rep. 2017;9(1):162–76.

49. Niu W, et al. In vivo reprogramming of astrocytes to neuroblasts in the adult brain. Nat Cell Biol. 2013;15(10):1164–75.

50. Heinrich C, et al. Directing astroglia from the cerebral cortex into subtype specific functional neurons. PLoS Biol. 2010;8(5):e1000373.

51. Wanner IB. An in vitro trauma model to study rodent and human astrocyte reactivity. Methods Mol Biol. 2012;814:189–219.

52. Tezel G, Hernandez MR, Wax MB. In vitro evaluation of reactive astrocyte migration, a component of tissue remodeling in glaucomatous optic nerve head. Glia. 2001;34(3):178–89.

53. Wang K, et al. TNF-alpha promotes extracellular vesicle release in mouse astrocytes through glutaminase. J Neuroinflammation. 2017;14(1):87.

54. Costa MR, Gotz M, Berninger B. What determines neurogenic competence in glia? Brain Res Rev. 2010;63(1–2):47–59.

55. Merkle FT, Mirzadeh Z, Alvarez-Buylla A. Mosaic organization of neural stem cells in the adult brain. Science. 2007;317(5836):381–4.

56. Wood HB, Episkopou V. Comparative expression of the mouse Sox1, Sox2 and Sox3 genes from pre-gastrulation to early somite stages. Mech Dev. 1999;86(1–2):197–201.

57. Manuel M, et al. The transcription factor Foxg1 regulates the competence of telencephalic cells to adopt subpallial fates in mice. Development. 2010;137(3): 487–97.

58. Martynoga B, et al. Foxg1 is required for specification of ventral telencephalon and region-specific regulation of dorsal telencephalic precursor proliferation and apoptosis. Dev Biol. 2005;283(1):113–27.

59. Rash BG, Grove EA. Patterning the dorsal telencephalon: a role for sonic hedgehog? J Neurosci. 2007;27(43):11595–603.

60. Marin O, Rubenstein JL. A long, remarkable journey: tangential migration in the telencephalon. Nat Rev Neurosci. 2001;2(11):780–90.

61. Li XJ, et al. Coordination of sonic hedgehog and Wnt signaling determines ventral and dorsal telencephalic neuron types from human embryonic stem cells. Development. 2009;136(23):4055–63.

62. Matsumoto K, et al. L3, a novel murine LIM-homeodomain transcription factor expressed in the ventral telencephalon and the mesenchyme surrounding the oral cavity. Neurosci Lett. 1996;204(1):113–6.

63. Manabe T, et al. L3/Lhx8 is involved in the determination of cholinergic or GABAergic cell fate. J Neurochem. 2005;94(3):723–30.

64. Ferri AL, et al. Foxa1 and Foxa2 regulate multiple phases of midbrain dopaminergic neuron development in a dosage-dependent manner. Development. 2007;134(15):2761–9.

65. Lin W, et al. Foxa1 and Foxa2 function both upstream of and cooperatively with Lmx1a and Lmx1b in a feedforward loop promoting mesodiencephalic dopaminergic neuron development. Dev Biol. 2009;333(2):386–96.

66. Nakatani T, et al. Lmx1a and Lmx1b cooperate with Foxa2 to coordinate the specification of dopaminergic neurons and control of floor plate cell differentiation in the developing mesencephalon. Dev Biol. 2010;339(1):101–13.

67. Yarygin KN, et al. Mechanisms of positive effects of transplantation of human placental mesenchymal stem cells on recovery of rats after experimental ischemic stroke. Bull Exp Biol Med. 2009;148(6):862–8.

68. Lee H, et al. Bone-marrow-derived mesenchymal stem cells promote proliferation and neuronal differentiation of Niemann-pick type C mouse neural stem cells by upregulation and secretion of CCL2. Hum Gene Ther. 2013;24(7):655–69.

Permissions

The contributors of this book come from diverse backgrounds, making this book a truly international effort. This book will bring forth new frontiers with its revolutionizing research information and detailed analysis of the nascent developments around the world.

We would like to thank all the contributing authors for lending their expertise to make the book truly unique. They have played a crucial role in the development of this book. Without their invaluable contributions this book wouldn't have been possible. They have made vital efforts to compile up to date information on the varied aspects of this subject to make this book a valuable addition to the collection of many professionals and students.

This book was conceptualized with the vision of imparting up-to-date information and advanced data in this field. To ensure the same, a matchless editorial board was set up. Every individual on the board went through rigorous rounds of assessment to prove their worth. After which they invested a large part of their time researching and compiling the most relevant data for our readers.

The editorial board has been involved in producing this book since its inception. They have spent rigorous hours researching and exploring the diverse topics which have resulted in the successful publishing of this book. They have passed on their knowledge of decades through this book. To expedite this challenging task, the publisher supported the team at every step. A small team of assistant editors was also appointed to further simplify the editing procedure and attain best results for the readers.

Apart from the editorial board, the designing team has also invested a significant amount of their time in understanding the subject and creating the most relevant covers. They scrutinized every image to scout for the most suitable representation of the subject and create an appropriate cover for the book.

The publishing team has been an ardent support to the editorial, designing and production team. Their endless efforts to recruit the best for this project, has resulted in the accomplishment of this book. They are a veteran in the field of academics and their pool of knowledge is as vast as their experience in printing. Their expertise and guidance has proved useful at every step. Their uncompromising quality standards have made this book an exceptional effort. Their encouragement from time to time has been an inspiration for everyone.

The publisher and the editorial board hope that this book will prove to be a valuable piece of knowledge for researchers, students, practitioners and scholars across the globe.

List of Contributors

Lei Wei
Department of Neurology, The Third Affiliated Hospital of Sun Yat-sen University, Guangzhou 510630, China
Department of Neurology, The First Affiliated Hospital of Sun Yat-sen University, Guangzhou 510080, China

Ming-shu Mo, Ming Lei and Limin Zhang
Department of Neurology, The First Affiliated Hospital of Sun Yat-sen University, Guangzhou 510080, China

Pingyi Xu
Department of Neurology, The First Affiliated Hospital of Sun Yat-sen University, Guangzhou 510080, China
Department of Neurology, The First Affiliated Hospital of Guangzhou Medical University, Guangzhou 510120, China

Li Ding
Department of pathology, The First Affiliated Hospital of Sun Yat-sen University, Guangzhou 510080, China

Kang Chen
Division of Clinical Laboratory, Zhongshan Hospital of Sun Yat-sen University, Zhongshan 528403, China

Yiwei Qian, Jiujiang Liu, Shaoqing Xu, Xiaodong Yang and Qin Xiao
Ruijin Hospital affiliated to Shanghai JiaoTong University School of Medicine, No. 197, Ruijin Er Road, Shanghai 200025, China

Guodong Gao and Qian Yang
Department of Neurosurgery, Tangdu Hospital, The Fourth Military Medical University, No. 569 Xinsi Road, Baqiao District, Xi'an 710038, Shaanxi Province, China

Bao Wang
Department of Neurosurgery, Tangdu Hospital, The Fourth Military Medical University, No. 569 Xinsi Road, Baqiao District, Xi'an 710038, Shaanxi Province, China
Department of Neurology, Beth Isreal Deaconess Medical Center, Harvard Medical School, 330 Brookline Ave, Boston 02215, MA, USA

Neeta Abraham
Department of Neurology, Beth Isreal Deaconess Medical Center, Harvard Medical School, 330 Brookline Ave, Boston 02215, MA, USA

Jing Pan and Huaibin Cai
Transgenics Section, Laboratory of Neurogenetics, National Institute on Aging, National Institutes of Health, Building 35, Room 1A112, MSC 3707, 35 Convent Drive, Bethesda, MD 20892-3707, USA

Bin-Yin Li, Ying Wang, Hui-dong Tang and Sheng-Di Chen
Department of Neurology, Institute of Neurology and the Collaborative Innovation Center for Brain Science, Rui Jin Hospital affiliated to Shanghai Jiao Tong University School of Medicine, Shanghai 200025, China

Rao Fu, Xiao-Guang Luo, Yan Ren, Zhi-Yi He and Hong Lv
Neurology Department, Outpatient of Parkinson's Disease, First Affiliated Hospital of China Medical University, 155# Nanjing bei streetHeping District, Shenyang 110001, P R China

Hui Sun, Qiong Cai, Jingxing Zhang, Yigang Liu, Liang Feng, Zhiyu Nie and Lingjing Jin
Department of Neurology, Shanghai Tongji Hospital, Tongji University School of Medicine, 389 Xincun Road, Shanghai 200065, People's Republic of China

Jianmin Fang
School of Life Science and Technology, Tongji University, 1239 Siping Road, Shanghai 200092, People's Republic of China

Ming Jiang
School of Life Science and Technology, Tongji University, 1239 Siping Road, Shanghai 200092, People's Republic of China
Biomedical Research Center, Tongji University Suzhou Institute, Building 2, 198 Jinfeng Road, Wuzhong District, Suzhou, Jiangsu 215101, China

Xing Fu, Yanxin Yin, Jia Guo, Lihua Yu and Yun Jiang
Biomedical Research Center, Tongji University Suzhou Institute, Building 2, 198 Jinfeng Road, Wuzhong District, Suzhou, Jiangsu 215101, China

Piu Chan
Department of Neurobiology, Neurology and Geriatrics, Xuanwu Hospital Capital Medical University, Beijing 100051, China

Beijing Key Laboratory on Parkinson's Disease, Parkinson Disease Center of Beijing Institute for Brain Disorders, Beijing 100051, China

Shu-Ying Liu
Department of Neurobiology, Neurology and Geriatrics, Xuanwu Hospital Capital Medical University, Beijing 100051, China
Beijing Key Laboratory on Parkinson's Disease, Parkinson Disease Center of Beijing Institute for Brain Disorders, Beijing 100051, China
Pacific Parkinson's Research Centre, Division of Neurology and Djavad Mowafaghian Centre for Brain Health, University of British Columbia and Vancouver Coastal Health, Vancouver V6T 1Z3, BC, Canada

A. Jon Stoessl
Pacific Parkinson's Research Centre, Division of Neurology and Djavad Mowafaghian Centre for Brain Health, University of British Columbia and Vancouver Coastal Health, Vancouver V6T 1Z3, BC, Canada

Xin-Ling Su, Xiao-Guang Luo, Hong Lv, Yan Ren and Zhi-Yi He
Department of Neurology, First Affiliated Hospital, China Medical University, China Medical University, 155 Nanjing North Street, Heping District, Shenyang 110001, China

Jun Wang
Department of Neurosurgery, First Affiliated Hospital, China Medical University, China Medical University, Shenyang, China

Maowen Ba
Department of Neurology, Yuhuangding Hospital Affiliated to Qingdao Medical University, Qingdao, Shandong 264000, People's Republic of China
McGill Centre for Studies in Aging, McGill University, Douglas Institute, 6825 Lasalle Boul, Montreal, QC H4H 1R3, Canada

Pedro Rosa-Neto and Serge Gauthier
McGill Centre for Studies in Aging, McGill University, Douglas Institute, 6825 Lasalle Boul, Montreal, QC H4H 1R3, Canada

Xiaofeng Li
McGill Centre for Studies in Aging, McGill University, Douglas Institute, 6825 Lasalle Boul, Montreal, QC H4H 1R3, Canada
Department of Neurology, The Second Affiliated Hospital of Chongqing Medical University, Chongqing 400010, People's Republic of China

Kok Pin Ng
McGill Centre for Studies in Aging, McGill University, Douglas Institute, 6825 Lasalle Boul, Montreal, QC H4H 1R3, Canada

Department of Neurology, National Neuroscience Institute Singapore, Singapore, Singapore

Min Kong
Department of Neurology, Yantaishan Hospital, Yantai City, Shandong 264000, People's Republic of China

Chaoyang Liu
School of Information and Safety Engineering, Zhongnan University of Economics and Law, Wuhan 430073, P.R. China

Chi Bun Chan
Department of Physiology, University of Oklahoma Health Sciences Center, 940 Stanton L. Young Blvd., Oklahoma City, OK 73104, USA

Keqiang Ye
Department of Pathology and Laboratory Medicine, Emory University School of Medicine, 615 Michael Street, Atlanta, GA 30322, USA

Bing Yu
Sydney Medical School (Central), The University of Sydney, Camperdown, NSW 2006, Australia
Department of Medical Genomics, Royal Prince Alfred Hospital and NSW Health Pathology, Camperdown, NSW 2050, Australia

Roger Pamphlett
Discipline of Pathology, Brain and Mind Centre, The University of Sydney, 94 Mallett St, Camperdown, NSW 2050, Australia
Department of Neuropathology, Royal Prince Alfred Hospital, Camperdown, NSW 2050, Australia

Qiongqiong Li and Suya Sun
Department of Neurology and Institute of Neurology, Ruijin Hospital, Shanghai Jiao Tong University School of Medicine, 197 Ruijin Er Road, Shanghai 200025, China

Shengdi Chen and Bei Zhang
Department of Neurology and Institute of Neurology, Ruijin Hospital, Shanghai Jiao Tong University School of Medicine, 197 Ruijin Er Road, Shanghai 200025, China
Laboratory of Neurodegenerative Diseases, Institute of Health Sciences, Shanghai Institutes for Biological Sciences (SIBS), Chinese Academy of Sciences (CAS) and Shanghai Jiao Tong University School of Medicine (SJTUSM), Shanghai 200025, China

Xingkun Chu
Laboratory of Neurodegenerative Diseases, Institute of Health Sciences, Shanghai Institutes for Biological Sciences (SIBS), Chinese Academy of Sciences (CAS) and Shanghai Jiao Tong University School of Medicine (SJTUSM), Shanghai 200025, China

Yaqian Xu, Jing Yang and Huifang Shang
Department of Neurology, West China Hospital, Sichuan University, 610041 Chengdu, Sichuan, China

Guo-hua Zhao
Department of Neurology, Second Affiliated Hospital, School of Medicine, Zhejiang University, Hangzhou 310009, China
Department of Neurology, Fourth Affiliated Hospital, School of Medicine, Zhejiang University, Yiwu 322000, China

Xiao-min Liu
Department of Neurology, Qianfoshan Hospital, Shandong University, Jinan 16766, China

Zhibin Wang and Xiao-Guang Luo
Neurology Department, The First Affiliated Hospital of China Medical University, 155# Nanjing Bei Street Heping District, Shenyang 110001, People's Republic of China

Chao Gao
Neurology Department, Ruijin Hospital, Shanghai Jiaotong University School of Medicine, Ruijin 2nd Road 197, Shanghai 200025, People's Republic of China

Brati Das and Riqiang Yan
Department of Neurosciences, Lerner Research Institute, Cleveland Clinic, 9500 Euclid Avenue/NC30, Cleveland, OH 44195, USA

Yuhuan Shi, Wanying Huang, Yu Wang, Rui Zhang, Lina Hou, Jianrong Xu, Hongzhuan Chen, Yongfang Zhang and Hao Wang
Department of Pharmacology and Chemical Biology, Institute of Medical Sciences, Shanghai JiaoTong University School of Medicine, Shanghai 200025, People's Republic of China

Zhuibai Qiu and Qiong Xie
Department of Medicinal Chemistry, School of Pharmacy, Fudan University, Shanghai, People's Republic of China

Ye Liu, Xiao-Ying Zhu, Xiao-Jin Zhang, and Yun-Cheng Wu
Department of Neurology, Shanghai General Hospital, Shanghai Jiao Tong University School of Medicine, No.100, Haining Road, Shanghai 200080, People's Republic of China

Sheng-Han Kuo
Department of Neurology, College of Physicians and Surgeons, Columbia University, New York, USA

William G. Ondo
Methodist Neurological Institute, Houston, TX, USA

Hyun Jin Cho
Department of Biochemistry and Biomedical Sciences, Seoul National University, College of Medicine, 28 Yungun-dong, Jongro-gu, Seoul 110-799, South Korea

Chengsong Xie and Huaibin Cai
Transgenics Section, Laboratory of Neurogenetics, National Institute on Aging, National Institutes of Health, Building 35, Room 1A112, MSC 3707, 35 Convent Drive, Bethesda, MD 20892–3707, USA

Rodolfo G. Gatto
Department of Anatomy and Cell Biology, University of Illinois at Chicago, 808 S. Wood St. Rm 578 M/C 512, Chicago, IL 60612, USA

Manish Y. Amin and Daniel Deyoung
Department of Physics, University of Florida, Gainesville, FL, USA

Matthew Hey
Department of Applied Physiology and Kinesiology, University of Florida, Gainesville, FL, USA

Thomas H. Mareci
Department of Biochemistry and Molecular Biology, University of Florida, Gainesville, FL, USA

Richard L. Magin
Department of Bioengineering, University of Illinois at Chicago, Chicago, IL, USA

Parisa Tabeshmehr and Mohammad Hossein Khorraminejad Shirazi
Student Research Committee, Shiraz University of Medical Sciences, Shiraz, Iran
Cell and Molecular Medicine Student Research Group, Medical Faculty, Shiraz University of Medical Sciences, Shiraz, Iran

Seyed Mojtaba Hosseini
Student Research Committee, Shiraz University of Medical Sciences, Shiraz, Iran
Cell and Molecular Medicine Student Research Group, Medical Faculty, Shiraz University of Medical Sciences, Shiraz, Iran
Stem Cell Laboratory, Department of Anatomy, Shiraz University of Medical Sciences, Shiraz, Iran

Haider Kh Husnain
Department of Basic Sciences, SRU, Riyadh, Saudi Arabia

Mahin Salmannejad and Mahsa Sani
Stem Cell Laboratory, Department of Anatomy, Shiraz University of Medical Sciences, Shiraz, Iran

Haifang Wang, Tao Wang, Meiling Qin, Puhua Bao, Ruiqi Wang, Yuwei Liu, Hung-Chun Chang, Jun Yan and Jin Xu
Institute of Neuroscience, State Key Laboratory of Neuroscience, CAS Key laboratory of Primate Neurobiology, Shanghai Institutes for Biological Sciences, Chinese Academy of Sciences, New Life Science Bldg, 320 Yue Yang Road, Shanghai 200031, China

Xin Jiang and Tao Zhang
Institute of Neuroscience, State Key Laboratory of Neuroscience, CAS Key laboratory of Primate Neurobiology, Shanghai Institutes for Biological Sciences, Chinese Academy of Sciences, New Life Science Bldg, 320 Yue Yang Road, Shanghai 200031, China
University of Chinese Academy of Sciences, Shanghai 200031, China

Ke Yang, Bo Shen, Da-ke Li, Ying Wang, Jue Zhao, Jian Zhao, Wen-Bo Yu, Zhen-yang Liu, Yi-lin Tang, Feng-tao Liu, Huan Yu, Jian Wang and Qi-hao Guo
Department of Neurology and Institute of Neurology, Huashan Hospital, Fudan University, 12 Wulumuqi Zhong Road, Shanghai 200040, China

Jian-jun Wu
Department of Neurology and Institute of Neurology, Huashan Hospital, Fudan University, 12 Wulumuqi Zhong Road, Shanghai 200040, China
Department of Neurology, Jing'an District Center Hospital of Shanghai, 259 Xikang Road, Shanghai 20040, China

Xiaobei Deng, Xiaohuan Xia, Zhaohuan Fan, Xinrui Qi, Yizhao Ma and Chunhong Li
Center for Translational Neurodegeneration and Regenerative Therapy, Shanghai Tenth People's Hospital affiliated to Tongji University School of Medicine, Shanghai 200072, China

Jialin C. Zheng
Center for Translational Neurodegeneration and Regenerative Therapy, Shanghai Tenth People's Hospital affiliated to Tongji University School of Medicine, Shanghai 200072, China
Collaborative Innovation Center for Brain Science, Tongji University, Shanghai 200092, China
Departments of Pharmacology and Experimental Neuroscience, University of Nebraska Medical Center, Omaha, NE 68198-5930, USA
Department of Pathology and Microbiology, University of Nebraska Medical Center, Omaha, NE 68198-5930, USA

Kangmu Ma, Yongxiang Wang, Yuju Li, Qiang Chen, Yunlong Huang and Changhai Tian
Center for Translational Neurodegeneration and Regenerative Therapy, Shanghai Tenth People's Hospital affiliated to Tongji University School of Medicine, Shanghai 200072, China
Departments of Pharmacology and Experimental Neuroscience, University of Nebraska Medical Center, Omaha, NE 68198-5930, USA

Hui Peng
Departments of Pharmacology and Experimental Neuroscience, University of Nebraska Medical Center, Omaha, NE 68198-5930, USA

Jianqing Ding
Department of Neurology and Institute of Neurology, Ruijin Hospital affiliated to Shanghai Jiao Tong University School of Medicine, Shanghai 200025, China

Index